Our Parents
IN CRISIS

Confronting Medical Errors, Ageist Doctors,
and Other Healthcare Failings

Ann G. Sjoerdsma

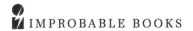 IMPROBABLE BOOKS

Published by Improbable Books, www.improbablebooks.com.
Please address all inquiries to 211 N. Union Street, Suite 100, Alexandria, Va.
22314; (703) 519-1226; or publisher@improbablebooks.com.

Cover and interior design by Tamira Ci Thayne, www.tamiracithayne.com.

COVER PHOTOGRAPHS: On front: 1) Fern and Al Sjoerdsma attend an
international scientific symposium in Milan, Italy, in 1964; and 2) relax on a
deck in their back yard in North Carolina in 2007.

On back: 1) The author celebrates her mother's 88th birthday with her parents
in 2012; and 2) Fern and Al Sjoerdsma examine an award that Dr. Al received
from the American Assn. for the Advancement of Science in 1958. Family
photographs are courtesy of Britt L. Sjoerdsma.

Manufactured in the United States of America
First Edition

10   9   8   7   6   5   4   3   2   1

Publisher's Cataloging-in-Publication Data
   (Provided by Quality Books, Inc.)

Sjoerdsma, Ann G., author.
      Our parents in crisis : confronting medical errors,
      ageist doctors, and other healthcare failings / Ann G.
      Sjoerdsma. -- First edition.
      pages cm
      Includes bibliographical references and index.
      LCCN 2014902303
      ISBN 978-0-615-19302-1

      1. Older people--Medical care--Moral and ethical
   aspects--United States. 2. Older people--Health and
   hygiene--United States--Popular works. 3. Aging parents
   --Care--United States--Popular works. 4. Patient
   advocacy--United States.   I. Title.

   RA564.8.S56 2015   362.19897'00973
                           QBI15-600142

ISBN: 13: 978-0-615-19302-1
LCCN: 2014902303

To my precious parents, with love

Also by
Ann G. Sjoerdsma

STARTING WITH SEROTONIN
*How a High-Rolling Father of Drug Discovery
Repeatedly Beat the Odds*

Through the Ages . . .

"We don't stop playing because we get old; we get old because we stop playing."

—GEORGE BERNARD SHAW (1856-1950)

"To get back my youth I would do anything in the world except take exercise, get up early, or be respectable."

—OSCAR WILDE (1854-1900),
in "The Picture of Dorian Gray"

"In spite of illness, in spite even of the archenemy sorrow, one can remain alive long past the usual date of disintegration if one is unafraid of change, insatiable in intellectual curiosity, interested in big things, and happy in small ways."

—EDITH WHARTON (1862-1937),
in her autobiography "A Backward Glance"

"I feel particularly inspired by the realization that aging is a transitional phase, rather than a phasing out. . . . I continue to realize that old age is a time of great fulfillment—personal fulfillment—when all the loose ends of life can be gathered together."

—MAGGIE KUHN (1905-95),
founder of the Gray Panthers

"Aging and death do seem to be what Nature has planned for us. But what if we have other plans?"

—BERNARD STREHLER (1925-2001),
USC biology professor and founding editor-in-chief of
"Mechanisms of Aging and Development"

Contents

Acknowledgments and Notes

I would like to thank the University of Maryland, the University of Virginia, and the University of North Carolina for giving me access to scores of medical journal articles through their health sciences libraries that I either could not obtain on the Internet or for which I would have paid a considerable amount to obtain. State medical school libraries are a fantastic resource for the public, and I hope these three continue to keep their doors open to those of us outside of the medical community who wish to do research. There is no substitute for primary sources.

I am also grateful to the Georgetown University School of Medicine for the mini-medical schools that it hosts twice a year and to the Georgetown faculty and Washington, D.C.-area physicians who teach the "mini" classes. This medical-education program for the public, which has become a popular tradition, is superb. I have attended four Georgetown mini-medical schools and plan to attend more. They stimulate and enlighten.

The Georgetown mini-medical school stands alone, in content and concept, but other medical schools offer comparable programs. I greatly benefited from a Johns Hopkins University mini-medical school on aging and from a class about aging in a U. Va. mini-medical school. All three schools also present lectures that are designed to educate the public about cutting-edge medicine. I thank the organizers behind these events for their community interest and outreach. I value your efforts.

In my narrative, I tried to acknowledge those people who reached out with expertise, kindness, educated advice, and other help to my parents, my siblings, and me during difficult times. I only named a handful of them. With these exceptions, the names of all physicians, nurses, caregivers, and other healthcare personnel in my book are fictional. I also used pseudonyms for friends and friends' relatives. My heartfelt thanks to the people who truly cared for us.

Outside of my narrative, I am grateful to my dear friends who gave me emotional and intellectual support during the times I describe, as well as during my writing trials: Jim and Mary Cary, Madeleine Fagan, Lynne Durbin, Ann Young, Karin Nelson, Jack Bowers, Carol Adams, Ann Cavanaugh, and my special journalist friend, Cate Kozak, who talked me up whenever I thought about quitting.

After I finished a solid draft of my manuscript, I received insightful assistance from my editor Carla Joinson, who has a sharp eye that complements my own, and from Dr. Julie Quinn, who medically vetted Chapter Twelve and sections of other chapters. Fellow lawyer/writer Michele Gatto and lawyer/publisher Bruce L. Bortz provided invaluable opinions on some key choices I had to make.

Thank you so much, one and all.

This book would not exist if my father hadn't encouraged me, advised me, and read some of my early chapter drafts, including Chapter Seven, which in its first version even put *him* to sleep.

"The book is great when you're reading the personal story," Dad said when he returned chapters to me, "but then you hit that aging science and stop dead in your tracks." At the top of my chapter-seven draft, he had written: "TOO ACADEMIC!" I got busy on a rewrite, one of several.

Dr. Al was my best reader and editor, as well as my inspiration. My heart is filled with love, gratitude, and admiration for him. I dedicate this book to my wonderful, one-of-a-kind father and to my beautiful mother, who modeled the grace and calm in a crisis that I learned as a child and later applied as an advocate.

Medical-scientific breakthroughs happen—not nearly as often as scientists and newspaper and other media reporters would lead you to believe—but they do happen. Medical guidelines and recommendations also change. At the time that I was writing, all of my medical claims were current. To be certain that some of those in a fast-evolving field are still the latest word, you may have to do a little homework.

—Ann G. Sjoerdsma

Preface

Old Age is Not
A DIAGNOSIS

So Get Your Ass Off The Cot

In his tell-all memoir, "Becoming a Doctor: A Journey of Initiation in Medical School," Melvin Konner recalls a lecture by a gerontologist who "had been brilliant, outrageous, and funny." The star lecturer spoke during Konner's preclinical years, when medical-school students are fire-hosed by information, but not yet burned out on patients and the demands of their upper-class clinical rotations.

This exceptional gerontologist, Konner relates, "used to shout at us, 'You think life expectancy is threescore and ten! You think old people are *supposed* to die! You're lying there at three A.M. in the on-call room and your beeper rings. There's a patient in the E.W. with chest pain. It's an eighty-two-year-old man! You do a lightning calculation. This guy's life expectancy is minus twelve years! You turn over and go back to sleep.

"'Well let me tell you something! This guy's life expectancy is not much different from that of a sixty-five-year-old. This guy's life expectancy may not be much different from yours! This guy is a survivor! He's here at eighty-two because he's tough! And he'll be here at ninety-two for exactly the same reason! So get your ass off the cot and down to the E.W. and save his goddamn life!'

"... This brilliant man," Konner reflects, "had indelibly impressed on us that old people are not sick because they are old. They are sick because they are sick. Our job is to find out what is wrong with them. Age has no bearing on how much someone deserves a diagnosis, and old age is not a diagnosis. Even the slightest shift in expectations, based solely on age, could bias us and become a dangerous, unprofessional, self-fulfilling prophecy."[i]

I have spent more than 12 years as a healthcare advocate, companion, sounding board, and watchdog for my parents. Thanks to these two remarkable people, I intimately understand that old age is not a diagnosis. I also know how hard it can be to get a doctor's ass "off of the cot" because of ingrained ageist thinking.

In my advocacy, I have encountered the expectations, biases, and dangerous and unprofessional prophecies that are rooted in medical ageism. I've also encountered the pitfalls of today's highly specialized and fragmented U.S. healthcare system: the disconnections between physicians; the lack of continuity in treatment; the costly errors and misdiagnoses, and so many more failings than even I, a skeptical lawyer, journalist, and daughter of two physicians, ever imagined.

If a doctor ever asks you, one of your parents, or another older loved one, "What do you expect at your age?," ask him or her, "What do *you* expect?," and then find another doctor. Life is hard enough without having to put up with ageist nonsense from people who should know better.

Old age is a fact in a story that differs among storytellers. Here is mine.

---

i. Melvin Konner, *Becoming a Doctor: A Journey of Initiation in Medical School* (Penguin Books, paperback, 1987), pp. 303-04. Konner was a 35-year-old Harvard professor of anthropology when he decided to pursue a medical degree and enrolled at (thinly disguised) Harvard Medical School. He never practiced medicine.

Chapter One

2002: Proceed Until APPREHENDED

Or You Might Lose Your Mother

My mother complained on Tuesday, May 28, 2002, of a "really bad" headache "in the front," she said. Mom rarely has a headache, nor does she complain.

"I think she's getting some kind of flu," my father suggested on the telephone that evening.

I had spent the Memorial Day weekend with friends in Charlotte and faced a week of work. At the time, I had a lucrative contract as a telecommuting legal-journal editor. I promised Dad I'd drop by tomorrow evening and wished my mother, who celebrated her 78th birthday on May 5, a quick recovery.

My parents and I live a half-mile apart in the lush woods of Southern Shores, a year-round community on the north end of North Carolina's Outer Banks. I moved there first, after taking a newspaper job in nearby Norfolk, Va., which I considered a dreary, never-in-a-million-years-would-I-live-there town. I preferred to live in North Carolina on the beach that I'd known since I was a child. I transplanted from Baltimore and knew that Mom and Dad intended to retire to Southern Shores; the only question was when.

I dropped by to see Mom Wednesday night and was dismayed to learn that she now had a severe sore throat and cough and still could not relieve her painful headache with medication. She lay on the floral sectional couch in the family room. "I'm just so tired," she said. Earlier, she had felt nauseous and vomited a bit. She also had stopped eating, claiming to have a bad taste in her mouth. Although her headache worried me a lot, I reasoned, optimistically, that the other symptoms seemed like an "everyday" virus. My parents agreed.

On Thursday evening, I found Mom sitting up and conversing. Dad knew of other people who recently had suffered debilitating headaches, including a repairman with whom Mom had contact. Something must be going around. Mom ate a dish of apple cobbler with ice cream and gave me a kiss when I left. Perhaps the worst was over. The next day I had a lively telephone conversation with her. My brother, Al, talked with her, also, and thought she had more energy. Mom paid some bills that day. She was getting better.

Over the June 1-2 weekend, I busied myself at home. When I saw Mom Sunday night, I was shocked.

SUNDAY, JUNE 2

When I think back on the early days of my mother's mysterious medical crisis, I am struck by two things: 1) the changeable course of her flu-like illness; and 2) the trust I had in my parents' ability to care for themselves. Not only did I lack necessary medical knowledge, I didn't know the lengths to which my intelligent parents would go to avoid acknowledging how sick Mom was.

Both were retired physicians. Physicians confront clinical facts, right? They deal with truths as they are, not as they wish them to be. Wow, was I off-base.

My mother was an introspective, warm, and unflappable psychiatrist, caring but reserved. Trained in Freudian analysis, she formerly treated adults of all ages and young children, whom she adored.

When my three siblings and I were growing up, Mom saw patients several nights a week in our home. This was the 1960s, before "patients" became "clients." The patient would ring our doorbell, enter the front hallway, which had been cordoned off from the living room by a folding door, and sit down to wait for the psychiatrist. After each consultation, Mom would type up her notes, and I would steal into her inner sanctum and read them. My violation of confidentiality aside, I viewed each patient as an individual with a problem that I felt certain my mother could fix, and I wanted to know his or her story.

My father was a prominent scientist-physician—and medical pioneer—whose clinical expertise I had long regarded as limitless. Trained in cardiology, internal medicine, and pharmacology, Dad had a textbook command of anatomy, physiology, and medicine. Interested in drug discovery, he earned a reputation during the 1950s and '60s as the Father of Clinical Pharmacology for his cutting-edge "rational" research in the National Heart Institute of the National Institutes of Health in Bethesda, Md.

Rational research was based on biochemical mechanisms—that is, on how the body works, on a chemical level, about which little was then known. When he started out, Dad wanted to *design* therapeutic agents—drugs—not engage in the time-worn practice of random screening with pharmacologically active plant extracts. He eschewed trial-and-error for rational theory.

Dad's first target was high blood pressure (hypertension), which regularly debilitated and killed people. He thought he might be able to lower pressure by blocking a key enzyme in the metabolic pathway of serotonin, which had been discovered, but not elaborated upon. This thinking, which did not prove to be true, nonetheless led to ground-breaking research on serotonin and other molecules, some of which, like serotonin, became known as important neurotransmitters, and to the breakthrough antihypertensive drug, Aldomet®.

After 20 years with the NIH during its "Golden Age of Research and Development," my father spent 20 years as an executive in the pharmaceutical industry, in Europe and the United States. His most recognizable drug achievement is probably the antihistamine Allegra®. Although no longer hands-on with research during its development, he initiated and oversaw the basic-science and clinical work that resulted in Allegra; without him, it would not exist.

Dad loved to brainstorm with other scientists and excelled at reason, logic, and creative thinking. If anyone could deduce what was happening to Mom, it would be my often audacious and tough genius father. But that proved not to be the case. Dr. Albert Sjoerdsma, M.D., Ph.D., was too emotionally involved to care for the patient in his own bed.

Still he was worried. When Mom could not recall any of the evening news she had watched Sunday, his worry became alarm. I, too, found her mentally confused, as well as lethargic. Again, she lay slumped on the sectional, but now her pale-blue eyes showed no life, no sparkle. She had become dead weight and couldn't move without assistance. Her body ached and shook with chills.

"Mom, you're much sicker than you think you are," I insisted repeatedly, as she scoffed at my suggestions to call 911 or to go to the hospital.

Dad, too, discouraged medical intervention, persisting in the belief that this mystery virus would run its course.

My older sister Leslie, a registered nurse in Florida, had speculated that Mom had viral meningitis, and it seemed obvious to me that an infection of some kind was affecting Mom's brain, altering her cognition. So why was Dad minimizing its seriousness?

I sized up our options at 9 o'clock on a Sunday night: We could take Mom to the emergency department (ED) of the newly opened Outer Banks Hospital (OBH) in Nags Head or to the ED at Albemarle Hospital in Elizabeth City, which was an hour away. Having no experience with either, each presented unknowns. The local press about the OBH had been sharply critical, so I hesitated to take Mom there, but a drive to Elizabeth City seemed worse.

Reluctantly, I yielded to my father's suggestion. We would transport Mom to the nearby Kitty Hawk medical center, an urgent-care way station, first thing in the morning.

That night, I went against my better judgment to act immediately, but I wasn't a doctor, and, even though Dad had warned me all my life to "stay away from hospitals and doctors. . . . They'll make you sick"—or worse: "They'll kill you."—I wasn't yet ready to substitute my judgment for a medical professional's.

I also didn't understand what it meant to my father, however brilliant, to see his wife of 52 years so sick. I didn't appreciate how grief and the denial he summoned to combat it clouded his reason. In the anxious days ahead, I would have to confront my powerful father and his altered psyche, as well as doctors whose knee-jerk perceptions and ageism prevented them from doing enough to save my mother's life.

My "caregiving" would require all of the intellectual chops and moxie I had acquired in life, and then some. Whatever I did, I owed it to my mother to pull out the stops.

MONDAY, JUNE 3

The morning of Monday, June 3, Mom sat for 90 minutes in a wheelchair, holding her sagging head wearily in her hand, as we waited for a bed to open up at Beach Medical in Kitty Hawk. I silently cursed every sniffle in the crowded waiting room. Urgent? Give me a break. My mother was nearly immobile.

I had helped Mom to wash, dress, eat breakfast, use the toilet, and walk to my parents' car. I also had packed an overnight bag for her and emailed Al, Leslie, and my younger sister, Britt, that Mom would likely be hospitalized that night. She was aware and communicative, but occasionally confused and very lethargic. The young nurse who assisted Mom curbside called her "hon" and spoke in that annoying sing-song voice that nurses and other healthcare personnel use with old people. Like they're talking to babies, not adults.

While I wanted medical answers that day, I had not yet assumed the leadership that I would. Needing to attend to some work and errands, I popped in and out of the clinic until early afternoon. When Dad called at 1:30 to tell me that Dr. Washburn,* the urgent-care physician, had diagnosed a urinary tract infection, I became furious.

Mom had a 102-degree fever. According to my father, Dr. Washburn, an internist with 25 years of practice, had ordered blood work, a urinalysis, and a chest X-ray. The urine sample that he obtained—which, Dad pointed out, was uncatherized and, thus, impure—showed pus, i.e., the presence of white blood cells, suggestive of a urinary tract infection, to which my mother, like many older women, was prone. Dr. Washburn prescribed Tylenol®, an intravenous administration of fluids (dextrose in water), and the broad-spectrum antibiotic, Rocephin®, which in generic form is ceftriaxone.

This was ridiculous, I thought. A *UTI?* Hadn't Dad explained Mom's symptoms in detail to the doctor? Didn't Dr. Washburn understand how seriously ill she was? What about the confusion, the lethargy, the headache? How could *all* of that be caused by a UTI?

I quickly called my R.N. sister: What can I do? Dad refuses to see how sick Mom is, and Dr. Washburn is blowing her off. I needed solid medical advice. The diagnosis didn't add up.

Encouraged by Leslie, I drove back to Beach Medical, found my mother hooked up to IVs and sleeping, and asked to see the doctor. My eye fell on a nurse's notation in Mom's medical chart: Patient complains of "aches in her head," it said.

In her normal state, my mother would never talk like that. That the nurse quoted her and apparently thought nothing of this unusual description suggested little-old-lady patronizing to me. My sister had instructed me to personalize Mom for the doctor and nurses, explaining: "They don't know who she is. They've never seen her before. You have to tell them about her." And so I tried.

---

*See note in Acknowledgments about names of people in the book.

I told Dr. Washburn he was seeing "a shell of my mother, 180 degrees from her usual self." I detailed the course of her symptoms since May 28 and sought to characterize her baseline, how she behaved before her illness. She swam every day, drove a car, walked her dog, cooked, read Dickens, played "Jeopardy!" She had never shown signs of dementia.

Concerned that he would dismiss me as emotionally overwrought, I measured my tone and remained calm: "I'm a rational person," I flatly told him. "I logically evaluate the evidence. I don't panic." My mother is *very* sick, Dr. Washburn, more than you understand. Please find out why.

His response crushed me. He offered to do a CT scan of Mom's brain and to "hospitalize her, if you want." If *I* want? What about *you*, the medical expert, what do *you* advise? During my head of steam, I had told Dr. Washburn how opposed my parents were to hospitalization, how they seemed to minimize the seriousness of Mom's illness. Didn't Dr. Washburn understand the pressure I was under? Apparently, he had no clinical opinion beyond the UTI diagnosis. I felt abandoned.

I authorized the CT scan, a process that involved my repeatedly informing the consent-form taker that I wasn't concerned about dementia. My mother might be old, but she was acutely sick, not demented. Why did people seem to doubt me? Were they all ageists, buying into a prejudicial stereotype that when older people have cognitive problems they must be demented? Or did they question my credibility?

A technician wheeled Mom off, and, after a restless wait, the scan came back "negative." I didn't press for details. Mom received IV fluids and Rocephin continuously until 7 p.m. and noticeably perked up. She regained color in her face and even ate a sandwich. Dr. Washburn further prescribed oral Cipro®, which had been in the news as the anthrax antibiotic, and he and my father agreed to watch Mom for the next 12 hours—meaning until 9 a.m. tomorrow. The nurse who wheeled my mother to the car instructed her: "Now eat, honey." More patronizing, more sing-song babytalk.

About two miles down the road, Mom lapsed into confusion, and my heart sank. I pleaded with my parents to turn around and drive to the hospital, but both dismissed the idea, my father admonishing me: "*You* don't get to decide."

I walked Mom to the front door of my parents' home and thought she seemed even weaker than she had in the morning. She stared in horror at me when I told her that I regretted the decision not to hospitalize her.

Once inside, she started having chills. I begged my father to call 911 if she deteriorated during the night, and then I left, wrung out from the day's confrontations. Thirty minutes later Al called, having learned about Mom's fever and chills and becoming desperately concerned. I agreed, but I couldn't fight with Dad any longer about hospitalization.

I considered driving Mom to Johns Hopkins, the University of Virginia, Duke, or Chapel Hill, but I couldn't do that alone. I went to sleep with a prayer in my head.

Please, Mom, please just hold on.

TUESDAY, JUNE 4

The paramedics arrived like a SWAT team around 9:30 a.m. on Tuesday, June 4.

Shaking with chills, Mom had slept fitfully during the night. Around 5 a.m., she fell off of the toilet, unable to rise without Dad's assistance. He called me about 7:30, and I rushed to see her, alarmed to discover how rapid her breathing had become.

Mom seemed somnolent, but mentally aware. I wanted to call 911 immediately, but Dad insisted on driving to Beach Medical and seeing the useless Dr. Washburn about a referral. My old-school doctor father believed in going through physician channels. Later he called home to report that Washburn had called Dr. Logan at the Outer Banks Hospital in Nags Head, and an ambulance would soon arrive for Mom.

I washed and fed my mother and explained to her what was going to happen. As I waited for the paramedic team, I accepted that I had two patients on my hands. My father had refused to call 911. He was either too shaken or too stubborn to be trusted. I needed to take advantage of his vast medical knowledge, but go over his head—and help him to cope.

During the paramedics' careful transport of Mom down the front-porch steps, an emergency-medical technician about my age commented on the "role reversal" that adult children experience with their parents. "They become the children," he said.

While I appreciate that he was trying to be empathetic, I don't agree with him and hate when people say this. There's no role reversal between aged parents and adult children. There's a role adjustment. The parent-child relationship, like all relationships, evolves.

Dad and I drove to the OBH in separate cars. We checked in at the ED, answering the usual paperwork questions, and waited "for the nurse, who will come get you." I never did that again. After 90 minutes, during which I presumed Mom was undergoing a battery of tests, I questioned the wait, received an apology, and went into the patient area. It was about 12:45 p.m. Now wearing a green hospital gown, my mother lay on a hard, narrow bed, exhausted and attached to IV fluids, but not to an antibiotic. I was astonished. Where were the life-saving antibiotics? Where was the doctor?

Remarkably, Dr. Logan had left, without consulting us about Mom's history or advising us about her condition. He apparently had obtained the records from Beach Medical, repeated the tests she had yesterday, and skipped out, without ordering any treatment except fluids. What was he thinking? Was this more ageism? More of the old woman hasn't been eating enough? Or was he just inept? Indifferent? Already, the OBH was living up to its reputation in the community.

Dad and I insisted on talking to a doctor, and Dr. Barnett obliged. Somewhat familiar with Mom's case, Barnett, who appeared to be about 30, had arrived recently from Michigan, my mother's home state. He listened politely as my father enumerated all of Mom's symptoms, mentioned meningitis as a possible cause, and suggested doing a lumbar puncture, a tap that would yield cerebrospinal fluid for diagnostic purposes.

Dr. Barnett also indulged my father's schmoozing about medicine and his own illustrious career in a ritual that I later dubbed the physician shuffle, a type of medical *pas de deux* without music.

Starved for intellectual stimulation in the Outer Banks, Dad eagerly "shuffled" whenever he met a fellow physician. During this particular exchange, Dad told Dr. Barnett the story of Big Jim Tatum, which was his way of asking the slight-figured, young physician to look beyond the obvious, as Dr. Washburn had not done.

Big Jim Tatum took over the football program at the University of North Carolina at Chapel Hill, Tatum's alma mater (and mine), in 1956, after coaching championship teams at the University of Maryland. He was turning the lowly Tar Heels around when he fell acutely ill and died, much to the puzzlement of doctors at Chapel Hill's esteemed N.C. Memorial Hospital, who suspected a viral infection, but never made a diagnosis. Tatum's mystery illness? Rocky Mountain spotted fever, which he contracted from the bite of an infected tick.

"I leave you with that story to think about," my emotionally spent father told Barnett before, gratefully, heading for home. The shuffler had exhausted himself. I was on my own.

As soon as my father was out of sight, I delivered my "shell of my mother" speech to Barnett and questioned Dr. Logan's failure to administer antibiotics. To my dismay, Dr. Barnett, like his colleague, didn't want to prescribe anything until he knew what he was treating. He gave me the medical party line about the overuse of antibiotics leading to an increase in resistant bacteria, as if that had anything to do with my mother's critical condition.

I next tried my "rational person, examining the evidence" argument on him and wanted to know his plan of action. Yes, I nodded, agreeing with him that medicine isn't black-and-white: Life isn't black-and-white. But with step-by-step research come results, clues, detection, a diagnosis that makes sense. Certainly, I reasoned, doctors must think like lawyers and journalists do, like all critical thinkers bent on solving a problem.

Please, Dr. Barnett, tell me what's next.

LATER ON JUNE 4

Dr. Barnett suggested another CT scan (!) and advised me to grab lunch while he studied the records and examined Mom. I went to a nearby supermarket and called Leslie on a cell phone from the parking lot, venting to her about Logan's disappearing act, the breakdown in care, and Barnett's refusal to start antibiotics. I urged her to call the young doc and communicate with him on a medical level. I didn't want to bungle this crisis out of ignorance.

Within 10 minutes, my sister reported back that Barnett had declined her call, having already spoken with "one Sjoerdsma sister." She left her name, number, and R.N. status with a nurse. Despite the stonewall, I felt reinforced, less alone, and was heartened to discover, upon my return to the ED, that Mom was receiving intravenous Rocephin, as a precaution. Dr. Barnett, bless him, had a plan.

Contrary to the results at Beach Medical (from the sample Dad said was impure), the ED urinalysis showed no evidence of infection. Because his earlier blood tests apparently had shed no light, Dr.

Barnett had ordered his own CT scan of Mom's brain, thus contributing to a pattern that I would see often during this crisis: repetitive testing, redundancy. Doctors refused to rely on *any* recent testing done by another doctor in Mom's treatment chain.

Barnett told me that he would be willing to scan Mom's abdomen as well, for a possible uterine abscess, if the family wanted. Mom had wondered recently whether she had a prolapse, which is a descension of the uterus into the vaginal canal. Based on his physical exam, however, Barnett thought that was unlikely. If the CT scan proved negative, he planned to perform a lumbar puncture and have Mom's spinal fluid analyzed, as we had been pushing.

Although I was frustrated by the repetition of tests, I felt encouraged by the emergency doctor's logical approach. I finally had his attention. To keep it, I had to be assertive, but not argumentative with him. With my reportorial and legal skills to draw on, I felt confident I could handle the situation.

Around 2 p.m., Mom had her brain X-rayed; at 3:30 p.m., someone tapped her spine. At 4 p.m., Dr. Barnett updated me: The CT scan showed only the "usual signs of age-related degeneration," and the puncture results would not be ready for another hour or so, by which time Barnett would be gone. Great. Another disruption in care. If the puncture proved negative for infection, Barnett told me, an OB Hospital internist would admit Mom overnight for observation. If it proved positive, Barnett's replacement would transfer her to Albemarle Hospital for treatment. I thanked him sincerely for his follow-through and approachability. He also filled Leslie in.

Dr. Logan, who had disappeared earlier, delivered the results of the cerebrospinal fluid analysis, his panicked look forecasting the bad news. My mother didn't have little-old-lady disease, after all. She had haemophilus influenzae meningitis, a highly infectious and potentially fatal disease.

Logan ordered the recommended antibiotic regimen for "H-flu," which included the toxic drug, gentamicin, and set about arranging a transfer, as soon as possible. He wanted to be sure that the hospital to which he sent Mom had both an infectious-disease specialist and a neurologist available for consultation. Albemarle Hospital in Elizabeth City lacked a neurologist, so Logan turned to Chesapeake General Hospital, 70 miles away in Virginia.

I stayed by my mother's side for nearly nine hours that day, leaving only during the tests that Dr. Barnett ordered, bathroom breaks, and cell-phone calls to my family. Although tired, febrile, and uncomfortable, my mother remained alert and carried on lucid conversations with me. I assisted with nursing tasks, helping her to the toilet and bringing her iced water and crackers, and I explained all of the medical goings-on, including the diagnosis. She seemed to appreciate its seriousness. I encouraged her to be strong and positive and asked her to promise me that she'd make it. She promised she would.

From the moment I received that promise, I never wavered in my belief that she would survive.

During our long wait for transportation to Chesapeake, a kind nurse named Jodie kept me apprised of what was happening. At last, at 9:30 p.m., I watched a young and energetic duo of male paramedics lift my beautiful mother into an ambulance. She blew kisses at me just before the door closed, and my tears finally came.

I didn't want to let her out of my sight, but I had another patient—my anxious father—waiting in the wings. Nonetheless, I only decided not to join Mom in the ambulance after she assured me she would not be lonely. That was very important to me. I did not want her to feel alone.

Despite the missteps, I still believed that the healthcare system would function as intended, to the patient's benefit. With Mom's paperwork being transported with her, I didn't see that I could lend much to Chesapeake's admissions process. I also would be without a car and personal belongings.

At midnight, I called the Chesapeake Intensive Care Unit, which Jodie said I should feel free to do. An unsympathetic nurse curtly informed me that Mom "was resting comfortably." I braced myself for tomorrow, June 5, the ninth day of my mother's illness.

WEDNESDAY, JUNE 5, TO THURSDAY, JUNE 6

The first thing I noticed about the Chesapeake ICU when Dad and I arrived was the noise. Nurses talked and laughed loudly, without self-consciousness or discretion, as if they were knocking back beers in someone's living room. My mother's nurse called her honey and sweetie and used that damn sing-song voice.

Even more upsetting was Mom's condition. Now in isolation, and despite nearly three days of IV antibiotics, she looked no better than she had the day before. She was still alert, but sluggish, and very, very tired. Her short-term memory faltered; she asked me about blue meningitis, instead of H-flu. She had managed to eat a little soup. Despite her malaise, no one had thought to catherize her. That she had struggled with a bedpan made me angry. My father and I quickly corrected that.

I had read up on haemophilus influenzae type b meningitis in "The Merck Manual" *(Merck)*, my medical bible, and talked about it with my father. H-flu is an acute bacteria-induced inflammation of the meninges—the surrounding membranes—of the brain and spinal cord. It is the most common cause of meningitis in children.

This seemed a strange diagnosis. Mom hadn't been exposed to children; and while she had experienced the fever and headache that characterize H-flu, she did not have the telltale stiff neck and some of the other symptoms. The progress of her illness only loosely fit with the *Merck* description of meningitis, which did not mention lethargy or profound fatigue. Dad and I eagerly awaited word from the consulting infectious disease (ID) specialist, but none came. Dr. Amble, the "hospitalist" in charge of Mom's case, had not deemed it necessary to bring in an ID expert *or* a neurologist.

We had never heard the term hospitalist before and were unsure of Dr. Amble's status vis-à-vis Mom, but, considering the emphasis Dr. Logan had placed on consultants when he made his referral, as well as the serious threat posed by bacterial meningitis to an older person, we viewed Dr. Amble's no-consult decision as a red flag. After Dad and I spoke with Amble, one of five hospitalists, or staff doctors, employed by Chesapeake General, we had further reason to question her care.

Dr. Amble was personable, but vacuous. Although he had spoken by telephone with Dr. Logan last night and had handled Mom's admission, he lacked familiarity with her case and acknowledged as much. He listened only politely, and with disinterest, I thought, to Dad's rundown of Mom's history. He took no notes; whereas I did. Again, I observed the "shell of my mother" and stressed that Mom had been high-functioning before this illness. Noting that she had elevated liver enzymes, Amble asked us whether she drank much alcohol! She did not and never had. He didn't pursue the issue further. I got the feeling he didn't believe us.

I asked Dr. Amble for a prescription for Rifampin®, which my father knew was a prophylaxis for bacterial meningitis, but Amble lacked the ability—and his supervisor was unwilling—to prescribe the drug. I didn't understand this. The recommended two-day Rifampin treatment would relieve Dad's and my anxiety over our own possible exposure to H-flu. When I asked him broad questions about Mom's prognosis and the course of her treatment, Amble did the physician shuffle with my father.

"Medicine isn't precise, Ann," they said, frosting me with that exclusive-club attitude unique to doctors. (Lawyers can frost, too, but they seem more like blowhards to me than Dr. Little Lord or Lady Fauntleroys.)

Maybe . . . but as I pointed out emphatically to Dad later, you can learn a lot by asking pointed questions and listening carefully to what is said and not said. You can apply reason; you don't need a medical degree to figure things out. In fact, as I was discovering, M.D.s were more often getting in the way.

In response to my queries, Dr. Amble estimated Mom's IV antibiotic treatment at eight to 10 days and admitted that he had treated only one other case of H-flu in 20 years of practice, and that patient had died.

When my father questioned him about the use of gentamicin, which can be toxic to the kidneys, Amble acknowledged the risk, adding, "It killed my grandmother." This floored me. I could do without such candor, but it provided valuable information about what we could expect at Chesapeake General.

Amble's medical position boiled down to a simple either-or proposition: Either the antibiotics would cure Mom or they wouldn't. Only time would tell. Her brain was fighting a life-threatening infection. She was old. She might die.

So unnerved was I by Amble's lack of authority and confidence that I emailed my younger sister Britt later: "We need to stay on top of her care and make sure no one screws up." Our mother wasn't going to die simply because Dr. Amble's grandmother had.

That night, Dad and I obtained a prescription for Rifampin from a former colleague of his and talked about moving Mom to a university hospital. Only Duke would satisfy my father. I suggested he start calling his influential friends for a referral.

At 11:30 p.m, Dad contacted Dr. Hayes, one of his clinical associates at the National Heart Institute in the 1960s and a former chief of medicine at Vanderbilt. Within an hour, an erstwhile resident on Dr. Hayes's Vanderbilt service, now an assistant professor at Duke and an infectious disease specialist, called my father. Without such clout, I'm not sure how I would have dealt with my apprehensions, which network I would have tried and how. But I would've done something. I felt certain that my mother's life depended on family intervention.

At 2 a.m. on what was now Thursday, June 6, Dad shared with me the results of his communications with the Duke Hospital transport department: An ICU bed may not be available, *and*, in any case, Mom would have to travel by ground, not air. Also, we would need a physician's referral from Chesapeake. We decided to suspend all talk of a move until 9 a.m. and mercifully got some sleep.

In the morning, Dad informed Dr. Amble by telephone of our intentions. The hospitalist, threatened by our end-run around him, beseeched: "Will you do me this favor? Will you see her before you make your decision? I think you'll find she's improved."

We agreed to hold off on arranging for the transfer until after we'd made the 75-minute drive to Chesapeake to see Mom.

Amble was right. Mom was more energetic and with it. She sat taller in bed and spoke more coherently. She told me that during the night, she had undergone *another* chest X-ray and brain CT scan, and before breakfast a new doctor—who turned out to be the ID specialist, Dr. Taft—had examined her. Dr. Taft decided to take her out of isolation. In fact, nurses told me, Amble was moving Mom out of the ICU, after about 40 hours, and into a private room on a nearby medical floor.

Whether our talk of a transfer to Duke prompted this flurry of activity cannot be determined from Mom's medical records, which I later obtained, because Dr. Amble made no notes. No notes. Not a single jotting. It was as if he didn't exist. But I don't think this transfer was coincidental. (Dr. Taft's report, which I read later, raised no red flags. He thought Mom's condition was consistent with bacterial meningitis.)

I was encouraged, but cautious. Just how sick was Mom? I walked beside her during the gurney transport to her new room and immediately sought out her nurses, filling them in on her illness and its progress. I was determined that Mom would be more than just an anonymous "78-year-old white woman." I placed family photographs on a bulletin board in her room, telling all visitors that Fern Esther MacAllister Sjoerdsma was a vivacious older woman with a full, happy life and many loved ones.

Soon, though, I learned that Mom would not be receiving consistent nursing care; the R.N.s would be changing shifts too frequently to permit that. Thursday's day nurse would not likely reappear on Friday.

Leslie urged me to assume nursing tasks, cautioning me in particular about the physiological damage that bed rest can cause, especially to elderly people. Reduced to its essence, the human body is made up of functions, the impairment of which can produce ghastly results. Prolonged immobility brings on such impairment.

Leslie drew up a two-page "plan of care," which she emailed to my siblings and me. Among other things, we would ensure that Mom regularly shifted position in bed, in order to guard against breakdowns of her skin (bedsores), and drank enough fluids daily to prevent dehydration. We also would be on the lookout for any new neurological signs indicating a brain infection: weakness of the extremities, drooping of the mouth, seizures.

When I left the hospital that afternoon, Mom was reading the newspaper funnies and planning to watch the evening news. She was still receiving intravenous gentamicin and ceftriaxone, the meningitis antibiotics. Her breathing seemed more rapid to me, but I hopefully assumed that all would soon be well. I put the Duke transport mentally on hold.

THE AFTERNOON OF JUNE 7

Throughout the week, I had kept Leslie, Al, and Britt informed by email and telephone of Mom's condition and medical treatment, and they had given me a lot of emotional support. Not knowing what the outcome of her frightening illness might be, each one wanted to see Mom.

Al Jr., a playwright in Ann Arbor, Mich., decided to fly in Friday morning, June 7, and left his return trip open-ended. Dad picked him up. Britt, a television editor in Alexandria, Va., outside of Washington, D.C., planned to drive down late Friday night. I booked a motel room for the two of us near the hospital. Leslie, married and the mother of two young children, checked flights for the weekend and was ready to leave at a moment's notice.

My father still suffered great distress. Although he had come through with the Duke contacts, he seemed to be in a fog. He blamed himself for not diagnosing Mom's illness and for believing that her mystery virus would simply run its course. Guilt and grief continued to color his thinking and made him vulnerable, especially while driving. I was grateful when Al arrived and could help me to look after Dad. On Friday afternoon, the two Als visited Mom and called me from the hospital parking lot.

Al Jr. was delighted to discover Mom so "with it." He had imagined her locked in an embrace with the grim reaper. Instead, they chatted happily about a variety of common interests. She laughed and teased him.

Al Sr., however, found his wife "unchanged" from Thursday and noted her shortness of breath and swollen feet. He had spoken with Dr. Frank, the Chesapeake General hospitalist who took over from Dr. Amble, about prescribing a diuretic, which would increase her flow of urine and thus reduce the fluid in her body. They also discussed precautions to guard against blood clots. A blood clot "thrown" from the leg to the lungs—at which point it becomes a pulmonary embolus—is a common and potentially lethal hazard of too much bed rest, especially for older patients with damaged circulation.

Dad liked Dr. Frank, who, he said, seemed "to have more on the ball" than Dr. Amble. My brother said Dad told Frank the Big Jim Tatum story in the hallway outside Mom's room.

"What's the Big Jim Tatum story?" Mom had asked about the Carolina football coach who contracted Rocky Mountain spotted fever.

I was concerned about the breathing difficulties that both Dad and I noticed and wondered if Mom should return to the ICU. I decided to assess her condition when I returned to the hospital that night and wished my father and brother a safe trip back to the Outer Banks.

Earlier, I had contacted a hospital lawyer friend of mine whose husband was a neurologist. Dr. Amble had not consulted a neurologist, and I wanted the opinion of a neurologist I could trust. Although Dad later informed me that a neurologist had in fact examined Mom and found nothing inconsistent with the meningitis diagnosis, I emailed my friend that I might call her husband, Dr. Roberts, that night.

I left home at 4:15 p.m., arriving in Mom's room about 5:45 p.m. In a million years, I never could have scripted the evening that lay ahead.

THE INTERMINABLE NIGHT OF FRIDAY, JUNE 7

My mother's appearance stunned me. She had deteriorated markedly in the 24 hours since I'd seen her. What in the world was going on?

Mom lay in bed, moaning and breathing rapidly and laboriously. Her whole body, especially her legs, seemed bloated. She failed to respond coherently to questions I asked and acted irritated by my attempts, scowling at me as she had after the day spent at the Kitty Hawk clinic. She was disoriented and withdrawn, listless, but also fitful. Dad and Al had left just two hours ago. What had happened? Was she having an adverse reaction to some medication? My mind raced. What should I do?

I grabbed the first hospital staffer who walked into the room, a nursing assistant who delivered the dinner tray. She deferred to the nurse, whom I sought, but could not find. I helped Mom drink some cranberry juice and water and tried to assess her condition better. She complained of pain on her side, circling with her hand an area to the right of, but below, her bellybutton. She made little sense, drifting off into incomplete non-sequiturs. Gibberish. I evaluated her as somnolent, but restless.

The nurse arrived, yet another new one, a "hon" sing-songer. I told her of the changes in Mom's condition, but she acted unfazed. She started the next round of IV gentamicin and sodium chloride (for fluid). When I inquired, she advised me that the doctor on duty was not scheduled to visit, but would "pop in"– with no notice. Still reeling, I told her I would like Mom moved on a regular basis, as per Leslie's instructions. She tartly replied that Mom "knows to move."

"Not anymore she doesn't," I said.

The nurse's indifference threw me. Maybe I *was* overreacting. I mentioned the visiting hours, scheduled to end around 9 p.m., and noted that I would like to stay later.

No problem, she chirped. "We're shorthanded tonight. We'd welcome the help. You can stay as long as you want."

My spirit sagged. My mother could be dying, and they're shorthanded tonight.

Cell-phone use was prohibited in the room, and I didn't want to disturb Mom by placing a calling-card call, so I went to the hospital lobby to call Leslie and Dad from a pay phone. Worried that we were losing Mom, I needed to understand what I was seeing. I needed medical opinions of people I could trust, and I had no faith in Chesapeake General's doctors or nurses.

My sister fired off scary terms like cerebral edema and third spacing, meaning Mom's brain and body had filled with a dangerous amount of watery fluid, and urged her immediate return to the ICU. Because of Mom's altered consciousness, Leslie wanted a neurologist called in, *stat.* I told her about Dr. Roberts, my friend's husband, and asked her to phone him, find out what he thought, and then call me back in the room. We concluded by agreeing that unless I sounded an alarm, Mom would likely be ignored, perhaps with disastrous consequences.

I then phoned my father to put him on stand-by. I might need his expertise in speaking with Dr. Frank. While I could describe Mom's symptoms, I couldn't begin to analyze them diagnostically and know the proper medical questions to ask. Unbeknownst to me, my call triggered my 77-year-old father's emotional collapse. Surely, the death he had feared all along would happen that night. He and Al Jr. grieved together—until I called later to assure them their mourning was premature, and they needed to get a grip.

These phone calls prepared and fortified me. I walked resolutely back to the floor and told the nurse in charge at the front station about my mother's deterioration and my grave concerns. I requested an immediate consultation with the doctor—who, much to my chagrin, turned out to be Dr. Amble, not Dr. Frank—and expressed a desire to transfer Mom to another hospital. I didn't want to threaten anyone, or be obnoxious, but I was determined not to be ignored.

In the 75 minutes that passed between this confrontation and Amble's arrival, a very competent nurse gave Mom a thorough examination, and I worked the phone, talking to Leslie, Dad, and Dr. Roberts. I no longer cared about the cell-phone rule or if my mother heard what I said on the telephone.

Naturally, Roberts was uncomfortable advising me about someone else's patient, sight unseen, so I presented my mother's case as a hypothetical one—a classic legal exercise—and sought only information, not conclusions. Suppose, I asked him, you had a patient with haemophilus influenzae meningitis, and she had shortness of breath and excessive fluid buildup . . . what would you think? What would you do? Roberts suggested that these "peripheral symptoms do not make sense in terms of the meningitis" and might be caused by another infection. He would consult infectious-disease, pulmonary, and cardiac specialists.

The new competent nurse had recorded a temperature of 100.6 degrees and a pulse of 106. A healthy, resting adult heart beats on average about 72 times per minute. Otherwise, Mom's respiration rate and blood pressure were normal.

"What does the infectious disease specialist think about her fever?" Dr. Roberts asked. I planned to ask Dr. Amble that as soon as I saw him.

～

Much to my amazement, Amble couldn't—or wouldn't—see the deterioration in Mom that was so evident to me. He described her as having "slight edema" and being more uncommunicative, but not that confused. When he questioned her about pain, she denied having any. I pointed out her stoical habit of minimizing her discomfort, but Amble attributed her fever and rapid breathing to the meningitis infection.

"She's very sick," he concluded. "Her brain is fighting a serious infection."

Yes, but caused by what? H-flu didn't make sense, and the therapy wasn't working. Not only had Mom's physical condition declined, but her personality had altered. A gracious, sweet person, she now snapped at us for making noise.

For the next hour, Amble calmly talked about Mom's worsening condition with me—as well as my father and Leslie, whom I called on the room phone at opportune moments—and resisted all of our suggestions. Under our questioning, he grew defensive. He acknowledged that my father and "his friends are very impressive," but Dr. Amble, too, was not to be lightly dismissed.

Amble adamantly refused my request to transfer Mom back to the ICU. If he did that, he asked me, how could he justify to his supervisor having moved her out just the day before? I didn't give a shit, but I was never anything but courteous with him. My brother, who listened in on Amble's stonewalling conversations with my father, remembers the Chesapeake hospitalist telling them: "She's getting better."

Lest I think he lacked medical muscle, Amble defended his credentials and staff status, telling me of his previous experience at a hospital whose reputation, I now knew, far exceeded Chesapeake's.

He also pointed out: "I know I'm talking to a lawyer."

Doctors don't much like lawyers—really, who does?—so I had made sure that Dr. Amble knew I was one. My opinion on medical malpractice notwithstanding, lawyers can hold doctors accountable. That status gave me leverage. Amble didn't have to know that I had stopped practicing years ago. But, if he actually thought I had a lawsuit even remotely in mind, he was way off-base. Families of critically ill patients don't want litigation after mistakes have been made; they want results while there's still time.

Despite my father's appeal for one, Amble wouldn't summon a pulmonary expert during the night. Any consult could wait until morning, he said. If we wanted to move Mom to Duke then, he'd be more than happy to refer her. I'm sure he thought we were the family from hell, but I wasn't liking him very much either.

Finally, Dr. Amble admitted to me: "I don't know what I'm treating."

But he failed to add what I thought *any* conscientious professional in *any* profession should add: "But I'll find out."

I challenged myself: How could I reach this placid, polite, yet intractable man? How could I convince him to take some action?

I never raised my voice or lost my cool. I searched for an angle, a way to break through to him. Finally, I asked Dr. Amble: "What would you do if you were in my position?" a question I have learned is *the* question to ask an obstructive doctor. I'll never forget his response.

"I'd kiss my mother, tell her I love her, and let the hospital take care of her," he said.

"Well, I can't do that," I replied. "I can't leave." This grandmother wasn't going to die because a doctor didn't know what he was treating.

Earlier, Dr. Amble had noted that the oxygen saturation in Mom's arterial blood was, at 60, a "little low."

"A little low!" Leslie had shrieked on the telephone. "He's crazy. That's dangerously low."

"What's normal?" I now asked Amble, being clueless about what the number measured.

In the 80s and 90s, he said, but elderly people run low.

"As low as 60?" I queried.

"No, usually not that low," he conceded, but he wasn't concerned.

I was horribly ignorant then. Sixty, indeed. A blood-oxygen saturation level below 90 percent is cause for concern.

Knowing that Mom's "PO2," as Dr. Amble called her oxygen saturation, was excessively low, I reached a compromise with him. I would cease and desist if he ordered more tests—of Mom's urine, blood gases, heart, lungs, and liver functioning, etc.—and call me if anything appeared abnormal.

"Would that make you feel more comfortable?" he asked.

"Yes, thank you," I said. "It would."

He agreed.

At 11:45 p.m., six hours after my arrival, I obtained a nametag from the nursing station, enabling me to re-enter the hospital later, and I left. I hadn't yet checked into the motel, and I wanted to be there, if possible, when Britt arrived.

No sooner had my sister entered the motel room, around 1:30 a.m., than Dr. Amble called. Mom's PO2 was now 57; her liver enzymes were "up a little," and she had become more confused. She might have a sepsis condition, an infection caused by pathogens in the blood. He was moving her back to the ICU.

Britt grabbed my nametag and flew out the door.

"Proceed until apprehended," I told her, echoing a phrase Leslie had coined when I expressed doubt about entering certain hospital zones. "Act like you belong."

I then hit the phone. We were transporting Mom to Duke. I only hoped it wouldn't be too late.

SATURDAY, JUNE 8

Throughout my mother's crisis I had this strong, but not wholly rational feeling that as long as I or another family member watched over her, she wouldn't die. It was a matter of control, I suppose, or connection. Thus, I felt comforted when I managed to reach Britt on a phone in Mom's room and learned that she planned to spend the night in the ICU. My sister's hospital presence freed me to send emails and place phone calls in preparation for tomorrow.

Leslie would be flying in from Florida. Al would be driving up from the Outer Banks. Dad would resume discussions with Duke. Britt would protect Mom, who by now was too far gone to recognize her youngest child. And Mom would hold on.

We finally would get competent help, and answers. But little sleep.

I didn't see Britt again until 10 a.m., when she returned to the motel to report that the pulmonary specialist, Dr. Kimble, had examined Mom and treated my sister rudely. When Britt tried to fill him in on Mom's condition, especially her mental status, he cut her off.

"I'm talking to her now," he said abruptly. "I want to know what she says, not you." When Britt asked about Mom's breathing, he explained that, because of the meningitis, "her brain is telling her to breathe in a shallow way."

"What can you do to make her better?" Britt wondered.

"Sometimes they don't get better," Kimble answered.

Why were these doctors so prepared for Mom to die? Because she was old? Or were they just irritated by our involvement?

After Kimble left, Britt said, a nurse asked Mom what month it was. She answered June. But she didn't know the year.

The rest of the day unfolded for my family in a series of assigned tasks: motel checkout; breakfast; *Merck* research into sepsis infections (I had my manual with me); a return to the ICU; a trip to the airport, where I met Leslie, who dissolved into tears on the arrival walkway, until I told her our mother was *not* going to die; phone calls to home, to Duke, to doctors at Chesapeake, to friends in Durham, N.C. Eventually, we four siblings converged on the ICU, waiting for the Duke helicopter to arrive. Mom had become delirious and was now receiving oxygen. She happily sang nonsensical songs and talked in a wispy childlike voice. "Whatcha doing over there?" she asked over and over.

That morning, Dr. Frank had taken over from Dr. Amble and been shocked by Mom's decline. He cooperated with the referral to Duke and consulted with doctors there, ordering two new antibiotics for her treatment regimen: doxycycline and Zosyn®, a broad-spectrum penicillin. He also called in a neurologist, who recommended another lumbar puncture and an MRI of Mom's brain. Dad consented to the puncture, but the neurologist couldn't execute the procedure. It was not as easy as Barnett at the Outer Banks Hospital had made it seem.

I never talked to Dr. Frank to find out what he thought was wrong. I just waited for the Duke angels to arrive and airlift Mom to safety. The wait was interminable—nothing happens quickly in a hospital, except disaster—but the angels, clothed in their medical flight suits, were worth it: Confident, efficient, friendly, optimistic. As soon as they took her out, relief washed over me like a refreshing swim. It was about 6 p.m., and Leslie, Al, Britt, and I had a three-and-a-half-hour drive ahead of us, in three cars, but we all felt euphoric. Almost giddy. Britt was firing off one-liners in her whimsical style, joking about "spending another night in the chair." For all its seriousness and our anxiety, that road trip to Durham felt like a reunion vacation.

Someone else could watch over our beloved mother for a while. Someone we could trust. Or so we hoped.

MIDNIGHT, DUKE INTENSIVE CARE

At midnight on Saturday, June 8, we sat in the darkened waiting room of Duke University Hospital's medical intensive care unit, expecting to meet with Dr. Roddick, whom Leslie had described, after a brief phone chat with him, as likeable and competent. When he arrived, Roddick wanted to know the full history of Mom's illness, from the onset of her "really bad" headache until the respiratory distress of the previous night and that afternoon's delirium. Not just what the tests showed, but what Mom had experienced over the past 11 days.

The young resident listened attentively to my account and then asked me some pointed questions about Mom.

Has she been out of town recently?

—Only to Washington, in April (when she attended Paul McCartney's Freedom concert at the MCI Center).

Has she traveled to Connecticut?

—No.

Does she live or walk in any woods?

—Yes.

Does she have a history of tick bites?

Ticks.

I knew of no recent bites, but I knew that, in walking her dog, Max, Mom would pick up ticks. She regularly checked herself for them. Max, too. The Outer Banks is a haven for ticks.

Roddick strongly suspected that Mom had contracted a *rickettsial* disease from an infected tick, either ehrlichiosis or Rocky Mountain spotted fever. Rickettsia is a genus of bacteria carried as parasites by ticks.

Oh, my God. Big Jim Tatum. Dad was right.

I had never heard of ehrlichiosis, but I certainly knew about RMSF.

"She's not going to die tonight," Roddick told us, but "she's very sick."

Very sick, indeed. I think it's accurate to say that our mother went away for a while. Just disappeared. She lost her ability to speak, to swallow, to move, to remember, and to reason, but she survived.

From June 8 to June 12, she lay in an ICU bed in a bewildered semi-comatose state. She opened her eyes, but showed no understanding or recognition. She was a blank slate, but she was safe. This ICU, unlike Chesapeake's, was a nurturing incubator, tended by efficient and kind nurses who spoke in hushed tones.

After Mom left intensive care, she spent 15 more days on one of Duke's medical floors, in an altered, but slowly improving mental state.

On Sunday, June 16, which was Father's Day and the eighth day of her hospitalization, she said her first words. She told a nurse: "I want to see my husband."

During her hospitalization and subsequent convalescence, Leslie, Al, Britt, and I stayed at Mom's bedside as close to around-the-clock as we could manage. When you come from a medical family, you know to be on the alert for hospital "never events," such as *nosocomial* infections, which are infections acquired in hospitals; adverse drug reactions; medical errors; and other undesired outcomes that should never happen in a hospital, but do. Many are possible. The one that we most feared for Mom was a fall.

We rented two extended-stay apartments in Durham and left our lease open-ended. I moved in; and the others came and went from their distant homes, rotating relief.

On June 21, diagnostic lab work confirmed what Roddick and my father's first Duke contact had suspected. Mom had ehrlichiosis, an infectious disease long known to exist in animals, but still emerging in people. The first human case in the United States was reported in 1986. The antibiotic doxycycline cures this disease, but only doxycycline or another tetracycline, not Rocephin, which Drs. Washburn and Barnett had administered—much less the anthrax-fighting Cipro.

JUNE 12 TO JUNE 27

The missed diagnosis, it turned out, was just chapter one in Mom's death-defying journey as we encountered missteps at Duke resulting from apathy, ageism, move-'em-out medicine, and over-zealousness. Once she moved from the womb-like ICU to a regular room, she encountered risks, both predictable and not, and we ran into obstacles.

Mom had the misfortune to be hospitalized at Duke shortly before one medical post-graduate training year ended on June 30, and another began on July 1. New interns, also called first-year residents, are just out of medical school and usually anxious, sometimes terrified, and always inexperienced. Their supervising residents have one or more years of post-medical-school training, but they, too, may be anxious and uncertain.

Medical professors at teaching hospitals, such as Duke, traditionally take turns serving as the attending physicians on the wards. Rotating attendings "attend" patients who arrive at the hospital without a physician of their own and also supervise the interns and residents, who are known collectively as house staff.* House staff is responsible for patients' hands-on medical care.

Because of June vacations and other scheduling conflicts, Mom had three attending physicians from June 12-27. In chronological order, they were conscientious and communicative (he left too soon); perfunctory and dismissive (he wanted Mom's bed); and grandstanding and arrogant (he avoided us). The latter—an I-walk-on-water psychiatrist named Gideon—is, hands down, the rudest, most egotistical, and biased physician I have ever met. He seemed determined to do harm.

Attending No. 1, who watched over Mom from June 8-16, eased our minds. Dr. Port was courteous, friendly, and generous with his time and knowledge. He explained Mom's condition and progress, discussed his judgments with us, and freely shared all test results. He was a gem.

Attending No. 2, Dr. Stevens, expressed more concern about cost than care and talked on June 17, his first day, about discharging Mom later that week. After a certain number of days in a bed, I learned, a recovering patient who requires little medical intervention becomes a losing financial proposition for a hospital. Too damn bad, I thought. Mom had spoken for the first time just the day before, but she was hardly mentally alert. She still had a feeding tube in her nose and couldn't move without assistance. Even more important, she was in the middle of a precious two-week intravenous treatment of doxycycline.

With Dr. Stevens threatening to discharge Mom to a nursing home/rehabilitation center, known in healthcare parlance as an SNF

---

* At teaching hospitals today, you may encounter hospitalists, who act as inpatient attendings, rather than traditional rotating attendings.

(skilled nursing facility), Al and I visited a number of such facilities in Durham. Mom's social worker arranged our appointments, and I prepared for them by doing Internet research and talking to a nursing-home-savvy acquaintance of one of my friends. From our interviews with SNF directors, Al and I knew they would not accept a patient who has an IV or can't swallow. Armed with this intelligence, we successfully resisted Dr. Stevens's bean-counting efforts, which continued through June 22, when he, too, departed.

Attending No. 3, the chanticleer Dr. Gideon, rebuffed both my introduction and my small talk the Sunday morning of his arrival. He then threw me out of Mom's room so he could talk alone with her and directly assess her "dementia," a diagnosis that he bluntly dumped on Mom behind the closed door, before asking for her permission to do a brain MRI.

Dementia? My poor sick mother had never thought of herself as demented. The word alone terrified her. She was scared for days. *Days.* This was patient care?

My father refused the MRI that Gideon wanted, but, unbeknownst to me, the cocksure attending ordered it anyway. I learned later, after obtaining Mom's medical records, that the interpreting radiologist found evidence of cerebral atherosclerosis, a vascular condition that can adversely affect cognition. There would have been no way, however, for Gideon to differentiate mental impairment caused by Mom's "hardened" arteries from impairment caused by the active infection in her brain, and she had been fine before her illness.

Nonetheless, as I also learned later from the records, Gideon administered a well-known 10-minute mental-status questionnaire to my critically ill mother and used its results to seal the deal on a "baseline dementia" diagnosis. I now know because of my study of Alzheimer's disease and other dementias that his clinical methods were both grossly inadequate and despicable. Considering her diseased state, the test score he obtained from Mom actually indicated a high level of cognitive aptitude.

In what was surely his coup de outrageous acts, Gideon put Mom on the potent anti-psychotic drug, Risperdal®, which is typically used to treat schizophrenics. My father, the drug expert, became furious when he found out, but he did not confront Dr. Ego. Instead, he intervened after Mom had been discharged to the rehab center that Al and I selected, easily convincing its on-call physician to discontinue the drug.

After our first encounter, when he barred me from Mom's room, I never saw Gideon or spoke with him again. He arranged his rounds so that he visited Mom at 6 a.m. during a gap in our family bedside coverage. We kept informed about Mom's progress through the resident on her case, young Dr. Susan Walker. Walker cared for Mom throughout her hospitalization and even visited her later at "Sunshine" Convalescent Center.

"Dr. Gideon doesn't like to meet with family members," she told us with a sly grin.

Like Dr. Stevens, Dr. Gideon ordered Mom's discharge before her IV doxycycline course was finished, and we again protested. I wondered if this alleged physician even knew that his patient had ehrlichiosis and what it was. He wanted Mom out on June 26, a mere day before her two-week doxycycline treatment was to end. Because of our resistance, our initial Duke contact, who had arranged for Mom's transfer from Chesapeake, called a meeting to mediate the dispute. Dad and I attended; Gideon did not. After observing that our family was unusually "actively involved" in Mom's healthcare, our contact agreed that a 24-hour delay made sense.

I readily admit that we were omnipresent and vigilant, but we were actively involved only because we felt we had to be. It wasn't personal for us until Stevens and Gideon made it so. It was just hospital business as usual: We knew how much could go wrong, so we took preventive action.

Despite our best efforts to ensure that nurses (and we) moved her around often in bed, Mom experienced a breakdown of skin on her buttocks—an ugly bedsore—and endured a hideous ordeal with impacted feces.

Fecal hardening and impaction are well-known consequences of the prolonged immobility occasioned by bed rest. The smooth muscle in the wall of the colon, which handles movement of solid waste, slackens, so that feces are not promptly evacuated. Instead, they build up, harden, and block.

One night the telephone rang at our rental apartment while Dad, Britt, Al, and I were eating a late dinner. Who in the world? Al answered. It was Mom calling! She had understood what we told her about the number we left by her phone and needed our help. She was trying to relieve a bowel impaction with her fingers, piece by piece.

Al grabbed the car keys and shot out the door. He spent the night in Mom's room, helping her to "pass" a massive fecal chunk.

Later, I saw what came out of my mother. It filled a toilet bowl. This disaster should never have happened.

Because Mom couldn't swallow, we had ruled out requesting a stool softener, but that didn't excuse the nurses from monitoring her bowel output. The nurse who assisted Al the night she called was already on my shit list (so to speak) because Mom's feeding tube became dislodged on his watch. I never believed his story that she yanked it out herself.

June 27 to Aug. 8

From June 27 until Aug. 8, Mom lived at Sunshine Convalescent Center in Durham, where she underwent physical, speech, and occupational therapy. Still mentally altered, and very weak, she had to learn to be human again.

The quarrelsome woman who had argued with me at the Chesapeake hospital emerged during the first week at Sunshine. I told the SNF caregivers: "This is not my mother. Her personality has changed." Please don't ignore her because she's difficult.

I also wrote an account of the crisis Mom had endured and posted it on the wall next to her bed, along with family photos. I wanted the nursing-home staff—the one registered nurse who supervised the medical care of all of the residents; the different therapists who helped to restore her functionality; and the certified nursing assistants (CNAs) who attended to her basic needs and had the most contact—to know who my mother truly was when her brain wasn't diseased.

"Mrs. Sjoerdsma did not have a stroke,". my tract announced at the top. "She does not have dementia." Too many of the typically 20-something CNAs assumed that because Mom was 1) old, at least by their standards, and 2) in a nursing home, where many of the residents were recovering from strokes, that she was cognitively impaired. The Sunshine center was an excellent SNF, but it didn't take long for me to observe that some CNAs ignored or took longer to respond to *certain* patients' call buttons.

We didn't know who Mom would be once she became well enough to leave the facility. Our initial Duke infectious-disease contact told us that, among severely ill ehrlichiosis patients he had known, only one had "come back" 100 percent. He cautioned us to expect some permanent mental damage. But he also told us her recovery would take months, even years. Mom had no memory of her hospital stay or of her first week at Sunshine, which was probably just as well.

I remember when I first realized that my mother was returning. She looked at me during one of my morning visits at Sunshine and said with great anguish: "What do I do now? I don't know what my life is anymore."

That she had such a strong sense of her self and her identity shouldn't have come as a surprise to me, but I think even I had fallen prey to thinking of her too much as a disease profile, rather than a person. She looked fragile, but her will was strong. She needed to process what had happened to her and figure out how she would go on.

While we were in Durham, I kept track of all of Mom's activities and coordinated the family's oversight.

During the day, my in-from-out-of-town siblings and I sat at Mom's bedside for hours, reading and watching over her. We also attended all of her therapy sessions—thus making sure that none was overlooked, and she was progressing—and walked with her through the hallways. To get well, she had to walk as much as possible, not just the short distance between her room and the physical-therapy gym. She started with a walker and gradually progressed to a cane as her strength increased. My siblings and I "spotted" her.

As Mom improved, we wheeled her outside for sunshine and fresh air and eventually down to the dining room for meals. I scheduled appointments for her with the Sunshine hairdresser; took her to see a gynecologist at Duke for a checkup; and even arranged for Max to visit. The Shih Tzu didn't recognize her.

At night, we entrusted Mom to two wonderful private-duty nurses whom we hired at $10 an hour. Leslie, knowing to cast about at Duke Hospital for CNAs who did outside contractual work, met Samantha there, and Samantha introduced us to her cousin, Carol. With Samantha and Carol on the job, Mom slept soundly every night (as did we) and had help whenever she awoke. They both had Mom dressed and walking each morning before breakfast, something we could not count on staff CNAs to do. Samantha gave Mom her first shower—a big step forward.

My mother had kept her promise to me, and, in so doing, she changed my life.

Chapter Two

Becoming An
ADVOCATE

And a Pox on Dad's Head

In the aftermath of Mom's near-death experience, I went on the journalistic attack, writing articles about the details of her crisis and her disease, which I published in several newspapers, including one of the local Outer Banks papers. Although I wrote the stories for *The Raleigh News and Observer*, the editor rejected them once she saw how critical I was of Mom's doctors. I refused to sugarcoat the facts.

Three doctors on the Outer Banks, an endemic area for ehrlichiosis, Rocky Mountain spotted fever, *and* Lyme disease, and at least six doctors, including an infectious disease specialist, in Chesapeake, Va., another endemic area, had examined my mother, and evaluated her lab tests and CT scans, and none had even considered a tick-borne disease. But, as we learned at Duke, the telltale signs were there: a low white-blood-cell count, depressed blood platelets, and elevated liver enzymes.

My mother wasn't a drunk, Dr. Amble. She was very, very sick.

Had Mom died on the Chesapeake hospitalist's watch, she would have been a victim of bacterial meningitis. His second in 20 years.

And if she had died, I would have failed as an advocate. I would have lost my campaign to protect her. Hers was not a hopeless cause. I had the skills and the determination to pull her through, if I always did my best.

In the course of interviewing ehrlichiosis specialists at the U.S. Centers for Disease Control and Prevention, Johns Hopkins School of Medicine, and Duke, among others, and reading on-point medical-journal articles, I became an expert in this disease myself. Ehrlichiosis lurks in the shadow of the much-better-known and feared Lyme disease. The knowledge gap exists, the experts said, because Lyme patients *live* and often are vexed by chronic crippling symptoms, whereas ehrlichiosis patients go undiagnosed and may die.

Human ehrlichiosis has several bacterial species. Its infection ranges from a mild febrile (with fever) illness, characterized by headache and malaise and suggestive of influenza, to a fatal illness. If untreated, vulnerable patients, such as those who are older or whose immunity is suppressed, can experience kidney failure, a serious bleeding disorder called disseminated intravascular coagulopathy, meningoencephalitis (brain inflammation), adult respiratory distress syndrome, seizures, coma, and death.

Three percent of patients infected with the type of ehrlichiosis that my mother had die because of meningoencephalitis or respiratory distress or both. Mom represented the worst-case scenario.[1]

After Mom's ordeal, my father informed Dr. Washburn about what had transpired. Washburn told Dad that he had never treated a patient for *any* tick-borne disease in his quarter-century of practice on the Outer Banks. Ha! I wonder how many other cases he's missed.

I adamantly believed that the urgent-care doctor dismissed my poor, pathetic wretch of a mother as suffering from a garden-variety urinary tract infection, albeit a serious garden-variety UTI, because he stereotyped her. "Little old ladies"– LOLs, in the medical-acronym dictionary–frequently get UTIs; ergo, Mom, being just an LOL in his filing-cabinet mind, had a UTI. The truth is older women don't get UTIs nearly as often as doctors diagnose them.[2]

Dad also thanked Dr. Barnett, who had performed the lumbar tap at the OBH, even though the young doctor, like Dr. Logan, his predecessor in the examination chain, had clearly given Mom the LOL brushoff until I started questioning him. Logan hadn't even bothered to talk to Dad and me. I thought they both owed us an apology.

Missing the Zebra

There's a wonderful maxim about medical diagnosis that goes: When you hear hoofbeats outside of the window, you should think of horses, not zebras. The maxim cuts to the core probability principle of diagnostic reasoning: It is more likely that hoofbeats will be made by the common horse than by the exotic zebra.

Zebras, I read, tend to be the province of medical students and inexperienced doctors who jump erroneously to the diagnosis of a recently learned condition. Having studied the improbable zebra and its peculiarities, they become predisposed to diagnosing it in a patient—achieving a sort of ego gratification. Those who hunt for zebras are thought to be showoffs.

But just as the medical neophyte may succumb to the sexy, life-or-death zebra diagnosis, more clinically experienced doctors, who have seen and treated a lot of horses and don't expect zebras to walk in the door (nor, perhaps, want them to!), may miss the stripes. Sometimes a severe headache plaguing a patient with a history of migraines is an aneurysmal subarachnoid hemorrhage, and the patient dies less than 24 hours after being treated in a hospital emergency department and discharged—without the on-duty doctor bothering to order a brain scan.

Missing the stripes is one thing; not recognizing or having heard of the zebra is quite another.

You might argue that ehrlichiosis is a *bona fide* zebra diagnosis, even for infectious-disease specialists. OK. I'm willing to grant that. So what, then, does the medical problem-solver do when the horse diagnosis does not respond to the standard treatment? How does the doctor proceed?

More to the point: Why didn't Dr. Amble reach outside of himself and discuss Mom's bewildering condition with other doctors who might know more than he does?

Apparently such common-sense behavior would have been an admission that he lacked knowledge, authority, intuition, or whatever medical Right Stuff he did not possess, not that he was a fallible human being who needed help. When I asked Dr. Amble about moving Mom back into intensive care, he immediately expressed concern that his supervisor would disapprove.

Why couldn't or wouldn't any of the doctors who treated Mom before her Duke hospitalization see what was so obvious to me? Why did I have to play doctor, as well as lawyer, in order to get them to respond?

I didn't see a lot of critical thinking going on in the medically trained minds I encountered. There was reaction, but little reasoning.

I had to wonder: Have doctors become so dependent on technology that they no longer see the clinical trees amid the forest of excessive tests? My father certainly thought so. Have they also forgotten how to listen well, or did they never know?

Or were these doctors sloughing my mother off because that was the easy thing to do? Or because they were tired, busy, lazy, apathetic ... *ageist?*

My beautiful mother, whose kind, gentle nature always buffered my father's dominating personality, was not going to die if I had any control over her fate. And I believed I did have control. Shit *doesn't* just happen.

Do most doctors tend to think that shit does happen? Or, perhaps, that shit happens to patients with whom they have no emotional connection? Or to people old enough that it's "all right" for it to happen?

And what about the Duke attendings who came in after the diagnostic blunders had been made? Why did two of them try to hustle us out, disregarding Mom's recommended treatment protocol? Were their attitudes indicative of more ageism? Or were they just irked that we were "actively involved" and did not regard them as all-knowing saviors?

I knew about the need for vigilance in a hospital: I had read that 300,000 patients die in U.S. hospitals each year because of errors, infections, and other preventable causes. (See Appendix One, "The Risks of Hospitalization," and Appendix Two, "Surgical Hazards.") But I never expected to encounter a physician who cared more about counting hospital beds or blinding the house staff with his brilliance than about his patient's well-being.

Heave-ho, out of bed you go—but before you go, kindly stop by the radiology department a few times so we can irradiate your brain for our gratification (and profit?).

And how could that abominable fecal impaction have occurred?

The answer to most of these questions was simple. The doctors and other healthcare professionals either weren't good enough or had performed inadequately under the circumstances. They failed us. I've met many more bad doctors, and posed many more questions, since then. I've also read accounts by other people of their harrowing hospital experiences. Hospital survival how-tos are virtually a genre of non-fiction.

"Going into a hospital as a patient," writes New York internist and rheumatologist Sheldon P. Blau in his book, "How to Get Out Alive," "is a death-defying act."

Blau's own crisis began with sudden unrelenting chest tightness and pain down his left arm. In short order, he underwent an angioplasty to open up a 90-percent blocked coronary artery, during which a technician ruptured the artery, necessitating emergency open-heart surgery. Before this second operation could occur, the 60-year-old Blau had a heart attack. After the surgery, he developed a potentially lethal staphylococcus infection and paralytic ileus, which is an obstruction of the bowel due to paralysis.

Everything that "I feared could go wrong, did. . . .," he writes. "My hospital stay continued to challenge my determination to survive."[3] Fortunately, the physician-patient had his wife standing watch during his 17-day hospitalization.

According to Blau, hospital patients fall into two groups: victims, who are passive and permit all of the errors that can befall them to occur, and survivors, who are not and, through action and control, do not.

Each patient, he somberly concludes, "is a potential morgue inhabitant."[4]

QUESTIONS, QUESTIONS

When my mother fell ill, I was 47 years old. For nearly 30 of those 47 years, I had been planning my future. I always had an eye on the next challenge, as well as today's. Now, suddenly, my life was just happening, and my priorities were crystal-clear. Simply because of aging—because of surviving—my mother and father had become vulnerable. If they needed protection, I had to protect them. I had to speak up. I couldn't let a physician's illogic, inaction, avoidance, bigotry, or any other failing or obfuscation within the healthcare system determine the fate of people I dearly love.

Could you?

I don't think any reasonable person could; but that doesn't mean that all reasonable people, by whom I mean clear-eyed critical thinkers, will act. Many such people automatically defer to physicians because of the latter's education, knowledge, and presumed intelligence and ethics. After all, doctors have spent most of their lives learning the mysterious how-tos and whys of the human body and its diseases. Laypeople can't begin to understand medicine and to make medical judgments.

Nonsense. You don't need a medical degree to "talk the talk" with physicians and "walk the walk" within the healthcare system. You just have to do your homework and be able to think and act like a reasonable person, often quickly and on your feet.

In his narcissistic coming-of-age book, "Intern: A Doctor's Initiation," Sandeep Jauhar, M.D., Ph.D. (in physics), who is the director of the Heart Failure Program at Long Island Jewish Medical Center, recalls an attending physician who categorized patients as either Kmart or Bloomingdale's shoppers.

Jauhar's attending, identified only as being at a "prominent" teaching hospital in New York City, preferred Kmart shoppers, he said, because they "have their own insurance, they don't pay cash, they're not going on the Internet, they don't ask a lot of questions, [and] they don't have a bunch of doctor friends secondguessing your decisions."5

In other words, in God they trust. (Note the elitist economic-class distinction.)

Jauhar did his internship in the late 1990s, before the Internet became everyone's go-to information source, The Patient Protection and Affordable Care Act ("Obamacare") became U.S. law, and Bloomie's scaled back the number of its stores. Substitute Saks Fifth Avenue, Nordstrom, or another upscale department store, if you prefer. Whichever you choose, I definitely shop there, and I can assure you that most doctors don't shop at Kmart or any other "mart." So why should you?

While I agree with Jauhar's attending that second-guessing physicians is a bad idea—absent compelling reason to do so—asking questions of them is important, even when you won't understand their answers. It's important that you *ask* questions, rather than interrogate. A doctor who acts annoyed by your questions or gives your family short shrift is a big red alert. The patronizing doctor, who does not consider you to have an intellect, also trips an alarm.

As I told my father repeatedly during Mom's ehrlichiosis crisis, when a doctor responds, you can evaluate his or her body language, facial expressions, attitudes, and other interpersonal signals. Good communicators know that communication encompasses more than mere words. It bears repeating: Sometimes what is *not* said is more important than what is said. (Your best doctors know this, too.)

In a medical emergency, you have to be concise; persuasive, but not aggressive; firm, but not angry. You must listen carefully and remain open-minded. But trust your own judgment and be prepared to act when action is required, even if you meet resistance. Be hopeful, but not unrealistic or naïve. If you tend toward denial, step aside. You're out of your comfort zone.

Never be a blowhard yourself; you could be wrong, too. Everybody is fallible. Rely upon logic and reason. Be courteous and respectful. Rudeness antagonizes people; it does me. But don't accept bald conclusions. Ask for the details that underlie them. Seek explanations.

It helps to have confidence and a familiarity with the medical world, but you can fake the former and acquire the latter. I had to acquire confidence, through the usual path of trials and errors in experience, but I came by the familiarity naturally.

GROWING AWARENESS

Unlike most people who first encounter a looming white-coated authority figure when they are small and insignificant, I never saw a pediatrician because I never had routine checkups. My father would shine a flashlight down my throat, feel my salivary glands, and send me to bed. Coca-cola and liquids in brown bottles seemed to cure everything that ailed me.

As grade-schoolers, my brother and I would page through our parents' thick medical books, pointing fingers and laughing uncomfortably at photographs of diseased naked people. The identity-obscuring black bars across their eyes only punctuated their otherness. These textbook cases were fully exposed—for the good of humankind, the advancement of medicine, or so I believed. I was proud of my parents' participation in such noble goals.

Still, it never seemed right to me that these sick people had to endure such humiliation and helplessness. I definitely was not doctor material.

Al and I had more fun skimming "Huber the Tuber," a sketch-filled tract about tuberculosis, and "Corky the Killer," a similar tale about the corkscrew-shaped demon syphilis. They were medical cartoon books for laypeople.

My father's NIH colleagues and medical luminaries from across the globe came to our suburban home for dinners and cocktail parties. They were real people—not mythic heroes—who ate with a knife and fork, laughed loudly, and sometimes drank too much; but they were undeniably elite in their profession. I was enchanted by their sophistication and loved to listen to their shoptalk.

Subject to these early influences, I developed a clinical approach toward illness. I am curious about diseases, diagnoses, and therapies and don't believe their understanding is beyond me. I also appreciate doctors as human beings, capable of fallibility (according to Dad, an alarming degree) and failings, as well as exceptional intelligence. I respect them, but not unconditionally.

I avoided science courses in high school and college, preferring English, history, drama, and just about anything but the domain ruled by my larger-than-life father. I should've learned chemistry; I didn't. I studied English literature and got into journalism, but struggled to find my professional niche, opting for law even though I knew I was a writer with my mother's empathy and my father's analytical and straight-shooting style.

A child of the 1960s and the '70s feminist movement, I wanted to advocate for people who couldn't effectively advocate for themselves and, I thought, deserved a voice. I believed I would do that by arguing in a courtroom, educating clients about their rights, or crafting a killer appellate brief. But in law school already, I felt like a misfit. I leaned toward mediation, not litigation, and didn't care for the grinding legal process or its practitioners. After practicing law for about a decade, I turned exclusively to journalism. Both of my parents furthered my evolving career with advice and more.

During my law studies, I briefly considered criminal law as a focus and attended a psychiatric seminar on the insanity defense as my mother's guest. As a journalist, I had often consulted Mom for the psychological angle on stories I was working: She gave me an insightful analysis of the Unabomber's psyche, for example, based on his writings.

Dad played a larger role. Over the years, he had been a source for free-lance medical stories that I had written. None of them dealt directly with his work, his special brand of research, however, until I wrote a "Perspective" cover piece in 2000 for *The Baltimore Sun* about a wonder drug discovered and developed under his auspices.[6]

Di-fluoro-methyl-ornithine (DFMO), approved by the U.S. Food and Drug Administration as the orphan drug, Ornidyl®, was a slam-dunk cure for a type of deadly African trypanosomiasis (tryps), which we know better as sleeping sickness. Because of incompetence, blunders, and bottom-line thinking, however, this Third World savior was no longer reaching dying patients. Since Dad's retirement, DFMO's manufacture had ceased, and its on-hand supply would soon run out.

To make matters worse and tragically ironic, American women troubled by excessive facial hair could get what desperate tryps-stricken Africans could not. The chief ingredient of Vaniqa®, a prescription hair-growth retardant launched by Bristol Myers Squibb in September 2000, was none other than DFMO, also called eflornithine. I decided to investigate DFMO's history and find out what had happened to it.

After he left the NIH in 1972, my father went to Strasbourg, France, to start a research institute for a U.S. pharmaceutical company. When he arrived, the construction of the building hadn't been finished, and for years he lacked what businesspeople called "critical mass" in staff—a concept that Dad ridiculed. He always figured that all he needed was one person to make a difference.

The first-ever director of the Centre de Recherche Merrell International hired a few young, promising chemists and challenged them to synthesize a compound that would stop cell replication, an investigatory focus that Dad had identified at the NIH. He then kept the research open-ended. If DFMO, one of the compounds that emerged, had a therapeutic effect in cancer—if it stopped mutated cells from growing—wonderful, but Dr. Sjoerdsma was fine with trypanosomiasis, too, or any other target.

Later, as director of Merrell International and National, and president of the Merrell Dow Research Institute in Cincinnati, my father made DFMO freely available to any investigator who asked for supply. He wanted the compound to find its use. Hundreds received DFMO for experimentation.

One of them, a U.S. university biologist, thought it might have an effect on trypanosomes, the single-celled parasites that cause the tryps infection carried by tsetse flies. It did. DFMO blocked their growth in culture and cured tryps-infected mice. After this discovery, Dad's team took over, doing all of the clinical research—even smuggling the compound into Africa so it would reach patients in the bush—and eventually securing the FDA's approval. So dramatic was DFMO's effect on comatose patients that it was dubbed The Resurrection Drug.

Shortly after my father made DFMO available widespread, the razor company Gillette asked for supply. Dad, thus, had known for quite some time about Gillette's hair-growth research and its eventual partnership with Bristol-Myers Squibb, which culminated in the cosmetic, Vaniqa.

Although angry about DFMO's abandonment as treatment for trypanosomiasis, Dad was nonetheless hopeful that Vaniqa, projected to be a $6 billion-a-year product, would be DFMO's salvation. I shared my father's outrage and knew the power of the press. I was not the first to expose the DFMO travesty, but I was the only journalist who had the inside story of the drug's R&D.

In May 2001, Medècins Sans Frontières (Doctors Without Borders) announced a pact with the World Health Organization, Bristol-Myers Squibb, and Aventis, which was a successor pharmaceutical company to the one for which my father had worked, to guarantee a five-year supply of DFMO. Dad considered his efforts to save DFMO his "last fight." For me, the fight was a beginning.

DOING HOMEWORK

The fascinating details of the DFMO story whetted my appetite for medical research. I also got to thinking about my father's accomplishments, especially those achieved when I was a child and unaware of what he was doing, and about his place in medical history. I decided to become my father's biographer.

Through long interview sessions, I learned everything Dad had ever thought and done as a physician-scientist-researcher-pharmaceutical company research chief and eventually knew more about his work than anyone in my family, including Mom. I read every article that he ever wrote. This research gave me the chance to relate to my father as a professional, and as an individual in various times of life, and to appreciate the depth and breadth of his full and rich *working* life, not just his family life.

In 2002, when my mother became ill, I had scarcely scratched the surface with Dad, whom I would interview extensively; and, despite my upbringing and education, I had never imagined becoming a healthcare advocate. I simply hadn't perceived the need. Still, my decision to advocate was a no-brainer. I had been training for the role my whole life. I knew how to do homework, to question, to think, and to proceed until apprehended. Homework, which anyone can do, is knowledge, and knowledge is empowering.

When I turn to the Internet for medical research, I usually consult the Mayo Clinic's website first for general knowledge and the National

Library of Medicine/NIH drug-information website for the basics about medications and their adverse effects.

After I obtain the Mayo Clinic's overview explanation, I often continue my research through both direct and free-associational exploration. Numerous medical-information websites exist now that didn't in 2002. If you have a discriminating mind, you can pick and choose from the most reliable sources, some of which appear in my endnotes, but you have to know when the oversimplification of complex subjects adds up to dumbed-down misinformation. Both trust and credibility are issues.

Like most journalists, I much prefer the expert or the near-expert human source, rather than the electronic one, when I can access him or her. Absent such a source, however, I have no hesitation in exploring medical topics and following my leads, either online or in a medical library. I read my *Merck.* I can always get the gist, even if some of the details elude me.

So can you.

A Pox on His Head

My first chance to be a spot-on medical advocate after Mom's illness and rehabilitation came about three months later, and I'm sorry to say that I dropped the ball. Despite the crisis with Mom, I still had faith in good people's good sense, and I still made assumptions that I shouldn't. Plus, I was back to working on other people's deadlines and not yet cognizant of how pervasive Murphy's Law is in healthcare.

By this time the former ehrlichiosis patient had resumed her full routine and showed no obvious signs of cognitive impairment. She again swam, drove, walked the dog, read Dickens, and solved puzzles. We figured Mom had dodged the proverbial bullet and hoped she would continue to do so.

On the day before Thanksgiving, Dad asked Mom and me to look at some blister-like lesions on his head that were extremely itchy and painful. The blisters started near the top right side of his forehead and went up into his scalp.

"They look like shingles to me," I said, sounding, and actually feeling, rather authoritative. "You need to see a doctor fast."

Several years before, a friend of mine had suffered an outbreak of shingles on her scalp. Theresa, who was in her early 40s, told me the clinical details about what she mistakenly, and with prejudice, bemoaned as "an old man's disease," and I could analogize Dad's lesions and other symptoms to hers.

Shingles is caused by the same virus that causes chickenpox, which most adults had when they were children.[7] Dad did, as did I. It is the varicella zoster virus. (The varicella vaccine, to prevent chickenpox, became available in the United States in 1995.)

After you contract the zoster virus, it lies dormant (resting) in your body's nerves, specifically in the sensory ganglia of your cranial nerves and in the spinal dorsal-root ganglia. Ganglia are structures that contain a number of neurons, also called nerve cells, linked by synapses. As you get older and your immune system naturally declines, the latent virus can reactivate.

People whose immunity has been weakened by cancer, human immunodeficiency virus (HIV), chronic disease, and certain medications, among other causes, are especially susceptible to a varicella outbreak. Prolonged stress, which my father recently had experienced, also may contribute. When the virus reactivates, it is known as the herpes zoster virus, or shingles. (Although shingles is one of the herpesviruses, it has nothing to do with herpes simplex, which causes cold sores (type 1) and genital vesicles (type 2).)

My freaked-out friend had told me that the drugs used to treat this viral infection are most effective when started within 72 hours after a rash appears. Theresa consulted her doctor immediately, took oral Valtrex® (valacyclovir), and quickly healed.

Dad contacted Mom's new internist, a young doctor who he thought would make a house call on a holiday weekend. Dr. Roland was an acquaintance of Dr. Walker, the resident who cared for Mom at Duke. A former Duke resident herself, Dr. Roland had moved recently to our Outer Banks neighborhood and agreed to drop by. Roland confirmed our suspicions, but did not prescribe Valtrex, *the* shingles medication, nor did she urge Dad to begin treatment. I thought she had. Instead, she passed him off, and I didn't follow the trajectory of her pass, so Dad lost precious time.

Never assume the appropriate followup will occur, even when it's obvious. Murphy is always lurking.

Because my father's vesicles were on his forehead, he feared damage to his right eye. He knew about herpes zoster *opthalmicus*, which results from an infection in the ophthalmic division of the trigeminal (or fifth cranial) nerve and threatens the orbit of the eye, including the optic nerve. Blurry vision, corneal ulceration and scarring, loss of sensation in the eye, and temporary or permanent blindness can result. Before the advent of the antiviral drugs in the 1990s, blindness was common. My parents had friends who had lost sight in an eye because of shingles.[8]

Dr. Roland referred my father on an emergency basis to an eye specialist who she thought was an ophthalmologist. Dad's own ophthalmologist, Dr. Bloomer, had a part-time practice on the Outer Banks—as do most M.D.s on the beach—and would not be available for at least another week. I took it for granted that Roland's referral was solid.

Unfortunately, the specialist Dad consulted the Monday after Thanksgiving—already past the 72-hour window—turned out to be an optometrist, who didn't know his zoster from first base. Optometrists are not medical doctors. During his examination of my father, Dr. Stone exited the room repeatedly, giving Dad the impression that he was consulting textbook sources. Eventually, the optometrist made the wrong call, prescribing an antibiotic, instead of Valtrex.

That I could recognize an eruption of shingles, but an optometrist could not, is a sad state of affairs.

After his appointment with Dr. Stone, Dad arranged to see Bloomer. He did not return to Dr. Roland or see his own primary-care physician. In retrospect, I should have insisted that he did. He suffered longer than he should have.

A seasoned pro, Dr. Bloomer had no trouble diagnosing shingles and prescribing the recommended dosage of oral Valtrex—800 mg. five times a day for seven to 10 days—and the steroid prednisone. In his examination record, Dr. Bloomer described the cornea of Dad's right eye as "crusty, scruffy, a little beat up."

Did the herpesvirus damage Dad's cornea? There was no way to know. In February 2004, however, when Dad had his right lens replaced at the Johns Hopkins Wilmer Eye Institute, the ophthalmologist put him on Valtrex and prednisone as a precaution before and after the cataract surgery. The last thing my father—and the surgeon—needed was a shingles flareup.

THE SHINGLES SCOURGE

According to the CDC, 30 percent of the estimated 90 percent of all adults in the United States who have had chickenpox will develop herpes zoster.9 This adds up to one million episodes of shingles occurring each year in the United States, the peak incidence being in adults ages 50 to 70.[10]

Shingles migrates along the paths of inflamed nerves to the surface of your skin, triggering severe burning or shooting pain, as well as tingling and itching. Within a day or two of these abnormal sensations, a rash of vesicles (blisters, for lack of a more apt non-medical word) appears, forming a band or clustered pattern.

Typically, the infection affects only one side of your body, usually on your chest or back, but sometimes it affects your neck, face, and head, as it had my father. In the most common case, vesicles form a single stripe around the left or right side of your torso, stopping in the middle. The word zoster comes from the Greek for belt or girdle; shingles comes from the Latin *cingulum*, also meaning girdle.[11]

The vesicles tend to scab after three to five days, and the rash usually clears within two to four weeks. During a shingles outbreak, you may experience fever, headache, chills, malaise, and/or some gastrointestinal upset. Neurological symptoms also may occur outside of the region of primary attack.

Herpes zoster can cause brain inflammation (encephalitis), Guillain-Barré syndrome, motor neuropathies, and other rare complications. In a worst-case scenario, the infection can lead to pneumonia and death.

Valtrex and the other shingles drugs, Zovirax® (acyclovir) and Famvir® (famciclovir), do not cure the infection, but they can decrease pain and other symptoms, speed healing, and stop the spread of the herpesvirus. This may not be the end of your suffering, however, as I discovered when I started doing my shingles homework.

Significantly, 20 percent of all infected people—and 40 percent of infected people over age 60—suffer from severe debilitating pain after the rash disappears. So-called post-herpetic neuralgia (PHN) is a nerve inflammation that can extend well beyond the area of the original rash and last for months, even years. The pain, which can be deep, throbbing, constant, and/or sharp, may be provoked by light touch or by changes in temperature and may persist even after the stimulus (e.g., cold air) is gone.

Zostavax®, the herpes zoster vaccine, became available in 2006. Dad elected to get an injection, even though recurrences of shingles constitute only 1 percent of all viral outbreaks. Both of my parents received their vaccines at a local pharmacy.[12]

A PERIOD OF CALM

For about three years, from 2003 into 2006, my parents and I stayed clear of hospitals that posed risks and doctors who did damage. Mom and Dad made a number of car trips to Baltimore, so Dad could have cataracts in both eyes removed, and Max, their dog, went along for the rides. I was able to be a writer again, and I traveled extensively to interview my father's former colleagues. By age 49, I had become a full-time free agent, having resigned from all free-lance jobs so I could work exclusively on my book.

When my parents marked their 80th birthdays in 2004, they were active and healthy, if reluctant celebrants: Mom wouldn't even allow us to mention the age. Dad took it more in stride.

"Eighty separates the men from the boys," he was fond of saying. Although Dad had struggled with some aging demons on his 70th birthday, he seemed to enjoy looking and feeling better than people expected at 80.

I certainly recognized that my parents were getting older, but I never thought of them as feeble or infirm. They had busy, independent, and enriching lives.

The irrepressible Dr. Al, as my father liked to be called outside of the family, was still "stirring the pot," challenging people on their political views and other assumptions and opinions that they might hold, just to evoke a response, and Mom was in her Zen state of peacefulness with the world. Dad was well-liked in our community for his great sense of humor and friendly agitation, and my mother charmed people with her warmth and kindness.

They made an interesting pair, and I enjoyed their company immensely. I always found it frustrating when a friend assumed that, because of their age, my parents were a burden to me. To the contrary, conversation in their household sizzled, and I loved to participate in it. My father kept the flow lively and filled with laughter. I never wanted it to end. But, of course, it would, despite our desires otherwise.

Chapter Three

2006: Bronchitis or a
MASSIVE BLOOD CLOT?

When Precautions and Primary Care Fail

Two years after their milestone 80th birthdays, my mother again experienced distressing respiratory symptoms, only this time Dr. Al didn't have to conjure up the spirit of Big Jim Tatum. It was fairly clear why she couldn't breathe. Or was it?

On May 22, 2006, Mom had her left knee replaced. Osteoarthritis had worn down the knee joint's cartilage to nothing—to "bone on bone," in orthopedic parlance—and she struggled with chronic pain and stiffness.

Osteoarthritis, which is associated with aging, but not caused by it, leads to joint instability and a decreased ability to withstand the stress of body weight. The amount of body weight pounding the joints makes a big difference—yet another reason to combat obesity. You may think of osteoarthritis as the chronic deterioration of joint cartilage.

This was knee surgery No. 2 for Mom. She had her right knee replaced in 2001 with no ill effects, but no resounding success either. She still favored it. She delayed the second surgery as long as she thought she could, often quoting the advice of her surgeon's chief assistant: "It's better to do it now than to wait until you're 90."

Although I was heartened that my 82-year-old mother contemplated reaching her tenth decade, I couldn't imagine any 90-year-old undergoing a knee arthroplasty. Joint replacements may be common, but, like all surgeries, they pose significant hazards.

In retrospect, Mom would have preferred to let the bum knee remain bum.

I visited my mother the day after her surgery at Sentara Leigh

Hospital, a 250-bed facility near the Norfolk-Virginia Beach line that specializes in orthopedic services, and was pleased to see her mindfully getting out of bed and moving. Immobility was again her enemy. I watched her do physical therapy in a rehab room and thought she seemed very motivated.

After a total knee replacement, a patient's risk of developing deep-vein thrombosis (DVT), which can lead to a fatal pulmonary embolus, is 50 percent or higher in the absence of pharmacological *prophylaxis*. Prophylaxis is prevention. This means that more than half of all knee arthroplasty patients who do not take an anticoagulating drug develop blood clots in their legs.[1]

Being sedentary for a prolonged period, as with bed rest, slows your venous blood circulation. DVT occurs when a thrombus (a clot) forms in a wall of one of your large veins, usually in your calf, in an area where the blood flow is slow or disturbed.

My parents knew the incidence of DVT in knee-replacement patients, so Mom took precautions. She was safe, right?

To understand why a thrombus in the leg can cause disaster in the lungs, you must know basic cardiovascular facts, including how and where blood circulates. I had only a rudimentary understanding of circulation when Mom had her knee surgery. I learned.

CARDIOVASCULAR BASICS

The heart is a hollow muscular pump, which, by contracting and relaxing (beating), controls the circulation of blood. It has two sides, left and right, each of which has two chambers, an upper chamber called an atrium and a lower chamber called a ventricle. The atria fill their respective ventricles with blood, which the ventricles then propel outward.

The heart's atria and ventricles are not arteries. They are cavities or rooms, if you will, made up of muscular walls. Confusion exists among laypeople about this, I think, because we so often hear, and worry, about blocked arteries, which supply the heart with blood, and not about heart muscle.

The two sides of the heart function independently of each other to pump blood into two different circulatory systems. They are the systemic circulation (left side) and the pulmonary circulation (right side). The heart also has its own circulation, which is served by the two main coronary arteries and their branches.

The left heart pumps oxygenated blood out into the body (the system), including the head and brain, through big arteries that eventually decrease in size until they end in microscopic capillaries that are wide enough for only one blood cell to pass. This is where the key exchange of oxygen, carbon dioxide, nutrients, and waste occurs in the tissues. Capillaries are vitally important. If you were to lay them end-to-end, these tiny vessels would stretch more than 50,000 miles.

Arterial (i.e. oxygenated) blood capillaries exist in beds with venous capillaries, such that you may think of a single capillary as having an arterial end and a venous end. By the time blood reaches the venous capillaries, it is deoxygenated. It flows from the venous capillaries into venules and progressively larger veins until it returns to the right atrium of the heart, thus completing the systemic loop.

The right atrium primes its ventricle with this return venous blood, which is not only lacking oxygen, but now contains carbon dioxide that must be expelled into the air. The right ventricle pumps this blood through the pulmonary trunk, which branches to form the right and left pulmonary arteries that go to their respective lungs. Through the respiratory exchange process, this blood releases carbon dioxide and receives oxygen. Oxygen-enriched blood then flows through the four pulmonary veins—two from each lung—into the heart's left atrium, thus completing the pulmonary circulatory loop.

Generally speaking, arteries carry blood away from the heart, and veins transport blood back. The pulmonary arteries, which carry deoxygenated blood from the right heart, and the pulmonary veins, which supply the left heart with oxygenated blood, are the exceptions.

Perhaps now you can better see that if a blood clot forms in a lower-body vein, breaks off, and travels in the systemic circulation, it can enter the heart through the right atrium and upon exiting the right ventricle get lodged in one of the pulmonary arteries.

It also helps to understand that pressure generated by the heart propels arterial blood, whereas skeletal-muscle contractions constrict the vessels to move venous blood back to the heart. Medium and large veins also have valves that keep blood from yielding to gravity and flowing backward. Thus, in addition to prolonged inactivity, a failure of muscle contraction and/or insufficient valves can result in blood pooling and clotting in the lower extremities.

Blood pressure is expressed as systolic arterial pressure over diastolic arterial pressure. Systole occurs during the heart's ventricular contraction, and diastole occurs during ventricular relaxation. The left ventricle is the Samson of the pressure system; it is much thicker and more potent than the right (pulmonary) ventricle. The atria also have systolic and diastolic pressures, but they are substantially weaker. (I take up the cardiac cycle in Chapter Five.)

Today, you may have your blood pressure recorded electronically and displayed on a digital device. Traditionally, however, a "gold-standard" pressure reading involved placing a rubber cuff on a patient's upper arm and inflating and deflating it to cause arterial constriction and relaxation, respectively. The cuff was connected to an instrument called a sphygmomanometer, which registered the patient's high and low pressures on a mercury column.

Generally speaking, blood pressure is considered normal when the systolic pressure is between 90 and 140 millimeters of mercury (mm Hg), and the diastolic is between 60 and 90 mm Hg.* Thus, both 120/70 and 90/60 are normal readings.

A constant systolic pressure of less than 90 mm Hg or a drop of at least 40 mm Hg for at least 15 minutes constitutes sustained hypotension (low blood pressure), which might signal a pulmonary embolus.[2]

DEEP-VEIN THROMBOSIS

A pulmonary embolus or embolism (PE) occurs when a fragment of a thrombus breaks loose from a vein wall and migrates through the systemic circulation to the lungs, where it blocks (embolizes) vessels encountered there. If the clot is large enough to obstruct one of the pulmonary arteries, sudden death can result. Collectively, DVT and PE are known as venous thromboembolism or VTE.[3] Anticoagulants, such as Coumadin® (warfarin), thwart clotting and, thus, keep blood flowing. Aspirin also inhibits platelet clumping, but it is not classified as an anticoagulant.

Although I had long been aware of the twin threats of DVT and PE, it took 39-year-old NBC reporter David Bloom's sudden death in April 2003 to shock me into awareness of their prevalence. Embedded in Iraq, Bloom slept in a Humvee, hunched over, with his legs folded under him. The next morning, a pulmonary embolus killed him.

---

*This measurement is still used even though mercury may not be.

My family strongly suspects that my mother's brother, my Uncle George, who had been known to have DVT, died suddenly at age 77 because of an embolus. A nurse in the Michigan hospital where he was being treated for severe depression returned to his room to find him sitting in a chair, dead.

In 2005, my brother Al absorbed stunning news when the chest pain and shortness of breath he had been downplaying for a month turned out to be a blood clot in the lower lobe of his right lung. Just 48, Al underwent a battery of tests to determine the cause of the thrombus. We feared cancer, but the tests all came back negative. The only trigger he could identify was a cramped 90-minute airplane trip during which he didn't get up to stretch his legs.

Dr. Johnson, my mother's surgeon and the son of the orthopod who performed her first knee arthroplasty, started her on intravenous heparin, an anticoagulant given only by IV or by subcutaneous injection, immediately after her surgery. Later that day, Dr. Johnson transitioned Mom to Coumadin, which is administered in a pill form.

The next day, my father, who disliked Coumadin's slow onset—its effectiveness is not immediate—persuaded Dr. Johnson to switch Mom to a different anticoagulant, so, on May 24, she started Lovenox® (enoxaparin). After her May 25 discharge, Dad injected her with Lovenox for 10 days.

Besides pharmacological blood-clot prophylaxis, knee-surgery patients may take mechanical precautions, which rely on physical forces. Elastic flesh-colored compression stockings, also called supportive or support stockings, are the most common. This tight-fitting hosiery applies graduated pressure on the lower leg and foot to increase venous blood circulation and thereby reduce clot formation. They are tightest at the ankle.

My Uncle George wore compression stockings for years, but I don't know if he was wearing some when he was stricken, nor do I know if he was taking an anticoagulant.

After her surgery, Mom faithfully pulled on her compression stockings every day. She also tried to sleep with her legs in a bulky device that stimulates blood flow by applying intermittent pneumatic compression (inflating and deflating air bags). She did not suffer this metallic bed partner lightly and soon quit it. After she successfully completed a month of physical therapy, I assumed that all of the precautions she had taken had worked, and we could relax. There would be no "complications." No worrisome clots.

I forgot about Murphy.

Bronchitis, Anyone?

During my mother's first post-operative month, I traveled out of town several times, conducting interviews, and busied myself at home with work and massages to relieve my own physical problem. I had been coping for five months with pain in my lower back, left hip, and left leg, and I could not sit comfortably—no matter what type of chair I used. Depending on the repetitive-stress motion in which I engaged, I suffered with muscle aches and pins and needles of nerve pain. Computer deskwork and long-distance driving were killing me and the quality of my life.

Because of my new disability, I didn't go with Mom to her six-week follow-up appointment with Dr. Johnson, nor did Johnson himself show. Instead, he entrusted my mother to his assistant who, my father told me later, examined her left knee, chiefly by bending it, and detected no problems. The assistant did not know, however, nor did I, that Mom had not been eating well and had been feeling weak.

Again, as with the ehrlichiosis, my doctor-parents thought Mom had a virus. My uncomplaining mother said nothing about her illness to Dr. Johnson's assistant, who perceived no need to check the pulse in her ankles, much less to arrange for an ultrasound of her legs. I don't know what Mom's blood pressure was, but I know she didn't have the telltale edema in her legs that occurs when blood flow is interrupted.

This type of edema results when venous blood flow backs up and the capillaries leak fluid into the surrounding tissues. Normally, the blood vessels and the lymphatic system maintain a balance of extracellular or "interstitial" fluid. Swelling associated with clots can be so extreme that skin breaks.

In the days after this followup, Mom's weakness and fatigue rapidly worsened, and her breath became shorter and shorter. Not being on the scene, *I* was caught short by her deteriorated condition. This was déjà vu. Both Dad and I feared a pulmonary embolus.

On Thursday, July 6, my parents visited Dr. Charles, Mom's Kitty Hawk internist, who had signed off on the arthroplasty. Now very concerned, I went with them, but I didn't go far enough. Reasoning that my presence in Dr. Charles's tiny examining room would be one too many bodies, I sat in the waiting room. What could possibly go wrong? All the doctor had to do was see Mom, listen to her recent history, and X-ray her chest, and he'd know that something was seriously wrong, right? Dad would advance the embolus theory, and the two M.D.s would consult. I would only be in the way of the physician shuffle.

Wrong. Wrong. Wrong. As it turned out, I would have been the only person to press the issue.

After an hour with Dr. Charles, my parents emerged with a preposterous diagnosis of bronchitis and an even more preposterous prescription for a common antibiotic.

If you don't know that antibiotics are ineffective against viruses—such as cold viruses—you should. Acute bronchitis is viral. A doctor may prescribe an antibiotic for a bronchitis patient if the doc fears a bacterial infection may develop in the patient's lungs, but this is the exception, not the rule.

I was incredulous. Mom hadn't even undergone a chest X-ray, which Dad now informed me "probably" would not reveal a clot anyway. (She would need a CT scan.) In that case, I asked, wouldn't the absence of disease be meaningful? Can't you rule out causes . . . such as bronchitis?

Despite Dad's naysaying, I implored my mother: "Mom, you have to have a chest X-ray." Exhausted on her feet—on the verge of collapsing—she begged off. I could coax *ad nauseum*, but I could not coerce. Nor could I pack her in the car and take her to the ED for a CT scan.

I just didn't get it. What had been the point of this visit? Dr. Charles had listened to Mom's chest, made his flaky diagnosis, and shown my parents the door. And they had allowed the brushoff.

Here again, it seemed, was another lackadaisical healthcare obstructionist in a white lab coat. Was he ageist, too? I figured him for his forties. Incompetent? I'd seen enough bronchitis in my lifetime to know this wasn't bronchitis.

The excursion to Charles's office had exhausted my 82-year-old parents. They could do no more.

That afternoon, I repeatedly asked my father: "Bronchitis? How in the world could Mom have developed bronchitis? She hasn't had a cold or an infection." Straining the limits of my disease knowledge, I stressed, "And she's never had bronchitis in her life. She's not even coughing!"

"Let's just see what happens in the next 24 hours," my father urged. But I knew he knew better. He just wasn't prepared yet to confront the stress of the inevitable.

"So, we'll take her to the emergency room on a Friday, in July," I protested, "with mobs of tourists!"

Fool me once . . . fool me twice. I was an idiot, and my parents were nose-deep in denial. Or maybe it was emotional shock? Or fatigue? I grew weary.

Thankfully, I had reason to hope we could avoid spending a day in the Outer Banks Hospital Emergency Department. The three of us agreed that if Mom needed further medical attention, she would see her cardiologist in the morning, and he would smooth her admission to the hospital.

How many times could I think it? *Hold on, Mom. Hold on.*

Stat to Radiology

As soon as Dr. Anthony's office opened on Friday, July 7, my father called to request an emergency appointment. Soon we were all congregated in one of Anthony's examining rooms, listening to Mom gasp as she related her symptoms. When the intense and fast-talking cardiologist, who treated both of my parents, asked if her shortness of breath had been progressive, and she answered, "No," I was very glad I was there.

"That's not true," I interjected. "You're much worse today than you were yesterday. It's gotten worse every day."

Wanting to be respectful of my mother's autonomy, I hesitated to speak for her. She always had been very independent and secure in her intelligence and reasoning. I did not want Anthony to start talking to me and referring to Mom in the third person—a poor habit of some physicians who examine older patients with their younger relatives present.

I needn't have worried. Not only was Anthony juiced—a force of nature in black scrubs—he was very good about looping Mom and Dad into the conversation. Mom was the patient. She was his focus, but he listened to me, too.

Anthony approached the problem logically, analyzing a "pyramid" of causes, at the top of which were the most threatening. This was where he started, not at the familiar bottom, as Dr. Charles had. Before considering the embolus theory, which Anthony thought likely, he wanted first to rule out an adverse drug reaction or interaction. With Dr. Al firmly shaking his head, Anthony did not tarry. Before I knew it, he was on the telephone arranging for Mom to be seen *stat* in the radiology department of the Outer Banks Hospital.

In the years since Mom's errant H-flu meningitis diagnosis, the OBH still had not earned my confidence, and I wasn't thrilled to be returning there. But I will always be grateful for Anthony's decisiveness. *Stat* meant *stat.*

My parents drove ahead to the hospital. By the time I arrived, Dad was finishing up the paperwork process in admissions. We hadn't had time to catch our own breaths before we were summoned from the waiting room. The technicians' worried eyes conveyed the severity of the problem that awaited.

Not only did Mom have a pulmonary embolus, she had a massive embolus. What they called a saddle thrombus was lodged in the space between the openings of the branches to her two pulmonary arteries. The clot was blocking the blood flow to both of her lungs!

The radiology technicians seemed stunned that Mom was still alive. But there she was, engulfed by a huge computed tomographic machine that I had never seen before, looking small but calm, her obstructed blood still circulating, barely.

Mom was receiving intravenous heparin, and, we were told, there were other clots in her legs. She could drop dead like Uncle George.

There was no question what would happen next: Mom would be transported by ambulance to a hospital in Norfolk or Virginia Beach, Va., at least 90 minutes away.

Since my mother's 2002 ehrlichiosis crisis, Dad and I had done our homework on the area hospitals and now knew that Norfolk Sentara General Hospital, affiliated with the Eastern Virginia Medical School (EVMS), was the best. Fortunately, it had an open bed. Mom would be admitted to the ICU through the ED—at just about the worst possible time during the calendar year. It was mere days after the new EVMS house staff had reported. Just as we had at Duke, we would face what I had come to know as the "July phenomenon," when teaching hospitals experience an uptick in patient deaths.4

Interns and residents have medical degrees, but they lack clinical experience and are best viewed as doctors-in-training. When contrasted with Dr. Charles, the bronchitis doc, however, EVMS's house staff looked pretty darn good to me. At least they would be fresh and eager to please their attendings. I looked forward to meeting them.

I did not look forward to the crowd in the ED, though. On a summertime weekend, there was bound to be a steady flow of victims injured in traffic collisions, fights, and crimes, including gunshot victims.

On my way home from the OBH to pack Mom's and my suitcases, I started calling my siblings, who had been in the dark about any problems.

"You're kidding me!" exclaimed Al, who had visited the beach just three weeks before. "How did this *happen*?"

Britt, too, was stunned. She quickly responded to my request that she drive down from Alexandria.

Leslie was the most alarmed. I couldn't answer many of her questions because I had no idea what would be done, but I assured her that Mom was stable and positive. She was very sick, but she didn't believe she was dying, and so I didn't believe she was, either.

"That could just be denial," Les said.

"If it is," I answered, "it's helping her to cope."

I had no idea when I would be home again. I picked up my "Merck Manual," along with my toothbrush and other essentials, and left for Norfolk.

THE EMERGENCY ROOM

At 4:30 p.m., I checked in at the reception desk of Sentara Norfolk's emergency department and received directions to Mom's room and a pass that allowed me to come and go freely through a locked entry door. I easily found Mom, uncomfortably hooked up to a heparin drip and a vital signs monitor in a room with a draw curtain, which gave her some privacy. This became important as the Friday-night patients started flowing in, and the stretchers lined the hallways.

Adrenaline masked my usual back and leg pain. My "on-it" clinical self couldn't help itself. I was charged. I found the ED exciting.

A resident dropped by at 6:25 p.m. to explain Mom's condition and her treatment options. She was empathetic and professional, and Mom communicated well with her.

I thought the monster inside my mother's chest needed to be broken up or removed post-haste, but the discussion centered on the possible insertion of a filter in Mom's inferior vena cava, the big vein that carries blood from the lower body to the heart's right side. The filter, which theoretically would prevent any more leg clots from traveling to her lungs, would be inserted via catherization. According to the resident, the implanted filter would look like an open, upside-down umbrella and could be removed later when no longer needed.

I knew that a younger doctor friend and protégé of my father's, Paul S., had suffered severe chest pains, suggestive of a myocardial infarction,* and undergone emergency thrombolytic therapy for a clot in a coronary artery. In plain English, doctors had eliminated his clot. I asked the resident about this therapy, and she advised me that it was not being contemplated for Mom. Nor were doctors considering an embolectomy (clot removal), either through open surgery or a transvenous catheter approach.

Dad had explained to me that thrombolytic agents—clot busters, I called them—work by promoting production of the enzyme, plasmin. Plasmin "lyses" or destroys a blood clot by breaking down its fibrin, a protein important in coagulation, and its fibrinogen, which converts to fibrin. Paul S. received an agent called tissue plasminogen activator (tPA), which rapidly catalyzes clot dissolution.

It was hard for me to accept that this jumbo-sized clot would remain in my mother's chest undisturbed, but the resident's explanations seemed reasonable. I didn't want Mom to undergo therapy that was inappropriately aggressive and would put her at more risk, and the filter furthered a safe-not-sorry ending.

As I found out later when I obtained Mom's medical records, the resident was as thorough and efficient as she seemed. Describing Mom's condition as guarded, she noted that she would check "a 2-D echo to evaluate for any right heart strain as the presence of right heart strain and some blood pressure instability [very low pressure] would warrant the use of thrombolytic therapy." Mom remained hemodynamically stable, so no clot-busting was necessary.

The ED nurses who popped in and out, checking on "Miz Fern" and keeping us updated on the ICU-bed status, helped to relieve the strain of the crisis. Upbeat, friendly, and conscientious, they gave me reassurance that we could trust the advice we received. I kept an eye

---

*An MI, commonly called a heart attack, occurs when a blockage in one of the heart's arteries prevents oxygen-rich blood from flowing to heart-muscle tissue, and the tissue dies. Myocardial connotes heart muscle; an infarction is tissue death.

on Mom's vital signs, helped with her basic needs, and was gripped by the purposefulness of the moment.

Periodically during my vigil, I exited, passing a growing crowd in the ED reception room, to make telephone calls in the parking lot. Sultry afternoon turned into sultry night. Britt was driving down from Alexandria that evening with her boyfriend. Leslie and Al were checking flight times. Dad was fielding my medical questions from home. My natural optimism held steady.

Around 7:15 p.m., I slipped away to find a hotel room for the weekend. Having worked at the daily newspaper in Norfolk, I knew that the nearby choices were two: 1) over-priced luxury hotel and 2) I-wouldn't-be-caught-dead-there dump. I also knew enough to ask the nurses and nursing assistants which of the lodgings offered a discount rate for patients' family members and received directions to the closest dump and better motels in nearby Chesapeake.

Someone referred me to the hospital's own guest rooms on the sixth floor of the main building. I could bunk at the hospital in a converted patient room and literally be on call whenever Mom needed me. After swinging by one of the luxury hotels, I convinced myself that antiseptic and convenient were the way to go. Each hospital guest room had two single beds, a chair, a telephone, a television, sink, and toilet. Residents shared showers and a kitchen that were down the hall.

It was perfect. I reserved two rooms.

At 10:45 p.m. two young nursing assistants wheeled Mom out of her ED room, past a gauntlet of patients on stretchers, to a back staff elevator, which transported us to the floor of the Intensive Care Unit. Everyone except the patient was giddy with the freedom inherent in this movement. We had a bed! By 10:50 p.m., my mother rested in it.

I met Mom's nurse and gave her my telephone number. I didn't know when Britt might arrive, or how much sleep I would get, but I knew this much: The octogenarian with the two titanium knees and saddle embolus was alive, cheating death yet again.

FILTER IMPLANT

At 9 a.m. on Saturday, July 8, 2006, Britt and I listened intently to a radiologist explain how she would implant the IVC filter. She said she would go in with the catheter (a tube) through Mom's right internal jugular vein, creating a slight wound near her neck. The whole process would take about an hour, and we would be able to talk to Mom in the ICU around 11.

My tired mind now had two images to reconcile: a big, brutish saddle blocking blood to Mom's lungs and a dainty cocktail umbrella, flipped upside-down. Neither was accurate, of course, but they helped me to process this unfolding drama, to deal with what seemed to me to be an ongoing threat. The saddle was staying put, to dissolve on its own terms, while the umbrella would prevent any other clots from joining it. The medical records I obtained later attested to evidence of a "left *totally occlusive* thrombus in distal femoral vein."

Translated, this meant Mom had another bad-assed clot in her left leg.

The records also revealed that, besides the saddle clot, she had "bilateral second, third, fourth order branch pulmonary embolus present." I took that to mean multiple small emboli in vessels of both lungs. If my Dad, who consulted with the EVMS resident by telephone, knew this, he never told me.

That damn knee replacement.

After her IVC surgery, Britt and I visited Mom in intensive care. She was in good spirits. The jugular-vein catherization, she told us, had been "so easy." A small bandage covered her neck at the point of entry.

The next day, Mom moved from the ICU to a room on a medical floor, and doctors transitioned her from heparin to Coumadin. As long as she was in the hospital, someone from my family stayed in the guest rooms. We attended morning rounds with the attending physician, the resident on the case, and other young house staff; put Leslie's hospital care plan into effect, this time checking up on Mom, rather than watching over her bedridden immobile body; and brought newspapers and changes of clothes.

We had her up and walking the hallway at least three times a day.

Both the attending, Dr. Ramses, who turned out to be a senior member of EVMS's Internal Medicine Dept., and the resident shared their phone numbers and made themselves available for consultation. There was no hospitalist. Nurses, who were uniformly personable and proficient, responded to any requests we had, all of which were minor. With the exception of the first two of Mom's roommates, who listened to television noise night and day, it seemed a dream hospitalization.

Even though I knew Ramses and his team were monitoring Mom's heart, lungs, and blood pressure, I continued to be troubled by the saddle embolus. But my tough and resilient mother never expressed any doubt. On July 17, she moved to a spacious room on the rehabilitation wing of the hospital and underwent concentrated occupational and physical therapy, which she had started earlier. She returned home on July 21.

According to Dr. Anthony, who saw Mom in his office on July 24, she would be on Coumadin for life, and, thus, would have the clotting capability of her blood lab-tested regularly. A test known as PT-INR, for Prothrombin Time-International Normalized Ratio, allows the clotting time of a Coumadin patient's blood to be calculated.

Coumadin antagonizes vitamin K, which is essential to the liver's production of blood-clot-promoting factors. Patients who take Coumadin, therefore, are advised to watch their intake of foods high in vitamin K, such as leafy vegetables.

I distinctly remember Anthony imposing the Coumadin life sentence on Mom, and my mother frowning. I was not present when Anthony changed his mind 3 ½ years later during a routine appointment.

The occurrence of an *acute* pulmonary embolus, I learned later, is rare in an orthopedic surgical patient who, like Mom, observes prophylaxis. Undoubtedly the precautions Mom took and her upright status influenced Dr. Charles's and Dr. Johnson's clinical opinions about her—the latter deciding not to bother even seeing her. Or maybe Johnson relied on Dad's judgment, inasmuch as he had yielded to his drug protocol. In any case, Mom was nowhere near as sick as PE patients can be.

I now know that the clinical presentation of a patient with acute PE ranges from mild dyspnea (shortness of breath) or chest pain to shock or sustained hypotension. A pulmonary embolus also can be asymptomatic and only incidentally discovered upon imaging for other purposes. Conversely, a massive PE can cause immediate death.[5]

When my elderly mother, who was experiencing obvious dyspnea and attendant symptoms after recent knee arthroplasty, presented herself in her Kitty Hawk internist's office for diagnosis, the *clinical* probability of her having a pulmonary embolus, despite the drug prophylaxis, was high.[6]

The way I see it, Dr. Charles should have assessed Mom individually, not just considered the overall likelihood of a PE—if that's indeed what he did. Surely, Mom met what should be a low threshold for undergoing additional studies, including imaging.

Charles need not have been an emergency-medicine specialist to ask himself: What's the worst-case diagnosis for this *particular* 82-year-old woman with unexplained shortness of breath? How do I guard against an adverse outcome, specifically, that she drops dead after leaving my office? He could have done what Anthony did the next day.

Instead, he diagnosed bronchitis. Give me a break.

Not long afterward, Dr. Charles disappeared from the beach, apparently fired from his job, or so the scuttlebutt went. Last I heard, he still practices in North Carolina.

DOING HOMEWORK: "THINK CLOT"

In preparation for this book, I decided to find out how rare a pulmonary embolus is for a prophylaxing knee-arthroplasty patient. I did some medical-library research, but I didn't find much.

The most illuminating article described a study by a team of orthopedic surgeons and critical-care physicians in India who examined 1,013 cases of total knee replacement performed in a New Delhi hospital from September 2006 to October 2008.

The team discovered that fewer than 1.0 percent of the patients who used anticoagulants developed pulmonary emboli. Among all of the knee patients, regardless of prophylaxis, PE occurred in between 1.8 and 7.0 percent, with fatalities occurring in 0.2-0.7 percent of the total.[7]

The explanation for this low incidence may be ethnicity. It is believed that people of Indian origin are less susceptible to thromboembolic disease. I had better luck with finding data about surgical patients, generally.

According to VTE heavyweight, Dr. Charles W. Francis of the University of Rochester's Department of Hematology and Oncology, and other experts whose articles I read, up to 65 percent of ALL orthopedic surgical patients who do not prophylax develop VTE. Even more shocking: One-third of all non-prophylaxing patients who undergo *general surgery* unrelated to orthopedics also develop VTE. [8] My parents may have underestimated Mom's risk of developing PE in the absence of prophylaxis.

Elsewhere, I learned that the fatality rate for all U.S. patients with *diagnosed* PE ranges widely in reported studies from less than 1.0 percent to about 60 percent. This is regardless of prophylaxis and precipitating factors such as prior surgery or illness. The fatality rate at three months after PE diagnosis is about 15 percent.[9]

Dissatisfaction with these wide-ranging data prompted me to look for whole numbers, which I thought might be more meaningful than percentages. What I discovered was that, contrary to popular belief, venous thromboembolism is not a freak or unlucky "complication" of surgery. VTE is a silent epidemic.

According to Drs. Francis and Victor F. Tapson, of Duke's pulmonary and critical care medicine division, more than 900,000 Americans suffer VTE each year. In 400,000 of them, the condition manifests itself first as deep-vein thrombosis; in the other 500,000, as a pulmonary embolus.[10]

As many as 300,000 people die annually in the United States from acute PE, *which is often not diagnosed until autopsy.*[11] These are not necessarily deaths from medical error, although it is likely that quite a few should be considered such. A chief factor in PE fatalities in the United States is a delay in medical intervention, and delay, a failure to act, constitutes error.[12] A chief factor in intervention delay is ignorance.

As I would learn, autopsies are rarely performed today. It is probable that tens of thousands of people not subjected to autopsy die every year from undiagnosed pulmonary emboli. Instead, their physicians attribute their deaths to an acute myocardial infarction or a ventricular arrhythmia.[13]

Other shocking figures:

Twenty-five percent of all venous thromboembolism cases are associated with hospitalization. Of these cases, nearly 80 percent occur in hospitalized patients on the *medical* service, not in surgery. In fact, 70 to 80 percent of the fatal pulmonary emboli in U.S. hospitals occur in medical patients.[14] Those who are at the greatest risk of clotting disaster include patients with congestive heart failure, acute respiratory failure, infectious diseases, active cancer, and acute strokes, especially strokes associated with leg paralysis.

As for surgical patients, all have an increased risk of VTE, regardless of the procedure they have. Even something as seemingly "routine" as rotator-cuff surgery may end terribly in a pulmonary-embolus death.

Medical Ignorance, Neglect

Despite a global effort of more than two decades designed to educate them, physicians remain woefully uncognizant of the risk or the symptoms and signs of VTE.

Since 1986, when the American College of Chest Physicians first promulgated guidelines for antithrombotic therapy, there has been no shortage of information about VTE, DVT, and PE—the whole bowl of alphabet soup.

The heavy hitters in the field, among them, cardiovascular specialist Samuel Z. Goldhaber of Harvard's Brigham and Women's Hospital and Duke's Victor Tapson, have repeatedly sounded the clarion call for increased prevention and better care. International patient registries also have been set up for the purpose of identifying factors associated with PE deaths and of assessing routine clinical practices in the provision of VTE prophylaxis to acutely ill hospitalized medical patients.[15]

Even though published studies show that proper prophylaxis—of the correct type and duration—can prevent in-hospital VTE, physicians grossly underuse such measures with at-risk medical patients who have no obvious VTE symptoms. In fact, fewer than 50 percent of all patients who are *diagnosed* and hospitalized with deep-vein thrombosis receive life-saving prophylaxis![16]

When my father's astute colleague, retired clinician Karl Engelman, M.D., formerly of the NIH and the University of Pennsylvania School of Medicine, underwent a hip replacement in August 2010, he, not his orthopedic surgeon, decided his prophylaxis regimen. After evaluating surgeons' practices and reading up on recommendations, Engelman, who was in his early 70s, settled on 30 days of low-molecular-weight heparin after surgery. (Experts recommend a minimum 10-day course of heparin for all at-risk orthopedic surgical patients.)

"You have to take matters into your own hands if you want decent medical care today," he told me.

Physicians regularly fail to use what Goldhaber at Brigham and Women's Hospital calls "simple, well-established, and effective methods of DVT prevention" because they:

1) are unaware of the risk [hello?];
2) assess the risk of DVT "differently"; and

3) perceive an unacceptable risk of bleeding with prophylaxis[17]

My good friend Jeff, a former investment banker, developed deep-vein thrombosis after surgery at New York's esteemed Sloan-Kettering Memorial Hospital for the rare cancer pseudomyxoma peritonei. During his convalescence, Jeff, then 57, not his doctors, noticed extreme swelling in his legs and brought it to their attention. ("What about my legs? Look at my legs!")

Jeff had not prophylaxed for clots because his doctors feared bleeding. As a consequence, he underwent an IVC filter implant, which stayed in place for nine months, and injected himself daily in the buttocks with an anticoagulant for six months. These injections, Jeff assures me, were as painful as you might imagine.

Citing clinical trials with different anticoagulants, Tapson and a host of other investigators insist that these drugs pose no significantly increased risk of "clinically relevant bleeding" to patients who do not have counter-indicative underlying medical conditions. Doctors, they say, are simply uninformed. (18)

To tip the scales more in favor of patients, Tapson, Goldhaber, and their professional peers stress:

✓ improving the standards of care for VTE prevention;
✓ enhancing physician training about VTE risk assessment, diagnosis, and therapy; and
✓ requiring "systematic practice-reinforcing interventions that go beyond publication and dissemination of consensus recommendations."[19]

In other words, they propose fixing a broken cornerstone of the huge and sprawling healthcare system.

Without a trace of irony, Goldhaber and his colleagues conclude from their analysis of 2,392 cases of massive PE worldwide that there is a need for "improved multidisciplinary collaboration to optimize the in-hospital management of patients with acute massive PE, involving vascular medicine specialists, intensive care or emergency medicine specialists, interventional cardiologists/radiologists, and cardiovascular surgeons."[20]

But you and I can't wait for the New York Yankees of critical-care specialists to descend on our 20- to 250-bed community hospital. We have to protect our elders now.

CLOT RISK ASSESSMENT

Whenever your parent is hospitalized–especially if he or she is acutely ill, such as with heart disease or cancer–you should think about blood clots. You should assess his or her risk. You can't count on physicians to make this assessment and suggest preventive measures. You have to do it.

If your Mom or Pop is a surgical patient, you can reasonably expect the surgeon to be tuned into prophylaxis, provided the procedure is orthopedic, especially a hip or knee replacement. But he or she may not know the best drug regimen for your Mom or Pop, as Dr. Engelman discovered in his research. Further, general surgeons performing major nonorthopedic surgeries are less likely than the orthopods to be aware of the DVT and PE threats.

In either case, medical or surgical, you must be a watchdog. I encourage you to independently evaluate your parent's risk of developing VTE and to discuss that risk with his or her physician or surgeon.[21]

The recognized precipitating or risk factors for venous thromboembolism are:

- ❖ Advanced age (especially 75 and older)
- ❖ Prolonged immobility or paralysis
- ❖ Stroke
- ❖ Previous VTE
- ❖ Cancer and its treatment (tumors can promote clot formation; chemotherapy is a risk)
- ❖ Major surgery (particularly, operations involving the abdomen, pelvis, and lower extremities)
- ❖ Respiratory failure
- ❖ Trauma (especially fractures of the pelvis, hip, or leg)
- ❖ Obesity (a body mass index of more than 30, where BMI is the patient's weight in kilograms divided by the square of his or her height in meters)
- ❖ Varicose veins
- ❖ Congestive heart failure and myocardial infarction
- ❖ Indwelling central venous catheters (those in blood vessels)

❖ Inflammatory bowel disease
❖ Nephrotic syndrome
❖ Post-menopausal hormone replacement (also pregnancy and the use of oral contraceptives by pre-menopausal women)
❖ Inherited predisposition for clotting[22]

According to a 2008 review by Duke's Tapson: "Total hip and knee replacement, surgery for hip fracture, and surgery for cancer impart particularly high risks, as do trauma and spinal cord injury."[23]

Markedly reduced mobility, such as occurs with the dreaded BED REST, "also confers an increased risk," writes Tapson, but the degree and duration of reduced mobility that trigger the increase "remain unclear, often depending on concomitant risk factors."

Other threats of thromboembolism, he continues, include "prolonged air or ground travel [and] a sedentary lifestyle and occupations involving long periods of sitting"–such as book writing or other computer-driven work.

There actually is such a thing as eThrombosis. It describes thrombotic events related to "extended periods of sitting at a computer terminal."[24]

Today's over-75 Moms and Pops generally don't have to worry about eThrombosis. That's one for my generation and those sitting on their butts after us.

Dr. Francis of the University of Rochester believes that *all* patients should be assessed for their VTE risk upon admission to a hospital and then reassessed when their status changes, such as after surgery. He supports prophylaxis for medical patients who are older than 40, have limited mobility for three days or more, and have at least one risk factor.[25]

If you think your Mom or Pop should be receiving a preventive anticoagulant, talk to the physician in charge. The American College of Chest Physicians' 2008 clinical practice guidelines suggest several strategies that have been shown to decrease DVT rates and recommend that every hospital develop a formal policy for VTE prevention. If you meet medical resistance, ask to see that policy and be prepared to proceed until apprehended.[26] Don't let the system's failure defeat you.

We, the patient's family, have a role in recognizing the risk of venous thromboembolism and in protecting our elders and other loved ones from that risk.

I was much gratified to read Goldhaber's and his colleagues' opinion that "an unexplained shortness of breath should trigger the suspicion of PE by *lay persons* and health-care professionals."[27]

I urge you to think clot.

VERTEBRO-TWINGE AND PLASTY

Mom decided she liked Dr. Ramses enough to start seeing him for her primary care, even though it meant driving to Norfolk for checkups.

The term primary care, which my father never used, became popular in the 1990s. It was first proposed in the 1960s to "clarify the importance and role of generalist medicine in an advancing era of technologically driven specialty care," according to University of Albany Public Health Professor Timothy Hoff, in his book, "Practice Under Pressure: Primary Care Physicians and Their Medicine in the Twenty-first Century."[28] I will use it here interchangeably with internal medicine, even though some primary-care physicians (PCPs) are family practitioners, rather than general internists.

Dr. Ramses had been personable and authoritative during Mom's hospitalization. That he and my mother were both from the same small Michigan town also gave them an unexpected affinity.

I hoped that we could relax for a while, and stay clear of the healthcare system, but less than six months elapsed before I was back in a physician's office with my mother, confronting another immovable object in a white lab coat.

In mid-December, Mom awoke with a "twinge" of pain in her back that would not subside. She treated herself with an analgesic—perhaps a prescription she had on hand, I don't recall—but it was not enough. What I *do* recall is trying to persuade the nurse in the local orthopedic surgeon's office shortly before Christmas to give Mom an appointment.

"All we want is an X-ray, so we know what we're dealing with," I insisted.

Because Dr. Turner was one of those medical specialists who live out of town and come to the beach for a day every week or two, our window of opportunity was limited. We adamantly did not want to spend hours at the OBH Emergency Department.

The nurse insisted that Dr. Turner "did not do backs" and only reluctantly scheduled Mom.

Sure enough, the doctor didn't do backs. He saw Mom's crooked spine and osteoporosis on X-rays, but he missed the compression fracture of her T-12 vertebra. I listened to his X-ray analysis and thought he was wrong, but you can't make a doctor see what he doesn't want to see.

Was this LOL bias . . . again? Or simply "I don't do backs," period, ever, and you can't make me?

My mother medicated her severe pain through the holidays and got a correct interpretation in January from a radiologist in Norfolk to whom Ramses referred her.

I derived some satisfaction from the shocked and mortified expression on the nurse's face when I returned to Dr. Turner's office for Mom's medical records and told her about the fracture. Oops.

Back pain is so common among older people, especially in the over-80 age group, that it rarely raises a medical eyebrow. After years of absorbing the wear-and-tear of walking, standing, bending, and other activities, muscles in the back may strain, and structural degeneration may occur. Nonetheless, a fracture should provoke some interest.

The spine is comprised of 24 small bones called vertebrae, which are connected by ligaments and, when stacked upon each other, create the spinal *column*. Between each pair of vertebrae is a disk, a soft, gel-like cushion that helps to absorb pressure and keeps the bones from rubbing against each other. Each vertebra has a hole in its center so that, when all are aligned, they form a hollow tube that holds and protects the all-important spinal *cord* and its nerve roots. .

The thoracic (T) area of the spine is in the middle of the column, between the cervical (upper) and lumbar (lower) spines. It supports your shoulders, arms, and trunk, and consists of 12 vertebrae, labeled T-1 to T-12.

When osteoporosis, a systemic skeletal disorder in which bones become porous, weakens vertebrae, they may fracture spontaneously as they slowly crumble or collapse (i.e., compress). Compression fractures usually occur because of downward pressure being exerted on the spine by gravity and body-weight stress. The vertebrae most often compressed are those at T-11 and T-12 and L-1, the first vertebra of the lumbar spine.

With age, bones slowly lose minerals and become less dense; they lose mass. The drop in blood-estrogen levels that women experience with the onset of menopause accelerates bone thinning and contributes to the development of osteoporosis. Just like osteoarthritis, osteoporosis destabilizes joints.

Although osteoporosis is typically associated with postmenopausal women, older men develop it, too, usually after age 70, when bone loss accelerates. Compression of vertebrae causes a loss of height and kyphosis, which is a curve in the upper back that you may know better as dowager's or widow's hump, despite the gender equality.[29]

At Ramses's suggestion, my mother underwent a vertebroplasty, an outpatient procedure in which a surgeon injects medical cement (polymethylmethacrylate) with a needle into a fractured osteoporotic vertebra in order to stabilize the bone.

My parents presented this surgery to me as a foregone conclusion before I even had time to consider its necessity or hazards. I yielded to their medical judgment, being especially influenced by Dad's lack of skepticism: Both were on board with whatever Ramses recommended.

Unbeknownst to me then, by early 2007, vertebroplasties had become common among elders—all the rage, you might say—because of local Medicare reimbursement. With more than 750,000 osteoporotic vertebral fractures occurring each year in the United States, they rang up some big-dollar numbers.[30]

I since have learned, however, that their efficacy is debatable.

A vertebroplasty's cementing purportedly decreases pain and increases function, and some physicians believe it helps to prevent further vertebral collapse. But recent clinical studies suggest that the vertebroplasty may offer little or no benefit and may even increase the likelihood of another stress fracture. The evidence is simply not there.[31]

Nortin A. Hadler, M.D., author of "Rethinking Aging: Growing Old and Living Well in an Overtreated Society," reserved special derision for vertebroplasties in a 2012 lecture that I attended at my alma mater about "Health Screening Gone Wild."

I have heard Hadler, a UNC medical professor whose specialty is rheumatology, speak twice. He strikes me as an arrogant, shoot-from-the-hip and play-fast-and-loose-with-the-facts attention-seeker, but I think he's right about vertebroplasties. They offer little therapeutic benefit.[32]

Hadler has emerged nationally as an opponent of the "medicalization" of normal aging-related conditions, such as menopause or even lower back pain. In an interview with *The Washington Post*, he encouraged patients to ask their doctors: "How certain are you that what you are offering me will produce meaningful benefits? What does the evidence show about the possibility of harm?"[33] Excellent questions.

Fortunately, my mother experienced no immediate ill effects from her vertebroplasty. Whether the procedure played any part in the T-10 compression fracture she suffered about three years later, no one can say. Mom's bones were porous, and she noticeably had lost height, but she was pain-free. As long as she remained standing—knock on wood—we figured she was fine.

Falling, it turned out, would be my father's propensity.

Chapter Four

DoctorThink and
NO-THINK

Psyching Out Misdiagnoses

In 2002, when I encountered Dr. Amble's clinical nearsightedness, I knew enough about psychology to know that he had found what he was looking for—a diagnosis he could accept and defend—and he wasn't going to look any further. He was satisfied; I was not.

Ditto with Dr. Washburn, who fit my mother's symptoms and test results into a familiar pattern he recognized and could treat—a urinary tract infection—and closed his mind.

Dr. Charles did the same in 2006 when he latched onto the cookbook diagnosis of bronchitis.

None of these doctors seemed to consider alternative diagnoses that conflicted with their conclusions, although Washburn did offer to hospitalize Mom.

It happens that there is a creative and vigorous debate going on in medicine today about clinical diagnostic reasoning and the nature of the errors that occur. The debate stems from the reality that 1) too many diagnostic errors are made, and 2) the physicians who make errors do not wish to acknowledge them, thereby appearing fallible (i.e., human) and risking a lawsuit.

So driven are the error-makers to deny or avoid fallibility that they may even succeed in convincing themselves that no error occurred. They somehow dissociate from reality.

I now share with you some of my homework on diagnostic theories and the frequency and nature of misdiagnoses.

No-Think

Notwithstanding physicians' perceptions and admissions, diagnostic errors accounted for 29 percent of all U.S. malpractice lawsuits filed between 1986-2010 that were decided in favor of the patient-plaintiff or his/her family. According to a recent analysis of successful U.S. malpractice claims, incorrect, missed, or delayed diagnoses accounted for 35 percent of all monies paid out and caused 39 percent of malpractice-related deaths.[1]

While I let it be known to Dr. Amble that I was a lawyer (albeit a non-practicing lawyer), and that fact made him uncomfortable (which gave me some bargaining leverage), I never threatened litigation, nor would I ever contemplate it unless an unconscionably grievous error occurred—something on the order of transfusing the wrong type of blood. In such a case, the defendants' insurance companies would be eager to settle, and your battle would be over dollars, not liability.

I view litigation as horribly stress-inducing and spirit-draining, and I urge you to avoid it at all cost. Instead, concentrate on communicating with medical professionals and on educating yourself so that you can maximize your communications. Misdiagnosis is a window into a physician's mind, which I believe you can and should psyche out.

Diagnostic reasoning, according to Dr. Sherwin B. Nuland, the late surgeon, medical historian, and author of "How We Die," among many books, "is every doctor's measure of his own abilities; it is the most important ingredient in his professional self-image."[2]

But this measure, asserts Dr. Mark L. Graber, a national figure in diagnostic-error research and theory and a senior scientist at RTI International in North Carolina, is likely to be imbued with overconfidence, which is "ubiquitous in modern medicine."[3] I refer to this overconfidence as the physician swagger, which is not to be confused with the amiable shuffle.

It has been my experience that once doctors form diagnostic judgments, they tend to reinforce them, not challenge them, and they may become defensive when questioned about their decisions and choices. In so doing, they exhibit a lack of open-mindedness, self-awareness, critical perception, and/or curiosity and initiative. Generally speaking, they are loath to admit that their diagnostic reasoning could be uncertain, much less wrong. They would rather appear as powerful soothsayers.

Too often, I believe, doctors fail to exercise critical-thinking skills and cognitive awareness. In particular, they tend not to stand back from a patient's situation and their immediate medical response to it, or their immediate emotional response to the patient. They don't reflect, and analyze their own thinking, especially their assumptions.

As physician Arthur Garson Jr. gently puts it in his book, "Health Care Half Truths: Too Many Myths, Not Enough Reality": "We health care professionals don't check ourselves and don't ask for help often enough."4

In contrast, lawyers are trained to stand back from a situation, perceive the big picture, and objectively evaluate all of the viewpoints, not just the one they're hired to represent. Lawyers have to be able to perceive all of the relevant facts and issues and to argue cogently from any side to a dispute. I am not a cheerleader for the legal profession, but I do appreciate the legal-reasoning process.

Unlike doctors, lawyers don't ask, what's the answer? We ask, what are the questions? And the one question that we pose in as many ways as we can brainstorm is: "What if?" What if I factor in yet another fill-in-the-blank factor in my equation?

Despite doctors' pride of expertise, the documented medical diagnosis failure rate, I've discovered, is alarmingly high. Goodness knows what the undocumented rate is. Before we look at *how* doctors form misdiagnoses, let's look at how often they do.

AUTOPSY STUDIES

A diagnostic error occurs whenever a diagnosis is wrong or a correct diagnosis is unintentionally delayed or missed, as detected by a subsequent definitive test or finding.

Medical-error researchers differentiate between those errors that result in "worsened patient prognosis," including the patient's death, and those that do not. Most diagnostic errors occur in family, internal medicine, and emergency-department practices.

Ever since 1912, when physician and social-work pioneer Richard Clarke Cabot performed an error analysis of 3,000 autopsies at Harvard's prestigious Massachusetts General Hospital (Mass General), autopsy results have been the gold standard for evaluating, or double-checking, clinical diagnoses.

Cabot, who worked in the Mass General outpatient department, compared antemortem (pre-death) diagnoses with diagnoses determined at autopsy and found an overall error rate of 40 percent.[5] Using the same method, modern autopsy studies have calculated diagnostic error rates ranging from 10 percent to 40 percent.[6]

Autopsy researchers usually compare several years' or decades' worth of antemortem and postmortem findings at a single hospital. Unfortunately, with a decline in the past 50 years of the number of autopsies being performed, doctors "are more often literally and figuratively burying our mistakes," according to one research team.

The U.S. autopsy rate is now estimated to be less than 5 percent of all deaths, down from nearly 60 percent in the 1950s and 30 to 40 percent in the 1960s.[7] This is a great loss of a learning tool, a quality-control measure, and "a check against *false security in new diagnostic technology*," write geriatric specialists at Harvard.[8]

One hundred years ago, Cabot surmised that doctors at the Mass General were correct in diagnosing *dying* patients less than 50 percent of the time. The modern rate of major missed diagnoses, which, if known, might have prolonged patients' survival, has consistently been 10 to 15 percent.

Since the 1950s, both the overall and major misdiagnosis rates, as detected through autopsy studies, have not changed with advances in laboratory and imaging technology. They have not improved with improved technology because human error affects technology's accuracy, too.[9]

According to a prominent review of autopsies performed at Harvard's Peter Brigham Hospital (now known as Brigham and Women's Hospital) from 1959-1980, 10 percent of the misdiagnoses resulted in "worsened patient prognosis."[10]

In comparison, a team of University of California at San Francisco (UCSF), Baylor University, and Stanford University medical researchers who analyzed 50 autopsy studies spanning nearly 40 years (1966-2002) established that between 4 and 8 percent of all deaths had "diagnostic discrepancies" that may have harmed the patient.[11]

Patient-safety advocate Dr. Lucian Leape claims that 40,000 to 80,000 patients die annually in U.S. hospitals because of misdiagnoses.[12] This jibes with the UCSF-Baylor-Stanford research, which concluded that 8.4 percent of the people who die in U.S. hospitals have clinically undetected major diagnoses, about half of whom might have survived to discharge if not for the error.[13]

The diagnoses most frequently missed are pulmonary embolus, myocardial infarction, cancers, and infections, particularly pneumonia.[14] These are big-time Mom-and-Pop afflictions.

Research shows that autopsy rates decline as patient age increases. Doctors tend to avoid asking for autopsies of their deceased over-65 patients, in part because they believe the postmortems will provide little additional information—the diagnosis being obvious. Remember, ubiquitous overconfidence, physician swagger. [15]

Doctors also fail to request autopsies because, among other reported reasons, they lack training in how to seek autopsy permission; become frustrated with delays in receipt of autopsy results; and do not trust the pathologists' opinions.[16]

While some doctors may believe that families would rather not have their deceased loved ones "desecrated," and some surviving relatives tell them so, there's also evidence that doctors often don't tell families they have the option to request an autopsy. Conversations with grieving survivors about autopsies can be emotionally intense and trying. Many doctors would just as soon avoid having them.

During the question-and-answer session of a lecture on pathology that I attended in 2012 at the Georgetown University Medical Center, I asked pathologist Dr. Mary Furlong why so few autopsies were performed today. I quoted the 5 percent figure. She summarily replied that, with modern diagnostic technology, autopsies were no longer necessary. Doctors "know the causes of most deaths," she said, not believing her security to be false.

Then real life intervened. A woman in the audience about my age voiced her extreme frustration with trying to have her hospitalized mother, who died suddenly, autopsied at a hospital *anywhere* in the Washington, D.C. area. She was prepared to pay whatever it cost, but hospital after hospital, including Georgetown, turned down her request: "We don't do autopsies," she was told.[17]

TEST FAILURES

In arriving at diagnoses, physicians typically rely on laboratory (blood, urine analyses) and imaging tests, such as X-rays and ultrasounds, to provide data about the patient's physiological status. The specialized computed tomographic machine that exposed my mother's saddle embolus, for example, led directly to life-saving medical intervention.

Technology is not always a magic wand, however. Indeed, it may be the poisoned dart that, upon impact, paralyzes a doctor's thinking. Studies show that the traditional patient history and physical examination (H&P) provide more conclusive information about an underlying medical problem than diagnostic technologies do, assuming they are done accurately and with thoroughness.[18]

The time-tested medical aphorism, *A patient will almost always tell a doctor what's wrong with him or her if the doctor is willing to listen*, still holds true today.[19]

Why is the H&P often superior to lab or imaging wizardry? Because errors can occur in the testing process—with test ordering, specimen processing, test performance, interpretation, and follow-up testing—as well as in how doctors perceive various tests.

Physician (mis)perception can short-circuit the testing process, such as when a doctor focuses on one lab finding, accepts it as the exclusive window into the diagnosis, and stops looking any further. Or when the physician lacks the knowledge to evaluate the tests properly, as happened with my mother's pre-Duke doctors, including the Virginia infectious disease specialist, who didn't know the telltale signs of ehrlichiosis.

Even worse for your Mom's and Pop's health are the doctors who just order images and ask the radiologist for a diagnosis.[20] These clinicians see little value in the evidence-gathering H&P and place undue emphasis on test results in lieu of other clinical data. They represent a new-school perspective that dates to the 1990s and permits "diagnosis at a distance," writes the prolific Sandeep Jauhar in a 2006 *New England Journal of Medicine* article.

According to Jauhar, these young (under-45) doctors "are increasingly open in their disdain for the quaint methods of their predecessors."[21] Uncomfortable with uncertainty, they combat it with overconfidence.

Unfortunately, radiologists, upon whom they chiefly rely, are often wrong.

For a diagnosis to be accurate, the selection and interpretation of tests, as well as the clinical *cognition* before and after the procedures, must be accurate. Alas, human fallibility intervenes.

IMAGING

Let's look at radiological testing.

Computed tomography (CT), also known as computerized axial tomography (CAT), uses an X-ray scanner to make hundreds of images of an area of the body by rotating 360 degrees around it. A computer then processes these images to produce three-dimensional cross-sections.

Positron emission tomography (PET) also generates 3-D images or scans by computer, but the technique employed is quite different. PET scans rely on glucose metabolism in the patient's tissues. (I delve more into this technology in later chapters.) Typically, a radiologist recommends a PET scan after he or she reads a CT scan that does not provide enough detail.

An MRI, an abbreviation for magnetic resonance imaging, relies upon a powerful magnet and radiowaves, rather than X-rays, to capture images, but it also produces three-dimensional cross sections of an area. The MRI technique is based on the amount of water in a given tissue; it provides a clearer and more refined view than an X-ray does.

According to the American College of Radiology, radiologists overlook or misread evidence of disease about 30 percent of the time. This would include false-negatives (your Mom or Pop actually has the disease, but the interpretation says otherwise) and false-positives (your Mom or Pop does not have the disease, but is informed otherwise).

Radiologists miss evidence of cancer 75 percent of the time on mammograms and up to 90 percent of the time on chest X-rays. In some cases, radiologists miss evidence that's in plain view because they're distracted or tired or overworked. At other times they see the evidence but draw the wrong conclusion.[22]

My eyes were opened to the extraordinary number of errors committed by radiologists by Harvard medical professor Dr. Jerome Groopman's marvelous best seller, "How Doctors Think."

According to Groopman, who, like Jauhar, is also a frequent contributor to *The New Yorker*, the best radiologists "are expected to have gestalt," enabling them to reach reliable conclusions from first impressions, just as top-notch emergency doctors "shoot from the hip." Naturally, they have pride of interpretation and, once they make an interpretation, will perpetuate an error simply because to acknowledge it is to undercut their professional- and self-worth. Or so they believe.[23]

And yet, the amount of imaging data generated by CT scans, MRIs, and ultrasounds (which use sound waves to produce images), writes Groopman, is "enormous." There may be more than 1,000 images per CT scan or MRI. When you consider that the number of such tests performed in the past 10 years has increased by 50 percent, it is small wonder that radiologists increasingly complain of blurred vision, eyestrain, difficulty in focusing, and headaches—all of which affect their accuracy and efficiency.[24]

In addition to physical limitations, radiologists exhibit cognitive tendencies that may cause them to make interpretational errors. A radiologist may miss things, Groopman explains, because, on a subconscious level, he or she has decided that the image being interpreted is simply not important. Preconceived notions or biases can literally blind an X-ray beholder to what is in front of him or her. Conversely, radiologists can begin to "see things that are not there" in order to gratify their hunches and reinforce their brilliance.[25]

Gail Van Kanegan, an Illinois nurse practitioner (NP) and author of "How to Survive Your Hospital Stay," suggests that you and I regard a diagnosis as "an educated guess."

This advice gives the doctor the benefit of any doubt and also factors in the probability of error. It is spot-on when the patient's symptoms are so vague, confusing, and/or numerous as to render any diagnosis uncertain. New evidence may change the diagnostic picture in the next hour, by nightfall, or by tomorrow.

"Tests are important at arriving at or confirming a diagnosis," writes Van Kanegan, who has been an NP for 30 years, "but they're not always definitive. . . . They can be done incorrectly, or the results can be misreported . . . [m]ore commonly, they produce a result that is ambiguous, is open to interpretation, or could support more than one diagnosis. That's where the doctor's judgment comes into play."[26]

THE HOW-TO OF DIAGNOSTICS

Just 40 years ago serious research into the how-to of the diagnostic process was nonexistent. Then psychologist Arthur S. Elstein introduced the now-classic hypothetico-deductive model of clinical reasoning.

Elstein and other researchers of the 1970s observed experienced clinicians and students at different levels of medical training interacting with standardized patients and asked them to "think aloud." They discovered that, upon encountering a new patient, a doctor generates a short list of diagnostic *hypotheses*, based upon early, often visual, clues. He or she then tests these probable diagnoses against the data gathered later about the patient, through the medical history, the physical exam, the lab tests, imaging studies, followup, and observation. She thus confirms or eliminates each hypothesis.[27]

A doctor's generation of hypotheses (solutions) occurs unconsciously as an act of memory association and may take only a matter of seconds. What seems to distinguish expert clinicians from novices, according to researchers, is not that they generate more or quicker hypotheses, but that they generate more accurate hypotheses.[28]

Since Elstein's presentation of the hypothetico-deductive method of diagnostic problem-solving, its use has been recognized as common, but error-prone. It doesn't take a Ph.D. in psychology to realize that goal-directed reasoning (essentially *proving* your own hypothesis) will be subject to bias. Most people want their first impressions to be correct.

In the 1980s and '90s, research into diagnostic reasoning shifted into the study of medical expertise, memory recall, and clinical experience. In a key 1990 *Academic Medicine* article, researchers theorized that medical expertise is a matter of progressive development.

According to this developmental theory, clinicians first acquire three kinds of knowledge:

1) Knowledge of basic science;
2) Formal knowledge of diseases and their probabilities; and
3) Experiential knowledge;

After which they learn, in chronological order:

1) Basic mechanisms of disease;
2) Illness scripts, defined as a "wealth of clinically relevant information" about disease, its consequences and context; and
3) Exemplars derived from experience. [29]

Over time diagnostics researchers gradually came to recognize expert clinical reasoning as a "consequence of an extensive and multidimensional knowledge base," not simply a trait. And while practice helps, expertise is not just a matter of practice, practice, practice. Some doctors develop it; some never will.[30]

In the diagnostic-reasoning process, knowledge unquestionably comes first. Every clinician must secure and store in his or her long-term memory a solid knowledge base of prototypical disease profiles that he or she can retrieve rapidly and readily during a new patient encounter.[31]

Beyond knowledge, the clinician must acquire the experience to be able to differentiate a Clydesdale (bronchitis) from an Appaloosa (pulmonary embolus) and to deduce when a horse is a zebra in a timely enough fashion for it to matter to the patient's recovery—during on-the-clock, flesh-and-blood decision-making. Horses have their exotica, too.

Beyond both knowledge and experience, expert diagnosis involves clinical cognition and reasoning, which sometimes may seem to the observer like intuition or even art. A diagnostician must synthesize and discriminate among his or her many impressions, perceptions, inferences, deductions, and much more within his cognitive grasp. When misdiagnoses happen, it is typically because of a phenomenon that I call How Doctors Don't Think.

Whether you are advocating for a Mom or Pop whose true diagnosis is a zebra (ehrlichiosis) or an Appaloosa (the clot), you should know something about how doctors think, even if they themselves do not. Don't leave all of clinical reasoning to "the experts." Form your own independent judgments.

PATTERN RECOGNITION

Theory aside, most analysts today recognize and promote diagnostic reasoning by one of two approaches and encourage a blend of the two. The approaches are: 1) pattern recognition, which is a nonanalytical process; and 2) analytical thinking, employed when pattern recognition fails.

Pattern recognition is reasoning by case analogy or similarity, by experience. The patient's clinical data coalesce into a pattern that the doctor identifies as a specific disease or condition: In other words, the doctor has seen the clinical problem before.

Pattern diagnoses are fast, automatic, and, because of disease prevalence, largely accurate. The doctor's thinking is nonanalytical because it occurs unconsciously, intuitively. In internal and emergency medicine, pattern diagnoses are horses, not zebras.

"Doctors are machines of pattern recognition," said Dr. Peter Rabins, director of the Johns Hopkins Division of Geriatric Psychiatry and Neuropsychiatry, whom I heard speak in 2012. Rabins frequently exercises diagnostic judgment when evaluating cognitively impaired patients, but he does nothing machine-like. (See Chapter Eight.)

When a doctor can't find a pattern, is puzzled, or is faced with a complicated or ill-defined problem, such as my mother's ehrlichiosis, he or she will (and should) engage in analytical thinking, systematically (re)considering the clinical features of the patient's presentation and their relation to potential diagnoses. This thinking is slower and more consciously deliberate. Ideally, the doctor carefully identifies and considers all key features before generating a probable hypothesis.[32]

It is not difficult to see that, while pattern recognition may serve most of the diagnoses most of the time, it also may transform a patient's unique narrative into a doctor's preconceived, and *erroneous*, illness script. Bronchitis, anyone?

Similarly, while analytical thinking may reduce the likelihood of a cognitive error that derives from evaluating a patient with a specific diagnosis in mind, it also carries its own baggage. The analysis is only as effective as the analyst: The expert knows what questions to ask and which findings are significant, but what about the non-expert?

Novice or early-in-their career medical professionals simply do not have the clinical memories of the experts, who have stored illness scripts and can recall knowledge as diseases, conditions, or syndromes that they relate to certain patients. They have not yet made connections between their knowledge and specific clinical encounters.[33]

To compensate for gaps in both expertise and experience, student doctors learn to engage in a technique called differential diagnosis, which Dr. Cabot, the autopsy analyst, introduced in 1912 at the Mass General. Cabot initiated hospital teaching conferences in which physicians generated lists of all of the *possible* diagnoses—not just the probable ones—that matched cues culled from patient data.

In initiating a civil lawsuit, lawyers frequently employ the kitchen-sink approach (as in "everything but . . . "), throwing every possible claim, no matter how far-fetched, into the complaint. Differential diagnosis is medicine's kitchen sink.

Young West Coast anesthesiologist Deb Faulk, quoted in the student self-help guide, "Med School Confidential," calls this diagnostic exercise "the key to life." Faulk advises medical students to "[s]tart thinking about this early in your training! Ask why and how about everything you can."

She continues: "I think medical school trains us well to memorize details for multiple-guess questions or to expand on the minutiae of a single disease process quite well. Patients, however, rarely present us with a single disease. More often, they present us with multiple vague symptoms and we must pick one of the several things that may be the cause. . . . The larger your differential, the less likely you are to miss something."[34]

Although Faulk makes a good point about medical-school training, and its over-emphasis on hyper-memorization, she misses a better point about differential diagnosis, which is the role of critical analysis.

Doctors need to know how to prioritize the diagnoses they brainstorm, a process that involves both nonanalytical and analytical thinking. They have to be able to evaluate and compare diagnoses on the basis of the clinical data, the typical presentations, and the relative probabilities. If their medical education, during both their undergraduate and post-graduate years, has not prepared them to engage in such an intellectual exercise, then generating a differential diagnosis may be little more than a time-consuming parlor game.

EVIDENCE-BASED MEDICINE

Medical-school educators know they have a problem with fostering in students the critical-thinking skills that underlie clinical decision-making and diagnostics. Since the 1990s, they have been experimenting with nontraditional educational methods to promote better analytical DoctorThink.

As a corollary to this movement, a new medical-practice paradigm called evidence-based medicine (EBM) emerged in an attempt to reduce dependence on an individual doctor's opinion and experience and to neutralize errors committed because of them. EBM focuses on the best evidence derived from actual clinical studies, on what has been shown in trials to be effective.[35]

As I understand it, a doctor or a medical student initiates the EBM approach by formulating a precise clinical question from a patient's problem. He or she then searches medical-research databases for relevant clinical articles about this question; evaluates the evidence she finds for its validity and usefulness; and implements the useful findings into her clinical practice and care of the patient. Thus:

Step One: Ask a clinical question.

Step Two: Search the medical literature.

Step Three: Critically evaluate the medical literature.

Step Four: Apply to your patient.

The questions asked may be general medical background questions, such as—and I'm quoting here from a recent article—When does cardiac rupture usually occur after an acute myocardial infarction?—or questions specific to a patient, for example, what is the expected benefit to a 60-year-old diabetic with normal blood pressure of beginning a particular type of antihypertensive therapy?

Apparently, medical students and residents who learn EBM diagnosis observe preset algorithms and practice guidelines in the form of decision trees. The patient's major symptoms or test results form the trunk of the tree, which is contained within a box from which arrows branch out to other boxes.

Groopman gives the example of a sore throat beginning the algorithm, followed by a series of branches with yes/no questions about associated symptoms. A lab test, such as a throat culture for bacteria, would appear farther down the trunk and have its own yes/no branches. Eventually, the branches should lead to the correct evidence-based diagnosis and therapy.[36]

Evidence-based medicine is the rage. It is au courant, and it makes sense.

Recently, I attended a lecture by Dr. Jeffrey Weinfeld of Georgetown University about the EBM process and health information technology. Still feeling unsure about how EBM applies to diagnosis, I asked Dr. Weinfeld to give me an example. He couldn't. He responded by saying that EBM decision-making mostly applies to treatment.

Detractors of evidence-based medicine fear its computer-based approach will eliminate the *art* or humanism of medicine, an elusive concept that can play an important role in diagnostics. While I believe in basing decisions on evidence, I think they have a point. The more detached a physician is from a patient's unique brand of humanness, the more likely it is that his or her diagnostic accuracy will suffer.

DIAGNOSTIC ART

Gifted diagnosticians are said to be able to eyeball "something intangible, yet unsettling in the patient's presentation" that others cannot perceive and make an astute diagnosis; or to "smell" the problem upon entering the examining room where a new patient awaits.[37] They are medical artists. Somehow they just *know*.

According to Dr. Perri Klass, a professor of journalism and pediatrics at New York University, the art of medicine flows from "your life experience, as a doctor and as a human being" and, in particular, from clinical experience, "which teaches you to ask the questions and to listen to the answers, and to listen for what is not said, or for what has not been asked."[38] This sounds a lot like the interview technique I used with Mom's doctors when I was seeking more than medical answers.

Klass regards clinical medicine as being "all about stories."[39]

Contrast her perspective with that of Georgetown University cardiologist David L. Pearle, who defined the art of medicine in a 2012 class I attended as "applying the science of medicine to a particular patient."

Pearle's definition omits much of the art of art, I think, but it seems simple enough. Suppose, however, that a doctor does not truly know his or her patient? Is the application of the wrong science art? Of course not. So, how does a doctor learn to *know*?

Being a person who appreciates the nuances of listening and the importance of story, I believe that in order to acquire a bounty of life experience to bring to bear on a problem, clinical or otherwise, a professional has to be open and receptive to other people, sincere and willing to risk vulnerability.

Author and Cornell clinical medicine professor Charles Bardes eloquently describes the ways that the best doctors, the scientists who practice art, just know:

"The physician knows biology, chemistry, and physiology, knows how they work in the human body, knows the results of clinical studies that argue for or against a given therapy. Less recognized, but equally important, is a second way of knowing: the physician accumulates stories, layer upon layer. . . . a vast accretion of personal and collective knowledge. The science is important, of course; but the stories too are important, and without them we know only halfway, and the leukemic patient goes to surgery, and dwindles in the ICU, and dies in the hospital sometime in late November."[40]

The art of medicine may be simply clinical experience and confidence or even spectacular skill at pattern recognition, but I think it involves a creativity, an insight, an intuition, and empathy that only the most sensitive possess. Many doctors with years of experience lack artistry, and I've met at least one 40-year-old doctor who I'm sure had it. I believe in the art of medicine and respect its masters.

THE HOW-TO OF ERRORS

OK, now that I've probed how doctors formulate diagnoses, let's look at how they formulate misdiagnoses. Today's leading medical researchers of diagnostic errors classify them by cause, of which there are three: 1) no-fault; 2) system-related; and 3) cognitive:[41]

❖ No-fault errors occur when a disease is "silent" or "masked" or presents in such an atypical fashion that you would not expect the correct diagnosis; or when the patient gives the doctor misleading or incomplete information, perhaps because of faulty memory or illness-induced deficits, and/or acts uncooperatively or deceptively.

❖ System-related errors encompass workplace conditions predisposed to error such as organizational flaws and equipment problems and/or technical failures.

❖ Cognitive errors trace to the doctor's thinking and implicate faulty knowledge, faulty data-gathering, and/or faulty synthesis. (My How Doctors Don't Think.)[42]

As you know, I've contended with no-fault errors: My breathless mother minimized the severity of her symptoms when Dr. Anthony asked her about their progression. I also have witnessed organizational breakdowns. But when it comes to misdiagnoses, I'm all over cognitive errors.

Prolific diagnostic-error expert Pat Croskerry, M.D., Ph.D., a Canadian medical professor and emergency physician, says that physicians' cognitive errors often stem from their "cognitive dispositions to respond to certain patients in predictable ways."

Cognitive dispositions to respond–"CDRs"–are basically shortcuts in doctors' problem-solving and clinical decision-making. CDRs explain why doctors fail to question their assumptions, why their thinking is sometimes closed or skewed, why they overlook gaps in their knowledge, and, in general, why they honestly believe errors are made by "someone else."

Cognitive psychologists call such shortcuts *heuristics*, a word that, like the word eureka, comes from the German for to invent or discover. When heuristics work well, which is in the majority of patients' cases (pattern recognition), they seem resourceful and effective. When they fail, when the outcome is adverse, they reflect cognitive biases and lapses in critical reasoning.43

Patient-safety advocate Dr. Lucian Leape captured the essence of CDRs in a 2009 lecture when he spoke of the "many ways in which we [doctors] don't think straight."44 An extensive medical literature now exists about CDRs in diagnostic reasoning. Let's check some of them out.

Stop Looking, Stop Thinking

Dr. Croskerry identifies 30 CDRs in his articles; Dr. Groopman expounds upon 15 in his book; and I key on five that are frequently associated with pattern recognition. My Big Five overlap substantially and boil down to this: *The doctor stopped looking and, therefore, stopped thinking.*

When asked on anonymous surveys to admit their own or to report other doctors' missed diagnoses and to explain how they happened, doctors typically offer such reasons as "It never crossed my mind," "I didn't suspect it," and "I didn't realize the severity of the patient's illness." Nothing evil or scandalous, just absent. See how these explanations jibe with my Big Five:45

1) **ANCHORING** is a doctor's tendency to fixate on specific

features of a patient's presentation (often first impressions) too early in the diagnostic process. Instead of considering multiple diagnostic possibilities, the doctor quickly and firmly latches on to a single one, certain that he or she has "cast his anchor" where it needs it to be. When doctors make anchored diagnoses, they see only the markers they expect to see and neglect those that should tell them they're wrong. Anchoring leads to a premature closure of thinking, which is dangerous when the diagnosis is wrong. (All of the doctors who blew my mother's diagnoses in 2002 and 2006 anchored their incorrect reasoning.)

2) **AVAILABILITY** (aka RECENCY) is the tendency to settle on a diagnosis that comes readily to mind. The doctor assumes that the evidence that is the most available, meaning the most recent in his or her memory, is the most relevant. Groopman offers the example of a doctor diagnosing a patient as alcoholic simply because the doctor is in an inner-city hospital populated by large numbers of alcoholics, and he recently has seen quite a few alcoholics. Nonavailability (out of sight, out of mind) occurs when the doctor pays insufficient attention to what is *not* immediately called to mind, i.e., the zebra.

3) **CONFIRMATION BIAS** is the tendency to look for confirming evidence to support a diagnosis rather than disconfirming evidence to refute it, despite the contrary evidence being more persuasive and definitive. Doctors who prematurely adopt a diagnosis cherry-pick symptoms in order to confirm what they expect to find: They selectively accept or ignore information. Confirmation bias follows anchoring.

4) **PREMATURE CLOSURE** (a biggie!) is the tendency to apply closure to the clinical problem-solving process before a diagnosis has been fully verified. Typically, a doctor accepts as definitive one of the several diagnoses he or she generated early in the case. Premature closure may occur because of anchoring features of the patient's presentation, or, according to Croskerry, it may "reflect a laziness of thought and a desire to achieve completion, especially under conditions of fatigue or circadian dysynchronicity." (Yes, their biological clocks may be off. Typically, this occurs with over-worked and sleep-deprived interns and residents.)

5) **SEARCH SATISFICING** (aka SATISFACTION) is the tendency to stop searching once something (a diagnosis) has been found. Unfortunately, there may be more to find. A further problem is that the doctor may have searched in the wrong place, in which case he or she will stop looking once he has found nothing. According to Groopman, search satisficing is common among radiologists.

Assuming that you've gotten into the CDR spirit, I briefly offer some others, courtesy of Croskerry and Groopman, that you should keep in mind:[46]

❖ **ASCERTAINMENT BIAS** occurs when the doctor ascertains from the patient what he or she expects to see or what the doctor hopes to find. Stereotyping and biases, including ageism and sexism, are examples of ascertainment bias. A doctor may diagnose a memory-impaired older person with early Alzheimer's disease, when, in fact, she has a severe vitamin B-12 deficiency, merely because he expects to find Alzheimer's.

❖ **ATTRIBUTION** is a doctor's tendency to blame the patient, rather than the circumstances, when things go wrong. Attribution, which can be similar to ascertainment bias, is based on negative stereotypes and reflects a doctor's lack of compassion and understanding. The danger is that it results in inappropriate or inadequate care. Many doctors have affective and cognitive problems with patients who seem to have "self-inflicted" ailments. They include alcoholics, heavy smokers, grossly obese people, or people who don't follow doctors' orders. Psychiatric patients ("nuts," "wackos") also fare poorly.[47]

❖ **CLINICAL PROTOTYPE BIAS** reflects "If it looks like a duck, walks like a duck, and quacks like a duck, it's a duck" thinking. This CDR underlies the pattern recognition theory of diagnosis: Common things are common. A doctor's familiarity with a clinical prototype can lead to a rejection of alternative diagnoses and result in delayed or erroneous conclusions.

❖ **DIAGNOSIS MOMENTUM** occurs when a doctor passes on to his or her peers and subordinates a particular fixed diagnosis, despite incomplete evidence, so that it gains momentum with them, crushing alternate theories. The patient is forever labeled incorrectly.

❖ **FRAMING EFFECT** describes the strong influence that the verbal presentation or framing of a patient's problem(s) by nurses, other physicians, and even the patient himself has on a doctor. The doctor follows the framer's train of thought.

❖ **SUTTON'S SLIP or SUTTON'S LAW** is a tendency to "go where the money is," i.e., for the obvious diagnosis. The name comes from Willie Sutton, the Brooklyn bank robber who, when asked by a judge at his trial why he robbed banks, allegedly said, "Because that's where the money is." Of course, if you go for the obvious diagnosis, you fail to look for other possibilities, engaging in search sacrificing and other CDRs.

❖ **VERTICAL LINE FAILURE** is your basic thinking inside the box. According to Croskerry, "routine, repetitive tasks often lead to thinking in silos—predictable, orthodox styles that emphasize economy, efficacy, and utility." The danger is inflexibility. "Lateral thinking" that breaks out of the ordinary can be vital for zebra diagnoses. The probing question should be, "What else can this be?"—which is more like legal "What if?" analysis. Sometimes, Croskerry notes, an MRI is the box. Its results constrain a doctor's thinking.

❖ **VISCERAL BIAS** describes the influence of affective factors, both negative (like attribution) and positive (such as sexual attraction), on medical decision-making. A doctor's emotional involvement with a patient may lead to diagnostic error, a lower standard of care, or other mismanagement, including an over-investigation of the case. (In his work, Croskerry distinguishes affective dispositions to respond (ADRs), or emotional influences on doctors' thinking, which can have a powerful effect on their actions. Doctors may experience affection, disgust, annoyance, respect, etc., toward patients, or they may allow their moods to color their medical perspectives.)[48]

❖ **YIN-YANG OUT** is the failure to think of a new direction with a patient who has been worked "up the Yin-Yang," because the doctor falsely assumes all ideas have been explored.

One more CDR bears mentioning, but it occurs during patient treatment, not at diagnosis. Groopman labels it the **SURRENDER** error and explains: "Instead of coming at the malady from a different angle, seeking its vulnerable point by adding other drugs or customizing a regimen, the physician, in essence, surrenders. He sticks with the same treatment, not taking the risk of devising a novel, individual approach when the condition is not improving because 'it's a bad disease.'"

Doctors surrender, Groopman suggests, because "they deeply dislike failure." I would add that they *can* surrender only when other medical practitioners would do so. Conformity and custom keep them safe from both uncertainty and liability.[49]

The medical literature reflects an ongoing discussion about how to "de-bias" physicians and to otherwise curb cognitive errors, such as through changes in clinical-medicine courses in medical schools. You and I can't reform medical education, but we can raise our awareness.

ERRORS IN THE ED

There is probably no place in which you need to be more aware, more alert to cognitive errors and ageism, which is the bias that concerns me the most, than in the emergency department of a hospital. Diagnostics expert Pat Croskerry, himself an emergency physician, characterizes emergency medicine as "a natural laboratory of errors," a petri dish of CDRs.

Up to 50 percent of the malpractice lawsuits filed against emergency physicians are based on misdiagnoses, as compared with a third of the alleged negligence claims filed against primary-care physicians in hospitals and outpatient settings.[50]

Studies estimate that 1 to 12 percent of all *admitted* patients who visit the emergency department are misdiagnosed. Of course, the vast majority of ED patients are not admitted: They are treated and discharged.[51]

"Nowhere in medicine," writes Croskerry, "is rationality more bounded by relatively poor access to information and with limited time to process it, all within a milieu renowned for its error-producing conditions. It is where heuristics dominate, and without them emergency departments would inexorably grind to a halt."[52]

Emergency departments, even the one in the small Outer Banks Hospital, pose circumstantial obstacles that do not exist anywhere else in hospitals, including:

* Constant distractions;
* A steady, sometimes heavy flow of patients;
* Relentless background noise; and/or
* Demanding trauma cases

Doctors and nurses, alike, may be fatigued, anxious, and/or irritable. If you're in the emergency department of a teaching hospital, you may encounter residents who are working long shifts and are suffering from exhaustion and that disruption in circadian rhythm that Croskerry warned about.53 (Thanks to mandatory reductions in residents' hours, however, today's resident is not as sleep-deprived as his or her predecessors were. See Appendix Three, "The Paradox of the Better-Rested Resident.")

Whether your parent is coming to the ED from home or from another facility, such as a nursing home, you must quickly size up the scene, so your Mom or Pop doesn't get overlooked. I've usually been able to identify a competent and keen nurse to whom I could turn for help: She (or he, but not in my experience) is efficient without being brusque and doesn't call anyone honey.

At the same time, I've accepted that doctors are available only fleetingly—and may disappear off-shift suddenly—so I maximize my minutes with them. If the doctor sees my parent before I've arrived, I seek him or her out, but only after making a polite inquiry of the nurse. Whatever the problem is, whether it is a progressive illness or a sudden disabling event, I have a written timeline or synopsis of what has happened, as well as copies of my parent's medical and prescription-drug histories, which each has prepared, and my healthcare power of attorney. I identify the salient features that I think the doctor should know about Mom's or Dad's condition, before and after the illness, fall, attack, etc., and the questions I'd most like to ask.

It's important to appreciate that all emergency doctors' working (short-term) memory for problem-solving may be seriously limited and to accept that your Mom's or Pop's diagnosis is an ongoing process.54

"Becoming a Doctor" author Melvin Konner describes the job of the emergency staff as "the immediate and temporary prevention of deterioration and death."55 This is what Croskerry calls rul[ing] out the worst-case scenario, or "ROWS." Before an emergency doctor can discharge this weighty responsibility, he or she has to recognize the seriousness of the patient's condition. Because of CDRs, prompted by no-fault, system-related, and/or cognitive errors, this is not as easy as it may seem.[56] This is where you come in.

Consider how your Mom or Pop will appear to ED doctors and nurses who are seeing her or him for the first time. What is likely to be their initial impression?

Did your Mom with the (currently undiagnosed) obstructed bowel arrive by car or by ambulance? Did she walk in or was she wheeled in? One means of transport may signal urgency to the emergency medical team, whereas the other may not. The visceral biases that doctors and nurses adopt–the attribution and other affective errors–start forming immediately.

Does your mother seem fine to someone who doesn't know her baseline health? Is she already on medication that may mask her symptoms? How effectively does she communicate? How does *she* "frame" her problem to the medical people? What kind of personality does she have? Is she hyper-critical, impatient, prickly, someone who might annoy or irritate medical technicians, nurses, and doctors, or is she even-tempered and courteous, even when in pain?

In the ED, you must be especially wary of your parent's framing and the no-fault causes that he or she introduces, such as memory lapses or even denial of symptoms, and the tendency for doctors to anchor to the easy-to-categorize-and-treat diagnosis and then to engage in vertical-line failure. They are eager and ready to move on to the next patient.

According to a major study of closed malpractice claims based on misdiagnoses, the four leading breakdowns in diagnostic reasoning in the emergency department are:

1) Failure to order tests;
2) Inadequate performance of the patient medical history and physical examination;
3) Incorrect interpretation of tests; and
4) Failure to request a consultation[57]

All four breakdowns apply to the brushoff my mother received at the Outer Banks Hospital before I stepped in. All four reflect How Doctors Don't Think.

TAKE ACTION!

In her fascinating series, "Medical Mysteries," *The Washington Post* writing contributor Sandra G. Boodman exposes physicians' diagnostic shortcomings. Boodman's mystery patients go from doctor to doctor seeking truth and wisdom. Not only do they not get answers, they sometimes get rebuffed.

"He acted like it was all in my head" is a frequent patient complaint about such doctors. This is ironic when you consider what may be in *his* head: He can't figure you out, he reasons, so *no one* can figure you out. How rational is that?

If you ever feel like a doctor is treating you or your Mom and Pop as if you, he, or she doesn't have a brain in your/his/her head, walk out *immediately*, if you can, or ask to see another doctor, if you can't. An illness may be in your Mom's or Pop's head, but smart, competent doctors don't trivialize illness, deride their patients, or dismiss very real symptoms. They don't make matters worse.

During a Mom-or-Pop crisis in the hospital, you may be time-, energy-, hope-, brain-, and/or voice-deprived. Weary and worried, you just may not have it in you to do medical homework, brainstorm your own differential diagnosis, and confront the doctor gaps. But if you do nothing else, at least pay attention to some basic warning signs, suggested by Gail Van Kanegan, the nurse practitioner, and amplified by me. If . . .

✓ Your Mom's or Pop's treatment isn't working the way the doctor has told you (or you think) it should; or . . .

✓ The doctor is defensive when you (politely and respectfully) question him or her; or . . .

✓ The test results seem out of whack with the diagnosis (OK, a little homework here); or . . .

✓ You have a feeling that things aren't right . . .

ACT. Do something. Talk to the doctor, and if he or she won't listen, ask to speak to the head of the department. Make some noise, without getting hysterical. Be firm and insistent. Proceed until apprehended.

Remember: Diagnosis is ongoing. Good doctors listen. Don't rationalize away your doubts and compromise your common sense. Trust your instincts. If you have time, get a second opinion, but bear in mind that second opinions can be wrong, too.[58]

Chapter Five

2010: Falls and
FRACTURES

Life Turned Upside-Down

My father's fall history dates back to September 1998, when he stumbled while stepping from a ladder to the roof of our family beach cottage and plunged 25 feet to the sandy ground.

Impatient waiting for my brother to help him with a shingle repair job, or so he claimed, Dad violated his own rule about never using a ladder without a spotter. When Mom and Al reached him, he cried out: "Don't call 911!" This was wishful thinking from a literally broken man who still clung to able-bodied autonomy.

Within 20 seconds, the full extent of the damage had settled over his body, and he corrected himself: "Never mind. Call."

I rushed from my home to the Kitty Hawk Regional Medical Center where I found my still-vigorous father, inconsolably and hideously contorted by pain. I had never seen him so undone. He couldn't stop moaning and wincing as he waited for the helicopter that would airlift him to Sentara Norfolk General Hospital. The Outer Banks Hospital did not yet exist. If it had, he might have been taken there first, a delay that could have caused disastrous consequences.

Two punctured lungs reduced Dad's breathing to labored gasps, and the pain from *10* cracked ribs pierced his chest. He felt so bad en route to Norfolk that he thought he would die. I worried that he would, too.

Scheduled to leave the day of Dad's accident for an intensive mediation course in Baltimore, I did not step up into what would become my customary advocacy role. I left town and trusted that my bewildered mother and brother would rally from their shock and keep me updated. But we didn't have cell phones in 1998, and we didn't have a crisis strategy yet.

"Go to the hospital *tonight*," I stressed to Mom and Al before I left the beach. And they did.

For many years before this near-fatal drop, Dr. Al had insisted—to the amusement of many—that he knew how to fall and could execute perfect fall form in a split-second. Of course, he meant on the ground, not off of a roof.

When you feel yourself falling, he would say, you have to convert the fall to a roll so that you avoid injury to your head—as well as your hands and wrists, which can be smashed if you instinctively reach out to brace yourself.

Although hip, back, and other non-head injuries sustained in a fall can be life-threatening—often because of risks presented during the post-surgical recovery period—the most frightening of all injuries is a brain trauma that results in either severe cognitive damage or death. Elders with fall-related head injuries often don't make it back.

AFTER THE ROOF DROP

Then 74, Dad quickly progressed at Sentara Norfolk General from the intensive care unit to an orthopedic ward, but that didn't mean, necessarily, that he was improving. Quite the contrary. He continued to struggle with his breathing, despite receiving supplemental oxygen, as well as with agonizing pain.

Angry at himself for his rooftop lapse in judgment and extremely anxious about his chance for survival, Dr. Al aggressively micromanaged his own care. He became patient *non grata* with the chief surgeon on his case, but healthcare-team members of lower rank, who perhaps had their own issues with said surgeon, regarded Dr. Al as "a breath of fresh air," or so they told me. Although my father had some good-behavior moments, he generally exhibited Difficult Patient Syndrome, my own diagnosis. He was cranky, critical, and caustic.

But his high-anxiety agitation also proved useful.

More than a couple days elapsed before anyone at Sentara with an M.D. figured out that the darkness in Dad's right lung, clearly visible on X-rays, was bloody fluid. Had he not harangued his healthcare providers, so that they could not ignore him, they might not have detected his life-threatening hemopneumothorax. Once they drained a *quart* of bloody fluid—a full 32 ounces—from his pleural cavity, his lungs re-expanded, and Dad could breathe easily again! No wonder he had trouble trusting doctors!

During this hospitalization, my father also developed an irregularity in his heartbeat. This wasn't his first episode of arrhythmia, but it was his first in many years.

One night about 45 years before this fall, Dad felt his heart beating abnormally fast while he was reading in bed. Being a physician, he knew he could slow it by stimulating his vagus nerve. When he first told me this, I had no idea what he was talking about. Only much later did I learn about the wonder of the vagus nerve, which is cranial nerve X. The 12 cranial nerves are designated by Roman numerals.

Actually, there is a pair of vagus nerves, as there are all cranial nerves, but you always hear about the vagus in the singular. It extends from the brain stem all the way to the abdomen via various organs, including the heart, lungs, stomach, and intestines, and plays a critical role in heart rate, respiration, digestion, and other important functions. It's a central switchboard in your body.

Dr. Al indirectly stimulated his vagus nerve by massaging one of the carotid arteries in his neck. This worked, but he worried: He didn't know if the tachycardia originated in the ventricles, which could be catastrophic, or the atria, with which he could live.

For years, whenever Dad felt an occasional premature heartbeat, he would pop a fast-acting quinidine pill. Quinidine is an old anti-malarial drug that also restores normal heart rhythm. One day while working at the National Heart Institute, he experienced the irregular beat and enlisted a colleague's help in wiring him to an electrocardiograph. The results showed that his rapid rate was caused by a premature atrial contraction.

Blood conduction in the heart is the result of a nerve-to-muscle electrical connection facilitated by ions, which are electrically charged molecules that include sodium, calcium, and the other electrolytes. Electrical currents act upon these ions, which move across muscle-cell membranes.

The heartbeat begins with an electrical signal that emanates from pacemaker cells of the sinoatrial (SA) node, a small mass of cardiac muscle fibers located in the rear of your right atrium. As the electrical signal travels from the right to the left atrium, it stimulates muscular contraction. A normally functioning SA node initiates the production of what is known as normal sinus rhythm.[1]

The impulse slows briefly at the atrioventricular (AV) node, which is another small mass of specialized muscle fibers, so that the atria and ventricles do not contract simultaneously, and blood flows effectively between the upper and lower chambers. The AV node delays conduction, allowing the ventricles to finish filling with blood before they pump it out.

Most of the blood that enters the left atrium and the right atrium flows into the left ventricle and the right ventricle, respectively, while the ventricles are relaxed (during diastole), having just contracted to propel blood out. Before the relaxation ends, the atria contract to push blood into their respective ventricles, so that the blood is there for their next contraction (systole). The two atria contract at the same time, as do the two ventricles.

I have just described what is known as the cardiac cycle. It consists of a first phase of relaxation when both the atria and ventricles are in diastole and blood flows into the atria; a phase two when the atria contract to fill the ventricles, and ventricular systole starts; and a phase three when ventricular ejection occurs. All of this happens within the span of just one heartbeat, which lasts only 0.85 second.

ATRIAL FIBRILLATION

According to cardiology specialists at Johns Hopkins, millions of heart muscle cells have the ability to "create their own electrical signals, [thus] disrupting the normal sinus rhythm."

If muscle cells "misfire," Hugh G. Calkins, M.D., and Ronald Berger, M.D., Ph.D., explain, the SA and AV nodes are preempted, and the heart may race from a resting rate of 60 to 90 beats per minute up to 200 bpm, and then slow down after just a few moments. "This irregularity," they say, "may occur hundreds of times a day, or only in several short episodes a year."

Electrical misfirings can result in premature or so-called ectopic heartbeats, meaning that a source other than the SA node is initiating them. If a "run" of such premature beats occurs, say Calkins and Berger, the atria may start to fibrillate, which means to quiver, rather than to contract forcefully. I have heard atrial fibrillation (AF) described as a "wormlike motion," an uncoordinated contraction that results in passive blood drainage into the ventricles. The heart's efficiency drops, but not enough to threaten a person's life.

Atrial fibrillation can lead, however, to an irregular and often rapid beating of the ventricles, whose contractions determine your pulse.[2] A few beats of ventricular tachycardia usually do not cause a problem, but if they turn into a sustained fibrillation, cardiac arrest will occur, absent medical intervention. To defibrillate the ventricles, and restore normalcy, an electrical shock must be applied to the heart.

A cardiologist friend of my father's suggested that one of his broken ribs might have caused his irregular heartbeat by interfering with his heart. If so, no one at Sentara detected the interference.

To treat the arrhythmia, the Norfolk doctors gave him digitalis, an old drug that is derived from the foxglove plant and used as a cardiac stimulant. Dr. Al had worked extensively with digitalis when he was a pharmacology graduate student, a post-graduate fellow, and a young researcher at the NIH. He pocketed the digitalis pills in his cheek and spit them out later. "That stuff can kill you!" he told me.

All together, he said, he had two AF episodes during this hospitalization, each lasting about eight hours. Both times his heart converted to normal sinus rhythm on its own.

Compounding his cardiac worries, Dad also "went off my rocker," as he recalled, becoming disoriented and hallucinating. He remembers seeing my brother in a corner of his room late at night and calling out to him. As I would learn later, a number of factors, including his extreme emotional distress, immobility, serious illness, and isolation from his family, made my father vulnerable to delirium. He attributed his altered cognition to the narcotic he was taking for pain.

Later when Dad was convalescing restlessly at home, he became paranoid and accusatory. Painkillers, stress, you name it, transformed him into a monster. Although he always apologized later for his erratic thinking and behavior, his unpredictability had everyone on edge. One night, I fainted dead-away at the dinner table, falling off of my chair and scaring the wits out of Mom and Al Jr., but not hurting myself. This was nothing compared to the stresses of my future advocacies. With every medical crisis, there is collateral damage to loved ones. I wish doctors took that fact more into account.

After his discharge from Sentara, my strong-willed father's body slowly mended, and he turned to Coastal Rehab in Kitty Hawk for physical therapy to restore his strength. I observed his recovery, but had no hand in managing it.

As Dad aged from his 70s into his 80s, it became clear that his balance was impaired. Increasingly, he showed up with bruises on his arms and legs, from stumble-falls in or around the house or garage. Mom also occasionally lost her balance and toppled, but she was better about using a cane, and, because of her knees, she walked slower.

In November 2009, my father, sans cane, lost his balance while walking down stairs at home and went hurtling into the living room.

Having just arrived from Florida for a long weekend, Leslie found him prone (face-down) on the floor, helpless and hurting. Again, he waved off a 911 call and denied any cause for concern, and again he reconsidered when the pain in his chest became severe. My sister handled the Saturday emergency-department honors at the Outer Banks Hospital. As suspected, he had cracked a rib. He treated the painful injury with an analgesic, as needed, and rest.

Dad had problems with what one fall expert, whose book I later read, calls static (standing) balance, as well as with dynamic (movement) balance. The idea that he could convert a fall into a roll, and protect his head, seemed remote in 2009, and yet he still had a strong presence that could convince you otherwise. Supreme confidence can carry a big load. But it can't deny a hip fracture.

THE NEXT BIG FALL

On Tuesday, Feb. 23, 2010, Dr. Al was home alone when his carpenter-handyman, Mark, arrived to talk about repair jobs. Mom had gone swimming with Britt, who was staying for an extended period in a nearby beach house.

Dad wanted to show Mark something outside, so the two exited the house and walked along the back deck, down some stairs, and onto a wooden walkway in the yard.

An animated talker who gestures with his hands, Dad not only wasn't paying attention to where he was walking but, true to form, he had left his cane behind. He was looking back over his shoulder at Mark while he walked absentmindedly ahead and . . . forgot about the step down in the walkway. He lost his footing and fell overboard, slamming his right side into the hard dirt.

Downplaying his pain, Dad told Mark not to call 911 (of course), but he did allow his young friend to carry him into the house and lower him into a chair at the kitchen table. After Mark left, Dad managed to walk on his own to a nearby sofa, where Britt found him about an hour later.

Insisting that he had only bruised himself, my stiff-upper-lip father asked Britt to help him walk to the bathroom and then get into bed. She obliged and then left. When Britt received the red-alert call about 7 p.m., Mom described Dad's pain as "excruciating."

The entire Southern Shores emergency management team apparently converged on my parents' house to move my now moaning father onto a stretcher and transport him by ambulance to the hospital. The paramedics had been in a training session when Mom called and, eager for action, they all had responded. Despite the "role-reversal" cliché I told you about, I have nothing but compliments for these efficient, unflappable, *and* compassionate volunteers. I respect them and the job they do.

Britt drove with Mom to the OBH Emergency Department where they ate the take-out dinners they had ordered before the 911 call and watched the winter Olympics on an overhead TV in the waiting room. According to my sister, the nurse who escorted them to Dad's curtained room in the patient area passed him off gladly, saying: "Now he can be nasty to you."

Difficult Patient Syndrome comes over Dr. Al whenever he is hospitalized because he feels, and *is*, out of control and does not trust anyone. *He* knows more; *he* knows better. And very often he does. But that only makes him more anxious and more impossible to be around. I've tried talking with him about his rude and hostile behavior, but he either doesn't remember it, or he convinces himself that it never occurred. When possessed by DPS, Dad's in survival mode.

Lest I confuse you, I should clarify that the "difficult patient" is not the same as the patient I've seen described in the medical literature as "hateful."

In a 1978 *New England Journal of Medicine* article that would never be published today, psychiatrist James E. Groves wrote about the "hateful patient," who, "by a variety of behaviors related to profound dependency[,] stimulates a series of negative feelings in most doctors. Dependent *clingers* evoke aversion. Entitled *demanders* evoke fear and then counterattack upon entitlement. Manipulative *help-rejecters* evoke guilt and feelings of inadequacy. Self-destructive *deniers* ... evoke all of these negative feelings, as well as malice and, at times, the secret wish that the patient will 'die and get it over with.'" (Groves's emphasis)3

Hateful patients, as defined, still exist today, and doctors still have negative reactions to them. My neurologist friend Dr. Roberts disappointed me greatly when he spoke about a needy 90-year-old patient whom he wished would "hurry up and die already."

A doctor's visceral biases can poison medical decision-making and action. Beware.

Britt got the word out to Leslie, Al, and me via the sibling call network: Dad had a right femoral neck fracture, a common hip fracture that leaves many elders, post-surgery, with chronic pain and serious disability. I have learned since Dad's fall that delirium affects 35 to 65 percent of patients after hip-fracture repair and is associated with poor functional recovery.[4] So, of course, is hospitalization.

The femoral neck is in the upper portion of the femur, which is the long bone of the thigh that extends from the pelvis to the knee. The neck is just below the femur's head. It forms the ball part of the ball-and-socket joint of your hip. Other possible hip breaks include the intertrochanteric region fracture, which occurs just below the femoral neck, where the bone juts out, and the rare subtrochanteric fracture, a break within the femur itself.[5]

According to Britt, X-rays taken of Dad's pelvic region had to be emailed to a radiologist off-site because no one with expertise remained at the OBH! This was 9 o'clock at night, not 3 a.m. After the results came in, a groundswell for next-day hip-replacement surgery overtook the emergency department staff, who contacted Dad's orthopedic surgeon, Dr. Faber. Faber tentatively agreed with this game plan.

My father was resting in his hospital bed, benefiting from a morphine drip, when I spoke to him that night.

I was in Charlottesville, Va., where I had started living part-time in order to transition gradually to civilization from my once sought-after seaside isolation. My book had been out in print for 18 months, and I was still "between projects." The day before I had undergone periodontal surgery—a tissue graft to my receding gum—which had left me feeling unexpectedly wretched. I planned to return to the Outer Banks on the 24th, after an overnight stay in Alexandria at Britt's condo.

I was astonished to learn that Dad had consented readily to a hip replacement, also called a hip arthroplasty. A hip arthroplasty is major surgery in which he would undergo general anesthesia, not a less risky spinal anesthesia.

Although I knew that surgery had to be done soon, to ensure

the optimum result, it seemed to me that everything was moving too fast. Did he really need a prosthesis and all of the problems that it presented? Can't we talk about this?

My Uncle Pete, Dad's brother, who is twelve years his junior, drove a truck for a living and has paid a physical and medical price for the many miles and hours he spent hauling cargo. He has had both of his knees and one hip replaced, after they wore out, and his hip replacement replaced because it cracked when he fell off of a ladder! One of Uncle Pete's legs appears shorter than the other, and he walks off-kilter, increasing his propensity to fall.

Contemplating a hip replacement for Dad, I worried about incidental damage during surgery to his hip joint, other bones, and nerves, and about the implant itself, albeit biocompatible, causing infection later, loosening, or dislocating.6 What if? What if? The lawyer part of my mind raced.

"I'm going along with what the docs here tell me, Ann," Dad said. "I'm trusting the experts."

Since when? Since the morphine kicked in?

The next day I was relieved when I learned that Dr. Faber had reviewed Dad's X-rays and decided that he could insert three metal screws into the femoral neck to hold it together while the fracture healed. This was possible because the bone was still aligned properly and in good shape. Faber might have considered withholding his judgment until the morning and, thus, spared us (me) some anguish.

Now 85, my father was so unsteady on his feet that he could be standing in front of you, stationary, lose his balance, and stumble. And yet, he was unusually strong and vigorous for his age. I credited his robustness to confidence, a can-do attitude, good genes, and golf, and hoped these assets would carry him through to a full recovery.

POST-OP HOSPITALIZATION

Thankfully, Dad's hip-repair surgery could be performed with a spinal anesthesia, so that we didn't have to fear a deep sleep from which he never awoke. The procedure went well and quickly became a secondary issue as Britt and I shifted into post-op vigilance.

We knew on Day One of Dad's hospitalization that he likely would be discharged after four days. A hip fracture rates four to seven days of hospitalization under insurance plans. That meant we had until

Saturday to prepare for the Outer Banks hurricane that we could not avoid: Our crippled father's return home.

The DPS-possessed Dr. Al made it clear immediately after his surgery that he would be rehabbing at home in his own bed. Thereafter, whenever he would act up and test my patience, I would tell him: "You're lucky we're not parking you [or a part of his anatomy] in a nursing home."

That's how I thought of it: parking. I would never leave my parent's rehabilitation solely up to an institution, regardless of its reputation. Not if I could help it.

Britt and I also knew about the precarious position Dad was in and wanted to do all we could to further his recovery.

Hospitalization can trigger "an often irreversible decline in functional status and a change in quality and style of life" for older patients.[7] Hip fractures bode even worse outcomes. I had seen lonely, displaced people in the Durham facility where my mother convalesced, incapacitated by hip fractures, their rehabilitative progress grindingly slow. I also had friends whose parents broke hips and "slipped away."

Later, I learned, that one-quarter of all people age 65 and older who fracture their hip do not survive a year. Twenty-five percent. Numerous studies published during the past 25 years show that between 14 to 58 percent of all hip-fracture patients in the studied populations died within the first year.[8]

Other medical estimates suggest that from 25 to 50 percent of all hip-fracture patients convalesce in a nursing home after their hospital discharge because they're either too frail to return home or lack sufficient care there or both.[9]

These numbers are wake-up-and-fix-the-healthcare shocking.

After Dad slept enough to regain his energy, Britt and I wanted to get him up and moving. We knew that Dad's disuse of his muscles, joints, and tendons would lead quickly to their deterioration. His bones would fast lose density. With every hour that he spent in bed, his functioning capacity would diminish. This decline would be in addition to the other well-known risks his immobility posed of blood clots, bedsores, respiratory and urinary infections, and the like.

We needn't have worried. After Dad learned that his rehabilitation might take months, he allowed himself some time to feel depressed— that was his word—and then he got busy. The nurses expected him to spend his first day in bed, but he refused. He stood up.

During his physical therapy the next day, Dad walked 35 feet with the use of a walker, and two nurses spotting him, and sat 75 minutes in a chair, until he couldn't tolerate the position any longer. You couldn't hold him back. He wanted to drive and play golf again as soon as possible. He was as persistent and motivated as he was demanding and whiney.

Britt and I visited Dad every day, but he never wanted to chat much, just boss us around. When we tried to inquire about his physical-therapy regimen or medical care, he said he didn't need our help. So we observed. I also befriended one of the nurses, who filled me in out of his earshot. Dad never seemed to "get" that Britt and I, not he, would be responsible for his home care. That would be an admission of dependency, which he loathed, so we prepared without his cooperation.

High on self-centered determination, our father held court from his hospital bed, ordering Britt and me to bring him things when *he* wanted them and to manage other household matters, as instructed.

"A *USA Today* first thing in the morning? Tough luck," I told him. The hospital wasn't an easy 10-minute drive away.

"You know," I would remind his deaf ears, "I have a life, too. And I have a mother who needs looking after."

Tough love was the only way Britt and I could survive his angst-ridden bullying.

Naturally, my father spread his cheer to others. He complained every time a nurse or certified nursing assistant, aka a nurse's aide, took his vital signs, which I agree is too often and shouldn't be at the expense of much-needed sleep. He also objected to Dr. Langard, the hospital's chief of medicine, initiating each of their conversations by asking his name.

"Come *on*," Dr. Al would say disgustedly to Langard, when he asked who he was. Other times, my father answered: "I don't know. Who am I?"

This was bad behavior, of course, but I understood his attitude. Dr. Langard had a humorless, aloof, and bureaucratic way about him.

Confirming patient identification is one of the safe practices that arose after the Institute of Medicine released a report in 1999 quantifying all of the fatal errors that occur in hospitals. (See Appendix One, "The Risks of Hospitalization.") Doctors can confuse patients with each other, and patients can become confused.

But when the same physician repeatedly asks a lucid patient whose identity is well known to state his name, it's form over substance. No one wants an automaton for a doctor. The Outer Banks Hospital only had 19 beds.

As for my father's ID, those nurses and CNAs who could see through his hard shell to the softer center called him Dr. Al. Others just referred to him as "201," as in room 201, which made me bristle. Is it a person or a number lying in the bed? How hard is it to remember a name for a few days? It's not like memorizing Shakespeare.

Dad received an intravenous antibiotic for several days to guard against infection and also breathed supplemental oxygen until his blood-oxygen saturation level was considered acceptable. His lungs contained a lot of fluid, probably, he reasoned, because he'd been lying in bed too long. Dr. Langard, however, was concerned about left-heart failure and pneumonia and ordered repeated chest X-rays and electrocardiograms.

Dr. Al scoffed at what he regarded as bottom-line medicine: ordering unnecessary and expensive tests. I thought it might be cover-your-ass medicine. God forbid something disastrous should happen to 201!

At the time, I wasn't as up to speed on Dad's heart health as I would become. Dad had been seeing Dr. Anthony, the same cardiologist who sent my embolus-stricken mother *stat* to the OB hospital, for about five years; but he kept his own counsel, and his own records, on these checkups. I knew the medications he was taking and why. I also knew that Anthony had diagnosed him with mild pulmonary hypertension, a diagnosis that Dad didn't believe.

To assess his patients' cardiac health, Dr. Anthony favored the echocardiogram over the electrocardiogram, which Dr. Al preferred. An echocardiogram (echo) is an ultrasound; it uses sound waves to create a moving picture of your heart. An electrocardiogram is a tracing that depicts your heart's electrical activity. Both are produced by an electrocardiograph, a machine that measures the rate and regularity of your heartbeats. An electrocardiograph also can be used to evaluate the presence of any damage to your heart or the effects from drugs or devices (e.g., a pacemaker) used to regulate it.

For an electrocardiogram, you lie supine (on your back), and a nurse or technician affixes electrodes from the electrocardiograph to your arms, legs, and chest. The heart's electrical activity can be detected in this manner because its impulses produce currents that reach the skin, the body's surface.

An electrocardiograph records your heart's electrical impulses as waves; an electrocardiogram, thus, consists of wavy lines that you can see on a computer monitor or a paper printout. Although different, the terms electrocardiograph and electrocardiogram get used interchangeably, and both are abbreviated as EKG—an acronym for the German word, elektrokardiogramm—or, more commonly today, ECG.

For an echo, you lie on your side while a transducer, a microphone-like instrument, is "placed on your ribs near the breast bone and directed toward [your] heart. . . . The transducer" sends out ultrasonic sound waves that move through your skin and other tissues to the heart where it "picks up the echoes of the sound waves and transmits them as electrical impulses. The electrocardiograph machine converts these impulses into moving pictures of the [interior of the] heart."[10]

The transducer's sound waves bounce or echo off of the heart's tissues and structures, particularly its valves. The heart has four valves that, by opening and closing, control the flow of blood and prevent its backflow or backward leakage. Although the valves themselves are silent, the turbulence of the blood as it moves through them creates muted sounds. (If they weren't muted, you couldn't sneak up on anyone.)

The mitral or bicuspid valve is located between the left-side atrium and ventricle and prevents backflow during systole. The tricuspid valve serves the same function on the right side. These valves act together. The sound their blood flow makes is known as S_1. (I am told by a physician friend that this is one of two hypotheses. One is enough for me.)

The aortic semilunar valve, so-named because it has a half-moon shape, is located between the left ventricle and the aorta, the big artery that carries blood away from the heart. This valve prevents backflow into the ventricle during diastole. The pulmonic semilunar valve is located between the right ventricle and the trunk leading to the pulmonary arteries. It, too, prevents backflow during diastole. The sound of these two valves acting together is known as S_2.

Dr. Langard called Anthony to inform him of Dad's post-surgical "congestive heart failure," so, about three weeks after his discharge, my father had a cardiac checkup. It produced the following results:

BP 114/58; HR 56; lungs clear; heart S1, S2, regular rate; no edema in extremities.

"Really he is doing well," Anthony wrote in the medical record, with a recommendation that Dad return in a year.

While in the hospital, Dr. Al requested the anticoagulant, Lovenox, to thwart clot formation, but he quit taking it after one day because Dr. Faber, the orthopedic surgeon, advised him that he could get by with aspirin. This bad advice drove me nuts, but I did not yet have much sway in my father's medical matters. Dad branded Dr. Langard and other OBH doctors—loudly, with his hospital-room door open—"deficient." I would say the same about Faber's postoperative treatment.

My father continued on morphine, even though it made him nauseous and that, in turn, led to an antiemetic, which is a medication to prevent vomiting. No matter what painkiller you take, constipation also will become a problem if you don't address it.

After Feb. 23, you could say that my life went temporarily into the toilet as Britt and I began monitoring Dad's bowel movements, and he kept track as well. We had done the same oversight during Mom's hospitalization for the embolus and asked the resident in charge to prescribe a stool softener to assist her. The nightmare of Mom's massive fecal impaction at Duke would not repeat, not if we could help it.

Dad had his own bowel-production schedule: Action by post-op Day Two and then every 48 hours thereafter.

Thanks to a potent colonic remedy mixed by Pam, one of the CNAs who had become fond of Dr. Al and his cantankerous nature, my father met his goals. Pam's milk-of-magnesia-and-prune-juice concoction cleaned out his GI tract with surefire gusto.

As Leslie had at Duke, I looked around the Outer Banks Hospital for certified nursing aides who might be able to freelance home-nursing care. CNAs, whose training and educational prerequisites vary state-to-state, assist patients with their "activities of daily living," aka ADL. They are caregivers with rudimentary nursing knowledge.

The most basic ADL are:

❖ Bathing
❖ Dressing
❖ Using the toilet

❖ Transferring (for example, from the bed to the walker)
❖ Feeding[11]

I think of them as the minimal acts required for the job of living: Getting out of bed in the morning; using the toilet; washing; dressing; eating.

Pam was receptive to my inquiry about in-home caregiving and said she had a friend, Marie, who could help. Thank goodness!

Mom's Meltdown

The truth is my mother concerned me more than my father.

Even before Dad came home to convalesce, Mom was not coping well. She had lapsed into a confused, vacant state, seeming sadly like the proverbial transfixed deer in the headlights.

Mom's diminished presence startled me. She lacked her usual energy, and I thought she, too, might be depressed. No, she replied, not depressed. Are you anxious, then? I asked upon my return from Alexandria. Yes, she was anxious: "I don't know how to do anything," she said softly. Worrying about how she would fill my father's shoes was keeping her awake at night.

I hugged Mom, told her that I love her, and promised her that "we will always take care of you. You never have to worry." But her affect didn't change.

My parents had been married nearly 60 years. While I am one of the last people who should analyze their relationship, I certainly have knowledge of it. It is safe to call their marriage traditional, and their roles within it traditional, even though my mother does not conform to a gender-identity stereotype. Dad has handled all of their financial affairs, including purchases of all real estate and investments, and has maintained their houses, yards, and automobiles. Mom's domain has been hearth and home *inside*.

Perhaps the arrival in the mail of bills and financial documents for my father unnerved my mother. She also depended on Dad for her medications and may have been confused about what to take and how to get her first-of-the-month refills. Lately, too, Dad had been buying the groceries. Mom's two knee replacements hampered her mobility, but it also was no secret to any of us that her memory was deteriorating.

Nearly eight years ago Duke's Dr. Gideon had diagnosed Mom

with baseline dementia on insufficient evidence. It now appeared that she could be headed toward that fate. Of all of us kids, I knew the extent of her cognitive decline. She no longer had the superb recall and reasoning on which we all had depended.

When we visited Dad during his four-day hospitalization, my mother sat meekly to the side, not saying a word, except to ask: "Can we go home now?" She broke my heart. Just as my father had "lost it" during Mom's ehrlichiosis crisis, my mother was melting down under the stress of this upheaval. We had to make sure that she didn't forget to eat or drink. She was fragile.

Suddenly, Britt and I were in a full-blown, 24-hours-a-day, seven-days-a-week crisis and would be for the foreseeable future. We needed help.

Mom didn't like Pam, who doted on my father, because she was loud, opinionated, and very direct. Nonetheless, we might have to call on her. We could take only so much of Dr. Al's DPS.

It didn't help my mindset that, because of my gum surgery in Charlottesville, I couldn't eat solid food or exercise for a week. Without gym workouts, I had no quick way to release my stress. My sinkhole deepened.

DISCHARGE DAY

On Saturday, Feb. 27, Britt and I arrived to pick up Dad at the appointed hour, and . . . he threw us out, refusing to talk with us and ordering us to come back later. It seems he was intensely preoccupied with his basic functions—better he than we—and we interrupted his single-mindedness. Of course, about a half hour after he dismissed us, he began asking for us to reappear. We knew enough to step out into the hallway and converse with the nurses and not to leave the premises.

While waiting for our summons, I met with the hospital social worker, who referred me to a local private home-care service, whom I'll call the "Sitters." She further instructed me on how to enlist the Dare County EMS's assistance in transporting Dad from my car to his bedroom. Because of a few stairs on the front porch of my parents' home, we could not wheel him in.

Your parent's hospital discharge day can be tediously long, as you wait around for something to happen, never quite sure for what, or whom, you're waiting.

I encourage you to ask a friendly nurse the day before discharge for a discharge time—a specific hour. But don't hold her or him to it. Morning or afternoon may be the best time estimate you can get.

You have to be flexible, so don't think you can pop over on your lunch hour. Clear out your day.

Well before the actual exit, I try to speak to all knowledgeable people—the physicians, nurses, medical students, CNAs, physical therapists, social workers. I've learned through trial and error that discharge summaries accompanying patients are often inadequate.

On this day, I perused the discharge papers and committed a PC faux pas when I erroneously assumed that the name of the discharging physician, whom I had not met, was Indian, and I said so.

Dr. Khalid, who appeared to be in his late 30s, icily informed me that he was Pakistani. When I asked him what his name meant, he said, "a kind person," then quickly added, "but I'm not one."

"That should come in handy in the medical profession," I replied, or words to that effect.

You gotta love doctors. What in the world would a Pakistani, an Indian, or any other ethnicity doctor practicing on the feel-good Outer Banks have to get testy about? I wanted to ask him, but I needed prescriptions and a signature first.

As it turned out, Dr. Khalid prescribed a medication that—I found out later at the pharmacy—didn't exist in the form he requested, and Dr. Faber, the surgeon, failed to order physical therapy because he wanted my father to rest in bed, mend for three weeks, and do no exercise! Leave it to a surgeon to focus on his own handiwork and ignore the patient's general well-being. Bed rest is lethal. Strike three for Faber. I never imagined that there would be no PT order in the discharge packet, so I didn't look for one. Wrong.

Langard also complicated Dad's discharge by ordering tests performed on him during the wee hours of the previous night: another chest X-ray, an ECG, more lab work. My sleep-deprived father hit the roof, but he couldn't stave off the invaders. These test results needed to be in hand before Khalid would sign off on the discharge.

When I asked my favorite nurse about the need for the tests, she demurred with a knowing glance.

We were in for a long day.

Fortunately, the transport came off smoothly. Pam wheeled Dad down to the main entrance curb, where I had parked my car, and showed Britt and me the proper technique for moving him from the wheelchair to the front passenger seat—which we already knew from Mom's hospitalizations, but a refresher didn't hurt. We helped Dad stand, turn slightly so that his back faced the seat, and lower his rear end.

"Butt first," Pam instructed.

We then lifted his legs and gently swung them into the car.

About 10 minutes down the road—and after a seeming eternity of back-seat driving from the front-seat passenger—I called the EMS to request assistance at home and arrived about a minute before the paramedics did. I had been advised by the social worker not to keep them waiting.

The EMS performed brilliantly, carefully lifting my father, who sat upright, harnessed in a special chair, into the house and transferring him to bed. He had a portable toilet at his bedside that he could use unassisted—although he was supposed to have someone nearby when he did. That was the good news. The bad news was that he now suffered from the more virulent at-home type of DPS. Every request he made came out like a command that had to be fulfilled immediately and in nit-picking detail.

No, not *that* spoon, *that* bowl, *that* glass. *I want, I want, I want.* My father's conversation consisted almost exclusively of complaints. He seemed determined to shrink our worlds to the size of his.

The next time I came over, Mom was calling Dad, "Your Majesty," and mumbling under her breath.

STRANGERS ON THE YARD

The day after Dr. Al's discharge, the home-care physical therapist arrived for an evaluation visit—as promised and without a nudge call from us. Yeah! Once again, the same paperwork that Dad had completed for the hospital needed to be prepared.

You would think that with computers in use, patient information would convey with the patient, being transferred easily, for example, from the emergency department to a medical floor in a hospital, and from a hospital to a home agency, but you would be wrong. Redundancy is the rule of the healthcare system. Information never transfers. This may change in the future with electronic records, but not for many years yet.

My father handed the therapist a copy of a list he had at the ready of his medications, surgeries, etc. The next day, Monday, he would begin seven weeks of PT. Our local Coastal Rehab was on the ball.

Dad's program consisted of progressive range-of-motion and muscle-strengthening exercises, as well as sitting and walking. A PT dynamo named Karen, who could go nose-to-nose with Dr. Al any day of the week, worked him out. She was firm, good-natured, and empathetic. He loved her and began to quote her as his authority.

Karen visited three times a week for an hour at a stretch and left homework assignments, which my father unfailingly did. Britt and I monitored his form, ensuring that he didn't put his weight on his healing right side, counted his exercise repetitions, and accompanied him on the prescribed number of walks around the house. He initially used a rolling walker, then graduated to a cane.

Karen also clued us in about modifications we could make to the house to protect our parents from falling again: grab bars in the shower, carpeting on the stairs, rugs either tacked down or removed, handrails in the hallways. These were all common-sense precautions that Dad and Mom had not wanted to think about. They now went for the grab bars and the carpeting, but not the rails. In clinical studies, home-hazard reduction appears to be most effective when it is targeted at older people with a history of falls or with mobility limits, rather than the older population in general.[12] It also is better if you safeguard the home *before* the fall occurs.

Dad made rapid progress and was walking up and down stairs, initially with assistance, in no time. Less than two months after he fractured his hip, he was driving. When his in-home Medicare-covered PT maxed out, he started visiting Coastal Rehab for outpatient workouts. Six months after he fell, he thought his right leg still wasn't as strong as it had been, but, otherwise, he could detect no falloff in his physical condition. With independence, he became much more pleasant to be around.

But I get ahead of the story.

Mom shadowed Dad during his walks with Karen—posing a fall hazard for both of them—and called out whenever she heard low voices emanating from another room. She wanted to know everything that was being done or said, lest she be uninformed or unprepared, and became uncharacteristically angry if she felt excluded. But her eyes revealed that she wasn't comprehending what we told her. According to Dr. Al, she was "decompensating." I now think she may have been delirious.

In medicine, decompensation refers to the functional deterioration of a previously working physiological system. Cardiac decompensation, for example, connotes the heart's failure to maintain adequate blood circulation after longstanding, but previously *compensated* (maintained) vascular disease. This degradation typically occurs because of fatigue, stress, illness, or old age. Similarly, in psychiatry, decompensation refers to a deterioration of mental health in a mentally ill person who previously has maintained a functional balance. Essentially, it's a worsening of symptoms. In response to a stressor of some kind, the patient is unable to call upon the usual defense mechanisms.

My mother was not mentally ill, but she had lost her psychological equilibrium, and her functioning had deteriorated. I assumed and hoped that her anxious confusion would be transient, and "normalcy" would return after Dad resumed his role in the household. But irony interceded instead.

For the first four days after Dr. Al returned home, Britt and I alternated caregiving and housekeeping shifts, helping with meals, medications, cleanup, and any attention that either Dad or Mom needed. We also ran household errands, handled the mail and any payments due, and walked the dog. When we broached the subject of hiring Pam and her friend Marie or one of the Sitters, my parents would protest that they didn't "want someone in the house." To reinforce their stance, they would recall my grandfather's objection to what he called "strangers on the yard."

A retired farmer who was able to live at home until his death at age 96 because he didn't have chronic, disabling ailments and didn't need a lot of help with his ADL—and my Uncle Pete checked in on him regularly—Grandpa considered anyone who wasn't a friend or family member a "stranger."

"We don't want strangers on the yard," Mom and Dad would say.

My mother also insisted that she could take care of Dad, and she *was* capable of some tasks, such as serving breakfast and emptying the commode. But not much more. While Britt and I appreciated that she wanted to continue her spousal support, we knew that she needed care, too.

On March 2, I emailed my good friends that my sister and I were caring for *two* patients and burning out. Dad behaved like a terror, and poor Mom was terrified. I saw my separate life disappearing and started taking an antidepressant to ease the despair that had settled in my head and knotted my stomach.

Finally Britt and I gave our parents no choice. We had to have help. Neither one of us was a nurse or a martyr.

Little did we imagine the harm that strangers on the yard could do.

HOMEWORK ON HIP FRACTURES

Studies suggest that early or prompt surgery after a fall decreases the scary 25 percent, one-year mortality rate of older hip-fracture patients, most of whom are women. To reduce their mortality risk, ambulatory elders who were living at home when they fell and fractured a hip should have surgery within two calendar days.

When delay occurs between your Mom's hospital arrival and her surgery, it is often because of a lack of available operating suites and/or surgeons and/or a perceived lack of medical readiness on her part. Patients on anticoagulants or with serious pre-existing medical conditions, for example, present surgeons with complicating factors that they must manage. Most hip-fracture patients do not have surgery within 24 hours of their hospital arrival, much less within 24 hours of their fall, as my father did.[13]

The timing of surgery after a hip fracture may affect 1) problems that occur during surgery ("complications"), 2) the patient's functional recovery and independence, and 3) the length of her hospital stay.

Keep in mind that, as I noted earlier, there are different types of fractures and surgeries, as well as different types of patients. The healthier a patient is before the fracture and the fewer problems that occur after surgery, the better she will fare in recovery.

But even among hip-fracture patients who are age 50 and older, and thus, presumably stronger than elders, Johns Hopkins reports that 40 percent remain unable a year later to walk without a cane or other assistance, and 60 percent still cannot perform basic ADLs, such as dressing themselves.[14]

It is a very short slide from the discharge of your Mom to a nursing home for rehabilitation of a hip fracture . . . to her residency at the home for a year . . . to a permanent move there. Up to 25 percent of all hip-fracture patients live in a nursing home for at least a year. That's criminally sad.

If your Mom only undergoes 15 minutes of physical therapy per day, or 30 minutes every other day, or whatever the nursing home's regimen is, how is she supposed to regain ambulation on her wasted muscles and weak, porous bones?

CNAs in nursing homes are typically running (or, depending on the SNF, taking their time walking) among patients, feeding, bathing, dressing, and transporting them, as well as changing their diapers, making beds, and responding to the call lights outside of each room. They will walk with a patient if they have the time, but don't count on them ever having time. It is also likely that your Mom's physical therapist won't work on the weekends.

If you or another relative cannot visit your Mom every day and ensure that she walks often to regain strength and balance more quickly, then you should investigate other options, such as a private-duty nursing assistant. You can never assume that the PT your parent is receiving at an SNF is sufficient or that your Mom is exercising between sessions. I know cost is an issue, and Medicare runs out, but this is so important to your parent's well-being and survival that I urge you to make it happen.

Just being at home and in her own bed can be a huge emotional lift for an elder whose world also toppled when she fell and cracked her hip.

HOMEWORK ON FALLS

According to the Centers for Disease Control and Prevention, one in three adults age 65 and older—about 13 million people—falls each year in the United States.[15] After age 80, writes Dr. Adam Darowski, author of the patient- and advocate-friendly primer, "Falls: The Facts," the fall rate is one in two.[16]

Of the 13 million, reports the CDC, 20 to 30 percent suffer "moderate to severe injuries that make it hard for them to get around or live independently, and increase their risk of early death."[17]

According to medical-journal articles I read, one in five falls among elders living in the community requires some medical attention—for bruising, lacerations, sprains, and the like—but fewer than one in ten results in a fracture.[18] In his 80s, my father's rate of bone-fracture-to-fall was about one-in-three, with the bone usually being a rib.

Regardless of which health or medical source you consult, two facts are clear: Falls can be life-altering, if not debilitating, for an older person, and the risk of a fall increases with age.

In 2007, 18,334 people age 65 and older died from unintentional falls. This constituted about 1 percent of all mortalities in this age group.[19]

Falls incur well over $20 billion annually in direct healthcare costs in the United States, the majority of them for hip-fracture care. (In people ages 65 to 75, wrist fractures are more common fall-related injuries than hip fractures.)[20] Direct costs are those fees and expenses that patients and insurance companies pay. They include fees for physicians, hospital and nursing-home care, rehabilitation, and prescription drugs.

Falls also incur incalculable indirect costs related to their long-term effects, such as disability, lost time from work, and a reduced quality of life.

Dr. Darowski categorizes falls as follows:

* Accidents, trips, and slips
* Falls due to an illness that causes weakness or unsteadiness
* Falls due to an innate tendency to fall
* Falls due to faintness (or dizziness) or loss of consciousness[21]

He attributes the causes of these falls to what he calls intrinsic factors, which have to do with the status of the person who fell (hampered, e.g., by a bad knee, muscle weakness, poor grip, cognitive impairment, or visual deficits), and extrinsic factors, which usually exist in the environment (a slippery floor, loose rugs, or poor lighting).

Typically, extrinsic and intrinsic factors combine to create a fall.

Some medically trained fall experts distinguish further between extrinsic and environmental factors. The most common non-environmental extrinsic factor is polypharmacy, when your Mom or Pop takes four or more prescription drugs. The combination of so many drugs can have an adverse effect on your parent's mental and physical health, making him disoriented, for example, or wobbly on his feet.

Darowski cites four fall-promoting circumstances that you should bear in mind in trying to fall-proof your Mom and Pop and their home(s):

* Collisions in the dark, usually on getting out of bed at night
* Temporary hazards around the home that they may forget

(e.g., an object left on the floor)
* Loose carpets on which they might slip or catch a toe
* Simple carelessness about the house [22]

To assess an older person's risk of falling for purposes of prevention, you really need to probe his or her intrinsic factors.[23] One of the most important is balance—my father's chief problem—which affects gait or walking style. According to Darowski, the balance systems of elders are "less sensitive, less rapid, less accurate, and weaker."[24]

As the fall-facts expert explains, balance control has to do with your ability to recognize your body's position in space and to restore your body to a balanced position when it becomes unbalanced, for example, after a stumble. This control involves both conscious decisions to move and subconsciously made movements.

Being "in balance," Darowski writes, means your body's center of gravity is kept within an area above the feet known as the base of support. Your brain knows where the body's "vertical" lies and where the body is in space at any time because of sensations it receives from 1) your eyes, 2) the organ of balance in your inner ear, and 3) nerves throughout your body. When these sensations deteriorate, as they do with age or illness, you lose your balance.[25]

Proprioception is your unconscious perception of your body's movement and spatial orientation. Proprioception arises and depends on your body's nerves carrying sensory information to your brain, specifically, to the cerebellum, which, in lay terms, is the center of movement and coordination.

Besides those associated with your inner ear and eyes, "balance" nerves come from all of your muscles, joints, and tendons and tell you where you are in space. Those in the soles of your feet, for example, tell your brain whether you are on firm or shaky ground. Nerves that tell you about skin sensations assist your balance nerves.

According to Darowski, older people fall more often than young people because of degeneration of the nerves of body sensation and/or degeneration of the connections within the brain itself, a condition known as cerebral small vessel disease. Cerebral small vessel disease occurs, he says, when areas of the brain experience damage to their blood supply. This damage leads to small areas of cell death and disruption to pathways carrying nerve impulses from one part of the brain to another.[26]

Weak, damaged, or painful muscles and joints (think arthritis), which commonly beset aging bodies, also affect the brain's ability to process sensory information. If the nerves that transmit impulses to the muscles are damaged, there will be some impairment of balance and an increased likelihood of falling.

Balance may be threatened by a variety of other factors, including:

* Inner-ear (e.g., vertigo) or visual impairment
* Disease (notably, Parkinson's disease)
* Infection
* Alcohol intake
* Certain medications (e.g., psychotropics, such as drugs for depression) as well as multiple medications (polypharmacy)
* Frailty
* Anxiety
* Depression
* Confusion
* Simple lack of concentration[27]

You should be able to recognize when your Mom or Pop is a "fall risk" and take steps to hazard-proof them and their environment. But don't storm their house and re-do their familiar floors and nail bars into their familiar walls, without their permission. The loss of steady, reliable movement and balance is the loss of independence and control. You must respect that loss and take initiative with your parents as a team. Start with installing grab bars in the shower and removing throw rugs, steps that are not intrusive, and gently point out other hazards while you gently resist any stubborn refusal.

You don't want to become another threat in your parents' home(s). It's their sanctuary, their safe haven. Don't ruin it.

Chapter Six

2010 Cont.: Confusion, Pain
AND DECLINE

When Bad Things Happen While Others Watch

When Mom fell, I again was in Charlottesville, having been relieved in North Carolina by my brother. It was St. Patrick's Day.

Yes, I said, when Mom fell. It was a double whammy. First, Dad. Now, about three weeks later, Mom.

As Britt related on the telephone that evening, Mom had awakened at 5 a.m. to use the toilet. While standing in the entranceway to the bathroom, she fell—not because she tripped over an object or because she lost her balance. She may have collided with the door jam, but she couldn't say. She just fell. No explanation.

It was dark, and my already foggy-headed mother had taken a potent hypnotic before going to bed. That she sleeps on the side of the bed farthest from the bathroom also factored into a fall analysis.

Britt was so overburdened by this time that she noted Mom's fall almost as an incidental event: "Mom fell this morning," she told me.

"WHAT?"

"But she's all right," my sister said. She apparently lay on the floor for hours (!) before my hearing-impaired father awoke and called for my brother, who was sleeping upstairs. Al lifted Mom and helped her back to bed. She then enjoyed what could be called a normal day, under the abnormal circumstances, and even rode with Al and Britt to the airport—a three-hour round trip—without an utterance of pain or discomfort.

OK, I thought. She's OK. Thank God.

But the next night, March 18, when I walked into my parents' bedroom, I saw deep pain etched in my mother's face.

I asked her how she felt—"Terrible. My back hurts, and I can't move."—and announced that I would be calling 911 and arranging for her transport to the hospital emergency department. She needed X-rays and pain treatment. Mom didn't resist.

I envisioned "another night in the chair," as Britt had characterized her bedside vigil in the Chesapeake hospital ICU nearly eight years ago, and that turned out to be largely true. I didn't leave the ED until after 3 a.m. Although I wasn't happy about the circumstances that I left, I never imagined the treatment that my mother would receive. For the first and only time in my advocacy experience, I used profanity with a healthcare worker, and I didn't mince words. I dropped the F-bomb. I was furious.

LOL BIAS AGAIN

Our experience in the ED should have been fair warning. I felt out of sync with most of the nursing staff; the doctor on duty, one Teflon®-coated Dr. Offish; and the radiology technician. A child whose wails reverberated off of the white walls distracted the easily distracted Dr. Offish and the nurses. The tech simply didn't want me around. Time-consuming errors occurred.

The paramedics who transported my mother had been terrific—exceedingly capable, kind, and careful. They handled her as if she were a newborn baby, tending to her every wince. But once she got to Emergency, the baby became a sack of potatoes. Mom described her pain as a 10 on a scale of one to 10, but the CNAs moved her around as if they didn't believe she had been injured. I had to ask them to be more gentle.

I repeated to Dr. Offish and the nurses all of the detail that I had painstakingly given to the EMTs—whose reports ED personnel never seem to read: WHY NOT?—and was frustrated by their response. Despite my request for a stronger drug, the doctor prescribed only extra-strength Tylenol for Mom's pain. Physicians on principle don't like to dope up patients, and nurses don't like to care for them when they are doped up, but, in my humble opinion, giving Tylenol to a presumptive fracture patient with agonizing pain is like prepping a surgical patient with aspirin instead of anesthesia.

Mom spent what I considered an excessively long time in her room before the radiology technician showed up to wheel her out. I rose to accompany them, but the tech discouraged me from coming. Rather than disagree with her—Really, who needs a confrontation in the ED? And why is there a bug up *her* butt?—I deferred, thinking: What can go wrong?

Mistake. Murphy's Law always applies in hospitals. I knew better.

What can go wrong? Answer: The technician can X-ray the wrong area of your Mom's or Pop's body! This happens more times than you may think. Friends of mine have experienced the same sloppiness in an emergency department with their elderly parents. Fractures get overlooked, and old patients get stereotyped as demented or pigeonholed as complainers with fantasy pain.

I have no idea what the doctor ordered and what my mother told the tech about the location of her pain. All I know is that after Mom had returned from Radiology and I pointedly asked about the holdup in treatment, the nurse informed me that the X-rays had shown no fracture. I insisted this couldn't be so and felt compelled by the nurse's lack of sympathy to tell her that my mother wasn't a malingerer. I also brought up referred pain, a possibility that she acknowledged. Baffled, I asked to speak with Dr. Offish, who added patronizing and dismissive to the list of adjectives I would ascribe to the professional demeanor we encountered that night.

The indifferent young Dr. Offish seemed to believe Mom had Little Old Lady Syndrome and not a legitimate injury. How else could she have fallen without knowing how or why she fell? And why did Mom wait more than 24 hours before she came to the hospital? Further, if the X-rays revealed no fracture, then no fracture could exist: *Ipso facto.*

Neither Offish nor the nurse was forthcoming about the scope of the X-rays, and it wasn't until I took Mom to see Dad's orthopedic surgeon, Dr. Faber, 10 days later that he confirmed what I suspected. The initial X-rays had not scanned the thoracic area of her spine, despite her history of osteoporosis and compression fracture.

Eventually, my mother underwent another round in Radiology, and Offish returned with a diagnosis, which she couched in vagueness about how sometimes X-rays don't give a refined picture. Yeah, right. My mother had a compression fracture of her T-10 vertebra of "less than 10 percent," the percentage, as I understood it, being a quantification of how much vertebral height (bone) had been lost. By then we had been in the ED for *four hours*. At last, Dr. Offish ordered a morphine drip for her patient's level-10 pain.

I was hopeful that Mom would be safely in a hospital bed before I left, but she spent the night in Emergency instead, no bed being available, or so I was told. How disgraceful is that? I slipped out at 3:15 a.m. Once home, I emailed all of my siblings about Mom's status and slept about two hours before returning to the ED at 8 a.m.

PAIN "MANAGEMENT"

To my chagrin, Dr. Langard was now on the scene. He explained that Mom would be admitted shortly and would likely stay for two days during which time she would receive pain medication and management and a PT consult.

Langard specifically said Mom's pain would be "managed." He also informed me that her fracture had been reassessed at 25 percent compression, which he viewed as an improvement, showing how uninformed either he or I was.

While awaiting Mom's transfer, Langard asked her, in his robotic style, if she wanted a DNR order. Knowing she was a doctor, he used the acronym rather than the words it abbreviates: Do not resuscitate. When Mom expressed confusion, I explained his question, and she quickly answered: "No. I want to be resuscitated."

Sensing my dismay, the medical chief proffered: "I have to ask this."

Really? I thought. For a compression fracture? And did you have to ask it in such a clumsy and thoughtless fashion? Without first ascertaining the psychological status of the patient? What ham-handed red tape.

In referencing whether a patient is DNR or not, doctors commonly speak about his code status. To code or not to code, that is the question: When a patient's heart or breathing stops (when cardiopulmonary arrest occurs), does he or she (or the family) want doctors and other medical-team members to take full emergency action in order to resuscitate him or her or not? To code the coding patient is to seek to revive him using all available heroic measures.

If a patient is a no-code, doctors will not aggressively intervene to save him, instead favoring "comfort-care" measures, which may be the more humane course of action. If the patient's condition is bleak, prolonging his life can seem cruel.

According to an operating-room nurse I know with 30 years'

experience, however, doctors can be callous to no-code patients, writing them off and not even offering comfort. Even code patients can be ignored. My sister Leslie told me about a doctor who upon arriving late to the hospital room of a code patient in severe distress scolded the nurses who had responded without her: "What are you doing? She's 81!"

Consider the glum advice dispensed by a physician to the wife of an advanced cancer patient who initially wanted "everything" to be done for him. In telling her how doctors code, the M.D., quoted by Dr. Sandeep Jauhar in his book, "Intern," sounds like an odds-savvy poker player who knows when to fold 'em:

"He will get intubated [for mechanical ventilation]," he explained. "Then we will not know his [oxygen] volume status, so we will have to insert a catheter into his lungs. He will get an infection. We will give him antibiotics. His blood pressure will drop. We will give him intravenous pressors. His kidneys will fail. He will need dialysis. And, despite everything we do, his cancer will not go away. Eventually you will make him DNR, but by then he will have suffered for no good purpose."[1]

Fortunately, I didn't have a tough DNR decision to make. My mother was old, but not at death's door. She certainly didn't need to contemplate coding.

The morning nurses, who calmed me down after my exchange with Langard, were like-night-and-day better than the crew I had met in the wee hours. One especially efficient and kind nurse, whom we knew from Dr. Anthony's office, took good care of Mom. I relaxed in her custody, but her custody didn't last long.

It was now Friday, March 19. After Mom arrived in room 202 and met her nurses for the day, the charge nurse, Sally, started asking questions about her medical history. This would be the third time in less than 24 hours that we filled in these blanks. I wanted "Miss Fern," as they called Mom, to take control of this exercise as much as possible, but Sally preferred to look to me.

Hospital patients typically have three nurses assigned to them daily: A CNA, an R.N. duty nurse, and the R.N. charge nurse who supervises the other two. You can glance at an erasable board on the wall of your Mom's or Pop's room and immediately learn the first names of all three. Unfortunately, as I noted during my mother's ehrlichiosis crisis, they change often, so continuity of care, which is especially important for cognitively impaired elders, is lost.

Sally asked a long series of familiar questions and entered all of our responses into a bedside computer. When she got to a question about Mom's "knowledge deficit," I felt conflicted. I didn't want to mention my mother's "decompensation" and faulty memory in front of her, but I also wanted the nurses to know that Miss Fern was in an altered cognitive state.

"Knowledge deficit," Sally loudly announced. "I always check that." I couldn't tell if my mother reacted to this, and I didn't like Sally's ageist presumption, but it fit in her case. Sally also asked if Mom had an advance directive, a legal document that, in North Carolina, states a person's desires regarding the receipt of life-prolonging measures when death is imminent and appoints a healthcare power of attorney to act for her when she can't make her own decisions. Mom did. I had her POA. I also had Dad's. (Advance directives are alternately called living wills.)

While I don't dispute the value of most of the patient information that Sally gathered, I do dispute the method of its acquisition, as well as its redundancy. This perfunctory exercise, which I've seen performed in other hospitals, makes me wonder how often healthcare personnel view the patient as more than a collection of data. Too often interpersonal communication skills and empathy are lacking.

Being an empathetic person myself, as well as an advocate capable of seeing "the other side," I also understand that during this exercise the good nurse may elicit valuable information not previously obtained, as well as establish a relationship with the patient. I am all for *useful* communication.

When I left the hospital, Mom was resting, pain-free. At 2:57 p.m., I emailed Leslie and Al from home:

Mom is now hospitalized in room 202 of the OBH, phone # (252) 449-5702. She'll most likely spend 1-2 days in the hospital, during which time she'll receive pain medication/management and a PT consult, then she'll be discharged to home. The consensus among the doctors, including Dr. Faber, Dad's orthopedic surgeon, and Mom's primary care physician, is that she will not need nor benefit from any surgical procedure. She just needs time to mend. Besides controlling her pain, the most important thing is to get her up ASAP. . . . [I then suggested ways in which we could care for both

Mom and Dad at home.]
    *I'm totally pooped, but expecting Britt to drop by shortly, so we
can go over scheduling concerns.*

Britt and I did that, and then I collapsed. I slept 17 hours. I, thus,
was well-rested for my big scene.

MORE F---ING NEGLECT

When I returned to the hospital Saturday afternoon to visit Mom,
I found a situation much like the one I had encountered Thursday
evening at my parents' home. My mother was in bed, unable to move
much and quietly suffering from atrocious pain. The doctor on her
case, Dr. Minor, had not "managed" her pain one iota, nor had Nurse
Susan, the most recent duty nurse, administered relief. Mom was now
taking ibuprofen. I-bu-*fucking*-profen.
    I was beside myself. What was the point of this hospital admission?
Of the long miserable hours waiting in the emergency department for
a no-brainer diagnosis? Of the uncomfortable night that Mom was
forced to spend in the ED because the hospital was too rinky-dink
to accommodate a 3 a.m. admission? Of putting up with people's
disinterested and uncaring attitudes?
    The point, I wanted to scream, was to relieve my poor, confused,
old, and very precious mother of PAIN. Pain, pain, pain!
    I grabbed the first figure in a nurse's aide uniform and demanded
to know—in a heated, but still rational manner—what was going on with
the meds. The CNA shrugged her shoulders. That only increased my
ire. With anger rising, I pointedly summarized the purpose of Mom's
hospitalization, ripped the medical staff for failing to achieve that
simple purpose and, therefore, causing needless suffering, and warned
that if appropriate pain therapy did not occur promptly: "I'm going to
file a fucking complaint."
    I thought I might explode like a firecracker from frustration. I
wanted to hurl other f--ks at people, but I restrained myself. Even
with my head bursting, I knew that one well-placed obscenity would
get action—especially when coupled with legal-type language—but
a tirade of them would not. If this is what it takes to get people who
are supposed to be paying attention to your ailing loved one to pay
attention, then this is what you have to do. Proceed until apprehended.

The targeted CNA gleaned the gist of what I said and beat tracks for help. Soon I got the full story of what had happened overnight, and Mom got a strong enough painkiller to make a difference. But that was only after an R.N. informed me that Dr. Minor, who had popped in earlier to spend a few moments with #202, could not be reached because "his pager probably wasn't working."

I thought it more likely that Minor himself wasn't working. Mom identified him as a young man in a T-shirt who didn't stay long. A T-shirt. Give me a break. How does an M.D. not understand the disrespect and detachment this half-ass attire communicates to patients? Too many doctors think they don the Golden Fleece when they slip on their white lab coats—presented, FYI, at the *start* of medical school, in a self-congratulatory ceremony, before they've attended a single class—but at least the coat conveys serious import and professionalism.

Fortunately, we didn't need to reach Dr. Minor. My mother's case file contained medical authorization for giving her Dilaudid® (hydromorphone) for severe pain. Jane, my favorite nurse from my father's hospitalization, had administered a dose of Dilaudid on Friday night before she went off-duty. When Susan came on, however, she suspended it and switched to ibuprofen.

According to nurse Emily, who responded to my "f'ing complaint" threat by dosing Mom again with Dilaudid, the drug can cause patients to become too fatigued or lightheaded to assist in their own care. Hence, they are more work (read: trouble) for the staff. Susan certainly didn't want more work.

I usually get along well with nurses, even the ones who "hon" me to pieces. I know nurses are the backbone of the healthcare system, as well as the most humanistic, honest, and approachable professionals encountered by patients. But the lovely Susan was an exception. She was hardened and defensive. Earlier, when Britt asked her about treating Mom's constipation, she answered: "She came in that way."

We didn't care *when* she became constipated. We just wanted help with the problem.

Minor heard about my angry confrontation—Eureka! The phone works!—and prescribed OxyContin® (oxycodone hydrochloride), every four hours, something he easily could have done in the first instance. Oxycodone, a powerful narcotic, can mummify patients, too.

Although my outburst achieved results, I left the hospital feeling like I had crossed the line of civility. I had snapped, lost my cool, and yet, I knew I had done what was necessary, and I would do it again.

Regardless of how I justified my lapse in composure, however, I couldn't shake my regret. My damn obsessive perfectionism plagued me. I'm a mediator, not a litigator, and I don't engage in power plays. I later apologized to the CNA for my language, but it wasn't until Jane, bless her heart, sought me out, that I let myself off of the self-scrutiny hook.

"Don't feel bad about what you did," she said. "I would've done the same thing if it had been my mother."

Thank you. Yes. My mother. I had to fight for my mother.

In the next few days, I would pull out more stops as I hurdled or eliminated obstacles that temporarily blocked me. Among them, Dad objected to Mom seeing his orthopod, Faber, as her follow-up physician, for reasons I really didn't buy. No, Faber wasn't a "back man"—is anyone?—but she needed someone medically expert to monitor her progress, and her primary-care physician, who was now Dr. Ramses, was too far away.

As it turned out, she might as well have seen her hairdresser. Seeing Dr. Faber was like seeing no one.

The out-of-touch Dr. Minor also complicated my life. He had written the oxycodone prescription without refills, because, of course, opiates are narcotics; doctors tread lightly with narcotics; and he wasn't Mom's regular doctor.

Naturally, when I called his office two days after Mom's discharge to inquire about refills, he already had left for the day. It was 1:30 p.m. And I know the man doesn't make house calls.

"CARE" IN THE HOME

At the heart of this crisis, which discouraged me more than any previous crisis, was guilt. My own. Mom probably would not have fallen, and the whole sorry ensuing mess probably would not have occurred, if Pam, Dad's private-duty CNA, hadn't rattled her so much. The stranger on the yard proved to be a meddlesome intruder.

Once Britt and I invited aides into our parents' home, we traded our healthcare advocacy for mediation of personality conflicts and drama-queen scenes. At least, I did. Britt wasn't interested in what she perceived as coddling the nursing aides. I saw it more as making the drastically altered interpersonal dynamics in our parents' household work. For the first time my sister and I butted heads over management style, and we suffered physically, each of us undergoing frequent massage therapy for our respective body pain.

Ironically, that's how we absorbed and then coped with our stress. We felt real pain. Mine was concentrated in my back and radiated to my legs. Britt had a mysterious fibromyalgia-like, full-body pain that eluded both diagnosis and relief.

Mom disliked Pam because she was aggressive, blustery, and loud—all of which worked with my straight-shooting father most of the time. Marie was softer, but she lacked the caregiving chops that Pam had. Pam, for example, installed the grab bars in the shower and helped Dad bathe. To her credit, Marie ably assisted me when I took Dad to his first follow-up appointment with Dr. Faber. She transported his wheelchair in and out of the car trunk, thus sparing my aching back, and gave me relief from my father's still uptight and controlling ways.

At home, though, Marie did more sitting than either of my parents could tolerate, and whenever she sat in their bedroom, they recoiled. Neither one would confront her about what they viewed as an intrusion, so any intervention was left to me.

In retrospect, I can see that had my already mentally unstable mother not been so shell-shocked by Pam's bombastic style and Marie's neglect of privacy, she would not have struggled so much with sleep and needed heavy-duty sedation and dot, dot, dot . . . fallen. But I wasn't there, amid the tension. I wasn't privy to the decision to medicate my mother so she could sleep soundly. I was still trying to have my own life out of town.

Just as you comparison-shop skilled nursing facilities, you should comparison-shop home nursing assistance. You may be desperate and exhausted. (We were.) You may not have the time or want to take the time to investigate. (We didn't.) You may not even have, or know you have, options to consider. (Our choices were limited.) OK, breathe deeply. Push past the desperation and exhaustion; take your time; ask around; ascertain the options. Trust me: *Caveat emptor.*

If I could do this situation over, I would remove my mother from the stressful environment that her home had become. Britt and I thought about it, but the two housing alternatives we had were problematic: Both my home and the rental cottage in which Britt was staying have steep stairway entries. In the long run, a hotel would have been safer and less traumatic for our second fracture patient.

With both parents in bed convalescing, we now had no choice but to bring in the Sitters, more strangers on the yard. Not only did we need twice the caregiving assistance, we had problems with the two whom we had already hired. Adding to her undesirability, Marie recently had informed us that she would require a week off to attend full-time training for a U.S. Census job.

On Sunday, March 21, while I handled Mom's discharge from the hospital, Britt met for a home assessment with Melissa, the Sitters' owner/manager, and her consulting R.N. My sister had discussed nursing coverage with Pam, so she knew which hours needed filling. I looked at the contract that Dad signed with the Sitters, but did not participate in the discussions about what the agency's aides would do for my parents. I assumed Britt and I could let down our guard once the Sitters stepped in. I was wrong.

The term home care is broad and refers to any diagnostic, therapeutic, or social support service given to a patient in his or her home by a variety of people. Physicians, nurses, rehabilitation therapists, social workers, dieticians, and other professionals may provide in-home post-acute care that lasts weeks to months. Personal-care aides, who may or may not be state-certified, typically provide long-term supportive care.[2] It is important to know that while CNAs can remind patients to take their medications, they legally cannot administer them.

THE BREAKDOWN

Before the Sitters arrived, Pam heavy-handedly made the point that she and Marie would require more money to care for two patients. That seemed reasonable to me, but her tactless and stiff-lipped insistence in front of Dr. Al, the check writer, alienated me. She also priced herself above the Sitters' going rate. (I'm talking $15-$20 an hour here.)

After the Sitters arrived, and my parents warmed to an aide named Sophie, Pam transformed into a green-eyed monster. The competition between Pam/Marie and Sophie, who was down on her luck and willing to do anything—feed and walk the dog, sweep the front porch, buy groceries, prepare meals—was absurd.

I ended up hearing a lot by phone from Pam and Marie, who had a penchant for venting their petty concerns. As much as possible, I encouraged them to talk directly with Dad and Mom, instead of putting me in the middle. I rued ever having given them my cell-phone number and knew it would be only a matter of time before they quit without giving us any notice. Indeed, Marie left us in the lurch. I persuaded Pam, who believed Sitters owner Melissa had deliberately undermined her, to stay long enough for us to make a transition.

Did I need this bickering? No, and you don't, either.

Meanwhile, Sophie, although friendly and eager to please, came with a lot of what you might call baggage, except her lack of baggage was also a problem. Sophie had no car, so her arrival and departure times depended on a third party. She survived on Pepsis and cigarettes, despite our entreaties that she eat while she was at the house; spent an inordinate amount of time on her cell phone, often talking to Melissa, who, we found out later, had hired the 60-year-old as a favor; and shared a troubling personal life that included estrangement from her children. Sophie also had a tendency to be sick and cancel at the last minute. Twice, she left us without coverage for the day.

Perhaps most relevant to this critique, however, is that Sophie did not consider oversight of my mother's diet and general well-being to be her responsibility. She viewed herself more as a homemaker than a health aide. As such, she insinuated herself into the household, acting like a confidante with Britt, but sometimes seeming to me like a gossip.

Britt and I argued about Sophie's dramatics, the way (I perceived that) she blew things out of proportion, and my sister, who was on the home scene more, took her side. After Melissa fired Sophie, the former aide became homeless and called Britt daily for rides, money, or a kind word. This "long story" reality show finally ended when Sophie moved out of state.

The Sitters were booked up when Britt initially contacted them, so we considered ourselves lucky to get Sophie. Other Sitters who later cared for my parents were superior in credentials and professionalism, but not necessarily in personality or work ethic. Ruth, a registered nurse, was very efficient, but also very opinionated. She clashed with Dad. Another, my father complained, "just sits on her ass." (Frankly, I didn't blame her. No sane person hurls herself into a raging inferno.)

If I were to have an introductory evaluation with a home-care agency today, I would stress three factors: the caregiver's experience; her scope of responsibility; and her likely compatibility with my parents. I would establish what the aide believes her responsibilities to be and how assertive she will be in carrying them out and be candid about my parents' likes, dislikes, habits, and personalities. It is better to anticipate an interpersonal conflict than to blithely ignore the possibility.

One day Sophie, who claimed to have been a one-time certified nursing aide in another state, confided to me that my mother had eaten only a cookie for lunch and wasn't drinking much water. I was stunned by this and asked her to *please* insist that Mom eat and drink. She didn't consider such directness part of her job and wasn't comfortable with coaxing. I didn't understand why she was averse to telling "Dr. Fern" to "eat up," and I didn't pay enough attention to her aversion.

On Monday, March 29, all of the angst and unease in my parents' house bubbled over when, upon returning with me from a checkup at Dr. Faber's office, Mom crumpled to the floor in a faint. Unbeknownst to me, she had been lightheaded lately upon rising, and Dad had correctly surmised that her orthostatic (standing) blood pressure was low.

Naturally, Dr. Faber had not taken her pressure during this followup, and I had not thought to ask him. (My bad.) My father prescribed food, water, and rest for Mom, and I left the next day for my out-of-town life.

In my absence, Dr. Al consulted from his sickbed with Dr. Ramses. Besides her hypotension, the two M.D.s were concerned about the possibility of blood clots in Mom's legs, which had become telltale swollen and shiny. When she showed little improvement over the next three days, they decided to hospitalize her at Sentara Norfolk General Hospital. My father was beside himself with worry, expressing concern by phone that "we're losing her."

On the morning of Friday, April 2–the start of another weekend–I learned that I would not be driving back home from Charlottesville, as I had planned. Instead, I would be rendezvousing with Britt and Ruth, the R.N. Sitter, in the Sentara parking lot. After transporting Mom to the hospital and overseeing her admission, which Ramses had authorized, my sister would be handing off her care to me.

From April 2 to April 13, my mother would reside in a treatment facility, first Sentara Norfolk and then a nursing home. It is safe to say that at no time during her stay did she ever comprehend why she was there.

DEHYDRATION AND CONFUSION

Mom suffered from dehydration, a common and potentially deadly problem for older people—and the reason doctors jump to LOL Syndrome diagnoses. Suspecting this, my father's fears were realistic. Studies suggest that, if untreated, 50 percent of adults 65 and older with dehydration will die.

Water sustains human life. Dehydration occurs when you lose more fluid than you take in, and your body doesn't have enough water and other fluids to function normally. This life-threatening condition happens disproportionately among elders living in institutions and, sadly, reflects neglect.3 My mother had Sophie to ensure that she wasn't neglected. So, what the heck?

Water makes up about 60 percent of an adult male's body weight, and 50 percent of a woman's, and is involved in all of your body's chemical processes, such as digestion, circulation, excretion, nutrient transportation, and maintenance of blood volume and body temperature. Although water is distributed throughout your body, the water content of adipose tissue (fat) is relatively low. Women generally have a higher percentage of body fat than men, hence the lower percentage of water in their body weight.

Your body's water exists in two different compartments. The intracellular fluid compartment contains all of the fluid inside your cells and makes up two-thirds of your total water content. This water is potassium-rich, oxygen-consuming, and metabolically active. The extracellular fluid compartment, which has special subcompartments, such as the cerebrospinal fluid and the humors of the eyes, contains all of the fluid outside of your cells and accounts for the other third.4

Your body continuously loses water, through:

* Your kidneys in the form of urine (excess water)
* Your skin in the form of sweat
* Your lungs as moisture in your breath, and
* Your gastrointestinal tract in elimination

You replace the water you lose by producing more on your own and by consuming foods and beverages.

As a young or middle-aged person, you may experience thirst, fatigue, weakness, queasiness, and discomfort with a 1 to 2 percent loss of fluid—maybe after being in the sun too long without fluid replenishment.

A 3 to 4 percent loss of fluid will cause you to experience impaired physical performance (e.g., weakness), dry mouth, flushed skin, reduced urine, and apathy. At 5 to 6 percent, headache, sleepiness, irritability, difficulty with concentrating, and adverse effects on body temperature and respiration occur. Severe dehydration, quantified as a 7 to 10 percent loss of body water, can lead to cerebral edema, seizures, kidney failure, coma, and death. It is unquestionably a medical emergency.[5]

Older adults' fluid intake and fluid losses are different. Some physiological events occur with aging that increase the likelihood of dehydration. Among the changes, an older person's sense of thirst becomes less acute, and his or her body loses some of its ability to conserve water. Older people, especially if they live and/or eat alone, tend to eat much less than younger people and may forget to eat or drink.

Changes in functional status, brought on by cognitive impairment, effects of medication, incontinence, mobility disorders, bed rest, etc., further put older people at increased risk for dehydration. The elder taking a diuretic (as my mother sometimes did) is losing water; the incontinent elder may be afraid of drinking; and the mobility-impaired elder may be unable to reach a water glass.[6]

Geriatricians at Harvard Medical School advise that dehydration in older people should be identified by a "rapid weight loss of greater than 3% of body weight." They estimate that the daily fluid intake requirement for adults 65 and older should be 30 milliliters per kilogram of body weight. Thus, a 160-pound person should be drinking between eight and nine cups of fluid per day.[7]

These same experts say that early diagnosis of a fluid and electrolyte crisis in an older person can be difficult because the classical physical signs may be vague, absent, or misleading. (I'll talk more about electrolytes, which are vital body chemicals, in later chapters.) Also, most elders who are hospitalized with dehydration have an underlying acute illness, such as pneumonia, influenza, gastroenteritis, or a urinary tract infection, which confounds a diagnosis.

Constipation is a common symptom among fluid-depleted elders. Abnormal declines in orthostatic blood pressure, as my mother had, also may signal dehydration.[8]

One sure way to gauge your Mom's or Pop's need for fluid is by the color of her or his urine. Clear or light-colored urine indicates good hydration; a dark yellow or amber color suggests dehydration. If there's little or no urination, your Mom or Pop may be in the danger zone, symptomatized by low blood pressure, a rapid heartbeat and rapid breathing, fever, and, in the most serious cases, delirium or unconsciousness.

My mother did not sufficiently hydrate herself, and Sophie did not consider it her job to monitor her water intake. Just like in the hospital, Mom had a water bottle at her bedside, but we did not check to ensure that she drank from it! We thought that was why we had Sophie. We also thought Mom could be trusted to ensure her own hydration. She could not.

When we asked later why she hadn't been drinking, Mom said either: "I wasn't thirsty" or "I forgot." This is an honest answer for an older person, regardless of his or her cognitive status. We had to wise up fast.

Hospitalization

Because Dr. Ramses, not the emergency department, admitted her to Sentara Norfolk General, Mom ended up on a quiet neurology wing in a private room. After she was settled and hooked up to intravenous saline, for hydration, her first duty nurse, Stacey, helped me to find a hotel in nearby Chesapeake, gave me her cell-phone number to call, and promised to contact me if anything happened.

Throughout my mother's hospitalization, I received support and cooperation from a number of superb nurses.

In the four years since her pulmonary-embolus crisis, major-chain hotels had opened near the Norfolk hospital, but they all had off-site parking lots, which meant that I would need an escort at night. No, thanks. I dropped by the hospital's guest rooms, but they were undergoing renovation.

Because Stacey did not call, I knew upon returning to the hospital after checking in at my hotel that the ultrasound technician had not yet scanned my mother's legs for thrombi. I felt relaxed, knowing that I would be in Mom's room when the imaging was done, and thus able to learn the results immediately and to communicate them to my confused mother and my worried family, or so I believed.

You see an assortment of people wearing green or blue lab scrubs in hospitals, most of whom are technicians. I am fascinated by what various technicians do, and by the equipment they employ, and always ask about their jobs, if they seem willing to talk.

The ultrasound technician that Friday night was a young woman with a quick smile and laugh. After we got to talking, she could not conceal her concern during Mom's ultrasonic exam, but she was careful not to tell me anything directly. Only the doctor could do that. Still, I knew. Stacey, too, was able to tell me that Mom had multiple clots in her legs, without actually saying so.

Since Mom's saddle embolus, I had learned that most pulmonary-embolus deaths result from recurrent emboli, not from the initial clot. In the years after a PE diagnosis, the risk of other emboli developing persists, and, thus, someone like my mother needs to remain on an anticoagulant past the minimum recommended three months.9

We thought she would be on Coumadin for life; Dr. Anthony actually said she would be. But the cardiologist changed his mind in January and discontinued the anticoagulant, switching her to aspirin. Now, three months later, that decision was haunting everyone, as we wondered: Was the inferior vena cava filter still doing its job?

Over the next five days, we got medical answers from a very efficient resident and a very sleepy medical student, who rounded mid- to late-morning with other peers. They all looked like kids to me—I was closing in on 55—like they were playing doctor, but they behaved like seasoned professionals.

The young doctors informed us that the clot-blocking filter was holding up fine, not having shifted from its place or having degraded. They transitioned Mom back to daily Coumadin and prescribed compression stockings for her legs, which by now were grotesquely swollen. (Later, a consulting cardiovascular surgeon on the Outer Banks advised us that the valves in her veins were irreparably damaged.)

I presumed everyone on the Sentara Norfolk medical team noticed my mother's forgetfulness and confusion, even though no one said so. I was surprised, therefore, when I learned later from her medical records that the team consistently assessed her as "cooperative and oriented," as defined by the Ramsay Sedation Scale. The Ramsay scale is typically used to characterize the rousability of a hospital patient who is under sedation or taking narcotic drugs, such as OxyContin.10

"Ramsay" may have thought my mother was oriented, but every time I visited her, she looked at me bewilderingly and asked: "What am

I doing here?" That hurt me a lot. I patiently explained how she had faltered at home and why she needed hospital care.

Besides treating Mom's dehydration with IV saline, the Norfolk doctors encouraged her to drink Ensure®, a protein supplement that she detested in every flavor. They also gave her medication for her fracture pain and a stool softener to counteract the inevitable constipation. In the medical records, they noted that Mom's T-10 fracture was 50 percent, not 25 percent. The radiologist also detected remote compression fractures at the T-2, T-12, and L-1 vertebrae.

Physical therapists showed up to get my nearly 86-year-old mother moving. Naturally, she had lost strength, endurance, and function, but, with assistance, she could rise and walk with a rolling walker. She was tough. Over the weekend, I walked with her several times a day, and Leslie did the same, when she arrived for a few days of relief.

CNAs were supposed to turn Mom in her bed every two hours in order to prevent skin breakdown, but it wasn't long before the chart outside of her room indicated that "self" was doing the turning. That was never true, but it was a minor negative blip on the hospital radar screen. I also never saw any of the CNAs use the hand sanitizer at the door to Mom's room, but the doctors and R.N.s always did.

By Wednesday, April 7, the day of her discharge, the veins in my mother's arms had been violated so many times by IVs and other needles that a phlebotomist seeking a last-minute blood sample had difficulty finding a good one. The blood was for a CBC, which is short for a complete blood count, a broad screening test that measures, according to the Mayo Clinic:

- ❖ Red blood cells, which carry oxygen

- ❖ White blood cells, which fight infection

- ❖ Hemoglobin, the oxygen-carrying protein in red blood cells

- ❖ Hematocrit, the proportion of red blood cells to the fluid component, or plasma, in your blood, and

- ❖ Platelets, which help with blood clotting.[1]

(I delve into all of these components in later chapters.)

To say that CBCs are excessively ordered in hospitals is a colossal understatement. When a CBC includes a "differential"—an order known as a "CBC with diff"—the lab will identify the five different types of white blood cells in a blood sample and count them separately. In the absence of a differential, it will only provide a count of the total number of WBCs.

The phlebotomist—she (or he) who draws blood from patients—was delaying our departure. After her second failed attempt, the wonderful nurse of the day told Mom, "You know, you can always refuse it."

Yeah! Patient autonomy. Now, *there's* a fast-and-loose term. But for today, it was perfect. We refuse! How refreshing.

Would that Mom's discharge had been equally as liberating.

Nursing Home Homework

My father didn't want my mother at home because he was convinced her needs would interfere with his physical recovery and emotional well-being. Her very presence made him anxious, and he was already over-the-top DPS anxious.

Oh, he *said* he thought she would receive better care in the Sentara Nursing Center, in Barco, N.C., a half-hour up the road from our home, but he was principally relieving himself of a burden—or so I believed. While I understood that he considered his plight a fight for survival, and he might be mildly depressed, that was as far as my understanding extended. Why should his claim to home be superior to Mom's?

According to her hospital records, Mom's doctors advised discharge to home. "The family," they wrote, requested the SNF discharge.

Medicare will cover up to 100 days of "skilled nursing care" in an SNF per "spell of illness," provided your Mom-or-Pop Medicare recipient had a "qualifying hospital stay" of at least three days (not including the discharge day) and entered the SNF within 30 days after that stay. You should know this if you have to rely upon an SNF for rehabilitative services.

The hospital social worker assigned to your parent's case can assist you with navigating the precise and often stringent requirements for Medicare coverage of SNF stays.[12] As I noted in Chapter One, she also can provide you with a list of available nursing homes and make appointments for you to visit them. In this instance, I only considered the one SNF in Barco. I had heard horror stories about the only nursing home on the beach.

Having passed the Barco center hundreds of time en route from the Outer Banks to Virginia and points north and back, I knew its institutional brick exterior and barren landscaping well. I also had an older acquaintance who rehabilitated there after a knee replacement, and he was god-awful miserable. Life, even temporary life, in a cramped, confined space with a stranger-roommate, especially one who prefers TV day and night or family gatherings when you prefer reading and solitude, can be stultifying. A mere 20 minutes can seem an eternity.

I argued the unfairness, the selfishness, the potential harm, and more to my convalescing father, but he would not relent. Absent more concrete evidence that Mom's discharge to the nursing home was a poor decision, I couldn't shake him.

Leslie checked out the facility, which had 25 acute-care beds and 75 long-term care beds, and pronounced it small, but OK. Officially, the center housed two private rooms, but tenant-patients who lived there permanently occupied them.

Constructed like a wheel with a central nurses' station serving as the hub and the residence halls as spokes, the center struck Les as functional and average. She did worry, however, about the space in the rooms. Only one person would be able to sit and visit with Mom at a time, and we planned on visiting every day for hours at a stretch.

Although the Sentara facility was not nearly as pleasant or as well-equipped as the much-larger Sunshine rehabilitation center in Durham, my R.N. sister thought it passed muster. I asked an elderly friend who had visited the knee-replacement rehabber there what she thought, and she called it "nice." Still, I hesitated. Her "nice" might not be my "nice." When Dad explained to Mom over the telephone why she couldn't come home, he didn't have to look into her confused eyes. I did, and I was sick at heart.

When you visit a nursing home, walk the hallways with an employee-escort, preferably the director, and peek into the residents' rooms to get a sense of whether your parent would feel comfortable in the environment. If mingling with dementia patients would depress your Mom or Pop, take note of whether such patients are sitting in their wheelchairs in doorways and common areas. You should be able to evaluate quickly whether your parent would thrive or wither in the facility.

Ask yourself: How would I feel about living in this nursing home? If it leaves you cold, cross it off of your list.

Be sure to talk with the director and the therapists about your parent's daily program and check out the rehab room. Is it a dump? Or does it seem to be well-stocked with fairly new equipment? You may not be allowed to observe residents undergoing physical therapy, as I did at Sunshine before Mom went there, but you still can pick up a sense of the mood among them, by hanging around a bit.

Depending on the reason for your parent's hospitalization (e.g., stroke), he or she may need rehabilitative therapy with an occupational therapist. The OT helps your Mom or Pop to reacquire, control, and execute the ability to perform her ADL and more complex tasks, such as preparing a cup of coffee or washing clothes, without assistance. OTs focus on your parent's physical and mental capacities and skills and work with her to achieve her highest level of independence.

Inquire specifically into the number of residents per certified nursing aide. This ratio will determine how much personal attention the CNAs can give each one. The number of registered nurses per nursing home may vary—there are never enough—but there is typically only one off-site doctor, whom you may never meet, for them to consult. This physician is likely to have a full-time family-medicine practice.

One of the Sentara Norfolk General Hospital nurses was helpful to me in coping with this discharge-transfer. Vicky liked "personal contact" with her patients and their families and always told me what she thought, when other nurses might hold back. I shared my reservations about the Barco nursing center with Vicky, and she analyzed my decision pragmatically. Her reasoning boiled down to "Why not?" Since Mom had been hospitalized for at least three days, Medicare would cover her stay in the Sentara SNF, and, if she didn't do well in the place, we could remove her.

Remove her, I thought, yeah, over my father's dead body. Still, I embraced Vicky's reasoning and told Mom that, if she didn't like the center, she didn't have to stay. She unhappily acceded to my father's wishes. Once I saw the nursing home firsthand, I started marking time with her.

"GET ME OUT OF THIS HELLHOLE"

It wasn't the wizened old man in the Washington Redskins jersey who sat outside the main entrance every day smoking cigarettes who bothered me. No, I was glad that he was safe and enjoying the warm spring weather, his smokes, and small talk with passers-by. It was after I entered the building and encountered many patients, some with obvious dementia, parked in wheelchairs around the nurses' station and filling the hallways that I felt differently. The facility was so crowded and unadorned as to be oppressive. A few plants or more wall art, anything cheerful, would have neutralized the dreariness.

A woman in her early 70s who was mending from a fracture and had the room across the hall from Mom's put it well when a CNA told her that she would soon have a roommate. "Oh, shit," she said, loudly. Oh, shit, indeed.

On the first day, I met with the nursing center's social worker, physical therapist, and nurse, acquainting each with Mom's history and current needs and making sure that they knew I would be the responsible on-the-scene family member. I walked the halls, getting my bearings, and tried to comfort my mother, who took an immediate dislike to her surroundings. I also was present when an aide weighed her and measured her height.

Throughout her adulthood, Mom had told people she was 5-foot-5, which was perhaps an exaggeration of a half-inch. She now stood 5-feet-tall, according to the SNF aide. The hospital, I discovered later, measured her at 5-foot-2.

Previously we had tried to convince Mom to carry a simple cell phone, or better yet, wear one, but she couldn't be bothered. Too complicated. No need, she said. Now she was pleased to have Dad's cell phone around her neck and quickly learned how to receive and place calls. That phone and the reading material that Leslie, Britt, and I brought were her only salvation in our absence. I hated to think of all of the empty hours she spent there.

Unfortunately, she could find no solace with her roommate, who presented a snapshot of how sadly a life can end.

In her prime, Miss Elizabeth, as the CNAs called her, had been a well-known and well-regarded business professional. But that once-proud, intelligent woman had been replaced by a thin and hollow substitute whose brain was hopelessly scrambled. Adding injury to the insult of Alzheimer's disease, Miss Elizabeth had fallen—under whose watch, we did not know, but she was well beyond self-care—and broken a hip. Now she was "rehabbing," which meant that the CNAs got her up, dressed her, fed her, strapped her into a chair in front of the television, and left her to "enjoy" her day.

I assume some range-of-motion therapy occurred when a CNA wheeled Miss Elizabeth out, but I never witnessed any. I did see her twice amid a group of residents assembled for an activity. She sat obliviously in her chair, her chin slumped on her chest.

Miss Elizabeth smiled vacantly and even spoke to us, in an amiable voice, but nothing she said had meaning. Incontinence furthered her tragic infantilization. She would urinate on the floor, while seated in her chair, looking somewhat embarrassed as the fluid trinkled through her diaper.

One day a CNA took Miss Elizabeth off to bathe, without first mopping up her puddle of urine, so that when Mom needed to use the bathroom minutes later, she didn't have a clear path. I found another CNA to clean up the floor, after which the first apologized to me. This is the sort of neglect that you encounter in a "good" nursing home. It's not malice; it's a failure to evaluate a situation thoughtfully and then respond well. It may be that housekeeping employees, not CNAs, usually deal with cleanups. How long would that urine have remained on the floor if I hadn't been there?

Each time I visited Mom, she would motion toward Miss Elizabeth and tell me that her roommate's mind was gone, as if this were a new revelation. That was when she wasn't telling me about how poorly she slept because of noise in the hallway and a crummy mattress, how unappetizing the food was, and how much she wanted to "get out of here."

I stressed the physical therapy that she was getting—which she claimed was minimal, at best—and made sure that we walked around the facility and went outdoors for fresh air. Britt and I even arranged to take her out to lunch at a nearby waterfront seafood restaurant, but the excursion didn't alter her affect much. She seemed defeated.

One day, she pleaded: "Get me out of this hellhole."

I felt sick. Every day I argued with Dad that she needed to come home.

THE "PRISONER" ON STRIKE

Monday, April 12, was to be a red-letter day for my mother. She finally would have her hair done, after weeks of bemoaning its state, and have a full PT session after a weekend off. When I arrived at her room at 1 p.m., I expected to see her happily coiffed and energized by the physical activity. Instead, she lay in bed, still in her nightgown, her hair unwashed and unstyled. I was shocked. What had happened to her appointments? Mom didn't know. Why didn't you see the hairdresser?

"They didn't come for me," she said.

This was my beautiful role model, the professional woman in the trim suit who had welcomed people in pain into her magical study and written copious notes about who they were and how she could help. Anger overtook me, and I went in search of answers.

According to Wendy, the center's sole registered nurse, with whom I had a friendly and open relationship, my mother had "rebelled" aggressively that morning. She had refused to get dressed, to eat, and to cooperate in any way with the staff. During her resistance, which Wendy labeled combative, Mom allegedly told her newly assigned CNA that she did not have a hair appointment, and she was not going to physical therapy. The CNA had left her to stew in bed.

"I never said that," Mom insisted. "I never did that." But I knew that she had. However her mind had processed her reality, there was no doubt in *my* mind that she was on strike. She was seizing control in the only way she could—by losing it.

I quickly hustled up the CNA, who showed renewed interest in my mother now that a family member was on the scene and apologized repeatedly. I asked her to check on the hairdresser and to help Mom get dressed, while I went to talk with the physical therapist. The hairdresser, a kind woman in her late 60s who visited every week or so, agreed to stick around, and she performed wonders with Mom's hair. This gave her—as it does most women—a big emotional lift. She then went through a brief PT session, which I observed and considered *less* than minimal. Granted, the therapist was fitting Mom into her afternoon, but the exercises she asked of her and the number of repetitions were insignificant. We could do much more for her at home and at Coastal Rehab.

Since arriving and finding Mom languishing in bed, I had begun preparing for her discharge. I asked the physical therapist: What would

Mom need to do before the therapist would sign off on it? The answer seemed to be to walk 50 yards, and that Mom could do. She had been doing more than that with Britt and me daily.

I then called my father: "She has to come home. She's getting worse." And she's not benefiting from anything that I would call therapy.

I told him about Mom's combative resistance and her inability to remember the morning's events. Dad didn't argue. If she's "decompensating," his word again, then we have to get her out.

I spent the rest of the afternoon speaking to the professionals who would facilitate Mom's discharge and canceling my own Tuesday plans. The Sentara social worker was especially helpful in advising me about ordering home medical equipment: Mom could (and did) get a hospital bed that was lower than her regular bed, so she could more easily swing her swollen legs in and out of it and protect her back. The SW also instructed me about other home-care services that Medicare would cover, including occupational therapy, which we later arranged. The home OT did a wonderful job of helping Mom to shower until she could manage on her own.

For the first time in weeks, I was able to give my mother good news. I would be bringing her home tomorrow. And we would manage just fine.

On discharge day I checked in one last time with Wendy about Mom's meds. Just as Jane had done at the OBH after my explosive scene, Wendy eased any doubts that I may have had about leaving.

"I hope if I ask my family to take me out of a nursing home," she said, "they'll do it right away, no questions asked."

She also assured me that Sentara Nursing Center is "one of the good ones." I hated to think about the others.

After my mother returned home on April 13, 2010, her mental cloudiness lifted, and she became more attentive and relaxed. Her wild-eyed frightened look disappeared, and she let go of the cares she'd had earlier about not knowing how to do things.

During the ensuing year, Mom and I drove past the nursing home many times. As soon as the building would come within sight, she invariably would say: "Oh, there's that awful place."

And sometimes she'd follow up with: "What was I doing there, again?"

And so I would explain the dehydration, the clots, the possible delirium, and, you know what? It *still* hurt. The only memory that felt good was the memory of getting Mom out of her hellhole and back home.

Vicky, the nurse at Sentara Norfolk General, had asked me: "Why not?" I now knew the answer, and it was exactly what I had feared.

Chapter Seven

Ageism and
AGING

A Study in Fear and Heterogeneity

Whenever my father ventured from home, he loved to engage people. He never outgrew the Illinois farm boy he had been and sought, in particular, to connect with working people. He had respect for anyone who applied him or herself to earning an honest day's wages.

Dad was a schmoozer, as well as a shuffler. He was an affable talker who sincerely wanted to know what was on people's minds. On the Outer Banks, the man known as Dr. Al had a reputation among workers at Food Lion, Ace Hardware, and Rite-Aid, the golf pro shop, the optician's office, and every other commercial establishment he frequented, as being a really great guy. So I was more than a little perplexed and angry one day when he passed along a "joke" that one of the Ace Hardware clerks had told him.

"Do you know what IHOP stands for?" the young man asked the Schmoozer.

"Sure," Dad replied, "International House of Pancakes."

"No," the youth answered with a grin, "It stands for I Hate Old People."

Ha-ha. Ha-ha.

Dad was dumbfounded, and a little wounded, by this insult. It had never occurred to him to be disliked because he was old. Why would it? Aging is a natural part of the human condition, and Dr. Al was intrigued by—and very knowledgeable about—the human condition. More than that, he rejoiced in it. To hate a person because he's old is to be ignorant and fearful about humanness. In short, to be a moron.

In 1968, psychiatrist Robert N. Butler (1927-2010) coined the term "age-ism" to describe a "deep-seated uneasiness" felt by young and middle-aged people about aging, which he further described as "a personal revulsion to and distaste for growing old, disease, disability; and fear of powerlessness, 'uselessness,' and death."[1]

Later in his career, Butler expounded on this bigotry, defining it as a "process of systematic stereotyping and discrimination against people because they are old," and analogized it to racism and sexism.[2]

All you have to do to appreciate how entrenched ageism is in mainstream U.S. culture is to skim the birthday cards in a drug store or watch programming on any television channel except "Turner Classic Movies." If you're not aging fabulously, according to card writers, you're drooping, dribbling, leaking, farting, shrinking, losing it, and otherwise becoming disgusting. On prime-time TV, you essentially disappear unless you're in a prescription drug commercial or you're Betty White.   ·

"We spent our entire youth making fun of old people," read the front of a birthday card I came across at Barnes and Noble.

"We are so screwed," read the inside punchline.

First, though, our parents are screwed, and we get to watch.

WHY SURVIVE?

Dr. Butler was a principal investigator in the National Institute of Mental Health's landmark longitudinal study of healthy elders living in the community. This research, conducted between 1955 and 1966, helped to establish that senility, a word derived from the Latin *senilis*, meaning old, is not an inevitable consequence of aging, as mental-health experts then believed, but rather a result of disease; and that older people's depression and other psychiatric conditions could be treated.

During his time at the NIH's NIMH, Butler also observed during visits to nursing homes that these facilities too often "warehoused" sick and infirm elders, as well as healthy elders who simply required assistance, and hired "undertrained" caregivers to attend to their residents. Further, doctors who cared for such elders knew little, and cared even less, about their needs. (Today, such doctors are largely voices on a telephone.)

Widely considered the Father of Modern Gerontology, Butler compiled his clinical and research observations into the 1975 book, "Why Survive? Being Old in America." The what's-the-point-in-living?

title is a biting indictment of American values, or lack thereof. The next year Butler became the first director of the newly founded National Institute on Aging, another NIH institute, and won the Pulitzer Prize for general non-fiction. In 1982 he left government service to found the first-ever geriatrics department at a U.S. medical school.

That the first medical-school geriatrics department dates back only to 1982 is shocking to me. Equally shocking is that, today, only about 5 percent of medical schools have a stand-alone geriatrics department.

As of 2010, Butler's department at Mount Sinai Medical Center in New York was one of only nine medical-school geriatrics departments in the country. Most medical-school geriatrics programs exist within another department, typically internal medicine, and are decidedly unpopular among medical students, the majority of whom are in their mid-20s and have an unrealistic concept of "old age." Fifty is ancient to them.3

When I was 48, I was taken aback by two 20-something Johns Hopkins dermatology residents who examined me and couldn't believe my age. I looked too good. After they left the examining room, I could hear these sheltered young things talking to the attending physician, who used the occasion to impress upon them the role that fitness plays in aging. I was then a buffed exercise fiend. But, come on, who thinks 48 is old? A 28-year-old, that's who.

Until his death Dr. Butler was an indefatigable and very public champion for elders, advocating, in particular, for changes in medical-school curricula that would ensure all future doctors a foundation in geriatrics, and identifying ageism in doctors' attitudes and in the healthcare system. Mt. Sinai, which takes a non-traditional approach to medical education, emphasizing cooperative learning over competitive learning, requires all of its students to complete a month-long rotation in geriatric medicine.

In "Why Survive?," Butler poignantly wrote:

"Old age in America is often a tragedy. Few of us like to consider it because it reminds us of our own mortality. It demands our energy and resources, it frightens us with illness and deformity, it is an affront to a culture with a passion for youth and productive capacity. We are so preoccupied with defending ourselves from the reality of death that we ignore the fact that *human beings are alive until they are actually dead.*" (my emphasis)4

All life deserves respect, but as long as physicians practice ageist medicine, elders won't receive it.

CHILDHOOD IN OLD AGE

According to Dr. Zaldy S. Tan, a Harvard geriatrics professor, the medical conditions associated with older people, such as frailty and immobility, strike young physicians-to-be, "as decidedly unchallenging, unappealing, and, well, unsexy."

Not only do "[y]oung doctors want to heal and to cure, not to be mere stewards of the incurable—doctors of none," writes Tan, but they learn in their undergraduate and post-graduate clinical training to regard older patients disdainfully. They're "crocks," which is medical slang for hypochondriacs whose physical complaints have no apparent organic basis. They suffer from "COPD," chronic old persons disease, which marks them as being persistently unwell from a non-specific and untreatable cause. At the very least, LOLs and "SOGs" (sick old guys) are a time-consuming drain on medical resources—including the young doctor's brilliance—that would be better spent elsewhere.

In the late 1990s, Tan himself was a "smug" resident who bought into the cynical and harmful stereotyping of older patients that hospital house staff and clinical faculty often perpetuate. Numerous medical "insider" reports that I've read in professional articles—which flow from questionnaires, situational studies, personal interviews, and other such data—support the proposition that not only does the medical-educational hierarchy preach and practice ageism, the culture cultivates and condones it. Medical schools also foster in students disillusionment and emotional detachment that contribute to such bias and animosity.[5]

Besides being concerned with "unsexy" and incurable diseases, geriatrics, writes Tan, "is the only specialty that actually causes a *decrease* in physician income with additional training." So older patients waste precious resources *and* cost doctors bigger bucks.

Not surprisingly, the specialty of geriatrics arose in response to ignorance and bigotry within medicine. Appalled by his instructors' view that old age condemned people to suffer, and, thus, that there was no point in treating older patients, Austrian-born American physician Ignatz L. Nascher founded geriatrics, and coined the term, in the early 20th century. It comes from the Greek, *geras*, meaning old age, and *iatrikos*, meaning "relating to the physician."

Suggesting that geriatrics covers the same field in "old age that is covered by the term paediatrics in childhood," Nascher, who was ahead of his time, but still of it, wrote in 1909:

"Senility is a distinct period of life having general features normal to it and abnormal at other periods of life. It is a physiological entity as much so as the period of childhood."[6]

Unfortunately, too often today physicians treat elders as it they were children.

One of my favorite stories about medical ageism comes from my hospital attorney friend Reagan, whose keen-witted mother lived past 100.

When Reagan's mother, Mrs. Middleton, was in her early 90s, she had her third colon resection for recurrent cancer. A firm believer in 24/7 vigilance, Reagan spent her mother's first night in the hospital, a Friday, with her. The next morning a man carrying a clipboard dropped by the room. He said he was Mrs. Middleton's anesthesiologist and wanted to know if he could ask her a few questions. Her mother turned to Reagan to see if that would be all right, and Reagan said, sure.

Mrs. Middleton then looked carefully at the alleged physician and asked him, very sweetly: "How do I know who you are?"

She explained: "You're not the anesthesiologist who took care of me for my surgery; you're dressed like you're going to play golf, and you don't have a name tag on."

"She was obviously more alert than I was!" Reagan recalled.

The anesthesiologist checked her chart and looked at her in amazement.

"Can you be Mrs. Middleton?" he wondered. "This says that you're 92 years old!"

To which Mrs. Middleton replied: "I may be old, but I'm not stupid."

GRANDPARENTS AND GOMERS

Today's geriatricians specialize in the study, diagnosis, and treatment of diseases and health problems specific to older adults. Gerontologists, who may be M.D.s, but are more likely to be Ph.D.s, study the biological, psychological, and sociocultural factors associated with old age and aging. Gerontology dates to the 1939 founding in Great Britain of the International Club for Research on Aging. That same year the U.S. research club that would become the American Gerontological Society in 1945 was organized.

Scientists working in the field of biogerontology engage in research about the biology of aging, whereas those in geriatric medicine do research related to age-associated diseases.[7]

Harvard's Dr. Tan chose to specialize in geriatrics largely because of his grandmother, whose final illness and death from liver cancer taught him "that when a cure is not possible, to relieve pain and to provide comfort . . . are equally worthy goals."[8] Dr. Butler also benefited from the wisdom and strength of his elders, having been raised from infancy by his grandparents.

Like these physicians, I, too, had relationships with my grandparents when I was young. I was especially close to my paternal Grandpa, who gave me my first real job and started me on my card-shark ways. I packed eggs in cartons at the chicken factory where Grandpa worked part-time when I visited my grandparents' farm as a 9-year-old. For my efforts, I earned $5.00, a box of Jujubees, and a lot of confidence. Grandpa also let me win at gin rummy until I was beating him fair and square.

My father, who was named for his paternal grandfather, grew up with the elder Albert and his beloved grandmother, living in their house during the Depression when his own father couldn't afford separate lodging and later living next door to them.

Albert Sr., a well-to-do country gentleman, was tough, but indulgent with his bright namesake. Dad's grandmother, a sweet, intelligent woman with oratorical gifts, encouraged his dream of becoming a doctor and praised him often. She was a midwife. Because of his vivacious grandmother, who starkly contrasted with his dour mother, my father developed a broad good humor and learned to play the piano.

As a child, my mother thought her 85-year-old maternal grandfather, who lived with her family, was "so old." But so were other people in her young life, she tells me. Aging seemed natural to her. "People just accepted aging," she says. Death, too, was part of her childhood. Although she didn't want to go, Mom's mother insisted that she attend funerals and pay her respects.

Familiarity with, and respect for aged people go a long way toward preventing bigoted notions from taking root in younger people's minds.

In the 1950s, Dr. Butler was shocked by how his Columbia University medical professors dismissed older patients' health concerns and insensitively labeled some of them crocks. After the pseudonymous Samuel Shem coined the pejorative term, gomer (or GOMER), in his 1978 medical-cult classic novel, "House of God," the floodgates on medical-ageist "humor" opened, and they have continued unabated.

Psychiatrist Stephen J. Bergman (b. 1944) wrote "House of God" to expose the punishing and abusive conditions under which interns then worked and lived. A gomer, which stands for "get out of my emergency room," is a patient that no sleep-deprived and overworked young intern or resident wants and will try to "turf" (get rid of or lateral) to another department.9

Bergman intended the term to describe a long-suffering, debilitated old patient who would rather die (and should die) than be cruelly resuscitated, but it has come to mean any sick old person, regardless of his or her mental state or prognosis. Medical professionals who defend its use typically do so by saying: "You need to laugh to survive."10 Ridiculing patients is par for the course.

During the Q&A of a 2011 mini-medical-school session at the University of Virginia, I asked Professor Diane Snustad, a geriatrician, if doctors still use the word gomer. Not being a big TV watcher, I didn't know that characters on the long-running medical sitcom-drama "Scrubs" regularly employed gomer-speak.

No, Snustad replied, she didn't think residents used the derogatory term anymore, but doctors and doctors-in-training do invoke "black humor." It's a way to "release stress and pressure," she defended, not a sign of "insensitivity" or a lack of caring.

Unquestionably, Snustad told me, there's ageism in the medical profession, just as there is in society at large. Too often, doctors attribute older patients' problems to "being old," she said, and when older people are sick, they look even older. Doctors don't ask for symptoms or explanations of how the old patient who says he or she feels sick, actually feels, she said—another failing. (Diagnosis: COPD.)

But gomer? No, she insisted, the term is passé.11

I wish Snustad had been with me when, several weeks after her lecture, I entered a U.Va. lab room just in time to see a neurology professor erasing the word gomer from a blackboard. He was about to brief us on the research he was doing with stroke patients—his own personal gomers. I was stunned.

In a 2000 internal medicine-journal article about "humor and slang in the hospital setting," a 25-year-old medical student recalls residents "talking about older patients as toads and frogs and gomes [a derivative of gomer] . . . It was 20 [physicians] sitting at breakfast together like a big football team and talking about patients in a way that was very disappointing."[12]

No, not disappointing, more like despicable.

"Nature did not wire into us the desire to take care of our aged," writes "Intern" memoirist Sandeep Jauhar. "Maybe that's why the contempt, the frustration, with gomers. They are heavy, dead evolutionary weight. They sap our resources. We don't want to take care of them. Baby shit doesn't smell. But gomer shit smells the worst."[13]

Who passes judgment like "dead evolutionary weight"? Doctors do.

Jauhar found it "almost comical," he further writes, "how [one older patient] cried out for us to leave him alone, to not hurt him, [or] punish him for his helplessness.

"This was a man loved by his family, a businessman or banker, perhaps, one who asserted his will on others," he continues, "and now he is a helpless child."

Wrong. This man was sick. He was only a helpless child to the haughty and disrespectful people who perceived him that way.

Ageism is about fearing the "Other" we will all be one day, if we don't die first. It's about ignorance and cowardice, which are both sad and despicable, and, in the medical model, inexcusable.

HETEROGENEITY

Adults age 65 and older currently make up 13 percent of the U.S. population, for a total of about 40 million people.

Sixty-five is the threshold to old age in our country, but it is an arbitrary designation that dates to the employment boom of the late-19th century Industrial Revolution. To accommodate the surplus of working-class people who flooded U.S. cities, employers originated forced retirement at 65 to thin out the workforce as well as keep it young and presumptively more able-bodied. To determine a person's actual aging, however, you must look at his or her physiological status, not chronological achievement.

Thanks to increased longevity and older adults' better self-care and fitness, today's *enlightened* geriatricians—not your average primary-care physicians—view people 65 and older in three categories: Those who are 65 to 74 years old are The Young Old; those who are 75 to 84 are The Old; and elders 85 and over comprise The Oldest Old.[14]

That the word "elderly" continues to serve in our society and public discourse as a collective noun for such an enormous group of dissimilar people is indicative of bias, insensitivity, and ignorance. I occasionally use elderly as an adjective, but never as a noun. I think the nominative use dehumanizes, devalues, and socially marginalizes older people.

Do you want to be a member of "the elderly"? Does age define you?

The truth about aging is that it is as complex as each individual who experiences it.

"Aging," according to Dr. Thomas A. Glass, an associate professor in the Johns Hopkins University School of Public Health, is "the study of heterogeneity." We're not all just indistinct peas in a common pod. We age differently.

Dr. Glass was the first speaker in a Johns Hopkins mini-medical school that I attended about aging and health. He got the class off to a rousing start by informing us that the human body's systems "peak" between ages 20 and 30 and that, every 8.6 years thereafter, our chance of death doubles as we become more susceptible to disease.[15]

"Chance of death"? *Doubles*? *Every 8.6 years*? Only an epidemiologist—which Dr. Glass is—could utter such statistical nonsense-speak. He might as well have said that humans age, and some die at younger ages than others. That's how meaningless his assertion struck me. But then he neutralized it with the nugget about heterogeneity. In other words, forget the 8.6 years. We're all individuals.

If you attend a track meet during a community's Senior Games, you'll keenly appreciate the variability in the older population. A senior athlete doesn't much resemble a diabetic, hypertensive, and obese 80-year-old who can no longer live independently.

Consider what 95-year-old Ida Keeling of the Bronx said when she became the world's "fastest running nonagenarian" in February 2011. After sprinting 60 meters in 29.86 seconds, an exuberant Keeling declared: "I feel younger now than when I was in my 30s and 40s!"[16]

Heterogeneity largely reflects physiology. Physiology is the branch of biology that deals with our *functions*; vital *processes*, such as digestion, circulation, and respiration; and various *parts* and *organs*. Georgetown pulmonologist, Dr. Robin L. Gross, calls it "physics in the body." While not much functional difference exists between one normal 21-year-old or one normal 30-year-old and the next, physiological functioning of people age 65 and older can differ widely.

Speaking physiologically, we have some say over how we will age by how well we take care of our bodies. Ida Keeling attests to that. Our aging is not just destiny, although some of it is genetically determined.

In Chapter Twelve, I delve into the nitty-gritty of our bodies' major functions and processes, and how aging affects them. This knowledge is important to have when you're evaluating an elderly parent in failing health, as my father would become. You'll be asking yourself: What's normal? Is this normal aging? Here I consider just what aging is, and how the medical-scientific perspective on it has evolved.

WHAT IS AGING?

In my medical research, I have seen aging defined as "[T]he sum of all changes, physiological, genetic, molecular, that occur with the passage of time, from fertilization to death."[17] If you accept this definition, then aging begins as soon as a sperm and egg unite into one cell. Most gerontologists believe, however, that biological aging starts after our sexual maturation, around the age of 22.

Dr. Snustad, of the University of Virginia, spoke for the majority view when she said that aging represents all of "the losses in normal function that occur after sexual maturation"—right up to the time of our maximum life span.

"Nature," explained Snustad, "wants reproduction." After we've ensured species survival by reproducing, she said, we "live on our bodily reserves until we run out."[18] Bodily reserves are physiological reserves.

The "hallmark" of aging, according to Leonard Hayflick, Ph.D., an influential U.S. microbiologist and gerontologist, "is an inexorable loss in physiological capacity."[19]

In 1962, Hayflick (b. 1928) made a breakthrough laboratory discovery: He observed in studies of human-cell cultures that normal cells have a limited capacity to divide. They do not proliferate continuously, living forever, as scientific belief had long held. (Cell cultures are colonies of cells removed from the body and maintained in a special nutrient medium in the lab.)

In contrast, scientists can keep cultured malignant (tumor) cells proliferating indefinitely: Their lines are immortal. (You may be familiar with HeLa, the code name for the first-ever cancer-cell line kept growing in a culture. Johns Hopkins scientists successfully harvested these cells from a dying patient's cervix in 1951; the line still exists today.)[20]

Normal cells eventually die, and, therefore, Hayflick reasoned, must undergo intracellular changes caused by . . . ? You guessed it: *aging*. The non-dividing, but still viable state of cultured normal cells is senescence or old age. His observation of their gradually diminished capacity came to be known as Hayflick's limit.[21]

After what Hayflick calls our "reproductive success"–when we are presumed to have contributed to our species' survival by procreating– we rely on our physiological reserves to enable us to continue living. Because those reserves differ from person to person, we differ in our aging.

In the wild, natural selection favors those animals that not only have the greater survival skills (the "fittest"), but also the physiological reserve in their vital organs to survive damage from predators, disease, accidents, and environmental hazards.

Humans no longer live in the wild and do not need excess physiological reserves to ensure reproductive success. Nonetheless, we have the potential for continued function well past both fulfillment of our goal of reproduction and nurturance of our offspring into adulthood. Why?

Pondering that question alone should be enough to convince you to set aside any ignorant preconceptions about old age being a time of suffering and decrepitude, disease, and disability. Stop thinking about death when you think about aging. Your Mom and Pop will appreciate it, and you just might wake up their physicians, whose treatment reflects their own age biases.

Instead, think about physiology and heterogeneity. Thanks to increased longevity, we can focus our attention squarely on both.

LONGEVITY EXTENDED

By 2050, adults 65 and older will make up about 25 percent of the U.S. population. This aging trend, fueled by declining fertility rates and increased longevity, according to Dr. Glass, represents a "silver tsunami" with which our healthcare system is not remotely prepared to contend.[22]

The world population seems headed toward the same dramatic change. The United Nations projects that people age 65 and older will outnumber children age 5 and under globally by 2016 for the first time in history. By 2030, the number of elders worldwide will surpass the number of children 18 and under.

While I don't dispute the U.S. and global population prospects, I would point out that they are speculative. Intervening factors, such as war, emerging infectious disease epidemics, reversals in fertility trends, and the like, may occur. In any case, I'd rather deal with the here and now, of which you and I and our parents are a part. This much we know now for certain: People are living longer.

Longevity may be defined in several ways, including:

❖ The average age at death of all members of a population
❖ The age to which the last 1 or 5 percent of a generation lives
❖ The maximum age to which any member of a population lives

The average age at death yields what is known as the life expectancy at birth. This is the total number of years that a human female or male, on average, can expect to live. Life expectancy is not always synonymous with longevity.

In 1900, the life expectancy from birth in the United States was 49.0 years for women and 46.4 for men. A high infant mortality rate accounted for these low *averages.* Infectious diseases for which there were no cures (typhoid, cholera, influenza) claimed many children.

In 2010, by comparison, the U.S. life expectancy from birth was 79.7 years for women and 72.6 for men. Epidemiologists project U.S. life expectancies from birth in 2050 of 82.9 years for women and 76.5 for men.[23]

The United States ranks only 28th among developed nations worldwide in life expectancy, even though it spends more in healthcare as a percentage of gross domestic product than any other nation. The top five long-living nations, in descending order, are: No. 1 Japan, then France, Italy, Spain, and Switzerland.[24]

Why does the USA have such a lowly ranking? Professor Glass ambiguously attributed it to "the way we organize ourselves," after rejecting class suggestions related to Americans' lifestyles.

I think it has to do with many factors, including lifestyle factors, and would implicate our ethnic heterogeneity, with its various genetic propensities for disease; our emphasis on individual interests over community welfare; our poor diets, sedentary habits, and increased obesity; and our workaholism and stressful, insane lives, which you can analyze every which way.

Life expectancy from birth first increased in the 20th century because of improvements in public health, specifically in sanitation and hygiene, which led to safer food and water supplies. Daily life on a subsistence level became cleaner and healthier. The advent of antibiotics and vaccinations in the 1940s-1950s further enhanced life expectancy, but not as profoundly as advances in public hygiene did.

Longevity received another boost in the 1960s-1980s, with the development of successful treatments for cardiovascular disease, in particular, drugs to control hypertension, which was my father's first research focus.[25]

At the NIH in the early 1950s, Dad recalls: "We saw people dying all over the place from high blood pressure, many in their twenties, thirties, and forties. When I went home at night, I would just keep my fingers crossed that none of my patients would stroke out before morning. They'd get strokes, and we couldn't do a damn thing."

Interestingly, despite extensions in the human life expectancy at birth, the maximum life span potential—the longest any human being *can* live—has not changed.

According to Hayflick, the maximum human life has been about 125 years for the past 100,000 years.[26] The U.S. maximum life span today falls short of that by about 10 years. Long-lived Americans tend to expire around age 114.[27]

For the record, the scientific consensus is that life arose spontaneously about 3.5-4.0 billion years ago from amino acids, nucleotides, and other basic chemicals of living organisms. Primates appeared 56 million years ago, and humans, such as they were, debuted 5 million years ago.[28]

For more than 99.9 percent of human time on Earth, writes Hayflick, the average life expectancy at birth was about age 20 or 30. Remains of prehistoric humans rarely reveal ages greater than 50.[29]

Frenchwoman Jeanne Louise Calment is reported to have lived the longest scientifically confirmed human life span: 122 years and 164 days. Born Feb. 21, 1875, Calment smoked two cigarettes a day for nearly 100 years (ages 21 to 117); regularly consumed port wine and chocolate, and shunned exercise. She died Aug. 4, 1997.[30]

MEDITERRANEAN DIET

Upon learning that four of the top five long-lived nations are in Europe and that the confirmed longest-living person was French, you might surmise that the European diet and lifestyle offer health advantages—and you would be correct. Ever since a 1950s study of the dietary patterns of long-lived Crete islanders, nutritionists have promoted the Mediterranean diet as the model of healthy eating.[31] Sixty years ago, Cretans had markedly low rates of heart disease and cancer.

The "traditional Mediterranean diet," according to a Greek epidemiologist and authority on the relationship between aging and nutrition, "is characterized by a high intake of vegetables, legumes, fruits and nuts, and cereals (that in the past were largely unrefined), and a high intake of olive oil but a low intake of saturated lipids, a moderately high intake of fish (depending on the proximity of the sea),* a low-to-moderate intake of dairy products (and then mostly in the form of cheese or yogurt), a low intake of meat and poultry, and a regular but moderate intake of ethanol, primarily in the form of wine and generally during meals."[32]

There are no Big Macs and greasy French fries on this menu. Europeans have much to lose if they trade their nutritious diet for high-caloric American fast food.

"The more often you visit the golden arches," joked Robert Blumenthal, M.D., cardiologist and director of the Johns Hopkins Ciccarone Center for the Prevention of Heart Disease, at a seminar, "the closer you get to the pearly gates."[33]

Long-term studies of Europeans elders (ages 70 to 90) consistently show that an adherence to a Mediterranean diet, in combination with other healthy practices (exercise, abstention from smoking), significantly lowers their risk of mortality from all causes, including cardiovascular disease.[34]

The plant-rich Mediterranean diet, which eschews saturated fats in favor of monounsaturated fats, served as the prototype for the low-

---

*Not coincidentally, the island nation of Japan, where fish is a dietary staple, ranks No. 1 worldwide in longevity.

sodium **D**ietary **A**pproaches to **S**top **H**ypertension or "DASH" diet, which U.S. cardiologists now recommend.35

Of course, diet is not the be-all-and-end-all of a long life. It is easy to recall historical Americans who reached ripe old ages long before public hygiene and biomedicine made a difference—and before we knew about the Mediterranean diet.

Born in 1841, U.S. Supreme Court Justice Oliver Wendell Holmes Jr. died just two days shy of his 94 birthday. Folk artist Grandma Moses (Anna Mary Robertson), born in 1860, made it to age 101, but of the 10 children to whom Robertson gave birth in the late 19th century, only five survived infancy.

These two Americans were intellectually and socially active people who engaged passionately in life. Grandma Moses took up painting in her 70s, after arthritis prevented her from continuing her first love of embroidery. Holmes, a jurist known as "The Great Dissenter," served on the Supreme Court from ages 61 to 90.

Regardless of how their activities and habits may have benefited them, you can safely assume that these historic elders possessed a resistance to disease that others of their generation did not. They possessed a physiological edge. This always has been true of people who lived to age 65. The big difference now is that, thanks to protective interventions such as antibiotics, many more people are reaching this milestone.

USUAL VS. SUCCESSFUL AGING

If you were a 65-year-old American in 1900, you were one of 3.1 million people age 65 and older, and your life expectancy was 76.7 years, if you were female, and 76.4, if you were male. In 2010, American 65-year-olds had life expectancies of 84.4 years and 80.4 years, respectively, an increase over 110 years of 7.7 years and 4.0 years.

My father has long said that "The older you get, the longer you live." This sounds absurd, but he's right. Once you reach age 65, you can expect to live to an older age than the age of your life expectancy at birth.

By 2050, the average life expectancy for a 65-year-old American is projected to be 86.5 years for women and 82.5 for men.36

Because of the seismic increase in the number of older adults, epidemiologists now calculate the Healthy Adjusted Life Expectancy at birth, which is the average number of years to be lived without disease, and the Active Disability-Free Life Expectancy. Your best physicians treat elders with a disease- and disability-free aging construct in mind. They seek to enhance life's *quality*, not just its quantity, so that increased longevity doesn't simply mean extended disability.

All human organ systems undergo normal age-related changes that make them less efficient and subject to problems. Physiological changes occur over time to everyone, but health differs substantially on an individual basis, a fact not appreciated by nearly enough physicians. Too many assume old age is a pattern-recognizable (white hair, wrinkles, stooped figure) diagnosis.

Modern gerontologists and geriatricians, however, distinguish among normal aging, usual aging, and successful aging–the latter two being recognized only within the past 20 years because of our increased longevity and obvious heterogeneity. Usual aging is what happens to people who, frankly, neglect their health. Their risk of disease or disability exceeds that of those who age normally, like my parents are doing.

According to physician John W. Rowe, co-author with psychologist Robert L. Kahn of the book, "Successful Aging," people who age in the usual manner undergo:

"[A] constellation of age-related or lifestyle-dependent changes such as increases in systolic blood pressure, abdominal fat, blood glucose, insulin, . . . that convey risk of disease or dysfunction. In addition to being risky, many aspects of 'usual aging' can be avoided or reversed."[37]

Avoided or *reversed*.

People who age successfully often have genetic factors in their favor, but they also have made smart choices about their health and environment. In general, an older person's functional capacity is closely linked to his or her nutrition, physical activity, and lifestyle habits throughout life, not just at old age. It is never too late, however, for elders to learn and practice new health "tricks." Tell your Mom and Pop that if they are using their age as an excuse for poor health or laziness.

Most adults 65 and older have two or more chronic diseases, such as heart disease, arthritis, diabetes, and osteoporosis. But this increased disease burden, as physicians call it, constitutes *usual* aging. It is not normal aging, much less successful aging.

Even with this increased burden, according to geriatrician Dr. Paulo H.M. Chaves of the Johns Hopkins Center on Aging and Health, older people "are still doing fine. . . . Survivors have resistance to disease. . . . Disability is not the norm." In fact, disability rates are falling because more elders are exercising regularly, foregoing smoking, keeping their weight down, and eating nutritiously.[38]

The prevalence of chronic diseases in the older population, reports U.Va.'s Dr. Snustad, is also declining.[39]

Dr. Chaves's approach to patient care differs from the by-the-numbers approach of frequent blood and screening tests favored by many primary-care physicians, including my parents'. His construct of healthy aging involves the whole patient and focuses on:

✓ Maintaining physical mobility and activity

✓ Keeping socially engaged and active

✓ Avoiding injury

✓ Preventing illness and disease

✓ Preserving cognitive vitality and avoiding dementia

Higher levels of activity, especially of physical exercise, associate strongly with improved function, longevity, *decreased* disease burden, and quality of life, Chaves says. Exercise, and the lack of it, contribute greatly to the heterogeneity that exists among older people–and among those of us in the next aging generation. It is "the single best intervention," according to Chaves. And the only magic pill.

In his geriatrics practice, Chaves focuses on compressing morbidity, that is, on decreasing the length and severity of illness that an elder experiences toward the end of his or her life. The idea is to keep the deleterious effects of aging to a minimum and to preserve function until senescence makes continued life impossible.[40] Avoidance–of disease, dysfunction, and *decline*–is his primary goal.

ANTI-AGING

Humans have long dreamed of discovering a fountain of youth that would reverse or eliminate the aging process. While we have succeeded in extending life expectancy, we have not found a cure for death, and we never will. Gerontologists postulate that even if the most common causes of death in old age—cardiovascular disease, stroke, and cancer—were eliminated, the human life expectancy (in the developed world) would gain only 15 years. Aging would become the leading cause of death.[41]

At least, that's the conventional medical wisdom.

In the 1990s, a contrary anti-aging movement arose that still has traction today and may change thinking tomorrow. It grew out of an enthusiastic response to a study reported in a 1990 *New England Journal of Medicine* article that showed men over 60 could increase their muscle mass by taking a biosynthetic form of human growth hormone (HGH).

Natural HGH plays a critical role in human development, especially in the height spurt of children. After age 30, however, its secretion from the pituitary gland declines. Most healthy older adults produce 50 percent less HGH than they did when they were younger.[42] This age-induced dropoff contributes to a loss in lean muscle mass and muscle strength that leads to weakness and can result in disability. Health-conscious elders know how important muscle-strengthening workouts are to their well-being.

Anti-aging advocates, thousands of whom are physicians, believe that aging can be slowed, reversed, or even prevented. Practitioners of anti-age medicine promote products and procedures for achieving these aims, chief among them, HGH. (See Chapter Twelve for the drawbacks to HGH therapy.)

Not surprisingly, traditional physicians liken these anti-aging practitioners to 19th century snake-oil salesmen.[43] Unquestionably, there are quacks and hustlers among them, but there also is good science happening in (anti-)aging research.

For now, at least, we all must age. But *why* do we age? I take a crack at answering that big, difficult, and loaded question next.

WHY DO WE AGE?

According to University of California-Berkeley molecular biologists Brian T. Weinert and Poala S. Timiras, most theories of aging can be categorized into one of two *modus operandi*: programming and error.

Programming theorists, such as Dr. Snustad, believe that there is something in our genetic "machinery" that leads us gradually to slow down and our bodily systems to wear out. We have an inborn aging process. A hard-wiring.

Over our lifetimes, Weinert and Timiras explain in elaborating upon this theory, our genes "sequentially [switch] on and off signals to the nervous, endocrine, and immune systems responsible for maintenance of homeostasis and for activation of defense responses."

Error theorists, in contrast, discount the existence of a pre-set biological clock. They believe that environmental insults at various levels, such as at the level of mitochondrial DNA, cause progressive damage that results in aging.44

Is it hard-wiring or accumulated damage? Whatever you believe, it's important to understand the basics about human cells, DNA (deoxyribonucleic acid), and homeostasis.

Cell division is a biological cornerstone. Human-cell development begins when a male sperm cell fertilizes a female egg (oocyte) to form a united single cell. This cell divides by mitosis to form two cells, which divide to form four cells, which divide to form eight cells, etc., etc., and so on.45

Embryonic cell growth occurs explosively; it starts to slow as cells become committed to specific functions within the fetal body. Many cells will continue to divide throughout the lives of our bodies, replacing dead or damaged tissues. Skin cells are the obvious example. Other cells, such as those in the heart and brain, stop dividing after they have reached a certain number.

Cellular division of labor is known as differentiation. Some cells, for example, produce a mineralized material that makes your bones hard, enabling them to protect your vital organs and to support your body's weight. Other cells produce and receive chemical and electrical signals that allow them to communicate with each other, such as when nerve cells communicate with muscle cells and cause them to contract. Our bodies are made up of many populations of specialized cells that determine the form and functions of our tissues and are critical to our survival.

Amazingly, *each* of our trillions of cells, no matter where it is, contains a copy of the genetic information that we receive from our parents. The nucleus of each of our cells contains 46 chromosomes, 23 chromosomes from each parent. Chromosomes are threadlike linear strands of DNA and associated proteins that carry our genes.

Each DNA molecule consists of two chains of nucleotides that, when joined to other DNA molecules, form strands resembling a twisted ladder. No doubt you've seen depictions of DNA's double-stranded helix. Each gene within the molecule has a sequence of these nucleotides, encoded with chemical instructions for making a specific protein. The human genome comprises 20,000 to 25,000 protein-coding genes in the chromosome and consists of more than 3 billion nucleotides.

Proteins perform numerous–*numerous*–functions in our bodies, such as enabling our muscles to contract and our blood to clot. Proteins are chains of amino acids. Because our bodies cannot synthesize all of the amino acids that we need to live, we must obtain other protein from our food.

Homeostasis is the internal equilibrium or stability that the human body must have in order to ensure normal physiological functions and processes. Our bodies need a relatively constant cellular environment, especially with regard to temperature. Water plays a principal role in thermal regulation, as well as in nutrient transport, waste removal, and other fundamental functions.

Stress and disease disrupt our homeostasis, causing imbalance. With age come a declining ability to respond to stress and other insults (injury, trauma) and an increasing homeostatic imbalance and incidence of pathology, i.e., disease and other abnormalities. The decline in homeostasis is why older people, when they get sick, recover more slowly than younger people.

The term allostasis, introduced in 1988, has been gaining recognition and use in addition to, or in lieu of homeostasis. Whereas homeostasis dictates biological stability through constancy, through maintaining, allostasis envisions stability through change, adaptation. The theory here is that aging and ultimately death result when allostasis fails.[46]

Theories of Aging

In 1951, Dr. Peter Medawar, a biologist who performed pioneering work in tissue grafting and transplantation and later received the Nobel prize, gave a lecture on aging at the University College London titled "An Unsolved Problem in Biology."[47] Ever since Medawar enunciated the "problem," hundreds of theories have been advanced for why–as contrasted with how–humans age. I will look at only a few.

FREE RADICALS

Three years after Medawar's talk, and while still engaged in postgraduate medical studies, Dr. Denham Harman, M.D., Ph.D., proposed the now well-known free radical theory as the basic chemical process underlying aging. As Harman explained: "The reaction of active free radicals, normally produced in [all living things during cell metabolism], with cellular constituents initiates the changes associated with aging."

To elaborate: Atoms or molecules that have an unpaired electron (and, thus, are free radicals) react with and alter the structure of other molecules that are critical for normal cell function. Free radicals occur as a *normal* part of metabolism and are oxygen reactive. Oxygen can be toxic. According to Harman, who was a chemist as well as a physician, free radicals largely cause the reactions involved in cell mutations, disease, and death.

"Metabolism" encompasses all of the chemical reactions in our bodies that are necessary to maintain life. We derive our energy from this vital process.

You may think of metabolism as being divided into those chemical reactions that occur during digestion and those chemical reactions that occur after the products of digestion are taken up by our cells. At normal body temperature, most metabolic reactions do not occur at a rate fast enough to benefit us. For this reason, special catalysts known as enzymes, which are generally protein in nature, exist to accelerate them.

According to the free-radical theory, metabolic activities involving oxygen create toxic reactive oxygen species (ROS) that damage cells. The effect of this damage is aging.

During early human life, Harman writes, a "relatively low free radical activity . . . permits growth and development of new offspring." In later life, however, free radicals damage the body and impair function by altering proteins, lipids (especially HDL, the "good" cholesterol), DNA, and RNA. Of particular import is the harm they cause mitochondria, which are rodlike organelles found in the cell's cytoplasm.

The mitochondria serve as the center of the enzyme activity that produces the essential nucleotide, ATP, or adenosine triphosphate. ATP is vital to the energy processes of all living cells, and, thus, to the repair of free-radical and other aging-associated damage. We inherit all or nearly all of our mitochondria from our mothers.[48]

In the 1970s, Harman, who was a biogerontologist on the faculty of the University of Nebraska Medical Center, recognized that the mitochondria are the primary source of O_2 radical generation in the cell. He discovered that the mitochondria *themselves* produce free radicals.

ANTIOXIDANTS

Thereafter, Harman tinkered with anti-aging. By adding antioxidants, such as vitamins C and E, to the diets of laboratory mice, he was able to increase the rodents' longevity, but not to lengthen their maximum life span. Eventually he concluded that the mitochondria, which were unaffected by the antioxidant supplements, determine the length of an individual life. He called them the body's "biologic clock."[49]

Each human cell has about 10,000 mitochondria, all of which have their own DNA. Damage to mitochondrial DNA (abbreviated as MtDNA), whether by free radicals or otherwise, escalates over time and cannot be repaired. Such damage causes faster cell replication and leads, cumulatively, to a lower energy state that can progress from fatigue to congestive heart failure to other vulnerable conditions eventually resulting in death.

The medical establishment ignored or discredited Harman's free-radical theory for decades before it gained even a nod of respectability. It now is one of the chief theories mentioned in physiology textbooks and mini-medical school lectures for why we age. And it has spawned the huge anti-aging business of antioxidant supplements, which purportedly cure all human evils from wrinkles to cancer.

Antioxidants donate electrons to free radicals, but data on their benefits are lacking.

While clinical evidence exists to support the belief that the consumption of fruits and vegetables rich in antioxidants prevents disease, there is no evidence that the consumption of antioxidant supplements will thwart aging and prolong life. According to my own expert, a distinguished medical professor emeritus at Vanderbilt who has studied oxidative stress, the only promising dietary antioxidant is resveratrol, which comes from the grapes used in producing red wines.

Resveratrol may prove "heart-healthy," in that it may help to increase levels of good cholesterol and protect against artery damage, but any definitive conclusions are years away. In addition, preliminary indications from resveratrol studies in mice suggest that a human being would have to drink over 60 liters of red wine every day to derive any benefit.[50] At that rate of consumption, red wine is certainly not the drinking fountain that Ponce de Leon sought in vain.

TELOMERES

Another prominent aging theory concerns biological material called telomeres, which molecular biologist Dr. Elizabeth H. Blackburn began studying in the 1970s when she was a postdoctoral fellow at Yale University. Blackburn, who subsequently joined the faculties of UCSF and UC-Berkeley, published her first article about telomeres in 1978. Thirty-one years later she and two other researchers received the Nobel Prize in Physiology or Medicine for their telomere studies.

Telomeres are repetitive DNA sequences that exist at the ends of chromosomes. Blackburn discovered that telomeres protect chromosomes from deterioration by acting as disposable buffers during DNA replication, which starts in the center of the strand. Telomeres are consumed during cell division, but later replenished by an enzyme called telomerase reverse transcriptase.[51]

Over time, however, because of continuous cell division, telomeres shorten or erode. In the process, cells reach their replicative limit, becoming unable to divide and progressing into senescence. Remember Hayflick's limit?

One of my Johns Hopkins mini-medical-school lecturers reduced the teleomere theory to its functional essence: "Senescent cells don't do what they're supposed to do."

As more and more cells become senescent or die off, vital organs deteriorate. Eventually this deterioration culminates in death.

THE KITCHEN-SINK THEORY

After reading about the main theories of aging, and listening to medical professors elucidate them, I have far more questions than I have answers. In part because of that, I have decided to endorse the viewpoint of Dr. Robin Holliday, a British molecular biologist-gerontologist who is currently a member of the Australian Academy of Science.

Many aging theorists advance a single cause. Harman wrote about his belief "that there had to be a basic cause which killed everything." Holliday doesn't buy this. He believes that since the late 20th century, scientists have been able to explain biologically and with certainty why we age, and the answer is multifactorial.[52]

In "Aging Is No Longer an Unsolved Problem," an article responding to Medawar's 1951 "Unsolved Problem" talk, Holliday enumerates what he considers to be the causes of aging, and I quote:

❖ The accumulation of genetic damage or mutations in genes, chromosomes, and mitochondria [genes are susceptible to radiation and other toxins];

❖ The deposition of lipofuscin and advanced glycation endproducts (AGEs) in many cell and tissue locations [such as in the heart];

❖ The cross-linking of collagen[*] and elastin, other abnormal modifications of proteins, and the accumulation of insoluble aggregates;

❖ Damage by reactive oxygen species in many contexts;

❖ Loss of immune functions and autoimmunity;

❖ A decline in muscle strength;

❖ Osteoporosis and osteoarthritis;

❖ Inflammatory damage to tissues;

❖ Hormone imbalance and a decline in homeostasis;

❖ Epigenetic abnormalities, including the loss or gain of DNA methylation; and

❖ A greatly increased incidence of tumors

While some of these events may seem more like effects than causes, all of them, Holliday writes, "can bring about a failure of major organ systems, such as the heart and major blood vessels, the brain and sensory organs, and so on.

"It is striking," he continues, "that the major theories of aging relate [only] to particular causes of aging, such as the free radical theory, the somatic mutation theory, the mitochondrial theory, theories that relate to the accumulation of abnormal proteins, the immunologic

---

[*]I discuss collagen, a fibrous protein, and cross-linking in Chapter Twelve.

theory, and several others. *If we accept the fact that there are multiple causes of aging, then it follows that many of the important theories of aging have some truth, and it is important to have a global view of both theories and causes of aging.*" (my emphasis added)53

Damage, loss, decline. That's what I read in and between these lines.

Essentially, Holliday is saying that aging occurs with progressive damage, not, I would presume, as a result of hard-wiring. Aging represents an accumulation over time of diverse, deleterious changes in our cells and tissues. We can repair the damage and degradation for only so long, and some of us, because of our physiological reserves, do a better job of repair than others.54

Holliday identifies 13 mechanisms that our bodies employ for maintaining cells, tissues, and organs. Some of them include: multiple pathways of DNA repair; defenses against oxygen-free radicals; methods to repair proteins; an immune response against pathogens and parasites; physiological homeostasis; wound healing, blood clotting, and the healing of broken bones and torn ligaments. All of the 13 depend on a large number of genes, but not exclusively so.55

The eminent Dr. Hayflick agrees with much of what Holliday observes, but he conceptualizes aging quite differently. Hayflick believes that humans "spend the first 20 years of our lives producing, ordering, and replacing our molecules with absolute fidelity. [Because of] natural selection, that fidelity must be maintained until reproductive success or our species would vanish."

I comprehend fidelity to mean structural integrity, like building a stone wall.

After reproduction, Hayflick contends, a "random downward spiral of molecular disorder" occurs that results in the cellular, tissue, and organ changes that we call aging. Ultimately, our body's loss of molecular fidelity exceeds its repair capacity and increases our susceptibility to pathology, such as cancers. Old cells are vulnerable.

Holliday agrees with Hayflick that "efficiency of maintenance" correlates with maximum life span, such that the more energy and metabolic resources that we invest in maintenance of function—as opposed to reproduction and basic metabolism—the longer we will live. Eventually maintenance breaks down, though, and all of the molecular and cellular events that Holliday characterizes as the aging process dominate.56

LONGEVITY GENES

While Hayflick regards aging as a random process—albeit, to my understanding, inborn—he views longevity as governed by the excess or reserve physiological capacity that humans, individually, have.

Genes "do not drive the aging process," he writes, "but they indirectly determine potential longevity."[57]

Research into so-called longevity or longevity-enabling genes is in the very early stages.[58] Studies have focused on genomic regions on specific chromosomes, as well as on putative genes and alleles, an allele being a part of a pair or series of genes. The ApoE4 allele, implicated in Alzheimer's disease (see Chapter Eight) and cardiovascular disease, has the distinction of being the most-studied for its effect on longevity—but as a deterrent to a longer life, not as a furtherance.[59]

While elderly twin and centenarian studies strongly suggest that there is a hereditary component to longevity, particularly exceptional or extreme longevity, such studies are still too few to form conclusions. Anecdotal evidence supports heredibility, however.

The Oliver Wendell Holmeses Senior and Junior lived exceptionally long lives for 19th century America, with Holmes Sr., a well-known physician and poet, dying in 1894 at age 85. His son, you will recall, lived nearly 94 years. The father of 122-year-old Madame Calment died just shy of his 100th birthday, and her mother lived to 86. An older brother of the Frenchwoman survived to 97.

I have extreme longevity on my father's side. My Grandpa died at age 96½ and might have lived longer if the attending physician during his final hospitalization had not overdosed him with an anticoagulant. Grandpa's bedridden legs had swollen grotesquely with fluid, but he bled to death.

My grandfather's mother, Dad's beloved grandmother, also reached 96½, and Albert Sr. lived to age 90. Both died at home.

My mother has lived a longer life than all of her familial elders. Her mother died of leukemia at 73, and her father's death at 82 was related to heart disease. I credit Mom's longevity to her physiological and cognitive reserves, optimism, an easy-going temperament, and the protection of her husband and children.

The number of 100-year-olds in industrialized nations is reportedly increasing at a rate of about 7 percent per year. With this surge in study subjects and their descendants and the development of less expensive and more powerful molecular genetic techniques, it is likely that scientists soon will achieve breakthroughs in aging determinants, both genetic and environmental.[60]

Will this help us to care better for elders? Will doctors, in turn, appreciate and respect them more? Will they listen more attentively to their concerns?

Will medical ageism be relegated to the past?

The IHOP creep at Ace Hardware apologized to my father for his offensive joke the next time he saw him, so there is always hope.

Chapter Eight

Memory
LOSS

Normal Aging, MCI, or Dementia?

I tried for more than two years to get my mother neuropsychologically evaluated, only to encounter resistance from both of my parents and from siblings who minimized the cognitive deficits I described.

Some people can and will find excuses for just about any mental deficiency you detect. This may sound harsh, but I view them as the head-in-the-sand legions who comfort themselves by not acknowledging the truth. Every family has them.

"Forgetting is normal," they will say, or "I do the same thing, and I'm in my 50s."

Yes, thank you, forgetting is normal, but there are different types of forgetting. The reliable person on the scene knows when memory loss is normal and when it is not. I quickly learned from being around her that Mom could not remember in the afternoon what I told her in the morning. EVER. This was not normal aging. Dad knew it, too.

Outside of my family, I found it staggering how many people would presume to know my mother's cognitive status better than I did and dispute my assessment.

"She's fine," a neighbor would say. "I talk with her on the street, and she does just fine."

Yes, that's because you do all of the talking, and Mom's a warm and attentive listener.

"I haven't noticed any problems," another acquaintance would say.

Yes, that's because Mom masks her confusion well, and you're not very observant.

These doubters also had no idea how superior my mother's functioning once had been. They knew her only as an older person, and they had low expectations.

Coping with a parent's cognitive impairment is difficult enough without having to contend with doubters and deniers. If a daughter or son shares with you her/his belief that a parent has experienced cognitive decline, just consider it fact and be supportive. Don't make the situation worse by second-guessing. False hope is not helpful.

MENTAL "LAPSES"

During a drive back to Carolina after seeing a dental specialist in Virginia, my mother made an observation that will stay with me always. "My memory," she softly said, "is not as good now, at 84, as it was at 83."

What an odd thought, I recall thinking: She can differentiate her cognitive status by consecutive ages. . . . And she was right. Her memory was deteriorating, and a year had made a difference. But it was only that year, from 2007 to 2008, during which I noticed a memory deficit. Duke's Dr. Gideon had been egregiously off-base in diagnosing dementia in 2002.

For more than five years, Mom had functioned at a relatively high level. It appeared that, despite the dire warnings we had received, the ehrlichiosis infection had not diminished her cognition. But now, her memory too often failed her, and she was less sure of herself. I could see doubt and surprise shadow her face whenever she learned of a clear act of forgetfulness. Had the ehrlichiosis caused this impairment?

Previously, Mom had complained about being treated "like a nitwit" at the dentist's office by well-meaning people who wanted me present whenever they talked about her treatment. The same had happened to my mother's Aunt Grace as she aged. A self-supporting, unmarried businesswoman her entire adult life, Grace had played the unwilling nitwit role, while her niece attended to all that was said and remembered for her.

Notwithstanding my objections to healthcare practitioners talking to their older patient's younger relative, instead of to the patient, and using a firm parent-to-child tone of voice with older patients, I appreciate their dilemma. No crisis has pained me more than my mother's altered cognition. I sometimes feel that she is slowly disappearing.

Mom had always been smart and perceptive, and her memory,

especially for numbers and facts, was outstanding. We never needed a telephone directory with Mom around; she could hear a number once and remember it forever. When she started asking me the phone numbers of my siblings, I worried.

My father actually was the first of my parents to exhibit what we thought were cognitive problems. I used to describe his struggle in terms of sequencing or processing information, but I now think it had more to do with his severely impaired hearing—his loss is about 60 percent—than his mind. You might say his auditory system was not decoding sound signals properly.

Dad stopped being able to follow dialogue in a TV show or movie without having captions on, and it wasn't because he couldn't hear the words. He heard them; they just didn't make sense. The same gap occurred in conversation. He rarely "heard" what a person said to him the first time around, whether he was wearing his hearing aid or not. Only when someone repeated the words would he comprehend their meaning. It was as if he hadn't focused on listening until the repetition.

According to Dr. Frank Lin, a Johns Hopkins otological surgeon who spoke during a mini-medical school I attended, hearing depends on 1) peripheral transduction, which is the mental encoding of an acoustic signal, and 2) central processing, which is the decoding of acoustic energy to a neural signal to be sent to the brain. As we age, our hearing threshold (the minimal stimulus) usually increases, and our frequency resolution deteriorates so that our ear "misses fine nuances," Lin said, resulting in "I can hear you, but I can't understand you."[1]

In this chapter, I share a lot of the homework that I did while trying to understand my mother's altered mental status. Unlike my father's cognitive changes, Mom's decline suggested predementia, a clinical state before the onset of Alzheimer's disease or another dementia, each of which is distinguished by pathological changes in the brain.

You start out in life with more than 100 billion neurons, a number that is fixed early because neurons, unlike other cells, do not divide. Neurons are the working units and inter-connectors of your nervous system, which I explore in detail in Chapter Twelve. When many neurons die in key parts of your brain, atrophy (tissue shrinkage) occurs, resulting in abnormalities in memory, thinking, and/or behavior, depending on the affected location.

Neuropathological links appear to exist among the three cognitive-impairment diagnoses that predominate in people 65 and older: dementia, depression, and delirium.

According to medical authorities, two-thirds of all elders who experience delirium have dementia; between one-third and one-half of all who are depressed have dementia; and as many as two-thirds of those with dementia will develop depression.[2] A fourth critical diagnosis, mild cognitive impairment (MCI), may be viewed as a precursor to dementia.

NORMAL COGNITIVE AGING

There is no question that as we age, our thinking slows down. Cognitive decline is natural, but its extent varies among individuals and among the cognitive functions that we perform. Decline should not be assumed; but neither should it be denied.

According to Ronald C. Petersen, M.D., director of the Mayo Alzheimer's Disease Research Center in Rochester, Minn., most people undergo a gradual cognitive decline over their lifetime, typically with regard to memory. This slowdown is minor and may be annoying, but it doesn't compromise your ability to function. Only one in 100 people, says Petersen, experiences "virtually" no decline. [3]

And don't we all want to be that one!

It is important to understand that intelligence is not the same as cognitive function, but intelligence does figure into cognitive aging.

According to my authoritative textbook, "Brocklehurst's Textbook of Geriatric Medicine & Gerontology" (*Brocklehurst*), an intelligence quotient (IQ) is a "derived score used in many test batteries designed to measure a hypothesized general ability." So-called "general intelligence," explain *Brocklehurst* contributors, Drs. Jane Martin and Michelle Gorenstein, can be thought of as our "overall ability on all types of intellectual tasks."[4]

General intelligence is subdivided into fluid intelligence, which measures the "degree to which an individual can solve novel problems without any previous training," Martin and Gorenstein explain, and crystallized intelligence, which is the amount of knowledge and information that a person brings to a testing situation.

Fluid intelligence eventually plateaus and declines with normal aging–between ages 49 and 92, according to studies–whereas crystallized intelligence, which increases from childhood into late adulthood, does not. Thus, an older person will have the benefit of youthful intellectual activities and educational pursuits—including school-based knowledge, vocabulary, and reading ability—to apply to a standardized cognitive test or an everyday cognitive challenge.5

Research strongly suggests that a person who possessed high childhood mental ability and engaged in intellectually demanding tasks and experiences as a child will show less cognitive decline with age than a person who did not. Such a person has a "cognitive reserve" that will buffer the loss when cognitive impairment occurs. The longtime pursuit of an active, socially engaged lifestyle also purportedly adds to this hypothetical reserve.

According to Martin and Gorenstein, the cognitive-reserve model suggests "that the brain actively attempts to compensate for the challenge represented by brain disease and hypothesizes that adults with higher initial cognitive ability are better able to compensate for the effects of aging and dementia."

Experts theorize that only after this reserve is depleted does an underlying impairment become apparent. People with brain pathology who have a superior cognitive reserve seem to compensate better than those whose impairment is of a similar degree, but who lack a strong early educational and intellectual foundation.6

Cognitive reserve is not the same as the "use-it-or-lose-it" hypothesis, which proposes that elders can slow the rate of age-related cognitive decline by engaging in mentally stimulating exercises. Although studies suggest that lifelong intellectual activities bolster old-age cognitive performance, use-it-or-lose-it is more of an "optimistic hope than an empirical reality," writes psychology Professor Timothy A. Salthouse, who is director of the Cognitive Aging Laboratory at the University of Virginia.7

Neuropsychiatric experts categorize cognitive functions by domain, which you may conceptualize as a realm of thinking. While each domain is distinctive, functional overlap exists among them and their respective operations. Memory, for example, consists of encoding, storing, and retrieving information, neural tasks that are influenced by our attentional ability, which involves both focus and concentration and the speed at which our brains can process information.

Experts base their understanding of how aging affects cognitive domains on studies of elders' performances on standardized intelligence and neuropsychological tests. Before cognitive profiles of older subjects can be compiled, they must take multiple tests of a given function. Because the scoring and evaluation of such tests can be tricky—at the very least, confounding factors such as fatigue, stress, and medication use must be considered—our understanding of cognitive aging lacks what you might call rock-solid conclusions. But you can count on some generalities.[8]

The most important domain functions are:

❖ Attention

Attention, according to the *Brocklehurst* authors, "is a complex process that allows one to filter stimuli from the environment, hold and manipulate information, and respond appropriately." It relates to your ability to focus and concentrate on a particular stimulus for a sustained time period.

Tests show that the effects of aging on a person's attention depend upon the complexity of the task presented. Even the oldest old can maintain attention for simple tasks, such as hearing and repeating a telephone number; but when tasks require older people to divide their attention, they tend to respond more slowly and make more errors.

Can your Mom or Pop answer questions you ask of them while they're watching TV? Mine can't, not without great effort. If yours can, is the conversation just small talk or more detailed discussion?

In general, normal aging causes a decline in *sustained* and *selective* attention—the latter of which requires screening out interference, such as a television—and an increase in distractibility. Intact attention is a prerequisite for healthy memory function.[9]

❖ Processing Speed

Processing speed is the rate at which you can process information. It, therefore, determines the amount of information that your brain can process at a given time.

Processing speed definitely declines with age and may account in large part for deterioration in memory and other cognitive processes, such as the executive functions (below). Not only does an elder's thinking slow, but his or her working memory no longer commands the same amount of information that it once could.

For decades, my father's big brain allowed him to carry on

numerous business and professional transactions without thinking twice, much less second-guessing himself. Now he labors over any correspondence that requires an accumulation of facts and relies upon me to double-check his reasoning. Completing a medical-history form for a new doctor requires the better part of Dad's day—which makes me want to yell: "What's the matter with you? Don't you understand what an ordeal your ridiculous paperwork is for older people?"

Apparently not.

According to Martin and Gorenstein, slower processing speed unquestionably accounts for the age-associated decline in fluid-intelligence ability, which includes both memory and spatial aptitude, the latter being your ability to perceive spatial relationships, such as between objects. Slower processing speed does not affect crystallized-intelligence ability, which controls verbal skills.[10]

❖ Verbal Abilities

Most verbal abilities remain preserved with normal aging.

The two verbal-skill areas that receive the most attention and testing in the older population are verbal fluency, which is the ability to retrieve words based on their meaning or their sounds (semantic and phonemic); and confrontation naming, the ability to identify an object by its name.

Your Mom or Pop may experience a slight natural decline in verbal fluency. In a typical test of this ability, an older subject must generate within a defined time period as many words as he possibly can that begin with a specific letter: Dog, doll, dart, dagger . . . You can see how memory would be implicated in such a test, too.

The tip-of-the-tongue or TOT phenomenon, which occurs when you know the name of a person or an object, but can't retrieve it, commonly affects the confrontation-naming ability. Older adults have significantly more TOT experiences than younger adults for proper nouns and difficult words. This is normal.[11]

❖ Executive Functions

Executive functions involve higher-order mental processes. According to Drs. Martin and Gorenstein, these functions "describe a wide range of abilities that relate to the capacity to respond to a novel situation."[12] They involve:

* Planning
* Decision-making
* Abstract thinking
* Initiating and inhibiting actions
* Monitoring and changing behavior
* Anticipating outcomes and adapting
* Troubleshooting

Your cerebral cortex is largely responsible for your higher brain functions, such as reasoning and memory. It forms the extensive surface layer of your cerebrum, which is what we tend to think of as the whole brain. The cerebral cortex is composed primarily of nerve-cell bodies and unmyelinated fibers and, because of its color, is called gray matter.

Your cerebrum is divided into two symmetrical halves called hemispheres, which are designated left and right. Each hemisphere, in turn, is divided into four lobes that are named for the skull bones overlying them: the frontal, parietal, occipital, and temporal. Because the brain-control center for the executive abilities is located in the prefrontal cortex, which occupies part of each hemisphere's frontal lobe, executive function is alternately known as frontal-lobe function.

The cerebrum encompasses all of the parts within your skull except your cerebellum (Latin for little brain), medulla oblongata, and pons. The cerebellum lies below the occipital lobes, which are in the posterior of the two hemispheres, and is responsible for the regulation and coordination of complex voluntary muscular movement and the maintenance of posture and balance. The medulla oblongata and pons make up the brain stem; the pons connects the cerebellum to the stem.

You need not know brain anatomy to know that normal aging is generally associated with a decline in executive functioning. This decline varies considerably from one person to the next, however, and fluid intelligence plays a part.[13]

* **Memory**

Your memory function erodes as you age, but research suggests that overall cognitive slowing, which includes reduced processing speed and slower information-retrieval time, and changes in attentional ability largely determine the extent of this erosion.

We laypeople typically distinguish short-term and long-term memory incorrectly, defining them as the recent past and the long-ago past, respectively.

Neuropsychological experts who test memory view short-term or, more precisely, *working memory* as the storage of encoded items for a few seconds up to two minutes. It is a temporary holding cell for information that our brains process and encode into long-term memory for later recall. To evaluate a patient's short-term recall, a test-giver may name three unrelated objects—a lamp, a cat, a turnip—and ask the patient to repeat the objects after just a few minutes have passed.[14]

Contrary to popular belief, long-term memory is not just the ability to recall past events and learned information. It also includes the ability to remember upcoming events, such as an appointment, and to keep track of information in the present, such as a conversation or a book you're reading.[15]

Normal age-associated memory regression or forgetfulness is usually minor and can be aggravating—misplacing keys, for example—but it does not compromise an elder's ability to manage daily activities. He or she still can prepare dinner, engage coherently in a conversation, shop for clothes, and do much more, independently and reliably. In evaluating cognitive impairment, independence is key.

LIFE IN THE MOMENT

After her observation in 2008 about her memory decline, Mom continued to function well within her small community orbit. She drove to weekly hair appointments and to her swim club and ran simple go-and-pick-up errands. Although she couldn't manage grocery shopping, Mom could shop for gifts. Dad paid the bills, but Mom still wrote an occasional check.

Despite her forgetfulness, my mother didn't miss a beat in managing her ADL, with one notable exception. She stopped remembering to take her medications, so my father became keeper of the meds. As time passed, the number of Dad's "take your pills" reminders increased. He also ensured that Mom's doctors renewed her prescriptions, and he picked up her drugs from the pharmacy.

Mom continued to solve puzzles on TV's "Wheel of Fortune" and to zing us with her "Jeopardy!" knowledge. She did word Jumbles® and completed exercises in a book of memory challenges that I bought for her, showing particular skill in those based on visual attentiveness.

Mom wrote letters to friends and went to bed at night with a book, but my father said she read the same pages over and over. She faithfully watched the TV evening news, but when asked about the headlines, she did not seem to recall much of what she'd seen or heard. She also read a daily newspaper, but how far she got beyond the comics was hard to determine. She never had much interest in politics, but she stayed abreast of pop culture. She paid attention to photographs of people.

Because of my faith in human mind-power (Dad's influence), and my empathy (Mom's) for those whose power is diminished, I've long been interested in Alzheimer's disease (AD), as well as other brain disorders. Years before my mother exhibited any cognitive impairment, I attended conferences held by the Washington, D.C.-area chapter of the Alzheimer's Assn. Thus, I knew quite a bit about AD and other dementias.

I had read about dementia patients who cannot retain information that they learned just minutes ago.[16] My mother's memory window was longer, but her retention was unpredictable. I learned that I could not confidently leave a telephone message with her, although telling her to write it down sometimes helped. If she didn't write it down immediately, however, she might not remember to do so after hanging up the phone.

I also learned that if I wrote something down to reinforce Mom's memory, she might forget to read the note later. So I started putting important events, such as the days I would be out of town or my siblings would be visiting, on her office wall calendar. She usually remembered to check it.

Apart from her memory loss, my father bemoaned the loss of the insightful, wise, and perceptive life partner whose judgment he valued and upon whom he had relied for nearly 60 years. I dearly missed that person, too.

Decision-making, troubleshooting, problem-solving . . . Mom struggled with these executive functions. She could never remember the topic, the issues, and the content of previous discussions, nor could she integrate, organize, and evaluate information that she received. Her brilliance and creativity faded, but sometimes, especially with her children gathered around, she could rise to an occasion.

Increasingly, life for and with my mother existed in the what-you-see-is-what-you-get moment.

MCI

The book, "Diagnostic and Statistics Manual of Mental Disorders" (*DSM*), published by the American Psychiatric Association (APA), serves as a clinical blueprint and standard dictionary for all psychiatric diagnoses, including those related to cognitive impairment.

During my research, *DSM* was in flux. The manual's fourth edition (*DSM-IV*™), upon which I principally relied, was undergoing revision.[17] The fifth edition (*DSM-5*™) came out in June 2013–months after I finished the bulk of my research–but I read about the anticipated changes.

Among them, *DSM-5* replaces the term, dementia, used in *DSM-IV*, with a new term: "major neurocognitive disorder."

According to the APA task force charged with revising the cognitive disorders section of *DSM-IV,* the term dementia was viewed by some medical specialists as pejorative, while others had ceased using it altogether in relation to non-Alzheimer's disease dementias. Still others liked the term, believed it had lost much of its earlier stigma, and protested its abandonment.

I agree with the latter, but I use dementia here for practical reasons. Referring repeatedly to a major neurocognitive disorder is too cumbersome. I also would be surprised if physicians start using the term regularly with their patients and their families.

A far more important change effective with *DSM-5* is the inclusion of the diagnosis of "mild neurocognitive disorder."

For years geriatrics specialists have conceptualized a transitional period between normal aging and clinically probable very early Alzheimer's disease or another dementia. This period, called mild cognitive impairment (MCI) in the medical literature, and by me here, has garnered much interest during the past decade as the emphasis in Alzheimer's disease research has shifted to the predementia phase of cognitive dysfunction, also called the prodromal or early warning phase.

DSM-5's recognition of neurocognitive disorders as either mild or major represents a huge step forward. It acknowledges a cognitive continuum, which, in turn, raises the possibility of predicting and preventing dementia and brings clinical subtlety to diagnoses that some physicians may have viewed as black-and-white. It also emphasizes the importance of the *severity* of a patient's functional impairment and, thus, better individualizes patients.

My worry was not that Mom had Alzheimer's disease or another dementia, but that her impairment would progress to dementia. I knew about AD's three stages, which range from mild forgetfulness to severe dementia, and I set out to learn more. Once I found out about mild cognitive impairment (MCI), I focused much of my research on it.

A Mom or Pop with MCI performs "worse [cognitively] than one expects with aging," explains Dr. Peter V. Rabins, director of the Division of Geriatric Psychiatry and Neuropsychiatry at Johns Hopkins, "but not as bad[ly] as a person with dementia."

While people with MCI are extremely forgetful, they do not exhibit dementia-associated functional decline, such as getting lost or being unable to pay bills.[18]

According to the Mayo Clinic's Dr. Petersen, a trailblazer who has largely defined this evolving disorder, 10 to 20 percent of all persons 65 and older in the United States have mild cognitive impairment. Researchers at the Duke University Medical Center Department of Psychiatry and Behavioral Sciences estimate that the incidence of MCI in this age group is higher: 17 to 36 percent.[19]

The authors of *DSM-5* describe mild neurocognitive disorder in terms of domain impairment and classify it, where appropriate, by the associated disease or other cause, such as Alzheimer's disease, vascular disease, or traumatic brain injury.

Far more helpful to me is Petersen's clinical subtyping of mild cognitive impairment as either 1) amnestic MCI or 2) non-amnestic MCI. As you might surmise, the former involves memory; the latter does not.

Patients with amnestic MCI (abbreviated aMCI) are increasingly and noticeably forgetful, but not yet exhibiting signs of domain dysfunction, such as impaired executive functioning. Except for "mild inefficiencies," writes Petersen, their other cognitive capacities are relatively preserved, and their functional activities are intact.

With time, Petersen explains, most patients with aMCI transition to Alzheimer's disease, vascular dementia, or another progressive dementia, but some remain stable. Those who have "reversible" aMCI due to depression, adverse effects of medication, hormonal changes, or a nonneurological cognition-affecting condition can improve.

In contrast, patients with nonamnestic MCI experience a cognitive decline that affects their attention, their use of language, and/ or their visuospatial skills, but *not* their memories. Less common than aMCI, nonamnestic MCI is a likely precursor to dementias unrelated to Alzheimer's disease, such as Lewy body dementia and frontotemporal dementia.[20] The latter describes a diverse group of uncommon disorders that primarily affect areas of the brain associated with personality, language, and behavior. It tends to occur in people between ages 40 and 75.

Memory loss associated with aMCI is far more prominent than age-related memory impairment. Nonetheless, distinguishing between MCI and normal aging can be a "challenge" for the clinician.

Typically, Petersen explains, aMCI patients "start to forget important information that they previously would have remembered easily, such as appointments, telephone conversations, or recent events [e.g., sports contests] that would normally interest them." Casual observers may not be aware of the forgetfulness, but the patients' loved ones and other intimates definitely are.[21] (Touché!)

According to Petersen, people with MCI range on a clinical spectrum from the very mildly impaired to the seriously impaired. It is a heterogeneous cognitive state. Not surprisingly, those with a high degree of memory loss or other deficits will progress more rapidly to dementia than those with a low degree.

When an MCI-diagnosed patient requires assistance with routine activities, he or she has crossed the "threshold" of dementia, says Petersen, noting that the "general rate" of progression among *all* MCI patients to dementia, not just Alzheimer's disease, is 10 percent per year. (I have heard other experts say between 10 to 15 percent.)

Significantly, however, more than 90 percent of *amnestic*-MCI patients in clinical trials who progress to dementia, progress to Alzheimer's disease. They have AD brain pathology.[22]

Petersen strongly discourages any physician from diagnosing an MCI patient with "early" Alzheimer's disease. The label can be erroneous, psychologically defeating, and, for the suicidal depressed patient, dangerous. I know it would devastate my mother.[23]

While I agree with Petersen that a rush to judgment is a mistake, I also exhort you not to pretend your Mom's or Pop's decline is not

happening. Your parent needs your help and understanding, not your
denial, or, worse yet, your anger. Far too often adult children take
out their own fears on their parent, either by looking the other way or
by giving vent to angry frustration. Always be kind. And . . . do your
homework.

AD AND OTHER DEMENTIAS

Although Alzheimer's disease is the most prevalent disorder
characterized by dementia, dementia is not synonymous with AD.

According to Dr. Rabins and psychiatrist Constantine G. Lyketsos,
director of the Johns Hopkins Memory and Alzheimer's Treatment
Center, about 75 diseases cause dementia. These diseases have in
common the destruction of brain neurons.[24]

Alzheimer's disease may be only "one-in-75," but it accounts for
up to 75 percent of all dementia cases. According to the Alzheimer's
Assn., one in 10 people age 65 and over and one in three people age 85
and over have the disease. Some experts estimate that the incidence of
Alzheimer's among people 80 and older is actually one in two.[25]

Considering how aware people are today of Alzheimer's disease
and its prevalence, it is shocking to contemplate that as recently as
the 1970s, physicians believed that most dementia in people 65 and
older resulted from cerebral atherosclerosis, what we commonly call
"hardening" of arteries in the brain. Alzheimer's disease came out of
"obscurity" in the late 1960s, writes one academic bioethicist, after
studies in England revealed that most dementia actually arose from
the same degenerative brain lesions that German psychiatrist Dr. Alois
Alzheimer described in 1907.[26]

It, thus, was not that long ago that physicians did not bother to
differentiate the causes of memory loss and other cognitive impairments
in older people. Confused elders were simply senile. Theoretically,
physicians today know better, but don't count on your Mom's or
Pop's primary-care doctor knowing much. Geriatric psychiatrists and
neuropsychiatrists, however, have come a long way.

According to Rabins, the most common age for an Alzheimer's
disease diagnosis is 82. Early-onset Alzheimer's disease, a diagnosis
applied to patients who are 65 and younger, exists, but early-onset
dementia, as a diagnosis, does not.[27]

Pathologically, the Johns Hopkins neuropsychiatrist says, "AD starts in a very specific part of the brain that has to do with smell." This is the entorhinal cortex.

The entorhinal cortex is the main interface between the hippocampus, a seahorse-shaped neural structure, and the neocortex, which is the outermost layer of your cerebral cortex. Rabins calls the hippocampus, which is beneath the cerebral cortex, "the center for new memory." Although neuroscientists always refer to the hippocampus in the singular, your brain has two hippocampi, one in each cerebral hemisphere. They play a role in spatial navigation and, if damaged, can cause disorientation.

"When you have Alzheimer's disease," Rabins points out, "you never feel like you're in a familiar place." You cannot connect your perceptions with your memories.

My mother lost her sense of smell (olfaction) years ago. I'm not sure when, but it was after her ehrlichiosis infection (age 78) and before her compression fracture and dehydration (age 85). Hyposmia, or smell deficiency, begins early in the course of AD, often many years before other symptoms arise, according to Rabins, who recommends a sniff test as part of the diagnostic process.

Scientists have identified two forms of Alzheimer's disease. The nongenetic or sporadic form accounts for 98 to 99 percent of all cases and can be diagnosed *definitively* only at autopsy by a microscopic examination of the deceased patient's brain. The telltale signs of AD evident in autopsied brain tissue are amyloid plaques and neurofibrillary tangles, which you may think of as abnormal brain deposits derived from proteins.

Clearly inherited or familial AD accounts for the remaining 1 to 2 percent of cases and often begins between ages 45 and 65. Accurate tests exist to determine whether a person has inherited any of the gene abnormalities that cause genetic AD.

Researchers do not know if the plaques and tangles cause sporadic AD or are simply a byproduct of some other cause, but for 20 years the amyloid hypothesis of AD has held currency. It posits that AD is triggered by the production, aggregation, and deposition of toxic, sticky plaques that contain the protein fragment, beta-amyloid, and lead to the death of brain neurons. Not all researchers believe this theory, however, and it may prove untrue.[28]

Genetics definitely plays a role in at least 30 to 60 percent of all sporadic AD cases, but just how has not been determined.

The presence of an allele called E4 on a normal gene known as apolipoprotein E (APOE) appears to increase by threefold a person's risk of getting Alzheimer's disease by age 75.[29]

Vascular dementia can result from any condition that damages blood vessels and reduces blood flow in the brain, thus depriving this vital organ of oxygen and nutrients and causing cell death. Usually this type of dementia develops after a person suffers a stroke—thus, its former name, multi-infarct (i.e., multi-stroke) dementia—but strokes don't necessarily cause dementia. A stroke's damage depends on its severity and on the area of the brain it affects.

With age come cerebrovascular wear-and-tear and the greater likelihood that vascular dementia will develop—usually not before age 65, but commonly in the 80s and 90s. Vascular changes in the brain can alter mood as well as cognition.[30]

It was only in preparing for this book that I learned Dr. Gideon had listed "arteriosclerotic dementia, uncomplicated" and "cerebral atherosclerosis" among my mother's secondary diagnoses. Despite my father's strenuous objection, he had succeeded in having Mom undergo a brain MRI. I'd had my mother's medical records since that crisis summer, but I'd assumed that Dad had thwarted the brain imaging, so I didn't look for MRI results.

The link between cerebrovascular disease and dementia is not as apparent as you might think. According to Rabins, diagnoses of vascular dementia are accurate only about 50 percent of the time, even "in the best of hands." I would never characterize Gideon's hands as the best.[31]

Lewy body dementia (LBD) is another common dementia, affecting about 1.3 million people in the United States. LBD patients have "tiny spherical deposits of a protein called alpha-synuclein" in their brains, say Johns Hopkins medical authorities. These protein deposits were named for Dr. Frederick Lewy, who identified them in 1912 while working in Dr. Alzheimer's lab. Because of changes in their brain chemistry, LBD patients develop both Alzheimer's-like cognitive problems and Parkinson's disease symptoms, such as muscle rigidity, a blank facial expression, tremors, and poor balance.

Unlike AD patients, people with LBD often have detailed and extremely vivid hallucinations early in their illness. They tend to show marked fluctuations in their cognitive functioning; fall asleep easily during the day; and have restless, disturbed sleep with behavioral acting out. LBD is difficult to diagnose.³²

Other common central-nervous-system conditions that cause progressive deficits in memory suggestive of Alzheimer's dementia include:

- ❖ Parkinson's disease
- ❖ Huntington's disease
- ❖ Subdural hematoma (a brain "bruise")
- ❖ Normal-pressure hydrocephalus
- ❖ Brain tumors

Some non-CNS-associated systemic conditions known to cause dementia are:

- ❖ Hypothyroidism (low thyroid)
- ❖ Vitamin B12, niacin, or folic-acid deficiency
- ❖ HIV infection

Depression also can produce dementia-like symptoms.³³

My Working Knowledge

Because of my earlier studies, I knew that the average Alzheimer's patient lives eight to 10 years after his or her initial diagnosis. Some patients die within three to four years, and others survive 20 years. Johns Hopkins researchers report that one-third of Alzheimer's patients do not decline at all during the first five years; one-third of them decline at a moderate rate; and the remaining one-third decline quickly.³⁴

If my mother has AD, I reasoned, she likely would be able to manage the first early/mild stage of Alzheimer's disease with our help. This stage is characterized by faulty memory of recent events and poor judgment and insight. The second middle/moderate stage and the third late/severe stage would pose tougher challenges.

In the second stage, Alzheimer's patients struggle with expressing themselves verbally and in writing and may be unable to handle simple activities of daily living, having to depend on others, for example, to dress and bathe them. They also may suffer delusions or hallucinations.

By the third stage, AD patients have lost all of their reasoning capacity and cannot assist in their self-care, depending completely on others. Most cannot walk or feed themselves. They develop physical symptoms, such as dysphasia, incontinence, and muteness, and become susceptible to other diseases, especially infections. Pneumonia is the No. 1 killer of AD patients.[35]

Eventually, when I had time, I would read what *DSM* had to say about diagnosing Alzheimer's disease. Until then, I principally relied on the Mayo Clinic's website and the Alzheimer's Assn. for my working knowledge.

A simplified checklist of Alzheimer's disease "signs" provided by the Mayo Clinic online includes:

✓ Memory loss
✓ An inability to learn or remember new information
✓ Difficulties with communicating, and/or planning and organizing, and/or coordination and motor functions
✓ An inability to reason
✓ Paranoia
✓ Agitation
✓ Personality changes [36]

At one of the D.C. Alzheimer's Assn. conferences, I picked up a brochure that I keep by my desk. Titled "Is It Alzheimer's? Ten Warning Signs You Should Know," it expands the Mayo Clinic's seven deficits into 10 and expounds upon them. For example:

❖ "Memory loss: One of the most common early signs of dementia is forgetting recently learned information. While it's normal to forget appointments, names, or telephone numbers, those with dementia will forget such things more often and not remember them later."

❖ "Difficulty performing familiar tasks: People with dementia often find it hard to complete everyday tasks that are so familiar we usually do not stop to think about how to do them. A person with Alzheimer's may not know the steps for preparing a meal, using a household appliance, or participating in a lifelong hobby."

❖ "Misplacing things: Anyone can temporarily misplace a wallet or key. A person with Alzheimer's disease may put things in unusual places: an iron in the freezer or a wristwatch in the sugar bowl."

I can't tell you how many times I've read all of these signs and assured myself that my mother didn't have AD. At least, not *yet*.

MEDICAL INTERVENTION

In January 2010, during Mom's regular six-month checkup, my father finally yielded to my request to ask Dr. Ramses for a referral to what then was known informally as the Memory Clinic at Eastern Virginia Medical School. The proper name is the EVMS Glennan Center for Geriatrics and Gerontology.

Dr. Al had resisted my efforts to have Mom tested because he believed that, even if she had first-stage Alzheimer's disease, she would not benefit much, if at all, from the medications available to treat the disease, and she might suffer loathsome effects.

The lack of treatment available for AD patients, as well as for MCI patients, is a huge problem. Even when effective, the current AD drugs only treat symptoms; they do not prevent or cure the disease.

My father is an expert in drugs that alter the synthesis of neurotransmitters, also known as chemical messengers. The top three Alzheimer's drugs inhibit an enzyme that catalyzes inactivation of the neurotransmitter, acetylcholine, and, in so doing, prevent its degradation. Brain acetylcholine is critical to memory and learning,

This enzyme is cholinesterase, and the AD drugs are called cholinesterase inhibitors, anti-cholinergic drugs, or simply anti-cholinergics. Acetylcholine exerts its chemical effects in the body through receptors that are described as cholinergic because of its action. A receptor is a site on a cell or a synapse that binds with substances such as neurotransmitters, hormones, or drugs. I always think of a receptor as a site of action.

As AD dementia becomes more pronounced, a person's levels of brain acetylcholine drop dramatically. The cholinesterase inhibitors boost these levels.

Other levels of neurotransmitters vital in brain function, including serotonin and norepinephrine, also decline in about half of all AD patients, but none of these neurotransmitters is implicated in the cause of Alzheimer's.

Dad had kept abreast of the clinical data regarding the use of cholinesterase inhibitors in Alzheimer's disease and didn't buy this therapy. He further argued that, even if the drugs had a marginal effect, there was little point in subjecting a then-85-year-old woman, with a limited life expectancy, to such toxic medication.

Clinical trials show that the anti-cholinergic drugs, donepezil (Aricept®), galantamine (Razadyne®), and rivastigmine (Exelon®), surpass placebos at improving symptoms of Alzheimer's dementia in only 15 to 20 percent of the patients who take them. Some doctors believe these drugs slow the disease's progression; other doctors do not.[37]

Unfortunately, the inhibitors can cause gastrointestinal problems, such as severe nausea, vomiting, diarrhea, and muscle cramps. (But when I asked Dr. Rabins about adverse effects in a Q&A after an October 2012 lecture at Johns Hopkins, he expressed little concern. It is the drugs' ineffectiveness, he said, not their unpleasantness, that usually compels people to quit taking them.)

A fourth medication exists for Alzheimer's, but it, too, lacks therapeutic punch, providing symptomatic relief for only some patients. Memantine (Namenda®) works on certain brain-cell receptors, not on acetylcholine. One authority I consulted described memantine as an "add-on" to a cholinesterase inhibitor, not as a solo therapy.[38]

Memantine also can produce GI distress, but, because of its mechanism of action, it typically generates agitation, headaches, confusion, and dizziness.

By early 2010, my friend Beatrice's father had been taking memantine for his early-stage Alzheimer's disease about four years. She did not believe the drug had slowed his cognitive decline, but he continued to take it. Why? Because his doctor prescribed it. In my view, this was futile "at-least-we're-doing-something" medicine, in which doctors commonly engage in order to give themselves purpose and placate patients and their families. "Doing-something" medicine is a major driver of healthcare costs.

The FDA has not approved any medications specifically for MCI therapy; and several placebo-controlled clinical trials of Alzheimer's drugs with MCI patients showed no significant reduction in the development of the dementia.[39]

Of course, if a patient's MCI is attributable to vascular or ischemic changes in the brain, he or she may take medications to control underlying problems, such as high blood pressure and diabetes. Many older people use a class of drugs called statins to lower their blood-cholesterol levels. Your Mom's or Pop's cardiologist would prescribe these meds.

Although I didn't disagree with Dr. Al about the Alzheimer's drugs, his argument frustrated me.

What if, I asked him, by age 88, Mom is in stage-two Alzheimer's, and she can no longer handle her daily grooming and dress? If the available Alzheimer's drugs would slow, even by weeks, the disease's inevitable timeline of deterioration and dependency, why shouldn't she try them? She could always terminate the therapy if the adverse effects proved intolerable.

Besides, Mom seemed interested in medication. Why shouldn't she be given the option to evaluate a drug's benefits and risks, with medical advice, and choose to take it, even though clinical trials, and patient experience, show it's not resoundingly effective? Suppose she could derive a placebo effect from one of the AD drugs? Wouldn't that be worth something?

Dad's approach was to help my mother maintain her current lifestyle as long as possible by keeping her in comfortable and familiar surroundings. But should she become dependent, he had no intention of being her "nursemaid." Remembering what happened with strangers on the yard, you can guess who would bear the responsibility for her care, as well as suffer considerable heartache in arranging it.

"If she ever gets lost driving home," a common problem for AD patients as the disease progresses and they lose their orientation, Dad would say, "we'll have a real problem."

Yes, *we* will.

PREPARING FOR MEMORY CONSULT

Mom's memory consult at EVMS was scheduled for March 8, 2010. In anticipation of it, she underwent a brain CT scan at Kitty Hawk Regional Medical Center. I went with her.

Dad showed me the results of the new images at Regional, but he never shared them with Mom, and she didn't ask. According to the interpreting radiologist, the CT scan revealed "mild cerebral atrophy," "atherosclerotic disease," and probable "microangiopathic disease," which is a narrowing of blood vessels caused by the atherosclerosis.

Although people without dementia of any type can have brain

shrinkage, almost *all* people with Alzheimer's disease have some degree of atrophy. Atherosclerosis, of course, is the primary underlying cause of vascular dementia.

My father fell and broke his hip after Mom had her CT scan, but before her Memory Clinic appointment.You might suppose that my mother canceled her memory evaluation, and you would be correct. But she canceled it on Jan. 25, the day of her CT scan—a full month before Dad's hip fracture. Why?

No doubt she disliked having her brain probed. But she also took one look at the cumbersome, unnecessarily detailed, multi-page questionnaire that EVMS sent for her to fill out before her appointment and said, "No way." And, besides, "my memory is not that bad." She tossed aside the paperwork and called EVMS to cancel. Needless to say, she never had a follow-up MRI.

The mother I have known all of my life would never have made such an impulsive call, nor acted so petulantly. Her personality had changed. She now got irritable, which was never the case before. She even told my father to "shut up"—language she never would have used, even in exasperation. I also noticed, sadly, that she didn't laugh as much. Her sense of humor had dimmed.

Nonetheless, I found it difficult to fault her disgust. Is it really that arduous a task for a geriatric neurologist or psychiatrist to interview a patient and just listen to her?

The prospect of a memory "consultation" understandably provokes anxiety and fear in people who already are worried about their forgetfulness. Why compound the stress, and risk alienation and distrust, by subjecting possible dementia patients and their families to rigorous advance questioning? We all know that these same questions will be covered later, again and again, in the doctor's office, and that doctors don't necessarily read patient forms.

The Memory Clinic physicians' failure to address my mother personally in their correspondence also alienated me. The signature on one form letter, which explained the purpose of the consult and instructed Mom to order all of her medical records, read "Sincerely, Memory Consultation Clinic," under which one M.D.'s name had been whited out and another's printed.

I didn't know the Ford Motor Co. was graduating doctors.

The Glennan Center asked Mom, or a family member, to submit a list of her medications, supplements, and allergies (this is standard), and to complete a five-page "Health History Form" and a one-page "Geriatric History Form."

Geriatric history? I'd like to meet the 35-year-old numbskull who came up with that clinical-speak title for a patient form. If there's any word that's guaranteed to elicit a negative response from an older person, it's geriatric. The frequent use of "geriatric" or "geriatrics" is another example of the insensitivity and cluelessness that too often characterize communications between physicians and their older patients.

The first question on this form was: "How long ago did family/ friends first notice memory problems?" That's a fair and important question, but it's better elicited in a more respectful and compassionate manner, such as "Please jot down the concerns you have about your or your loved one's memory. When did you first notice problems?"

As for EVMS's Health History Form, consider page three, which is devoted to "Safety." It consists of a series of yes-no questions under five red-alert, in-your-face categories: driving, fire safety [!], drugs, wandering [!], and accidents. None of the categories is preceded by an introductory phrase such as, "Do you ever find yourself . . .," or a qualifying question such as, "Are any of the following of concern to you?"

How do you suppose a cognitively impaired person who is clinging to her independence would answer the following truncated questions in the driving section?:

* Going too fast?
* Needing navigator?
* Accidents?
* Failure to observe signals?
* Going too slow [sic]?
* Getting lost?
* Violations?
* Changing lanes frequently?

I could predict my mother's responses: No . . . no . . . no . . . no, etc., etc. Yes-no. Demented-not demented. Give me a break.

Although discouraged by Mom's rejection of the Memory Clinic, I understood how she felt and didn't argue with her. I didn't want to overrule her self-determination or cause her emotional distress.

Further, I now doubted EVMS's assembly-line memory doctors, as well as Dr. Ramses, who never followed up on his referral. If the latter supposed that my father would bring it up at Mom's next appointment, he didn't know Dr. Al very well. In any case, Dad wasn't his patient; Mom was. He let her down.

I needed to do more homework. I had to read the *DSM*.

DSM SYMPTOMS OF DEMENTIA

DSM-IV defines dementia generally as "the development of multiple cognitive deficits that **include memory impairment** and at least one of the following cognitive disturbances," all of which reflect damage to the cerebral cortex:

- ❖ Aphasia;
- ❖ Apraxia;
- ❖ Agnosia; or
- ❖ A disturbance in executive functioning. [40]

According to the *DSM-IV*, therefore, memory impairment is the *sine qua non* symptom of *all* dementias, including AD. Without it, dementia cannot be diagnosed. Such impairment could be in your Mom's ability to learn new material or her ability to recall previously learned material.

Aphasia is a deterioration of *language*, both in articulation and comprehension. People with aphasia often have an abnormal difficulty in coming up with the names of familiar people and objects, such as a spoon, and may speak in a vague or empty fashion, excessively using indefinite terms, such as "thing" or "it." They may be unable to comprehend either or both spoken and written language and unable to repeat language that they've just heard.

Apraxia is an impaired ability to execute the *motor functions* required for a task, even though the person has intact motor and sensory abilities and comprehends the task. People with apraxia have difficulty pantomiming the use of objects, such as a comb, or executing known motor acts, such as waving goodbye. They may lose the ability to bathe or dress or perform other familiar activities.

Agnosia is a failure to *recognize or identify* objects, using sensory functions, even though these functions are intact. People with agnosia have normal tactile sensation (touch), but they cannot identify objects placed in their hands. They also may be unable to recognize family members or their own reflections in a mirror.

It is far more likely that you will first notice problems with executive functions. Common tests for deficits in these high-order mental abilities include asking the patient to count to 10, to recite the alphabet, to name as many animals as possible in one minute, and to subtract serial 7s, backwards, starting with 100: 100, 93, 86, etc.[41]

To establish dementia, *DSM-IV* further specifies that the cognitive deficit(s) must be "sufficiently severe to cause impairment in occupational or social functioning and represent a decline from a previously higher level of functioning."[42] *DSM-IV* differentiates dementias by type, one of which is the Alzheimer's type.

DSM-5 eliminates the requirement of a memory disturbance in *every* case of major neurocognitive disorder and reduces the emphasis on the cortical abnormalities. It is consciously less AD-centric, describing the cognitive domains (complex attention, language, learning and memory, executive function, etc.) in which impairment commonly occurs and then subtyping disorders as being "due to" Alzheimer's or another disease or cause.[43]

A diagnosis of Alzheimer's-associated major neurocognitive disorder requires prominent memory impairment, as it did in *DSM-IV*, and deficits in at least one other cognitive domain.[44] I otherwise leave the new *DSM* "fine print" to the experts.[45] Regardless of whether you apply the *DSM-IV* or *DSM-5* approach, independence continues to be key to assessing impairment.

When I heard him lecture at Johns Hopkins, Dr. Rabins used the term, dementia, not major neurocognitive disorder, and summarized the stages of Alzheimer's disease as:

1) Memory decline [typically with executive-function impairment]
2) Cortical symptom phase [aphasia, apraxia, and agnosia]
3) Physical decline

Contrary to the popular belief that if you are aware of your memory loss, then you don't have Alzheimer's, "two-thirds of AD patients," he said, "never know they are ill, and one-third are painfully aware." One-third of patients in the first stage, he further noted, undergo a personality change.

As for vascular dementia, *DSM-IV* requires a diagnosis to be based on evidence of cerebrovascular disease that a physician judges to be etiologically related to the patient's cognitive disturbances. This evidence may consist of "focal neurological signs and symptoms," such as abnormalities in a person's gait or weakness in one of his extremities, or of laboratory results.[46]

DSM-5 refers to a major or mild vascular neurocognitive disorder, the clinical features for which are "consistent with vascular etiology," as suggested by an onset of deficits *temporally* related to a cerebrovascular event, such as a stroke, or by a prominent decline in complex attention and frontal-executive function.[47]

DIAGNOSING ALZHEIMER'S

Before diagnosing Alzheimer's disease, Dr. Rabins advises, a physician must establish that *there is no other cause for the patient's cognitive deficits.* AD is considered a diagnosis of exclusion. The physician, therefore, engages in a process of elimination, the extent of which naturally depends upon his or her expertise.[48]

Only two types of laboratory tests, known as ADmark Assays, currently exist that *may* assist in the diagnosis of Alzheimer's disease or in its prediction.

One test identifies the variation of the APOE gene carried by the patient, and, therefore, assesses the *probability* that a person's dementia is due to AD. As noted, the presence of the E4 allele on this gene is associated with an increased risk of developing Alzheimer's. The test, therefore, is not definitive.

The other assay measures beta-amyloid and tau protein in cerebrospinal fluid (CSF) and requires a physician to perform a lumbar puncture on your Mom's or Pop's back to withdraw a sampling. A low level of beta-amyloid and an elevated level of tau in the CSF, which surrounds the spinal cord and brain, have been associated with the development of AD dementia.

Both ADmark Assays lack reliability and accuracy and are not routinely recommended by diagnostic physicians, but that may change in the next decade.

Much of the recent AD and MCI research has been directed toward identifying biomarkers, which are indicators *in vivo* (in the body), that might enable scientists to establish the presence or absence of AD's neurodegenerative pathology and/or to predict a person's risk of developing the disease later. A CSF biomarker that would suggest the level of beta-amyloid accumulation in the brain would be very useful indeed.[49]

There also currently exist specialized imaging techniques that can reveal information about the structure, function, and biological changes of areas of the brain affected by Alzheimer's disease. A type of PET imaging can detect beta-amyloid content, for example, and so-called quantitative MRI can measure hippocampal volumetry, and thus, the amount of atrophy that this vital memory center has undergone.

I leave this promising area of research to the high-tech scientists. So, far, the benefit of these techniques remains unproven.[50]

Dr. Rabins's own diagnostic process consists of gathering information on the patient's history, administering neuropsychological exams to her/him, and interviewing the patient, family members, and friends over a period of weeks.

Even though only an autopsy can confirm the disease, "Diagnoses based on this type of clinical information," he writes, "are accurate about 90 percent of the time."[51]

AD specialists have at their disposal numerous standardized mental-status tests, which separately target various aspects of memory and other cognitive functioning.

You may have heard of the Mini-Mental State Examination (MMSE®), a 10-minute test developed by Johns Hopkins neuro-psychiatrists 40 years ago to evaluate a person's cognitive status.[52]

The first five questions of the MMSE address orientation to time, posing: What is the year? Season? Date? Day of the week? Month?

The next five focus on place: Where are we now: State? County? Town/city? Hospital? Floor?

Succeeding questions test the patient's registration, which is a memory function gauged by asking your Mom to repeat numbers or words immediately after she hears them; attention and arithmetic calculation; recall; language; and repetition. Executive functioning is not addressed, *per se*, but the last question involves a complex command: copying a picture that depicts two pentagons intersecting.

A patient score of 24 or lower out of 30 possible points is considered evidence of impairment, with nine or below signifying severe impairment. Our favorite psychiatrist, Dr. Gideon, obtained a score of 23 from my mother when she was hospitalized at Duke—not bad for someone with encephalitis.

Many experts today believe the test lacks sensitivity for early impairment, especially in well-educated and/or highly intelligent people, like my mother.53 Their crystallized intelligence and their cognitive reserve enable them to perform well, despite their deficits.

Besides the MMSE, a physician may use other quickie cognitive assessments, including:

❖   The clock-drawing test: The patient must draw a clock with all of the numbers represented and the hands pointing to a specific time of day. The more distorted and inaccurate the drawing is, the more likely the patient is to have dementia.

❖   The change-making test: The patient must count out a dollar's worth of change from three quarters, seven dimes, and seven nickels, within three minutes. He or she is allowed two attempts to complete this simple math task.

❖   The category fluency test: The patient must name all of the animals he or she can think of in one minute. Fewer than 15 suggests a cognitive problem.54

Although it may appear to some families that certain tests discriminate against mathematically-"challenged" patients or those who habitually lose track of the date, neurologists and geriatric psychiatrists take such factors into consideration. No one makes a diagnosis of Alzheimer's disease lightly.

Beware the primary-care physician who attaches the Alzheimer's label to an older confused and memory-impaired patient without doing the requisite investigation. In fact, when it comes to dementia, beware the primary-care physician, period. Consult a specialist.

SOUNDING THE ALARM

After my father's hip fracture, Mom's vertebral break, her dehydration, and subsequent hospitalization—in other words, after the s--- hit the fan—I found it easy to back off from the memory consult. But I still thought about it.

On April 27, 2010, two weeks after my mother's discharge from the Sentara nursing-home hellhole, I was scheduled to attend a lecture on Alzheimer's disease at Georgetown.

The week before, I had taken Mom to an appointment with her cardiologist, Dr. Anthony, and Britt had accompanied Dad to his last follow-up appointment with Dr. Faber, the orthopod. Anthony referred Mom to the vascular surgeon, who diagnosed the peripheral valve defect I mentioned earlier and added compression stockings to her daily wardrobe. Dad was cleared for driving on his own. We were making progress.

Mom called me on my cell phone during my drive to Washington and asked about my itinerary, which I had written on her wall calendar.

My trip covered about three days and four nights of activities in two different locations, so it wasn't actually straightforward, but no matter how many times (four-five) I repeated it, Mom couldn't follow my explanation. It wasn't that she didn't understand what I would be doing; it was more that she couldn't put the pieces together into a whole picture—or hold them all in her brain. I was alarmed.

Should I advocate again within my family for an evaluation?

After his lecture that night, I approached Dr. R. Scott Turner, director of the Georgetown University Memory Disorders Program, and told him about the disturbing phone call. He encouraged me to bring Mom to Georgetown for an evaluation and CT scan (I didn't mention her earlier X-rays) and expressed confidence in the ability of the cholinesterase inhibitors to slow down the progression of Alzheimer's disease so as to benefit a patient of my mother's age, if, indeed, AD was her diagnosis.

Later I would learn that Dr. Turner had run afoul of one of "Finucane's laws," promulgated by Dr. Thomas E. Finucane of the Division of Geriatric Medicine and Gerontology at the Johns Hopkins Bayview Care Center. Finucane's fourth law is: "If a professor pronounces enthusiastically in favor of Alzheimer's drugs, then, number one, that person doesn't take care of patients as a primary care physician. Number two, that person receives emoluments [fees, perks] from the drug companies."

Most patients who take the cholinesterase inhibitors and/or memantine, according to Finucane, can't tell the difference from placebo, and neither can their families and caregivers.

"I told you so," my father said when I passed this information along to him. "I know!" I responded.55 But I still wanted to try.

I discussed the Georgetown evaluation with Leslie, Al, and Britt, whose Alexandria home would serve as a base, and they all endorsed it. No one denied Mom's cognitive problems now. I also asked my mother, and she seemed amenable, too. My father disapproved, but agreed not to stand in our way. I would have followed through on the appointment if I lived in the Washington area, but, instead, I allowed hardship to defeat me. I needed hands-on help. Just getting Mom packed, transported, and settled in Alexandria seemed overwhelming. Even Britt's townhouse condo, with its four flights of stairs, presented an obstacle.

Six months later, in October, I felt a chill go through me when I listened to a voice message left by Mom on my home answering machine.

"Where *are* you?" she asked plaintively. "Is Oliver here?"

I used to leave my cat Oliver with my parents when I went out of town, and I had dropped him off that morning, while my mother, unexpectedly, was out. The previous night I had checked in personally with her, told her the time I would be stopping by, and written my itinerary on her calendar. She had forgotten everything and been bewildered when she saw cat food in her refrigerator.

A YEAR LATER

In May 2011, Mom, now 87, again complained about how bad her memory was. Extended family had visited that month, so she had more people with whom to interact and more situations in which to trip up. I asked her if she wanted another referral to the EVMS Glennan Center for Geriatrics and Gerontology, reminding her of how she had disposed of the last.

"I didn't think my memory was bad then," she replied, but I could tell that she didn't remember the appointment.

I also offered to call the Glennan Center, which I knew had a new director, and to assist her in every step of the application and evaluation process. I would help her to fill out the damn questionnaire or do it myself. Mom seemed prepared to go forward, but in time she lost interest and became anxious whenever I brought up the subject. I settled for her seeing Dr. Ramses at the end of July, even though he had dropped the ball before. I insisted that she talk alone with her primary-care physician, instead of having my father remain in the examining room and talk for her.

It took me weeks to convince Dad to step out; he wouldn't even consider letting me accompany Mom in his place. He viewed my advocacy as interference. I think I threatened the psychological status quo in his marriage, as well as his everyday life. I was stepping on my parents' shared intimacy. Maybe Dad, too, was using denial to cope.

About three weeks before her appointment with Ramses, I found myself alone with Mom at my house and seized the opportunity to test her memory. Previously she had "passed" my informal serial-7 counting test, a test of executive function, by counting hesitantly backward by sevens from 100. I had been eager to give her the Mini-Mental State Examination that I had picked up at Georgetown.

Amazingly, Mom aced the MMSE. She scored 30 out of 30.

But she couldn't tell me a lick about the "Masterpiece Mystery!" show we had watched the previous night on TV.

I had not learned yet about cognitive reserve, but I intuitively understood that Mom had drawn on her superior intellect and education to blow away the MMSE.

Despite her perfect score, Mom didn't want to talk about her memory loss. She pointedly told me that she did not want to be reminded of it ever again. I agreed.

Later Mom confided her concern to Dr. Ramses, but he told her that she was doing fine and not to worry. According to my father, the internist could see no change in Mom's mental status since her checkup six months before.

Was Ramses playing the age card? Was he head-in-the-sand oblivious? Or was he just too busy to be bothered with a wheel that didn't squeak loudly?

Later I read that, according to psychiatrist Constantine G. Lyketsos, director of the Johns Hopkins Memory and Alzheimer's Treatment Center, primary-care physicians miss two-thirds of the Alzheimer's cases they see.[56]

Two-thirds. That's Alzheimer's, *dementia*. Not its precursor, MCI.
What's a daughter to do?

One thing I was committed to doing was to minimize the distress that my mother felt. As much as I wanted to procure medical relief for her, I knew Mom couldn't just take a pill and be all better. So I sought instead to comfort her. I did not want her to lose her peace of mind or any sleep over anxiety, nor did I want her to struggle with depression. Since her cognitive status changed, she had been depressed.

GETTING THE FAQ

Not long after I gave Mom the Mini-Mental State Examination, I came across the well-known Functional Activities Questionnaire, aka the "FAQ," that family members and caregivers can use to evaluate the cognitive status of a loved one. I rated my mother's ability to perform 10 complex, higher-order tasks on a scale of zero to three, as follows:

- ❖ Zero signifies "normal" or "never did the activity but could do it now";
- ❖ One represents "has difficulty, but does by self" or "never did the activity and would have difficulty doing it now";
- ❖ Two signifies "requires assistance"; and
- ❖ Three means "dependent"

The activities were:

- ❖ Writing checks, paying bills, and keeping financial records;
- ❖ Assembling tax records and making out business and insurance papers;
- ❖ Shopping alone for clothes, household necessities, or groceries;
- ❖ Playing a game of skill (e.g., bridge or chess) or working on a hobby;
- ❖ Heating water for a cup of coffee or tea and turning off the stove;
- ❖ Preparing a balanced meal;
- ❖ Keeping track of current events;
- ❖ Paying attention to and understanding a television show, book, or magazine;
- ❖ Remembering appointments, family occasions, and medications; and
- ❖ Traveling out of the neighborhood (e.g., driving or arranging to take buses)

I tallied nine points for Mom. I didn't give her any threes—

in part because she has never prepared a tax return or handled insurance papers— but I assigned two twos, on paying attention to and understanding a TV show or book and remembering appointments, family occasions, and medications. This was July 2011.

While many neuropsychiatric experts regard nine points as the cutoff for impairment, the Mayo Clinic's Petersen says people with mild cognitive impairment usually score around a four and those with mild dementia may score from 10 to 13.[57]

I was able to put Mom's score into perspective when I gave my friend Kathy the FAQ in order to evaluate her mother, who then lived alone with daytime assistance from a young, untrained, and not-very-astute caregiver. One of Kathy's three brothers lived nearby and checked on her occasionally, but she did not receive daily family care.

Kathy said her mother, who was in her early 80s, couldn't manage any of the functional activities. None. She couldn't remember something she'd heard just 10 minutes before. She had forgotten how to operate a simple room thermostat. When she "packed" for an out-of-town wedding, she brought sneakers to wear with a very old dress.

Her mother acts "more like a child and fixates on the dog," Kathy said. Fixates, but then forgets to feed him.

Soon after this assessment, Kathy and her brothers arranged for their mother to visit a small church-associated assisted-living facility in the Midwest, halfway across the country from her longtime New Jersey home. The brother who had been looking out for her no longer could, and the siblings, all of modest means, decided to move her as close as possible to a brother who could.

Their mother did not fare well in her new environment, becoming more frail, agitated, and argumentative. When Kathy visited her, she often did not recognize her daughter and had little interest in her staying. She clung to the dog that Kathy's brother brought for visits.

The four adult children had their mother evaluated by a neurologist. His diagnosis came as no surprise: Alzheimer's disease, well into the second stage.

Within less than a year after her move, Kathy's mother fell and fractured her hip, an injury that never healed. She died of pneumonia, letting go of life only after she knew that all four of her children were at her bedside.

Chapter Nine

2010-11: A Plumbing
NIGHTMARE

The High Price of Botched Repair

The memory-clinic rejection, the falls, the fractures, the dehydration, the nursing-home revolt . . . they consumed just the first half of a truly hideous year for my parents and me. Just like "The Godfather's" Michael Corleone, whenever I thought I was out, "they" pulled me back in.

During the summer Dad intimated that my brother would help him in September with a "male problem" he was having. I figured it had to be benign prostatic hyperplasia (aka hypertrophy), or "BPH," which is the medical term for what we laypeople call an enlarged prostate. Dad hinted at surgery. I offered to be his advocate, but he declined, insisting on his privacy and autonomy. Having had my fill of Difficult Patient Syndrome, I didn't argue.

Besides, I reasoned, Dr. Al is on top of things. He knows the potentially life-threatening problems prostatic hyperplasia can cause. He rescued his own father.

Grandpa had such severe BPH-induced urinary obstruction at age 80 that his kidneys shut down. He went into uremia, a toxic condition created by the backup of urinary waste products. A prostatectomy to remove the cell overgrowth interfering with his bladder's outlet saved his life. This was in 1981, before the development of drugs to treat the symptoms associated with BPH—one of which I knew Dad had been taking—and before most of today's surgical treatments.

My brother didn't insist that our father schedule his prostate surgery during his Outer Banks vacation or even investigate the status of Dad's "problem" when he was visiting. Al left everything up to Dad, who seemed prepared to delay the inevitable as long as he physically could.

Just when I thought the year couldn't get any worse, Dad's urine flow shut down, my brother was long gone, and there we were again, in crisis.

How could *this* have happened?

Although Dad had known for months that "something was wrong," as he recalled, his total bladder outlet obstruction (aka BOO)—a term that I learned much later—"came on suddenly." He could not void (urinate). On Oct. 19, 2010, he had to be catheterized—immediately.

By then, he says, he had been "waiting weeks" for his urologist, Dr. Naylor, an Outer Banks part-timer, to schedule BPH laser surgery. During this wait, Dad's urinary flow had trickled off so that his final pre-catheter stream could best be described (and generously) as a dribble.

Estimates of how much urine a human bladder can hold vary, with some sources saying from 600 to 800 milliliters and others citing a maximum for a distended bladder of 1000-1200 mL, which is more than a quart. (Of course, it depends on the size of the bladder, but I was surprised to find such a variance among my sources.) The nurse who catheterized my father drained 800 mL of urine from his bladder, "two days' worth," said Dr. Al. A normal retention is about 300 mL.

From Oct. 19 until Nov. 11, 2010, when Dr. Naylor finally operated, Dad's urine drained into a Foley catheter, a thin sterile tube inserted into his bladder, via the penile opening and urethra, which is the channel through which urine flows from the bladder, and secured there by an inflatable balloon. The catheter emptied the urine into a clear bag strapped to Dad's leg. This plumbing work-around would seem to be indignity and discomfort enough for my 86-year-old father to bear, but it was only the beginning.

WARNING: Your Pop needs to be very circumspect when deciding whom he will trust with his plumbing. Urologists are not created equal.

Until January 2013, when I obtained my father's medical records from Dr. Naylor's office—in order to write this chapter—I did not know that Dad first consulted him Nov. 3, 2009, nor did my father remember. I thought his initial appointment was in early May 2010, after he had recovered sufficiently from his hip fracture.

Thus, it was nearly a year after Dr. Naylor first prescribed BPH medication for Dad, not just five-and-a-half months, that he experienced a total bladder obstruction.

In hindsight, with the advantage of these records, I question how Naylor treated my father, and I will address some of his decisions later in this chapter.

In the long dreadful months that were to come, I would often hear Dad say: "You were right. I screwed up. I made nothing but mistakes."

I wish I could disagree.

THE PROSTATE

The prostate sits directly beneath a man's bladder and in front of his rectum—close enough to the anus for a urologist to feel some of its mass during a digital rectal exam, also known as a DRE. (Abbreviations and acronyms abound in urology.) Chiefly composed of glandular and smooth-muscular tissue, a normal prostate is the size and shape of a walnut.

As a man ages, a nonmalignant proliferation of certain prostatic cells often occurs, resulting in benign prostatic hyperplasia. When so enlarged, the size of the prostate may suggest a lime, a lemon, or even an orange. Such overgrowth is not cancer.

The prostate surrounds the top of the urethra, much like a doughnut with a hole in it. It is not part of the urinary system, however. The prostate serves the male reproductive function, most significantly, by producing and pumping into the urethra a milky, alkaline fluid that combines with sperm from the testes and fluids from other glands to make semen, which a man ejaculates during orgasm.

For years, my father had been diligent about seeing Dr. Evans, another part-time Outer Banks urologist, for regular checkups. I had kept up with Dad's prostatic health during this time and knew that his PSA blood levels had always been below 2.0 ng/mL. I also knew, as Dr. Al would remind me: "Every man age 80 and over has cancer of the prostate, some malignant cells, but they don't do anything."

Case in point: Grandpa had widespread metastasized prostate cancer when he died 16 years after his BPH surgery, but the cancer didn't kill him.

PSA stands for prostate-specific antigen, an enzyme produced by the prostate and secreted during ejaculation into ducts that empty into the urethra. Usually, only tiny amounts of PSA are present in the blood, but abnormalities of the prostate can create an opening for more to pass. Since its FDA approval in 1994, urologists have used a blood test for PSA to screen for evidence of prostate cancer.

PSA is measured by nanograms (ng) per milliliter of blood, a nanogram being a billionth of a gram. High blood levels of PSA may indicate problems, such as cancer, BPH, infections, and other conditions—or they may not.[1] The PSA marker is not cancer-specific: Many false-positives occur, as do false negatives. A PSA blood level below 4.0 ng/mL, is usually no cause for concern, but a man with prostate cancer may test low.[2] Because of these and other problems associated with it, the U.S. Preventive Services Task Force (USPSTF) recommended in 2012 that the PSA test not be used *routinely* for cancer screening. (See Appendix Four, "The PSA-Test Controversy.")

U.S. men have a 17 percent chance of being diagnosed with prostate cancer during their lifetimes, but only a 3 percent chance of dying from it. Most prostate cancers grow slowly and need not (depending on the circumstances, *should* not) be treated with surgery, intensive radiation, and other interventions that can cause urinary incontinence, erectile dysfunction (ED), bowel damage, and other serious harm.[3]

Upon retiring in 2006, Dr. Evans advised my father, "At your age [82], you have nothing to worry about," and recommended discontinuing PSA testing. Dad, therefore, was without a urologist when, more than three years later, he started having a weak urinary stream and other bothersome symptoms.

UROLOGY 101

In 2010, I had a decent understanding of prostate and urinary-system basics. Since then, I've studied up. Perhaps my homework will save you some time in your own Pop crisis.

The human urinary system has two tracts: the upper and the lower. The upper urinary tract (UT) consists of your two kidneys and their ureters, the long ducts through which the urine produced by your kidneys flows into your bladder. The lower urinary tract (LUT) consists of your bladder, your urethra, and other parts that handle urine storage and elimination.[4] Urologists refer to lower urinary tract symptoms, such as Dad's reduced stream or an "overactive" bladder (urge incontinence), as LUTS.

Urine normally flows continuously through your ureters to your bladder at a rate of about 1 mL per minute. Peristalsis (regular waves of smooth-muscle contractions) in the ureters produces the force that compels the kidney-to-bladder urine flow.

Your bladder is muscular and hollow. When it fills with urine, its walls stretch, compressing the ureteral openings. With this expansion, mechanoreceptors within the walls transmit increasing numbers of sensory impulses to the sacral region of your spinal cord. As a result (I'm skipping the neurological details), once your bladder has stored a few hundred milliliters of urine, its walls activate a reflex that causes it to release most of your urine into your urethra.

The motor function responsible for this expulsion is known as detrusor contractility because the detrusor muscle, which is the thick middle layer of the bladder's three layers, contracts. Detrusor contractility is essentially an involuntary push downward. When bladder contractility is uninhibited, detrusor overactivity occurs, and you void too frequently. Conversely, low detrusor function can result in insufficient bladder emptying.

Before your bladder can empty, your internal urethral sphincter must open. This sphincter, which acts involuntarily, is the result of thickened smooth muscle of the bladder that surrounds the urethra at the junction where the two connect, also called the bladder neck. As the bladder fills, its shape changes from an inverted pyramid to a sphere. During bladder emptying, aka micturition, the bladder's detrusor contraction and its stretched shape pull the internal sphincter open so that urine passes into the urethra.

Your external urethral sphincter is quite different. Made of skeletal muscle and located in the pelvic floor, which is the supportive area beneath your pelvis, this sphincter surrounds the muscular, tubelike urethra and acts voluntarily—meaning, you exercise control over it. In order to void, you must consciously relax your external sphincter. To hold your urine, and, thus, keep your urethra closed against strong bladder contractions, you consciously constrict it. Eventually, if you ignore "nature's call" too long, your bladder will overpower your resistance.

Some experts argue that the concept of internal and external sphincters is anatomically imprecise. They say the sphincter mechanism is "more accurately divided into factors intrinsic and extrinsic to the urethra itself."[5] Regardless of how you view sphincter control, it is critical to your urinary system and your quality of life, as my father unfortunately would discover.

In men, the 8-inch-long urethra extends to the end of the penis, where it opens to the outside. In women, a much-shorter urethra–only about an inch and a half–opens into the vestibule anterior to the vaginal opening.

The male urethra is divided into three parts. The only one that concerns me here is the uppermost, the prostatic urethra, which passes through the prostate. Because of its location and the age-related pathological changes it may undergo, the prostate can cause a myriad of urinary problems.

BPH AND THE FACTS OF LUTS

Benign prostatic hyperplasia may or may not produce LUTS. When it does, it's called clinical BPH. Prostatic cell overgrowth that does not cause symptoms–so a man is unaware of the change–is known as histologic BPH.

Histologic BPH is present in about 8 percent of all men age 31 to 40; 25 percent of men age 41 to 50; 50 percent of men age 51 to 60; 70 percent of men age 61 to 70; 80 percent of men age 71 to 80; and 90 percent of men age 81 and older.

Clinical BPH usually does not manifest until men reach their 50s. Its prevalence is: 26 percent of men age 51 to 60; 33 percent of men age 61 to 70; 41 percent of men age 71 to 80; and 46 percent of men age 81 and older.[6]

By age 80, according to Brian R. Matlaga, M.D., M.P.H., of Johns Hopkins's renowned James Buchanan Brady Urological Institute, "some 20 to 30 percent of men experience BPH symptoms severe enough to require some form of treatment."[7]

Anatomically speaking, the prostate is divided into three (or more) lobes and three zones. Urologists agree that the prostate has a central lobe and lobes on either side of the center, usually called the anterior or lateral lobes, left and right, but some break down the gland into more locations. The zone designations refer to tissue function and have more meaning to a pathologist than a urologist.

BPH begins in the transition zone, a small area of the inner prostate. This ring of tissue encircles the uretha. When it grows, it goes inward, toward the prostate's core. Hence, it constricts the bladder's outlet.

In contrast, prostate cancer, says Matlaga, usually starts in the peripheral zone, which accounts for 70 percent of the gland's size. The cancerous cells grow outward from the prostate and rarely produce any symptoms. When cancer "escapes"—when it metastasizes—it attacks nearby bone.[8]

In between these zones is the central zone, which makes up about 25 percent of prostate tissue, contains the ejaculatory ducts that move semen through the urethra, and is rarely associated with disease.

A urologist's DRE can be useful in assessing the shape (are there any irregularities?) and texture (lumps? hardness?) of your Pop's prostate—which may suggest cancer—as well as the size. But the gloved expert finger can only reach the gland's peripheral zone, not the transition zone, so enlargement is difficult to estimate.

The fully developed prostate of a young man weighs about 20 to 25 grams (between 0.71 and 0.88 ounces) and measures about 1.25 inches long. Clinical study data show that when a man's prostate is over 30 to 40 grams, a transrectal ultrasound, a test that uses sound waves to create an image of the prostate, provides a better estimation of its size than a DRE.[9]

An ultrasound also can be used to detect abnormalities in the kidneys or bladder, to determine the amount of residual urine in the bladder, and to detect the presence of bladder stones. The amount of residual urine in the bladder is known as postvoid residual or PVR. During his crisis, my father had repeated ultrasounds to measure his urine retention.

Clinical BPH is distinguished by a progressive development of LUTS that are variable and typically range from:

❖ Nocturia (excessive nighttime urination);
❖ Incomplete bladder emptying (the feeling that the bladder, after voiding, is not empty);
❖ Urinary hesitancy (trouble starting);
❖ Weak urinary stream;
❖ Frequent urination; and
❖ Urinary urgency to . . .
❖ The development of acute urinary retention (bingo!).[10]

Many urologists ask their new LUTS patients to complete a questionnaire designed to evaluate the nature and severity of their symptoms. Created in 1992 by the American Urological Assn. (AUA), the International Prostate Symptom Score (IPSS) enables physicians to rapidly diagnose, track, and treat LUTS. It consists of seven questions that address four obstructive and three storage symptoms

Originally (and alternatively) known as the AUA Symptom Index or AUASI, the IPSS yields a score on a scale of zero to 35, with zero to seven indicating mild symptoms; eight to 19, moderate symptoms; and 20 to 35, severe symptoms.[11]

Generally speaking, patients with mild symptoms do not need treatment; watchful waiting suffices. Moderate symptoms "usually call for some form of treatment," Dr. Matlaga of Johns Hopkins advises, "and severe symptoms indicate that surgery is most likely to be effective."[12]

Obstructive voiding, according to Aruna V. Sarma, Ph.D., and John T. Wei, M.D., of the University of Michigan Medical School's urology department, manifests as "urinary hesitancy, delay in initiating micturition, intermittency [in stream], involuntary interruption of voiding, weak urinary stream, straining to void, a sensation of incomplete emptying, and terminal dribbling." Storage symptoms include "urinary frequency, nocturia, urgency, incontinence, and bladder pain or dysuria [difficult or painful urination]."[13]

I also have seen obstructive symptoms distinguished by whether they indicate voiding or postvoiding dysfunction. Matlaga categorizes LUTS as obstructive or irritative, not obstructive and storage. He adds sexual dysfunction to Sarma and Wei's list of obstructive BPH symptoms and gives as examples of irritative symptoms frequent and urgent need to urinate day and night and leakage of urine before getting to the bathroom.[14]

Although BPH therapy is not one-size-fits-all, both the AUA and the European Association of Urology (EAU) publish guidelines for BPH management based on IPSS scores. These guidelines, as well as the IPSS, are available on the Internet. Check them out.[15] According to David R. Paolone, M.D., a prominent urologist at the University of Wisconsin School of Medicine and Public Health, the "current recommendation" is to use the IPSS.[16]

Regardless of a man's IPSS score, a thorough evaluation of his LUTS should begin with a medical, neurological, and urological history. Bladder dysfunction may be occurring because of bladder cancer, interstitial cystitis (inflamed bladder wall), diabetic neuropathy, or one of numerous other causes. Clinical BPH should not be assumed, and obstructive symptoms do not necessarily signal BOO.[17]

If your Pop ignores his LUTS, as do so many stubborn and/or stoical men (like my Grandpa), who would rather suffer with plumbing deficiencies than see a doctor, he will irreparably harm his bladder.

After months of chronic bladder outlet obstruction, during which the bladder "works against the resistance of the prostate," writes Matlaga, the organ will no longer function properly. Its walls will thicken, thus reducing its capacity to store urine. A "muscle-bound" bladder is elastic and flabby, a deterioration that leads to some of the LUTS.[18]

My father recalls having a weak stream, incomplete emptying, and dribbling—obstructive symptoms; the latter two related to postvoiding— but he also was getting up frequently during the night. Men with BPH-related nocturia may rise to void every hour-and-a-half to two hours. A normal adult should be able to sleep six hours without being awakened by bladder fullness.[19]

NORMAL LUT AGING

If you grew up in mainstream U.S. culture, you may believe that plumbing problems are inevitable with age. Not so. *Being* old doesn't mean your Pop will be getting out of bed repeatedly at night to urinate. Or, in the female case, that your Mom will be rushing to reach the bathroom before she has an "accident."

The following physiological changes occur in the lower urinary tract because of aging:

❖ The bladder becomes less expansive (less stretchy) because of changes in connective and elastic tissues. It stiffens.

❖ Smooth and striated muscle thickness and fiber density in the bladder and the urethra usually diminish, causing weakness.

❖ Urethral length and strength tend to decline in women, because of estrogen loss, just as prostate size increases in most men.

❖ Bladder capacity, contractility, and the ability to postpone voiding *may* decline, because of tissue and muscle changes.

Older people frequently experience impairment in their

neuromuscular detrusor and sphincteric functions, but, according to *Brocklehurst*: "[T]he relative contributions of aging have yet to be disentangled from those of the menopause, pelvic organ prolapse, bladder outlet obstruction, and comorbidities (obesity, cardiovascular insufficiency, dementia, diabetic and other neuropathies)."

Brocklehurst also suggests that age-*associated* pathologies, especially of the central nervous system, may disturb LUT processes more than is currently understood.[20]

Reported clinical studies attest to wide variability of LUT function among elders, so don't let your Mom and Pop presume that they will have toileting problems as they age. But, if they do have symptoms, bear in mind that, as St. Louis University geriatrics professor Julie K. Gammack, M.D., writes: "[M]edications, environmental factors, lifestyle choices, and acute and chronic diseases can contribute to [their] severity and frequency."[21]

Urinary incontinence is definitely not part of normal aging. According to my "Merck Manual of Geriatrics": "Urinary incontinence is abnormal regardless of age, mobility, mental status, or frailty."[22]

Incontinence–the inability to control leakage of urine–can be categorized by duration of symptoms, by clinical presentation, or by physiologic abnormality. Urge incontinence, for example, which is characterized by a frequent, sudden urge to void along with little control of the bladder, may be a symptom of a urinary infection or may result from injury, illness, or surgery.[23]

Even the stress incontinence that many elders, particularly women, experience when they cough, sneeze, lift heavy objects, or otherwise put stress on their bladders, is abnormal. Such leakage, also known as outlet incompetence, occurs because of laxity and poor function in the pelvic-floor muscles that support the bladder or control the release of urine and can be treated.

Vaginal childbirth can result in tissue and/or nerve damage that diminishes a woman's pelvic muscular control. Your Mom's bladder may drop. Not surprisingly, multiple vaginal deliveries are associated with a higher risk of stress incontinence, but so is obesity, a condition of many older women. Excess weight unquestionably increases pressure on the bladder.[24]

If you have a Mom or Pop with continence issues, you need to take her or him to a urologist who specializes in female or male incontinence, respectively.

While there's no denying that the *prevalence* of overactive bladder, nocturia, incomplete emptying, frequent or urgent urination, and other LUTS, among both men and women, increases with age, the answer to why this is so depends on more factors than merely age. Every body is different. In general, the more physically fit your parents are, the more fit their lower urinary tracts will be.

So don't let TV ads for Depends® or ignorant and tasteless jokes about old people in diapers psyche you out or dumb you down.

COUNTDOWN TO DISASTER

One of my father's golf buddies referred him to Dr. Naylor, who was, then, the only urologist on the Outer Banks. Naylor traveled to the beach from Edenton, N.C., 90 minutes away, to see patients every two weeks. The golf buddy swore by the good-ole-doc, who had treated him for prostate cancer, but Dr. Al never got along with him.

Although Dad grew up on a Midwestern farm and likes to mix it up with "the boys," he talks a different talk away from the golf course. He and Naylor never clicked. "He was hostile toward me from the beginning," he says.

Apparently it did not help their relationship that Dr. Al had studied under Dr. Charles Brenton Huggins (1901-97) at the University of Chicago and told Naylor so. "Charlie" Huggins, a prostate-cancer pioneer, is the only urologist to receive the Nobel Prize for Physiology or Medicine.

In the 1940s, Huggins, a Canada-born U.S. physician and researcher, discovered that cancerous, as well as normal, cells of the prostate depend on the male sex hormone, testosterone, and its active metabolite, dihydrotestosterone (DHT). DHT, a potent androgen, stimulates prostate cell growth.[25]

"Huggins was the first to show a hormonal relationship to cancer," says Dr. Al.

While I know my father can be demanding, and his background can intimidate doctors who are not secure in their own expertise, he generally glad-hands with fellow physicians. He reaches out to them, trying to connect. Remember the Physician Shuffle? He loves to schmooze. Dr. Naylor did not. When I finally met him, I thought he seemed pained to be in the same room with Dad.

Naylor called Dad, Big Guy, which was what one of the local

veterinarians, who bore a resemblance to the beefy urologist, called my mother's Shih Tzu.

"I guess I overwhelmed him," the Big Guy ruefully reflects.

Dr. Al also had difficulties with Naylor's supporting cast. The nurse who checked Dad's bladder-retention level during appointments and also catheterized him treated him brusquely—rudely and impatiently, he says. When I learned this, I was livid, but I couldn't convince my father to see another physician.

Too late, he said. "I'm not going out of town."

When a man's prostate is cancerous, a surgeon may excise the entire gland in a radical prostatectomy. The goal of a BPH prostatectomy is to remove only the tissue that is obstructing the bladder.

In the days before my father's prostatectomy, I tried to learn more about it. Dad told me that a laser would be used; that he would be hospitalized overnight; and that he would be able to void on his own within 24 hours after the procedure. He didn't know any more than that, and he didn't want to talk about it. He trusted Dr. Naylor, who had given him an instructional DVD to view (on June 15), but Dr. Al wasn't watching any DVD. He was doing whatever Naylor told him to do, Ann. That's enough. End of story.

I didn't understand his bullheadedness. What did Dad actually know about Dr. Naylor's experience and expertise? Or about this kind of surgery? The two had clashed. Bad feeling existed between them. You don't have to love your surgeon, but shouldn't you at least be on the same team?

I also questioned the surgical venue. Dad was being "greenlighted" or "TURPed"—two procedures he mentioned to me—at Edenton's Chowan County Hospital, a small community hospital that made the rinky-dink Chesapeake General look like the Mass General.

Dad refused to consider most of my questions about Naylor, Chowan County Hospital, the nuts and bolts of the surgery, its risks, his recovery, anything. His reaction was testier and more disagreeable than usual—not the psychological profile you want for a surgical patient. He seemed to be tapped out, anxious, and exhausted. He was 86, after all, and the year had been brutal. My psyche wasn't in very good shape, either.

I did Internet research on prostatectomies and learned that GreenLight® surgery uses laser energy to vaporize (ablate) the prostatic tissue obstructing the bladder outlet. The urologist inserts a cystoscope, a tubular instrument with a light and camera on it, into the urethra, and then introduces the laser fiber through the scope, directing it toward the prostatic tissue overgrowth.

I surmised from my research and what Dad told me that he was, in fact, having the GreenLight, also called photo-vaporization treatment or PVP, but he kept calling it a "laser TURP," so I was confused.

At the time, I didn't know that the PVP had been on the market only since 2001.

To make a bad situation worse, on Tuesday, Nov. 9, two days before the surgery, Dad had trouble with his indwelling catheter and became soaked in urine during a golf game. Because Dr. Naylor's office was closed, he went to the Outer Banks Hospital Emergency Department to get a new catheter inserted and returned with a large, bedside collection bag strapped to his leg. The ED didn't have a smaller bag in stock!

When I later learned that Naylor had recommended a quaint bed-and-breakfast for our overnight accommodations, and Dad had booked two rooms without consulting me, I almost lost it. Why not just release a swarm of hornets into a house filled with people and no exit? My agitated father in a B&B? Talk about a home invasion. We weren't going on vacation, for God's sake. We needed the predictability of a chain hotel: a firm mattress; a hot breakfast in the lobby; vending machines; an elevator, ramps. Mom was along for the ride, too.

I tried to explain to Dad how uncomfortable a bed-and-breakfast might be, but he refused to change his reservation: He was doing whatever the surgeon recommended.

I had not met Naylor and, thus, did not have a firsthand impression of him, but I seriously questioned this referral and his motivation. Was Naylor getting a commission from the innkeeper? Were they friends, relatives, lovers? Or was he just clueless and lacking in sympathy and "people skills"?

And on that latter point: How can a doctor not know that 86-year-old people often don't travel well? Why hadn't the doctor or one of his nurses provided lodging options, with my parents' physical limitations and low tolerance for stress in mind? Once again, I noted that medical care had nothing to do with a patient's well-being.

I hit the computer and found a room for myself at a new Hampton Inn. The tightly wound B&B innkeeper, who was already reeling from my very-hard-of-hearing and over-the-top-anxious father's phone calls, tried to dissuade me from canceling, but I couldn't sit on pins and needles *and* eat homemade cookies in the parlor. Something had to give.

WEDNESDAY, NOV. 10

Sure enough, the man with the bedside Foley bag strapped to his leg hadn't been in his B&B room more than two minutes before he started complaining about the heating system in the big, drafty house. "What the hell? It's freezing in here," and more protests issued from him, as he kicked up a loud fuss, and I traipsed behind him issuing explanations, apologies, and thank-yous.

The innkeeper relocated my parents to a different room, and I left to find my hotel and steady my nerves. I returned in a short while to pick up Dad and drive to Dr. Naylor's office to get the surgery paperwork.

Dad remained in the car while I checked in with a young receptionist, who struck me as unusually chilly. I turned on the charm to compensate for what I assumed was my father's DPS reputation. The instructions in Dad's packet described his surgery as "transurethral resection of prostate," without specifying the technique. In hindsight, I wondered if Naylor was so new to laser surgery that he hadn't updated his forms?

After picking up Mom, we drove to the hospital, where Dad spent about an hour in preoperative registration and consultation. All of the employees and volunteers in the ambulatory-surgery center were so helpful and good-natured that I managed to exhale.

My father would be Naylor's second patient the next morning, the first being a "complicated" cancer case. He would have a spinal anesthesia, so we didn't have to fear eternal sleep, and no sedative. I was attending to my mother when the surgical nurse and the anesthesiologist briefed Dad, so I missed my chance to ask about his procedure and to inquire about the first case. Dad was told to report between 9:30 and 10 a.m. I figured it would be a long day.

Nonetheless, as I stretched out on my hotel bed that night, wishing I had brought a bottle of wine with me, I dared to think that maybe things wouldn't go badly. Maybe all of my worry would be for naught. Maybe, just maybe, Murphy would be busy elsewhere.

Thursday, Nov. 11

The next morning, I swung by the B&B to pick up Mom and Dad, who was still anxious, but subdued, and we arrived at the hospital at 9:15. My father always insisted on being early.

It is preferable to be a surgeon's first patient of the day, when he or she is presumably fresh and rested and not yet behind schedule. Not having this advantage, we waited restlessly in a cramped pre-op examining room for 3½ hours, not knowing when Dad's turn would come. I tried not to feel annoyed, but I failed. Why not do the "easy" surgery first? Again, I noticed the lack of concern Dr. Naylor had for my father. Fortunately, the nurses were efficient, attentive, and empathetic.

My father finally went into surgery at 12:50 p.m., and Mom and I retired to a waiting room. After about an hour, Naylor came in, said things went "beautifully," in that "I-deliver-nothing-less" boastful way that some surgeons have, and exited. He didn't introduce himself or shake our hands and spent less than a minute with us.

Mom and I went to a restaurant for lunch while Dad was in recovery, waiting for the spinal anesthesia to wear off and his legs to regain sensation. Around 4:30 p.m., we dropped by his hospital room, arriving in time to hear some of the history questions that Nurse Gina asked at his bedside, her computer at the ready.

Just like at the OBH, it was honey-this and honey-that as Gina robotically went through her litany, which included asking Dad about his urinary habits! What habits?

Gina refused to allow Dad to lower a bedside guardrail so he could swing his legs around and sit up. Fortunately, another nurse, more mindful of the advantages to post-op movement and patient autonomy, and more practical about assessing Dad's fall risk, overruled her.

During our visit, both nurses and other patients' visitors stood outside Dad's room, loudly chatting and laughing, and even dancing. I considered this behavior bad form and a bad sign. I'm very noise-sensitive. Being hearing-impaired, my father is not. If the fooling around continued into the night, his impairment would come in handy.

I talked with Gina about Dad's care and the anticipated time tomorrow for his discharge. Both of my parents were exhausted. Because Mom had complained about being in Edenton, I had canceled the second night of our lodgings. I needed to drive her home and catch some sleep before returning for the big test: Could Dad void?

Friday, Nov. 12

The first thing my father told me when I walked into his hospital room the next afternoon was: "It didn't work."

"What didn't work?" I asked.

"The surgery didn't work," he said.

"How do you know?"

"I couldn't void."

My father had "flunked" his voiding trial. His catheter had been removed that morning, and he had attempted to void. No luck.

According to the hospital records I obtained later, Missy, the licensed practical nurse who assisted him, noted that he voided 50 mL of "pink urine" (i.e., it was bloody), and his ultrasound PVR (the postvoid residual in his bladder) was 480 mL, which is a lot. She notified Dr. Naylor and inserted a new Foley catheter.

I also learned that Dad had vomited up his dinner and breakfast and slept poorly during the night. Post-op vomiting is common, so it didn't worry me. What did concern me A LOT is that Naylor had severely chastised my demoralized father that morning after he resisted Missy's attempt to give him an enema. Now all Dad wanted to do was to get the hell out of Chowan County Hospital.

As far as I could tell, the upshot of Naylor's scolding—"The SOB really reamed me out"—was that Dr. Al had embarrassed the urologist, who obviously had ordered the enema, and distressed Missy, who clearly had complained. You can imagine how I received all of this news: What the ----?

I went by the urologist's office to talk with him about the failed voiding trial and the ream-out, intending to do damage control and gather intelligence. Instead, I listened to the doctor air his frustrations. He ventilated, big-time. Naylor was more solicitous of the nurse's feelings than my father's welfare.

"*I* have to work with these people," I can still hear him saying. "*I* have to keep them happy."

He was so vehement about the offensiveness of Dad's behavior that I began to think he might be mentally unhinged, not just another surgeon with a lousy bedside manner.

A large, fidgety man of about 50, Naylor went off on my father, complaining about how he schmoozed about his NIH background, his drug discoveries, and even Charlie Huggins. Clearly, Dad's professional pedigree rattled him. I saw a volatility in him, which I tried to extinguish with explanations about my father and his nature and with a kiss-ass apology. (Yes, I will kiss ass when the tactic benefits the home team.) This mediation wore me out.

As for the failed voiding trial, Naylor wasn't concerned: That sometimes happened, he said. Dad had a follow-up appointment on Tuesday, Nov. 16. He should remove his catheter 12 hours ahead and try again to void.

I headed back to the hospital determined to accelerate Dad's discharge. Thankfully, I found a cooperative nurse and, together, we worked the process. She gave us a spirited escort to the parking lot, but once again, Dad left a small North Carolina hospital with a big bedside catheter bag strapped to his leg because a smaller bag could not be found. Apparently, the urologist's mindfulness about his team did not extend to its equipment.

THAT EVENING

Dr. Naylor's demeanor struck me as so intensely odd and his priorities as so misplaced that I decided to check him out on the Internet that night.

Whoa. . . . Damn. Even with my misgivings, I was shocked. You must be kidding.

Licensed by North Carolina in 1999, Naylor, a 1986 medical-school graduate, had run afoul of the N.C. Medical Board because of continuous prescription abuses dating back to 2001 and other reckless behavior, including an arrest for drunken driving during which he had been "Do-you-know-who-I-am?" resistant with the police. In 2006, the Medical Board suspended his license, an order it stayed, subject to probation.

Here, with some explanatory annotations, is how I hurriedly summarized his "unprofessional conduct" in an email to my siblings:

"Basically, [Dr. Naylor] was taking drug samples for himself [e.g., Zoloft®, Ambien®, and Cipro®*], without keeping a record [a legally mandated "controlled substances log"], and also self-prescribing

---

* In order, these brand-name drugs are a popular antidepressant; a powerful sedative-hypnotic; and the anthrax antibiotic.

for a variety of diagnoses, including hypogonadism. Further, he was prescribing for a woman with whom he was emotionally involved, but who was not his patient [referred to as Patient A], and not keeping a record on her either. He blew a 0.18 when he was stopped for DWI [in 2003] and acted belligerently with the cops. He claimed at his hearing before the N.C. Medical Board that a psychiatrist was treating him for chronic post-traumatic stress disorder, but no cause of [the stress] was mentioned."

Dr. Naylor, I concluded, was (had been?) a loose cannon. If I'd known about his disciplinary action the night before my father's surgery, instead of the night after, I never would have allowed Dad to go to Edenton. And he couldn't have gone without me.

It was bad enough that they didn't get along. But this?

Hypogonadism translates to low testosterone. According to the Medical Board's findings, Naylor diagnosed himself with hypogonadism in 2001 and self-prescribed Depo-Testosterone® (testosterone cyp-ionate) and straight-up testosterone, which a "member of his staff" regularly injected in him from 2001 to 2005! I wondered which of his peachy nurses assisted with this task. These would not be shots in his arm.

Naylor also had prescribed the powerful sleep aid, Ambien, for Patient A, as well as alprazolam, which is the generic name for Xanax®, a popular anti-anxiety medication; hydrocodone, a narcotic painkiller; and ketorolac, a non-steroidal anti-inflammatory drug for short-term relief of severe pain. Quite a boyfriend, our big guy.

I certainly didn't begrudge Naylor therapy for any disorders he might have, whatever their nature. But the urologist had been irresponsible, opportunistic, and reckless with prescription meds and generally had behaved self-indulgently and arrogantly. He was more than obnoxious: He was potentially dangerous.

In April 2009, after a little more than three years, the Medical Board lifted Dr. Naylor's probation. Less than seven months later, my father walked into his office.

SATURDAY, NOV. 13

None of my siblings wanted me to tell Dad about my sleuthing, but I figured he had a right to know and would want to know. I decided to wait, however, until after the Nov. 16 appointment. The weekend was for rest and recovery. But even in Dr. Naylor's absence, we found more reason to distrust him.

Naylor had prescribed a relatively new antibiotic for Dad to take to thwart a urinary tract infection. After reading the extensive FDA-required black-box warning on the package insert that came with the drug, however, Dr. Al refused to take Levaquin®.

Named for the black border surrounding it, a boxed warning alerts patients and their physicians to serious adverse effects or risks associated with a medication. The black box is the sternest FDA warning that a medication can carry and still remain on the market in the United States. It must appear on the drug's label, package insert, and all other literature.

Levaquin (levofloxacin), a fluoroquinolone antibiotic first marketed in 1997, poses a risk of tendonitis and tendon rupture to *all* patients; but that risk greatly increases in patients over age 60. The FDA required manufacturer Ortho-McNeill to add Levaquin's black-box warning in 2008. By then it had become a go-to antibiotic for many urologists, who prescribed it for prostatitis and urinary tract infections.[26]

My friend Beatrice's 82-year-old father suffered a torn Archilles' heel tendon after his urologist prescribed Levaquin, so I knew the drug was bad news and reaffirmed Dad's decision not to take it.

Why did Dr. Naylor prescribe it instead of another antibiotic? Probably because he had a sweet deal with the drug company. Levaquin salespeople drop by urologists' offices peddling samples and offering giveaways and other perks, and the docs start writing scripts.

TUESDAY, NOV. 16

At 10:30 p.m. on Nov. 15, Dad removed his catheter and successfully voided on his own. He told me the news the next morning, and I jubilantly emailed my siblings:

"The waterworks are flowing. The surgery was a success.

"We're headed to the urologist's office shortly. I can't tell you how relieved I am. I had a big knot in my stomach this morning about the what-ifs, and then Dad called. . . ."

You might say this was premature ejaculation.

In his medical records, Dr. Naylor summarized his Nov. 16 appointment with Dad as follows:

"Dr. Sjoerdsma underwent cystoscopy and laser ablation of the prostate on 11-11-10. He did very well. However, he failed his voiding trial. A Foley catheter was reinserted. He took it out last evening as instructed. He last voided around 9:30 [a.m.], and it is now 11:30. He is unable to give a urine specimen. However, there's only 125 [mL] in his bladder and it's not unusual to not be able to initiate a stream at that level. Given that he voided two hours ago, I feel very comfortable that he has a minimal postvoid residual."

On the diagnosis line of this form, he wrote: BPH "with lower tract obstructive symptoms culminating in urinary retention with excellent results from laser ablation of the prostate."

Excellent results?

I sat in the examining room with Dad during the five collective minutes that the elusive Dr. Naylor, who multi-tasked among rooms, spent with him, and the message I got wasn't "excellent results." It was "things can take time." He scheduled Dad's next postoperative visit for Dec. 29. In his notes, he described it as the "final" check.

Later I told Dad about Naylor's prescription abuse, DWI, and medical probation, and my unpredictable father gave him a pass, saying that he liked him better knowing that "he's a little wild." After all that he'd been through, Dad thought that he and Naylor had "bonded."

Amazing. In his hopefulness, he was forgiving. I left town that afternoon on a long-planned trip.

Then the leaking began.

SATURDAY, NOV. 20

By Saturday, Nov. 20, my father had become so convinced that he wasn't voiding sufficiently—he still had no control over his flow—that he feared another shutdown. He decided to go to the Outer Banks Hospital Emergency Department to have his retention level assessed and called me before he and Mom left. I was driving home from Raleigh that day and arrived at the hospital about a half-hour after my parents did.

The three hours Dad invested at the OBH that afternoon were not among his or the healthcare system's finest. Again, I mediated.

The two nurses assisting my father had never used an ultrasound bladder scanner before, and could not figure out its operation, even after reading written instructions. They finally gave up. They also had trouble inserting a Foley catheter into Dad's bladder, succeeding only after two attempts.

Outside of his examining room, the nurses whispered about Dad's incontinence and his refusal to acknowledge it, intimating that he was cognitively impaired. This was the usual knee-jerk ageism. Had anyone even bothered to obtain a history?

My hearing is so good that I always overhear people who think they're out of earshot. I patiently explained the circumstances of Dad's recent surgery to the nurses, but they didn't get it. Fortunately, they managed to drain Dad's PVR: He was not retaining.

Dad kept asking to see a doctor. Belatedly, one popped by to refer Dad to Dr. Carlson, the OBH's new affiliated urologist. It seems Dr. Naylor had competition. Dad arranged to see Carlson on Monday.

Having learned my lesson about Naylor, I Googled Dr. Carlson that night and crossed my fingers about the 60-something-year-old urologist. He had graduated from a Mexican medical school and found it necessary to be licensed in six states, including Virginia and now North Carolina. What was next?

Monday, Nov. 22

Dr. Carlson turned out to be supremely loosey-goosey, a personality trait that I would ascribe to five of the six urologists whom I met and consulted during Dad's extended urological crisis. I left his office that day, feeling emotionally spent, utterly drained. I never wanted to return.

Carlson started by calling Dad, "Your Honor," thinking he was a lawyer, then got defensive when my father, who likes to provoke, told him we knew about his licenses. Carlson's explanation for his wanderlust had to do with preferring employment and a salary over private practice and the wait for insurance monies. (Give me strength.)

The two talked feverishly AT each other, neither one seeming to listen. "Doctor, let me finish," Dr. Carlson often protested, when Dr. Al interrupted. "I'm the worst patient, and you're the second worst," the urologist added. This ego-driven, chaotic conversation was helpful to me only insofar as I learned about the intrinsic sphincter. This would be the involuntary sphincter, not the one you can control by holding your urine.

I finally hit my ejection-seat button when Carlson moved to examine Dad before I had stepped out of the room and chided me for being modest. He thought I was Dad's wife!!! God, did I look 85? I certainly wasn't a trophy. Hadn't Loosey-Goosey heard me call Dad *Dad*? Not *Daddy*.

Carlson removed Dad's Foley and gave him a "treatment plan," which I dutifully wrote down. It amounted to doing pelvic-muscle (Kegel) exercises and keeping a record of leakage and the number of pads Dad used. Dr. Al refused to be "scoped" by Carlson or scheduled for any testing. Because the new-to-town urologist did not have an ultrasound machine yet, we would have to return to the OBH for a PVR reading! Dad refused to do that, too, instead arranging to see his old friend, Dr. Naylor, in a week. (More strength.)

TUESDAY, NOV. 30

I begged off on Dad's appointment with Naylor, having had enough of urologists for a while. According to Big Guy Naylor's written report, he "reassured [my father] that his symptoms should improve . . . [and] *thoroughly* reviewed Kegel exercises to strengthen the sphincter to his satisfaction."27

This sphincter would be the *external* sphincter, the *voluntary* sphincter, over which Dad might have some control.

He *thoroughly* reviewed? I doubt it. When I asked Dad the next day about Naylor's advice, he told me that the urologist had instructed him to stop and start his urine stream while standing at the toilet voiding. This is one of the methods by which a man can *locate* pelvic-floor muscles that help to control urination.

Alas, therein lay the rub: My father could no more find his pelvic-floor muscles than he could find a spider in a dark room. He did well just to squeeze his obvious sphincter muscles. Beyond that, he tried valiantly, but he was at a loss.

The diagnosis Dr. Naylor cited in his record of this appointment was: "Status post laser ablation of the prostate for urinary retention with urinary incontinence."

Say what? No status was recorded.

TUESDAY, DEC. 28

Dad last saw Dr. Naylor on Dec. 28, again without my (or my visiting siblings') participation.

"He is having *very mild stress incontinence*," Naylor concluded in his file report.

But Dad's incontinence wasn't leakage just when he sneezed or laughed or stood up, and it wasn't mild. He had stress incontinence *plus* leakage in all other circumstances, except during the night when he slept, and despite his daily Kegel exercises. He now wore Depends 24 hours a day and spent his awake time mopping up with wads of tissue.

His urinary channel was wide-open. His Dec. 28 ultrasound showed a PVR of just 6 mL.

Dr. Naylor and my father discussed his taking an alpha-receptor stimulator, such as Sudafed® or Advil Sinus®, to "help increase his [internal] sphincter tone." But that didn't work. Advised to return in six weeks for a "symptom check," Dr. Al finally wrote Naylor off. No more.

The leaking continued.

～

Between Nov. 3, 2009, and Oct. 19, 2010, my father saw Dr. Naylor six times. Dad may have blotted out memory of his two 2009 appointments because 10 days after the first one he took the header down the stairs that I described in Chapter Five and cracked a rib. Then in February, he broke his hip. I now wonder if the BPH drug that Dr. Naylor prescribed impaired his balance and mental alertness. Flomax® is known to cause dizziness and low blood pressure.

Unfortunately, I belatedly wonder a lot about Dr. Naylor's treatment. What follows is my hindsight critique of how he managed my father's case.

NOVEMBER TO DECEMBER 2009

During Dad's initial appointment, Dr. Naylor performed a DRE, and his nurse did an ultrasound of his bladder. He also ordered some other tests in an examination that constituted minimum standard procedure. He omitted the IPSS, the LUTS questionnaire, and did not suggest that Dad keep a voiding diary to ensure accuracy in his recall of urinary symptoms. As Dad's problem, he cited "lower tract obstructive symptoms."

Red flags appear in Naylor's Nov. 3 report, including:

One, he cites a retention level of 444 mL, which is high. Two, he estimates the size of Dad's prostate to be "15-20 gm.," which, according to my reading, is the size of a boy's!

Not being a urologist, I couldn't figure out this size business, but why isn't Dr. Naylor more concerned about the high postvoid residual?

Answer: Probably because the figure is a typo. In his follow-up report of Dec. 1, 2009, Naylor cites a previous PVR of 144 mL, not 444. Typos connote sloppiness to me. Naylor's failure to correct the discrepancy connotes the same.

Considering the small size of Dad's prostate, is it possible that his retention was caused by a disorder other than BPH? A problem with his detrusor function or his urethra, for example?

I have no way of knowing, and Dr. Naylor did not consider the possibility. He did not conduct even a simple neurologic history and exam.

Naylor also did not perceive a need to perform or schedule more testing, such as a *diagnostic* cystoscopy, in which he would use an optical device to visualize the bladder, urethra, and prostate. He describes my father, for the first and only time, as a "very pleasant 85-year-old gentleman."

Naylor instructed Dad to take a 0.4 mg. dose of Flomax (tamsulosin hydrochloride) twice daily and gave him samples of the drug. In treating moderate-to-severe obstructive LUTS, urologists tend to start with tamsulosin or a less selective alpha blocker and then go from there, depending on the results.

Originally developed as antihypertensive drugs, alpha(α)-adrenergic receptor blockers or "alpha blockers" were first used to treat BPH in the late 1980s. Alpha blockers exert their effect on receptor-mediated activities in the sympathetic nervous system.* They reduce obstructive LUTS by blocking receptor-mediated contraction of the prostatic smooth-muscle cells and bladder neck. In other words, they relax the muscles impinging on the outlet.[28]

Alpha blockers, I learned while writing this chapter, work quickly and are most effective with smaller enlarged prostates that weigh around 30 to 40 grams. Within a day or two, my father should have seen improvement in his urinary flow and have felt less need to void. Absent immediate results, however, Dr. Naylor should have considered other medication.[29]

---

*I explain the sympathetic nervous system in Chapter Twelve.

Urologists can prescribe BPH drugs that have a different mechanism of action, but none of them offers a cure. They only diminish symptoms, and, it is hoped, obviate the need for surgery.[30]

Among them, 5alpha-reductase inhibitors (5-ARIs), like alpha blockers, are first-line therapy for obstructive symptoms. These drugs inhibit the enzyme, 5alpha-reductase, which converts testosterone to its metabolite dihydrotestosterone. Unlike alpha blockers, however, 5-ARIs treat the prostate enlargement, not its symptoms: They shrink the prostate and reduce further growth.

The FDA has approved two 5-ARIs for BPH: finasteride (Proscar®) and dutasteride (Avodart®). Since it takes three to six months or longer to shrink a prostate, both 5-ARIs require long-term use.

Recent studies show that combination therapy with an alpha blocker and a 5alpha-reductase inhibitor is more effective than monotherapy with either agent, but poses a higher risk of adverse effects, such as erectile dysfunction.[31] Dr. Naylor never discussed finasteride or dutasteride with my father, who did not worry about ED.

In his report of Dad's Dec. 1 appointment, Dr. Naylor diagnoses BPH with lower tract obstructive symptoms that have "improved with Flomax." He does not elaborate on this assessment, however, except to note that Dad's postvoid residual is 150 mL. Perhaps my father reported improvement. They do not discuss other treatment options. Naylor recommends a followup in four months.

MAY TO JUNE 2010

The next time Dad sees Dr. Naylor is May 4. His PVR is 288 mL. In his report, Naylor notes that Dad "has noticed that he still has no obstructive symptoms as well as postvoid dribblings."

But Dad went to see him *because* he had symptoms. I assume the insertion of the word "no," which makes the statement meaningless, was a typo. More sloppiness.

Again, Naylor notes that Dad's "prostate is 15 gm.," which would be an undersized prostate, not an enlarged one. What gives? Could he possibly be referring to only the section of the gland that he can feel?

After this appointment, Dr. Naylor never does another DRE. If he obtains an estimate of Dad's prostate size from an ultrasound, he never mentions it in his reports.

The urologist confirms his diagnosis of "benign prostatic

hypertrophy with lower tract obstructive symptoms," but doesn't specifically cite any.

Dad's PVR has nearly doubled after six months of tamsulosin. How does Dr. Naylor respond to this development?

Does he prescribe a 5-ARI or, perhaps, try a combination drug therapy?

No.

Does he suggest a cystoscopy or specialized urodynamic tests in order to assess the condition and functioning of Dad's bladder and his urinary flow? A high PVR can indicate detrusor failure.

No.

What does he do? He doubles the Flomax prescription! Quick-and-easy, no-brainer medicine.

Of course, the double-dose has no effect. Why would it?

Six weeks later, Dad is back in Naylor's office for a followup. This time, he has a postvoid residual of 423 mL, three times the volume that he had six months before. In his report of June 15, Naylor notes that Dad "has done better with Flomax than he did with Uroxatral," and amends his diagnosis to read: BPH "with lower tract symptoms and incomplete emptying on maximum Flomax."

Does Dr. Naylor even know whom he is treating? At no time did my father take Uroxatral® (alfuzison), another alpha blocker. I confirmed this with Dad and his pharmacist's records. Is this more sloppiness or blatant neglect?

Naylor's all-purpose drug has failed. Surely, he has other tools in his BPH plumber's toolbox. Which is his next tool of choice?

Answer: He continues Dad on the ineffectual Flomax, discusses a "laser-ablation type of prostatectomy" with him, and puts him off for another eight weeks.

AUGUST TO OCTOBER 2010

By his Aug. 10 appointment, my father has a urinary retention of 450 mL, but, according to Dr. Naylor's report, he has "no voiding complaints."

Naylor claims they discuss the laser-ablation prostatectomy—no cystoscopy or urodynamics; no other treatments or surgeries—and concludes his file summary with: "We will see him in three months for a symptom check, urinalysis and postvoid residual but sooner if there's a problem."

My father didn't make it three months.

IF there's a problem?

Hmmm. Let's look at his PVRs and figure that out:

12/6/09: 155 mL
5/4/10: 288 mL
6/15/10: 423 mL
8/10/10: 450 mL

Dr. Naylor's tool—the all-purpose let's-just-up-the-Flomax-dose-and-see-how-things-go wrench—results in 10/19/10: 800 mL and catheterization.

If your Pop is diagnosed with BPH, I urge you to ask his urologist about the results he or she has achieved with his drug(s) of choice in patients whose BPH profiles (LUTS and IPSS scores) are similar to your Pop's. Find out the effective doses and time needed to achieve improvement. Also reassure yourself of the diagnosis by asking the doctor about urodynamic studies, which are the most definitive tests for determining the cause of voiding dysfunction and LUTS.

And, finally, find out which tools the doctor has for opening up your Pop's channel. A urologist in a small-town solo practice is not going to have them all. You should know what they are and start looking elsewhere if important ones are lacking.

Belatedly, I did some homework.

THE BPH TOOLBOX

If a BPH drug does not relieve your Pop's LUTS, his options fall into two categories, according to Johns Hopkins urologist Brian Matlaga: 1) minimally invasive treatments and 2) surgical procedures.[32]

You will see laser-surgery techniques advertised and promoted by urologists as "minimally invasive," but Matlaga and the American Urological Assn. use the term only to describe heat therapies that destroy prostatic tissue overgrowth. The most popular are the transurethral needle ablation (TUNA) and transurethral microwave thermotherapy (TUMT).

In a TUNA, the urologist places interstitial radiofrequency needles through the urethra and into the lobes of the prostate. In a TUMT, a catheter inserted through the urethra delivers microwave energy. Each therapy can be performed on an outpatient basis, under local anesthesia, in your Pop's urologist's office.

The downside to TUNA, TUMT, and other minimally invasive treatments is that LUTS take longer to improve with them than they do with surgery. It is also more likely that men who undergo heat therapy will need further treatment, which may include surgery.[33]

I don't know enough to express an opinion about the TUMT or TUNA. I simply advise you that some urologists—most likely, in large practices or at academic medical centers—have them in their toolboxes. (They did, when I wrote this chapter.)

Transurethral resection of the prostate (the TURP), which was first performed in the 1930s, has long been the gold-standard prostatectomy for men with moderate-to-severe LUTS-BPH.

Laser surgery dates to the early 1990s, but it is only since 2000 that new and better techniques of this technology have challenged the TURP for supremacy.[34] Medication, starting with alpha blockers, also has resulted in a dramatic decrease in TURPs.[35]

THE TURP AND ALTERNATIVES

In a TURP, the surgeon inserts a resectoscope into a patient's penis that passes through his urethra to his prostate. This long, thin, camera-equipped instrument has a wire loop on its end that cuts away the obstructing tissue piece by piece and seals (coagulates) blood vessels with an electric current—or more recently, with laser energy. The prostate tissue is cut and then physically removed.[36]

Men who undergo a TURP may have a spinal or general anesthesia. They usually remain in the hospital for one to two days and have a Foley catheter for one to three days post-surgery. Their full recovery typically takes up to three weeks. One percent of TURP patients experience permanent incontinence, and 5 to 10 percent suffer from ED, because of nerve damage. Unique to the TURP is the serious risk of an electrolyte disturbance called TURP Syndrome, which occurs when the body absorbs glycine, an irrigation fluid that may be used during the surgery.[37]

The "open" prostatectomy, like my grandfather had, involves incisions in a man's abdomen, bladder, and prostate, and, thus, is more invasive than the TURP. It also is more effective and durable, experts say. Most surgeons today reserve the open prostatectomy for patients whose prostates exceed 80 to 100 grams.

The open prostatectomy requires a general anesthesia; catheterization for at least three to seven days after surgery; and hospitalization for up to seven days. Full recovery may take up to six weeks, and the incidence of incontinence and ED is higher than with a TURP.[38]

A third less common non-laser surgery is the transurethral incision of the prostate (TUIP), which is performed using an electocautery blade to divide the bladder-neck fibers and the prostate at one or two locations. Tissue is not removed.[39]

According to the American Urological Assn., TUIP is an outpatient endoscopic procedure limited to the treatment of prostates that are less than 30 grams. It results in symptomatic improvement comparable to that attained after a TURP, but there is a higher rate of secondary procedures. The adverse effects include those seen with the TURP, except for the syndrome.[40]

There are two basic types of laser prostatectomies: Laser ablation melts away tissue, and laser enucleation cuts it away.[41] Laser techniques and systems differ and are fast-changing. In 2011, the holmium laser was popular.[42]

The appeal of these procedures–the advantages that urologists extol in their offices and on their websites–is that they can be done 1) with a spinal anesthesia and 2) on an outpatient basis or with a shorter hospital stay; and that, as compared with the TURP, 3) the recovery time is faster; and 4) the risk of ED and incontinence is lower. Patients usually have an indwelling catheter for one to three days.

Although clinical data evaluating the effectiveness and the risks of the laser techniques are encouraging, the evidence cannot yet be considered long-term.

When asked in 2009, what he would do if he were a 65-year-old man who had been taking BPH medication that "hadn't worked as expected," and now had "bothersome" LUTS, Matlaga replied that he would make an appointment to have a TURP.

"The reason I would choose a TURP over a minimally-invasive therapy or a laser surgical procedure," he continued, "is that doctors have better experience with TURP; the long-term data are there, and they are good. We just don't have the data with any of the laser ablation therapies. Finally, I would make sure I had the procedure done by someone who had performed hundreds of them."[43]

WARNING: There's a learning curve associated with the TURP

and all of the 21st century surgical techniques, and your Pop's urologist may not yet have slam-dunk skill.

Before your Pop commits to any LUTS-BPH treatment or surgery, make sure that his urologist is using a familiar tool.

Chapter Ten

2011: Concurrent
PROBLEMS

Lung Nodules and Fatigue

It was beginning to rain and to pour on my beleaguered father. Shortly before he experienced his pre-Halloween BOO, had a Foley catheter rigged to his bladder, and underwent his botched laser prostatectomy, Dad saw his internist/PCP, Dr. Buchanan, who ordered a chest X-ray as part of a routine checkup. Subsequently, the radiologist, Dr. Exeter, reported a new 5-millimeter "nodule" of "unclear" etiology in the upper lobe of Dad's right lung.

This would be the same lung that was pulverized when Dad fell off of the beach cottage roof, the same lung that filled with a quart of bloody fluid before physicians at Norfolk Sentara General Hospital figured out it needed draining so he could breathe.

Now this lung had a nodule. Could it be cancer?

My father had smoked for decades, but quit 30 years ago. What was his risk of developing smoking-related lung cancer?

Although Dr. Exeter's report cited cough as the "admit diagnosis," Dad did not have a cough, shortness of breath, or any other respiratory symptoms. This was a routine exam ordered by an internist whose timing turned out to be astoundingly awful. Dr. Al's anxiety grew.

Exeter compared this new Oct. 18, 2010 series of X-rays with some plain films of Dad's chest from 2007 and recommended a CT scan to "better evaluate the density" of this small and "smooth" nodule, which he alternately called a granuloma.

But Dad had no time to think about a CT scan. In 24 hours he would have his bladder drained of nearly a quart of urine.

"Dr. Sjoerdsma believes that the urinary problem takes precedence over the lung at this point," Dr. Naylor understatedly wrote in his report on that unpleasant Oct. 19.

If only Dr. Sjoerdsma had known how long "precedence" would take. He would have kept the catheter and discarded the urologist.

What this mystery nodule meant for me, as an advocate, is that I had another problem to keep an eye on, a concurrent medical issue to track that might turn out to be a co-morbidity. Co-morbidities are concomitant, but unrelated pathological or disease processes. Whether an issue or a co-morbidity, the number of medical specialists in Dad's life—ologists, I call them—would be expanding.

OLOGISTS

The urologist, the cardiologist, the pulmonologist, the gastroenterologist, the neurologist, nephrologist, etcetera, and so forth, *ad nauseum* ologist.

The more co-morbidities your parent has, the more medical-specialty, -subspecialty, and -subsubspecialty ologists, he or she will see, and, therefore, the more likely it will become that breakdowns in healthcare will occur. Being a Mom-and-Pop advocate/watchdog becomes a matter of communicating and coordinating with "ologists."

"Patients with several chronic conditions," a description that fits most adults 65 and older, "may visit up to 16 physicians in a year," writes Professor Thomas Bodenheimer of the University of California-San Francisco Center for Excellence in Primary Care, who describes coordinating healthcare as a "perilous journey."[1]

"A patient with anything but the simplest needs is traversing a very complicated system across many handoffs and locations and players," agrees Dr. Donald M. Berwick, then president of the Institute for Healthcare Improvement in Cambridge, Mass., in a 2006 *Time* magazine cover story titled:

"Q: What Scares Doctors?"

"A: Being the Patient."[2]

Traversing is a good verb to describe patient movement within the Hydra-like U.S. healthcare system. There is a lot of crossing over and through. Multiple handoffs, multiple sites, multiple players. Crossovers and handoffs result in disconnection and dysfunction, fumbles and mistakes that cause inconvenience, neglect, and disaster.

In contrast to primary-care physicians, your general internists, ologists typically focus on physiological systems, such as the cardiovascular or neurological system, not on the whole body or the general welfare of a person. In helping your Mom and Pop, you should be aware of ologists' not-my-area-of-expertise boundaries and not count on them for more—not unless you push, and even then, they may ignore or dismiss you.

Generally speaking, medical specialization, which has enabled new and better therapies and breakthroughs in biological understanding, has spawned healthcare fragmentation: Each ologist attends to only one "fragment" of your Mom's or Pop's healthcare, and no systemic oversight exists to ensure care coordination and continuity among them. If you think that your Mom's or Pop's primary-care physician has the time, much less the incentive, to coordinate her/his care among multiple ologists, think again.

Modern U.S. healthcare is a multi-specialty-compartment locomotive that conspicuously lacks a dedicated conductor or even assistant conductors to keep the passengers informed and on track. The passenger-patient and his/her advocate must conduct the train.

Among the fundamental lapses that occur in our fragmented healthcare system: "Referrals from primary care physicians to specialists often include insufficient information," writes Professor Bodenheimer, "and consultation reports from specialists back to primary care physicians are often late and inadequate." You also can expect multiple errors in the consultants' reports, some of them initiated by the PCP!

Your Mom's and Pop's visits to multiple healthcare providers, Bodenheimer warns, can result in "wasteful duplication of diagnostic testing [running up costs], perilous polypharmacy, and confusion about conflicting care plans."3 I can, and will, attest to all of these systemic failures.

A breakdown in care coordination can occur not only among multiple and diverse providers, including all physicians, diagnostic data sources, and emergency departments, but between physicians and their patients and families. Bodenheimer cites studies showing that up to 50 percent of ALL patients, not just those with an impairment that affects their comprehension, such as deafness, leave an office visit with their doctor not understanding what they were told; and 75 percent of physicians do not routinely contact patients about normal diagnostic test results.4

Sound familiar?

CYA RADIOLOGY

The radiologist is an unusual person on the healthcare locomotive. He or she may drive a diagnostic process—determine the route, if you will—but lack the expertise or willingness to evaluate his own direction. Case in point, I found Dr. Exeter's charts very frustrating.

Whenever unexplained spots turn up on X-rays of older people's lungs, radiologists tend to think first of cancer and second of the patient's smoking history. Such thinking reflects two realities: 1) Smoking accounts for 80 percent of all lung-cancer deaths[5]; and 2) a radiologist's failure to flag a lung abnormality as potentially cancerous could subject him or her to a malpractice lawsuit.

You should know that an error in medical judgment is not the same as legally actionable negligence or "malpractice." A missed cancer diagnosis can be reasonable—in the sense that the physician acted in conformity with applicable medical-care standards—and, thus, not malpractice, even though the patient suffered as a result of the judgment. That skilled trial lawyers and a sympathetic plaintiff can persuade a jury to view a reasonable error in judgment as malpractice does not change that fact.

The prospect of liability influences both the language and content of radiologists' reports and recommendations.[6] Radiologists "cover their asses"—a ploy well known in legal circles as CYA, with the Y signifying your—by being both vague and broad in their interpretations. They avoid specificity. While I don't necessarily disagree with a CYA approach, I do take issue, as you'll see, with the information that a radiologist chooses to impart and explain, or not. I particularly questioned Dr. Exeter's information and explanations.

My father smoked on and off for about 33 years, sometimes quitting for a year at a time. He favored cigarettes, smoking about a half-pack per day, before he belatedly switched to cigars. Dad finally went cold turkey in 1981 a few months before his 57 birthday. After 30 years, hadn't he dodged the cancer bullet?

Dr. Al had read study reports over the years suggesting that after 10 years of cessation, a former smoker's risk of lung cancer declines. He didn't believe he had lung cancer, but being a rational person, he couldn't rule it out. Drs. Exeter and Buchanan couldn't or wouldn't tell us about the relative risk of smoking-related cancer, and I didn't have time then to do any research.

Dr. Al reviewed the chest X-rays and the radiologist's findings with Dr. Exeter himself and was predictably unimpressed. To me, he scoffed: "Five millimeters? Come on, that's really small."

How small? Only half a centimeter or about 2/10 of an inch. A centimeter equals 0.393701 inch.

But what did we know about nodule size? More important, what did Dr. Exeter know?

Dad floated the idea that this granuloma could be the vestige of an old fungus infection, such as histoplasmosis. During his farming childhood, he had tended chickens, whose droppings may become contaminated with the spores that cause *Histoplasma capsulatum* infections.

Histoplasmosis? I did some quickie research. According to the American College of Chest Physicians, the most common causes of *benign* solitary pulmonary nodules are healed or nonspecific granulomas; active granulomatous infections, such as tuberculosis, coccidioidomycosis, cryptococcosis, aspergillosis, and histoplasmosis (consult your medical dictionary); and hamartomas, which are malformations of normal cells. Less common causes include nonspecific inflammation and fibrosis, lung abscesses, and bronchogenic cysts.[7]

Dad's nodule could even be scar tissue. Because of his rooftop fall, his right lung is substantially scarred, and his right hemidiaphragm—the right half of his diaphragm—is paralyzed and does not move during respiration.

CT SCAN NO. 1, OCT. 27

On Oct. 27, 2010, while waiting for Dr. Naylor to schedule his laser surgery and at Dr. Buchanan's urging, Dad underwent a CT scan of his chest with contrast. This time, Dr. Exeter found multiple small, "indeterminate" nodules in different regions of Dad's right lung, not just the upper lobe. In his report, he did not address the smoothness of these new nodules, as he had the initial solitary nodule, an inconsistency that I found irritating.

As I explained in Chapter Four, computerized tomography links an X-ray machine with a computer. When you undergo a chest CT, you lie supine on a narrow table, called a gantry, that slides into the center of the large doughnut-holed scanner. The scanner emits thin X-ray beams that rotate around your chest and produce many two-dimensional pictures of the same area from different angles. Each full scan takes about seven to 15 seconds, during which time you lie still and hold your breath because movement can produce blurred images. After the CT computer receives these data, it generates three-dimensional, high-resolution images of your lungs and chest cavity.[8]

Radiologists use contrast agents, also called media or dyes, to highlight specific organs, blood vessels, or tissues. Contrast material, such as iodine or barium, blocks the radiation and appears white on the images.

Patients who have thoracic CT scans typically receive contrast agents intravenously; contrasts used to highlight the abdomen and gastrointestinal organs are given orally or rectally. Once in your bloodstream, the contrast circulates through your veins and poses a threat to your kidneys. Radiologists, therefore, insist that patients have tested normally for creatinine and blood urea nitrogen (BUN), two indicators of kidney functioning, within the past three months. But they don't contact patients before scans to ensure that these lab tests have been done. That's not their department.

In fact, it's fair to say that patient contact is not radiologists' department—and quite possibly, one of the reasons they went into radiology. After all, they spend their days in dark rooms poring over "film."

To fully comprehend Dr. Exeter's CT findings, I needed a sophisticated knowledge of both computerized tomography and lung anatomy. Lacking both, I still could surmise that the nodules he identified were spread out in the periphery of Dad's right lung, in the upper lobe, as well as the middle and lower lobes. The right lung has three lobes; the smaller left lung, below which sits the heart, only two.

This could not be good, but I wondered: Was this pattern characteristic of cancer? Surely there are known cancer patterns. Lung cancer is not a new kid on the block.

According to Exeter, none of the nodules measured more than 5 mm. He observed, however, that "one solid component associated" with an area in Dad's right lower lobe spanned "some 10 x 14 mm in size." Ten-by-14-millimeters equates to 1.0-by-1.4 centimeters or about 4/10-inch-by-about-6/10-inch. I understood the sizing, and I figured solid couldn't be good, but the term, "component" struck me as meaningless. He might as well have said "part."

My father again sought out Exeter and sat elbow-to-elbow with him, reviewing the CT images. Even though Dad has considerable medical acumen, knowledge, and experience, not much came of this. He was still as removed from a diagnostic answer as a layperson who depends on his or her primary-care physician's verbal explanation of the radiology specialist's written interpretation.

What do PCPs like Dr. Buchanan know from nodules and components? Depending on their patient population, experience, inquisitiveness, and initiative, some may know a lot; others, not so much. I had reason to believe later that Dr. Buchanan fell into the latter category.

As important as CT-scan reports are, I thought, why don't radiologists give patients more guidance? Surely, they must adhere to common standards of practice when they evaluate and characterize nodules and then suggest how internists and other referring physicians should manage them. The multitude of Drs. Exeters across the country can't all be flying by the seat of their pants; they must have evidence-based guidelines to go by, guidelines that they could share with patients.

I would have liked an explanation of variations in nodule size, shape, appearance, and content, and the related odds of cancer with each, insofar as clinical studies suggest. What makes a nodule seem indeterminate to a radiologist rather than benign or malignant?

By my count, Exeter noted five indeterminate small nodules in his findings, about which he speculated: "They could possibly be associated with old granulomatous disease. The larger density [i.e., the solid component] . . . is more indeterminate for underlying neoplastic process. It could possibly be associated with the patient's previous trauma. It is larger than normally seen with old granulomatous disease."

"Neoplastic process" connotes cancer, a neoplasm being an abnormal new growth that proliferates more rapidly than normal cells would. But what should I make of Exeter's assertion that the solid component is "more" indeterminate for cancer? Does that mean less likely? Do radiologists have a sliding scale of indeterminateness?

"He's hedging," Dad said, when I asked. CYA-ing.

The existence of more than one nodule raised the grim possibility of metastasized cancer. Cancerous cells from a "primary tumor" elsewhere in Dad's body—in his kidney, for example—could have spread to his lung, in which case he did not have lung cancer, smoking-related or otherwise. He had a metastatic cancer.

Metastatic cancers have the same name and same type of cancer cells as their original tumors. Kidney cancer that spreads to the lungs, for example, is metastatic kidney cancer, not lung cancer, and would be treated as such.

I wondered if studies had been done that would help us to evaluate Dad's CT images. Question: How often do nodules that look like my father's nodules on CT imaging turn out to be malignant? How probable is it that he has metastatic cancer?

Dr. Exeter concluded his report with the suggestion that it "may be worthwhile" to perform a follow-up PET scan, the next stop in the diagnostic checkout line. Dr. Al still was not impressed, and, thanks to his rising floodwaters, I had no time to do a fast study of nodules, lung cancer, metastases, and what all else to give me context. Focused on his urinary distress, Dad decided that a PET scan would have to wait.

R.I.P., MARCUS WELBY

To a great extent, my father, being his own doctor and the only one he trusts, manages his own care, but, as Chapter Nine illustrated, he is not always successful. Also, as he has aged, he has become more anxious. Anxiety distorts his perceptions.

Since 2010, I have tried to stay focused on his big-picture needs, and to follow up on important details, but I often run into healthcare-system "business as usual," with both ologists and PCPs, that leaves me frustrated, angry, or just plain flabbergasted. Dad's incontinence and nodule "sagas" are cases in point.

The American College of Physicians represents physicians in general internal medicine and related subspecialties, such as pediatrics. According to the ACP, primary-care medicine, the "backbone" of the U.S. healthcare system, has been in crisis for at least 20 years and "is at grave risk of collapse due to a dysfunctional financing and delivery system."[9] The United States now has a shortage of primary-care doctors.

Much has been written about the many encumbrances that affect healthcare delivery by PCPs.[10] One of the worst, says UCSF Professor Bodenheimer, a national advocate for reforming the "healthcare model" to save primary care, is what he calls "the tyranny of the 15-minute visit."

Thanks to fee-for-service reimbursement by third-party payers, which rewards quantity—the number of patients PCPs see—over the quality or outcome of care that they deliver, primary-care doctors book patients every 15 minutes and then rush through their exams. In one study that Bodenheimer cites, physicians interrupted their patients' initial statement of their problem in an average of 23 seconds![11]

If you're old enough to remember TV's Marcus Welby, M.D., then you know the physician ideal of the kind, wise, all-knowing, and *unhurried* general practitioner who listened to his patients and made house calls. That ideal, personified by Dr. Welby, has been missing in action since the 1970s.

An older family physician, Welby—played by actor Robert Young, the television father who knew best in the 1950s—approached general medicine with common sense and compassion, not technology and specialty knowledge. While we wouldn't want to sacrifice technological advances and ologists' expertise, and we no longer embrace the elite white-male archetypal physician, most of us would like our doctors to be more Welbyesque. We want professionals, not businesspeople. M.D.s with M.B.A.s in healthcare economics need not apply.

As Professor Timothy Hoff elaborates in his book, "Practice Under Pressure: Primary Care Physicians and Their Medicine in the Twenty-first Century": "[Dr.] Welby sought to know and have relationships with his patients, understand the psychosocial backdrops for their illnesses, and through this connection he had the key to successful diagnosis and treatments."

In short, Welby cared about his patients. Besides treating their symptoms, he tried to understand who they were and how they lived.

R.I.P., Marcus Welby.

Judging by doctor TV shows popular since "Welby"—such as "ER," "House" (which I can't stand), and "Grey's Anatomy" (ditto)—today's "best" and "coolest" physicians are "superspecialists interacting . . . within hospital settings that are fast-paced, exciting, and attractively quirky," writes Hoff. [12]

These people are as unreal in your Mom's and Pop's healthcare lives as Marcus Welby would be.

Today's young doctors graduate from medical school with enormous debt and view the primary-care worklife as posing three strikes and they're out: Strike one, being constantly overwhelmed; strike two, being grossly underpaid; and strike three, having to know "too much." According to a 2013 report by the ACP, "grossly underpaid" translates to a gap of more than $100,000-$135,000 between the median annual subspecialist income and that of a primary-care physician.[13] The number of new PCPs has been dwindling for years.

"Right now, we're spending about 70 times more on the production of specialists than we are on the production of primary care physicians," said Dr. Barbara Starfield of the Bloomberg School of Public Health at Johns Hopkins University in a roundtable discussion about redesigning primary care. "That absolutely has to change."[14]

With their narrow expertise, ologists may be able to solve highly circumscribed and esoteric problems, but, in so doing, they may create other problems and miss some healthcare-giving opportunities. I remind you of the oncologists at Sloan-Kettering who surgically removed my friend Jack's appendix cancer, but failed to notice the edema in his legs. They underestimated the threat of an embolus.

None of the *many* urologists my father would consult ever inquired into his mental health or offered any advice for how he could cope emotionally, or practically, on a day-to-day basis, with his incontinence. They left his general outlook, attitude, well-being, whatever you want to call it, to him to manage. Not their department.

Ologists tend to regard patients as "discrete parts" and administer to them "in an impersonal manner," writes Hoff, of the University of Albany public health school. In my experience, they are disinterested in "the status of the patient," which is my father's phrase for describing general health and well-being.

In theory, Hoff notes, primary-care medicine treats each patient as "a living, breathing organism with a specific lifestyle, work and home environment, and biological risk profile." PCPs deal with patient "status." But theory is not always reality.[15]

"DEATH" BY DROWNING

By January 2011, it was clear that Dad was 100 percent, free-flowing incontinent, angry, and deranged. He hated his life and talked about dying.

"I'd rather die than live like this," he told me repeatedly. But before he did, he wanted to take out Dr. Naylor.

"It would almost be worth it," he would say, "to kill the bastard and go to jail. I know he did this deliberately."

So much for bonding with the Wild One.

I loved my father a lot, and I felt terrible that he was suffering so much, but I got so I dreaded answering his phone calls. He was decompensating—his own word for deterioration brought on by extreme mental distress. As time passed, he became more depressed, detached from reality, and abusive. I had to push back when he pushed, otherwise, I thought I would disappear. I also had to protect Mom. The only time I felt at peace was when I was out of town.

In February, two of my good law-school friends died, one of them taking her own life. Jennie's death tormented me and will hurt forever. In July, I lost a beloved canine friend after his long decline. These were bleak days.

It wasn't fair that Dad was hurting those he loved, but I understood why he was. He had trusted Dr. Naylor, and now he was wearing my mother's nursing-home diapers and filling up trashbags with Kleenex®. In time, the tissue gave way to pads that multiplied in the number he used daily. The Kegel exercises had next-to-no effect. Who wouldn't be miserable awash in urine?

Afraid that I would lose him, I told Dad that I would go with him anywhere he wanted: Duke, Johns Hopkins, the Mayo Clinic, anywhere. All he had to do was say the word. I would see this crisis through with him.

Thanks to a referral from Mom's internist at Norfolk Sentara General, we started closer to home. The ologists were multiplying.

THE FIRST LIFE-SAVING ATTEMPTS

Between Feb. 23 and Aug. 17, 2011, my father had seven appointments at a Virginia Beach urology practice associated with Sentara. I went with him four times. Two urologists with respected national reputations thoroughly examined, tested, evaluated, and advised him. He also underwent physical therapy with biofeedback.

None of these appointments accrued to his long-term benefit.

The paperwork that Dad completed before his first appointment at Urology of Virginia included the International Prostate Symptom Score, which I described in the previous chapter. I recall him responding to this symptom-screening tool again during at least one follow-up visit.

The Virginia urologists, Drs. Farrell and Smith, used a questionnaire with an eighth quality-of-life question that was added to the IPSS, but not to the AUA Symptom Index. It asks: "If you were to spend the rest of your life with your urinary condition just the way it is now, how would you feel about that?"

My father selected the "Unhappy" response, second only to "Terrible" in dissatisfaction among the six choices offered.[16]

On March 18, Dr. Farrell did a cystoscopy of Dad's urethra and performed two hours' worth of urodynamics tests designed to assess his LUT functioning. These tests, some of which Dr. Naylor might have used for diagnostic purposes, but did not, focused on the relation between pressure in Dad's bladder and the volume and rate of his urinary flow.[17]

Dad told me afterward that he had a lot of urinary leakage with "valsalva," which is the maneuver performed when you close your mouth, pinch your nose shut, and then try to exhale as if you were blowing up a balloon. You can use this technique to unclog your ears and stop hiccups.

The Valsalva maneuver—named for a 17th century Italian physician whose chief interest was the ear—is useful in diagnosing intrinsic sphincter deficiency (ISD), which is what Dr. Farrell told Dad he had when we met for a consultation after the tests. Dr. Naylor's GreenLight laser ablation had permanently damaged my father's internal sphincter, his involuntary faucet control.

I think my father stopped listening, or ceased hearing, after that pronouncement. When we talked later he had no recollection of Dr. Farrell's discussion of treatment options.

Besides continued physical therapy, the Virginia urologist told us about two devices that could be surgically implanted to prevent his incontinence: 1) a urethral sling; and 2) an artificial urinary sphincter (AUS). Dad adamantly opposed the sphincter, which operates with a pump, saying, "No way." But he did agree to see Dr. Farrell's colleague, Dr. Smith, who was the resident ISD expert.

I later obtained my father's medical records and read Dr. Farrell's March 18 notes. In his cystoscopy report, he describes Dad's urethra as normal, except at the prostatic segment, which is "somewhat irritated, irregular, and friable [brittle]." It appears to Dr. Farrell that the surgically "ablated area involved the [internal] sphincter somewhat." All of the urodynamics tests lead him to "suspect ISD," and his bottom-line assessment is "Pt. Is a 86 yo ISD after PVP."

Dad was told that the earliest Dr. Smith could see him was August, a delay that irritated him. No one in crisis wants to wait, but he soldiered on, continuing his Kegel exercises and his PT, which he didn't like, understand, or buy into; ranting about killing Dr. Naylor; and refusing—as always—to consider psychiatric help.

By now I knew that my father responded to illness and disability with extreme anxiety and despondency, which he either failed or refused to acknowledge, much less treat. Understanding the why of his behavior, however, didn't always make it easier for me to tolerate the how, which came in the form of frequent complaining, *obsessive* negativity about all subjects, and a "What have you done for me lately?" attitude.

Dad behaved abominably, and I felt terribly burdened, but I never felt belittled. He always held himself together in public. If he started bitching or naysaying while I was visiting him at home, I would leave. I'm not a martyr or an abuse victim. When I left, though, I hurt Mom, who longed to see me, and so I struggled.

Although he often would apologize the next day for the previous day's assault or offense, Dad couldn't (or wouldn't) stop himself from committing that day's assault. He couldn't (or wouldn't) let go of his anger. He was losing his grip.

"You were right. I made nothing but mistakes," he would say. "I have no one to blame but myself." His own failure, as he saw it, was eating him up, costing him his ability to reason and his will to live. I couldn't convince him to take an antidepressant—he didn't want to alter his (already altered) brain!—so I got medical help for myself.

This was misery.

ENDURANCE

In toto, my father endured six months of dispiriting and unproductive high-tech PT sessions in Virginia Beach. I knew that the sincere young physical therapists' "pelvic-floor muscle exercises with electromyography assistance for strengthening"—"electrodes in the ass," according to Dad—would never work, but I left it to him to terminate his increasingly shorter and futile sessions with them. After two PT visits, I'd had enough. He would never find that dark-room spider or his pelvic-floor muscles, and he was miserable trying. His incontinence just got worse.

On June 7, Dr. Carlson, the new local urologist, provided Dad some relief in the form of a Cunningham penile clamp, whose use enabled him to play 18 holes of golf again. My father now measured the value of his life by how often and how long he could play golf, and the clamp gave him hope.

But . . . a penile clamp is exactly what you think it is. Worn for too long, it starts to hurt the appendage it is clamping. My father considered it a godsend, though, and elevated Carlson's status for giving him one. Chalk one up for old-school medicine.

Because of an unexpected opening in Dr. Smith's schedule, Dad was able to see him on June 29—just before Smith was to travel to Chile to perform miracle surgery. Dr. Smith was a grandiose big shot who operated in overdrive. His big-shotness and lack of time alienated my father. Having come across Smith's name in my research, however, I was inclined to respect his counsel, despite his arrogance.

According to my notes, Dr. Smith described Dad's incontinence as "mild" and presented three options: The first was to do nothing and use the clamp; and the other two were the surgeries Dr. Farrell had mentioned. We focused on the sling, because the artificial urinary sphincter seemed too invasive. But, in truth, Dad wasn't mentally up to considering either seriously. He was too depressed and anxious.

Implanted under the urethra, and attached to muscle tissue or pubic bone, a synthetic mesh sling prevents leakage by elevating and compressing the urethra. Dr. Smith told us that 60 percent of men who receive a sling are cured of their incontinence, and 80 to 90 percent achieve some improvement after six to eight weeks. Although sling surgery is a short outpatient procedure, Smith recommended that Dad, because of his age, stay overnight in the hospital.

He also informed us that the risk of incontinence with a TURP is 1 percent, confirming what I had read, but he didn't mention the GreenLight, the "laser TURP." Much later I read in one of Smith's reports that Dad's detrusor contractility was low and "injury to [his intrinsic] sphincter [existed] at 5 o'clock." Low detrusor contractility meant that his bladder wasn't completely emptying even though he was incontinent.

In his summary about the laser surgery, Dr. Naylor had written that he ablated the left lobe of Dad's prostate from the 12 o'clock to the 5 o'clock position, and the right lobe from the 12 o'clock to 7 o'clock position.

All I know is, Dad's clock was cleaned.

Like the unstable Naylor, neither Dr. Farrell nor Dr. Smith provided "status of the patient" care. It would have benefited my father so much if one of these hotshots had expressed some "I can imagine what you're going through" empathy for his plight. He used to be a hotshot, too. But that was too much to ask—so, apparently, as I found out later, was considering his prostate beyond the role it had played in his incontinence.

My father last saw Smith and his physical therapists on Aug. 17, 2011. He discussed a home physical-therapy program and asked more questions about the sling procedure. That was the direction I assumed, and hoped, he would go in. What I had read about the artificial urinary sphincter caused me much consternation.

CHRONIC FATIGUE

My father's incontinence devastated him, but his health ills didn't end there. Besides his leakage and angry depression, his lung nodules weren't going away on their own. Although he downplayed them, I think Dr. Exeter's ambiguous chest CT findings added to his despair—another reason for radiologists to offer objective and clear diagnostic standards to their patients, not vague speculation.

That autumn Dad started sleeping on the living-room couch for several hours in the afternoon—after having slept 10 or more hours the night before. He began describing himself as "chronically" fatigued, and we thought again about his lung.

Could the fatigue be related to an underlying disease that had produced the "multiple small nodules" in his right lung? Could he have cancer?

Or, alternatively, were the stress and strain of his urological ordeal decreasing his resiliency and physiological reserves? Dad was chronically anxious and in denial about his anxiety. Maybe his mental disconnect was exhausting him.

Who knew? Certainly not his PCP, Dr. Buchanan, who, I believed then, was well-meaning and not of the old-age-as-diagnosis school of medicine. Dad said he had an excellent rapport with Buchanan, a man in his 60s, but Buchanan was no Marcus Welby. He wasn't going to launch a diagnostic investigation beyond the standard medicine by-the-test-numbers approach. He deferred 100 percent to Exeter on Dad's lung disease.

Perhaps I should have intervened.

I am a big believer in sitting unobtrusively in the examining room with my mother or father to ensure that the physician receives an accurate representation of any symptoms they might be having–and my forgetful parents have a written record of what was said. I try to be a fly on the wall. But I never did this with Dr. Buchanan, whose office was an hour's drive away. Dr. Al managed his own checkups and medications. After Dad told him about his generalized fatigue, the PCP ordered blood tests. Numbers.

A vitamin B-12 deficiency is an obvious possible underlying cause of fatigue. Vitamin B-12, also called cobalamin, helps your body make healthy red blood cells, which carry life-sustaining oxygen from your lungs. In recent years, Dad had been slightly anemic. His hematocrit, hemoglobin, and other red-blood-cell test results consistently came back low, but he'd never had a low serum B-12 result.

A hematocrit shows the percentage of red blood cells (RBCs) in a person's total blood volume. RBCs contain hemoglobin, a protein that transports oxygen from the lungs to the tissues. (See Chapter Twelve.)

In this latest round of bloodwork, Dad's B-12 level was normal, and his thyroid was fine. But he still had anemia. To my knowledge, Dr. Buchanan never made anything of Dad's anemia. It just *was*.

Besides his fatigue, Dad now walked with marked unsteadiness, with what doctors call ataxia, or uncoordinated movement. For many years he had tolerated numbness in the sole of his right foot, which he could relieve by lying down. He now had numbness and tingling in both of his hands and feet. He developed a tremor in his hands, too, but I don't recall if it dated to this time. He and I discussed a neurological workup, but, to my knowledge, Dad didn't bring these symptoms up with Dr. Buchanan until months later, and Buchanan didn't ask.

Less than two years before, my father had defiantly stared down disability from a hip fracture. Now, if he fell and broke his hip, he might not make it back. He had lost considerable strength, vigor, and fight. Concerned about sarcopenia (muscle decline) and frailty, I preached exercise and more exercise–walking in the neighborhood, playing golf for as long as he could, lifting weights at the local rehab center–but he was more often begging off from any physical effort.

We considered the possibility that a drug or a multiple-drug interaction was causing his fatigue, as well as some of his neurological symptoms. I was especially concerned about his dependence on Ambien, which Buchanan first prescribed for him in August 2009. I knew from acquaintances that Ambien was highly addictive and often left users with foggy-headiness and lethargy the morning after they took it. It seemed to me to be a bad drug choice for an elderly person.

I remember talking with Dad on Oct. 25, 2011, about arranging for the PET scan Dr. Exeter had suggested, but he was too tired to think about it. Eventually, he rallied, and on Nov. 14, just three days past the one-year anniversary of his botched laser surgery, he had another thoracic CT scan with contrast. This time, Exeter described his diagnosis as 1) "ABN X-ray," as in abnormal X-ray, and 2) chronic fatigue.

CT Scan No. 2

According to the radiologist's findings, all of the preexisting nodules had grown and now measured between 8 mm. and 9 mm., which, if you're with me on the basic math, is still less than a centimeter.

While I understood that growth is a bad sign, I didn't know how to evaluate this interpretation. It bothered me that the same pair of eyes was estimating the growth, which purportedly ranged from 1 mm. to 3 mm. per nodule. Having read Jerome Groopman's "How Doctors Think," I was aware of how *often* preconceived notions or biases influence a radiologist. It stood to reason that once Dr. Exeter typecast these nodules as potentially neoplastic, he would be predisposed to perceiving an increase in their size. Call it confirmation bias: People want to prove themselves right, not wrong.

But I also recognized that I had incentive to prove him wrong, so I kept tabs on my own bias.

This time Exeter found nodules in both of Dad's lungs, a point he had not made clear (not to me, at least) in his previous interpretation, and a new 4-mm. nodule in his right lung. He characterized two of the preexisting nodules as smooth, but otherwise did not comment on the nodules' appearance, thus being consistent in his inconsistency. He now called the right lung's solid component an "irregular density," making it seem more cancer-like, but he did not detect a change in its size. This area, you'll recall, bore the brunt of Dad's catastrophic fall.

Bottom line, Dr. Exeter concluded that the change in the nodules "has to suggest underlying active disease. *Metastatic disease is a leading consideration.*"

Metastatic disease. Cancer. But he didn't say cancer. He would never say cancer.

I parsed the words: A leading consideration? *A*, not *the*. What did that mean? How about giving us some other "leading considerations"? Dr. Buchanan, Dad's PCP, didn't have any to offer, either.

My logical mind told me that medicine should have come a lot further by now than this, *this* being having a patient submit to one test after another, undergo repeated exposure to radiation, and then try to make sense of vague interpretations. There's little care in such a process. Whether they actually talk to them or not, radiologists do work for patients, not for the physicians who refer them. They should be held more accountable for the impact their opinions have, and I don't mean in a legal sense.

Again, Dr. Exeter advised: A PET scan "may be of some help in defining a primary neoplasm." So why, I wondered, did Buchanan order another CT scan first? Was he another distracted PCP operating on automatic pilot? Did Buchanan benefit financially from these redundant tests?

"He's always in a hurry," Dad said when I asked him about Dr. Buchanan. "He only gives me 15 minutes."

Knowing the basics of cancer metastasis, my father did not believe his pulmonary nodules were metastases. But he's not an oncologist, nor are Drs. Exeter and Buchanan, so I did some quickie research.

Cancerous cells apparently spread from a primary neoplasm through your lymphatic system and your *venous* (deoxygenated) blood circulation, which, as you'll recall, is the blood returning to your heart and lungs. The most common sites of cancer metastasis, according to the online National Cancer Institute, are the lungs, the bones, and the liver, which have high *vascular* flow, but this does not mean that cancer always metastasizes to these sites first.[18]

Tumors of the breast, colon, kidney, skin, ovaries, uterus, pancreas, prostate, rectum, stomach, and thyroid, the NCI says, *can* metastasize to the lungs. Among them, breast, kidney, and thyroid tumors and melanomas commonly metastasize *first* to the lungs. The most common sites of metastasis for colon cancer, the NCI informs, are, in "descending order," the liver, the peritoneum, and the lungs. For pancreatic cancer, these sites are the liver, the lungs, and the peritoneum. With prostate cancer, it's bones-lungs-liver.[19]

This information struck me as just enough to be dangerous. To put it in a meaningful context, I needed better sources, like a real flesh-and-blood oncologist. I could do medical-literature homework, but I'm not sure how far it would get me, and, besides, I, like my father, was exhausted.

Although fatigued, Dad still had no respiratory symptoms: No persistent, worsening cough; no wheezing or shortness of breath; no chest pain. During his inactivity, he had put on weight, not lost it.[20] He also had no symptoms that would suggest a cancer elsewhere, such as blood in his urine or his stools.

THE PET SCAN

The much-anticipated radioactive imaging of my father's "whole body"—from neck to pelvis— occurred on Dec. 3, 2011, at the Outer Banks Hospital. More than a year had passed since Dr. Exeter's solitary-nodule report. The short answer to what this test revealed was: Nothing.

Nothing.

A Greenville, N.C., radiologist read the PET images, not Dr. Exeter. He identified "multiple bilateral pulmonary nodules" that "measure up to 8 mm. in diameter" and are "concerning for metastatic disease"—which, in proper English, means they suggest cancer (when did concerning become an adjective?)—but he could not "confirm" a primary neoplasm.

No neoplasm. No primary tumor. But the Greenville ologist did observe "mild hypermetabolic activity" in "several" of these nodules.

We had returned to radiology Never-Say-Neverland.

Positron emission tomography is the chief image-based detection method for tumors. It is also used in diagnosing heart disease and brain disorders. The PET test uses tracer radioactive material to illuminate how your tissues and organs are functioning on a cellular level. The type of radioactive material and its delivery method depend on which of your tissues or organs are being studied.

My father received an injection of radioactive deoxyglucose and then waited 45 minutes to an hour for the tracer sugar, which has a short half-life, to be absorbed by his body. Similar to the CT scan, he lay supine on a gantry, but this one slid him into the doughnut hole of a PET machine, which generated computerized pictures of his cells metabolizing (breaking down) the sugar.

"Because cancer cells use sugar faster than normal cells," the National Cancer Institute explains, "areas with cancer cells look brighter on the pictures."[21]

While it is true that cells that metabolize the radioactive sugar quickly are more likely to be cancerous, not everything hypermetabolic is cancer. Infected tissue tends to be hypermetabolic as well. Thus, the detection of "mild hypermetabolic activity" in several nodules—"mild" on what scale, if you please?— added up, once again, to "indeterminate" bupkis, and you can't treat, nor should you ever try to treat, bupkis, indeterminate or otherwise.

"Everybody is hedging," said Dr. Al, about his chest X-ray, CT scan, and PET scan interpretations. Dr. Exeter and the Greenville radiologist don't know, so "they're covering the bases and their asses."

I didn't know what to make of this. How could there not be established patterns of metastasis to inform radiologists in their assessments? Haven't enough people died of known metastatic cancers and been autopsied? Why don't "we" know more? Or do we? Just how au courant were the North Carolina radiologists?

According to the online NCI, sometimes a primary tumor cannot be found, despite extensive testing, because it "is too small or has completely regressed."[22] Fine, but don't radiologists have some idea of how often a negative PET scan turns out to be cancer? Aren't there data in the literature? I intended to find out, as soon as I had time.

Because I had no contact with Dr. Buchanan or Dr. Exeter, and Dad didn't welcome talk about cancer, I felt stymied. The next stop in the diagnostic checkout line was a lung-tissue biopsy, which I knew my father would never allow.

At Christmastime 2011, Britt, Al Jr., and I brainstormed alternate explanations for Dad's nodules. I had long favored a home investigation for toxic materials, but which toxic materials might exist, and why Dad would show effects *now*, I hadn't a clue. Al went in a different environmental direction, and before you could say, "kitty, kitty," he had branded my cat Oliver Felina Non Grata.

For nearly 10 years I had been leaving Oliver with my parents whenever I left town. Because Oliver roamed and slept in Dad's office and an adjacent bedroom during his stays, his dander clearly infiltrated Dad's atmosphere. Could cat dander cause lung nodules like the ones he had? Britt found some support for this theory on the Internet, and Dad liked it, even though it lacked anything close to scientific evidence, and he had never shown an allergic reaction to Oliver or any other cat.

Did Dad have a cancer that had metastasized to his lungs, lung cancer, or kitty dander disease? Had my father seen an oncologist now, it's likely that lung cancer would have been ruled out as an option, at least for me. If my father knew, based on his medical knowledge, that he didn't have lung cancer, he didn't tell me. Fortunately, whatever was happening pathologically in his chest was happening slowly.

The same could not be said of his urinary incontinence, which, by December, had become intolerable.

Having ignored the negative feelings he had for Dr. Naylor, Dr. Al was not going to make the same mistake with Dr. Smith, whose jet-setting unavailability rubbed him the wrong way. He decided he would go to Duke for any surgery, even though he dreaded the travel. The prospect loomed as a major hardship for me, but I was on board for the duration. I wanted my father to be well again, if possible, and I believed he could be. I had no idea what a challenge that would be.

On Tuesday, Jan. 3, 2012, I called Duke, hoping to make an appointment with renowned urological surgeon George D. Webster. I had read some of Webster's articles online and thought if anyone could fix Dad's plumbing, this master of urinary incontinence with 40 years of experience could.

Alas, the guru urologist had retired recently; we missed him by mere months. Upon being assured by Mary, the friendly and competent voice of the Duke Urology Clinic, that Dr. Terse, Webster's protégé and successor, more than filled his shoes, I scheduled a Jan. 25 appointment and got busy on hotel arrangements. The advocate was now a travel manager. Nine years after Duke saved my mother's life, we again were turning to the university medical center for salvation.

~

Chapter Eleven

Depression and
DELIRIUM

A Complicated Picture

When my father told me after his hip-fracture surgery that he was depressed, I knew he was reacting to his debilitated condition and the long recovery that lay ahead, and I figured his mood would be transient. He was a resilient person, a fighter. Still, I watched for signs of a more severe psychological change. They never materialized.

A year later, when Dad sank into a deep depression because of his post-BPH laser-surgery incontinence, he didn't always articulate a depressed mood. Instead, he seemed increasingly confused, forgetful, agitated, and irrational. He worried about his cognitive status, which made him anxious and more agitated. His despair had a mental snowball effect.

I did not see a fighter then. I saw a defeated and bitter man who had lost hope in his ability to regain the quality of life that he considered minimal for survival. Fortunately, he rallied, but his extreme anxiety may have exacted a physiological toll.

Certainly his altered mental state hurt me. I stopped writing for two months and took an antidepressant to regain and then maintain *my* emotional equilibrium. I was fading fast. I also worried about the effect my father's despondency would have on my mother's mental health.

Depression in older people is complicated. To be an effective advocate, you have to understand that your Mom's or Pop's depression can be an illness itself; a sign of another illness; or a psychological reaction to illness.

In 2009, when I was trying to have Mom neuropsychologically evaluated, she became severely and frighteningly depressed. I described her then as a paper cut-out of her former self.

Cerebrovascular disease, which was revealed by the brain CT scan that she underwent before her memory-clinic appointment, is a risk factor for dementia *and* depression, but so are some of the psychosocial factors that weighed on her. She knew she was mentally declining and losing her self-sufficiency.

According to the National Institute of Mental Health, 1 to 5 percent of older adults living independently in the community have major depression, as do 13.5 percent of those who need home healthcare and 11.5 percent of those who are hospitalized.[1]

The Geriatric Mental Health Foundation (GMHF), which was established by the American Assn. for Geriatric Psychiatry, estimates that about 15 of every 100 adults 65 and older suffer from major depression.[2]

Major depression is a "mental disorder" that *DSM-IV* defines as "a clinically significant behavioral or psychological syndrome or pattern that is associated with present distress (e.g., a painful symptom) or disability (i.e., impairment in one or more important areas of functioning) or a significantly increased risk of suffering death, pain, disability, or an important loss of freedom." The *DSM-5* definition is more complex than this, but not substantially different.[3]

A mild or moderate depression is considered a subsyndromal (i.e., sub-major) depression. Although less severe, subsyndromal depression is a risk factor for major depression.[4]

Just as cognitive impairment is not an unavoidable consequence of aging, neither is depression. Being old does not mean being depressed. That's 1950s-era thinking. Old people do not, simply by virtue of their age, spend days ruminating over their mortality. They also don't normally experience fatigue, loss of appetite, disturbed sleep, and other symptoms of depression.[5] To believe otherwise is ageism, to which too many trained medical professionals fall prey. Don't you do the same.

MOM'S DEPRESSION

I do not exaggerate when I say that I could feel Mom's depression, her gloom, when I walked into my parents' house. Her energy level and initiative precipitously fell off, and the life vanished from her eyes. She moved heavily and slowly, spoke without any animation, and showed scant interest in her daily activities. I saw nothing but pain in her face:

She was profoundly sad.

There are no psychiatrists on the Outer Banks, so my mother, with my father's and my urging, sought out a local clinical psychologist. This professional encouraged her to buy a laptop computer and to use the online community to help relieve her sense of isolation—which Mom apparently (and, I assume, genuinely) identified as the cause of her mood.

Social isolation has long been considered a psychosocial risk factor for depression, regardless of a person's age. Other depression stressors for older people include:

- ❖ An empty nest
- ❖ A move into an apartment, retirement facility, or nursing home
- ❖ Declining health
- ❖ Impending surgery
- ❖ The death of a spouse or friends
- ❖ Chronic and/or severe pain
- ❖ Disability
- ❖ Loneliness, and
- ❖ A loss of independence and control[6]

Although well-meaning, the psychologist's advice was ridiculous, and we knew it. My mother is a reserved and solitary person, not someone desirous of much social interaction. If she were, she never would have moved to the Outer Banks. She has an artist's sense of separateness. She also is technophobic.

Nonetheless, we put skepticism aside and bought Mom a laptop, setting her up with an email address and instructions on how to navigate the Web. She didn't take to it. Her memory failed her. We told her repeatedly how to create, send, and receive email and how to maneuver on and off websites, but she never remembered any of our instructions. I painstakingly wrote the processes down, in step-by-step detail. That didn't help, either. Instead, Mom felt stupid. This inadequacy fed her depression.

My mother regained her emotional well-being and, thus, her life, only after Dr. Ramses prescribed the antidepressant, Cymbalta® (duloxetine). There are more than 20 antidepressants on the market. If Cymbalta had not worked, he had others to try.

Because she was then very concerned about her forgetfulness, and both depression and antidepressant medication can cause memory impairment, Mom quit taking Cymbalta for a while and became depressed again. Not surprisingly, her cognitive problems also continued, so she resumed taking a small dose of the drug. She has taken 20 milligrams of Cymbalta daily ever since as maintenance.

When I would ask Mom why she was depressed, she usually told me that she felt grief-stricken, not depressed, and cited the loss of so many family members, friends, and even beloved pets over her long lifetime. Still sounding like the psychiatrist she was, she spoke of "collecting" grief: A death today would cause her to ruminate over so many deaths of yesterday.

Grief is a normal response to loss. It is a *temporary* state of mental and emotional distress and impaired social, occupational, or other functioning. We expect and culturally accept grief; we do not consider it to be a mental disorder. Being "down in the dumps" or feeling the blues temporarily is also normal.

I keenly appreciate the difference between grief and depression. But I also know that heavy grief can develop into a clinical depression, which is a life-threatening condition, and so I acted upon my mother's "grief."

In a major change from *DSM-IV* that incited some controversy, *DSM-5* attempts to distinguish grief from bereavement that is more accurately characterized as a major depressive episode. "In grief," *DSM-5* advises, "the predominant affect is feelings of emptiness and loss." If a bereaved person experiences a "persistent depressed mood and the inability to anticipate happiness or pleasure," he or she is more aptly described as depressed.

Those who take issue with this change point out, perhaps cynically, what a boon it is to the pharmaceutical industry to diagnose grief as depression.[7]

The most obvious life threat to a depressed person is suicide. In 2004, according to the U.S. Centers for Disease Control and Prevention, adults 65 and older committed 16 percent of all suicides in the United States, even though they then accounted for only 12 percent of the population. During the same time, the GMHF estimated elder-suicide at 25 percent of the total.

Regardless of whether the rate is 16 or 25 percent, adults 65 and older have the highest suicide rate of any U.S. age group. According to the National Institute of Mental Health, men account for 85 percent of all over-65 suicides: Among them, those who are white and over 80 pose the greatest risk to themselves.[8]

With Mom, I worried more about what I call mind-body connection damage than about suicide. I feared that her depression would lead to fatigue, sleep deprivation, loss of appetite, dehydration, a shutting down of functions. Depression can take a big toll on an older person's physiological reserves.

If your Mom or Pop is grieving someone's death or another significant loss, give her or him time to do so, but also keep a watchful eye. If you think the grief is excessive, either in duration or intensity, seek medical intervention. According to *DSM-IV*, bereavement that persists for more than two months or is "characterized by marked functional impairment, morbid preoccupation with [one's] worthlessness, suicidal ideation, psychotic symptoms, or psychomotor retardation" constitutes a major depression.[9] You don't want your loved one to slip away while she mourns.

"MAJOR DEPRESSION"

DSM-IV sets forth a two-part diagnosis for major depression.[*] A patient must experience one of the following symptoms most of the day nearly every day for two weeks:

- ❖ A depressed mood, or
- ❖ Markedly diminished interest or pleasure in all, or almost all, activities [this is called anhedonia]

PLUS four or more of the following seven psychological or somatic symptoms nearly every day during the same two-week period:

- ❖ Clinically significant weight loss in the absence of dieting or weight gain (e.g., a change of more than 5 percent in body weight in a month) or a decrease in appetite
- ❖ Insomnia or hypersomnia [excessive sleep]
- ❖ Observable psychomotor agitation or retardation

---

[*] A person with depression symptoms as well as a history or symptoms of mania may have bipolar disorder. The Mayo Clinic website, www.mayoclinic.com, provides an easy-to-understand explanation of this disorder, also known as manic depression.

❖ Fatigue or loss of energy

❖ Feelings of worthlessness or excessive or inappropriate guilt

❖ Diminished ability to think or concentrate, or indecisiveness, and

❖ Recurrent thoughts of death, recurrent suicidal ideation [meaning, the idea of suicide occurs to the patient] without a specific plan, a specific plan for committing suicide, or a suicide attempt[10]

My mother showed both a depressed mood and anhedonia. She stopped doing all of the activities that once interested her. She managed to get out of bed, dress, and prepare a cup of coffee, but after that, she retired to the couch, a sad and listless lump. She didn't even care to watch television. I observed psychomotor retardation, a loss of energy, and a diminished ability to think—three of the seven symptoms above, but I didn't need a fourth to be convinced of depression.

DSM-5 abandons this two-part diagnosis. It instead requires that a patient experience five of the nine symptoms listed above nearly every day during the same two-week period, with at least one of the symptoms being depressed mood or anhedonia. It also qualifies all of the symptoms, in particular, specifying that the depressed mood and anhedonia may be as indicated by "subjective report" or by "observation." Thus, a person who does not feel "sad, empty, or hopeless" may be diagnosed with depression.[11]

Mom had the requisite five. Beyond that, I do not wish to get entangled in *DSM-5*, which was not my guide when I tried to understand my mother's mental state.

The Geriatric Mental Health Foundation advises that depressed older people are less likely to appear sad or to talk about a depressed mood than depressed younger people are.

According to the GMHF, depressed elders more commonly complain about "vague aches and pains" that do not subside with treatment and exhibit "frequent demanding behavior." They tend to suffer insomnia, memory loss, and confusion; to appear irritable; and to withdraw from social situations.[12]

"Demanding behavior" falls grossly short of my father's acting out during his incontinence depression—if, indeed, depression is what it was. He was definitely irritable and often confused and forgetful. But he never crossed the line that divides demanding jerk from mean son of a bitch. I've seen the SOBs in clinic waiting rooms, haranguing their rattled daughters or daughters-in-law as the latter attempt to sort out an appointment or test snafu. They're not depressives; they're abusers.

The GMHF's description of elder depression also fits with how Dr. Constantine Lyketsos of Johns Hopkins distinguishes Alzheimer's-associated depression, which he describes as more like an affective disorder.

Its signs, Lyketsos says, include "irritability, anxiety, worry, agitation, but not necessarily sadness."[13]

DEPRESSION-DEMENTIA INTERFACE

Some geriatric psychiatrists believe there is an "interface" between depression and dementia in older people. They speak of a brain-disorder "continuum" from late-life depression to mild cognitive impairment to dementia.

By late-life depression, they mean late-onset depression, a term that applies to people who experience depression for the first time at an advanced age, the lower limit of which varies in studies from 45 to 65 years old. If they are to be believed, this describes both of my parents. Mom treated scores of depressed people during her psychiatric career, but she claims to have never experienced the illness herself. My father, however, has long struggled with anxiety. My mother's counsel apparently kept him on an even keel during the many struggles that occurred in his long and high-powered career.

Clinical evidence suggests that deficits in cognitive performance occur most consistently among older people with late-onset depression rather than those with early-onset depression. These elders, who frequently have medical comorbidity, such as with cardiovascular disease, have a higher relative risk of later developing some form of dementia.[14]

Does this mean that depression is a risk factor for dementia, particularly Alzheimer's disease? Or perhaps a prodromal symptom of dementia? Maybe.

Just what role does depression play in what clinical and epidemiological researchers refer to as predementia syndromes?

The verdict on the interface/continuum/role theories is still out and may always be. But clinical studies unquestionably implicate a neuropathological connection between depression and dementia in older people.

According to Drs. Rabins and Lyketsos, disabling psychiatric symptoms such as depression, delusions, and agitation "*almost universally* occur in persons with dementia." They attribute the high prevalence to "the same underlying brain processes that cause the cognitive symptoms." In other words, depression appears to be a feature of the patient's brain disorder.[15]

Let's look closer at this disorder.

ILLNESS-RELATED DEPRESSION

Before diagnosing major depression, your parent's psychiatrist or other physician should determine whether illness or another non-psychiatric cause, such as alcohol abuse, an adverse reaction to medication(s), or a general medical condition (hypothyroidism), might be responsible.

Depression occurs more commonly in elders with physical health problems than in those without such concerns and may come on after a stroke, a coronary bypass operation, or . . . a hip fracture.[16]

There is considerable medical literature on the subject of depression in heart patients. Clinical studies since the 1930s have borne out that 15 to 20 percent of all patients with coronary artery disease suffer major depression. Roughly 20 percent of patients who undergo bypass surgery feel depressed afterward; and most of them were depressed before their operation.[17] You can imagine the destructive feelings that a despondent elder with a bad heart might inflict on himself: paranoia, anxiety, agitation, irritability, anger, fear.

After an episode of atrial fibrillation in 2012, my father experienced what he described as "cardiac neurosis." He was obsessively afraid that he would "stroke out."

Blood from fibrillating atria moves slower and less efficiently into the ventricles and, therefore, can pool, making it more likely to clot. Within just two days of AF onset, a clot can form in the heart—typically in an area of the left atrium—break off, and travel to the brain, causing a stroke. Hence, people with atrial fibrillation typically take an anticoagulant.

Experts have identified a syndrome peculiar to older adults who suffer from cardiovascular disease and late-onset depression. It is called vascular depression, also known as depression-executive-dysfunction (DED) syndrome.

Compared with other profoundly depressed people, patients with DED syndrome exhibit "greater suspiciousness, diminished interest in activities, psychomotor retardation and disability, but a less pronounced vegetative [state]," according to Dr. George S. Alexopoulos, director of the Cornell Institute of Geriatric Psychiatry, and his associates, who first proposed DED syndrome.[18]

Physicians at the Harvard Medical School, who studied DED after the Cornell team, characterize its symptoms as "prominent anhedonia, psychomotor slowing, executive dysfunction, and high levels of disability, often with an absence of guilt or depressed mood and with limited insight into their condition."

Vascular depression, they say, arises from the "disruption of frontal-subcortical brain circuitry by white-matter lesions and other brain abnormalities" and can be more resistant to drug therapy than "standard" major depression.[19]

Because vascular depression, like all depressions, is multifactorial, psychosocial risk factors, such as social isolation, can trigger it.[20]

Regardless of its cause, depression can worsen the prognosis of a patient with any type of cardiovascular disease. Depressed cardiovascular patients hospitalized for acute myocardial infarctions, congestive heart failure, or bypass surgery are more likely to be re-hospitalized for cardiovascular causes and to die from them than are heart patients who are not depressed. Even more unnerving, according to the Harvard team, depression increases the risk of cardiac disease among previously healthy people![21]

Depression also affects how well a patient with cardiovascular disease will take care of himself and heed doctors' recommendations about diet, exercise, stress reduction, and medication. The disorder may induce harmful physiological changes in patients and increase the incidence of cardiac events, as well as the risk of death.[22]

Bottom line: Depression can disable and kill.

UNMASKING DEPRESSION

If you suspect that your Mom or Pop is depressed, the following questions, based on *DSM* criteria, will help you to determine if your suspicions are justified. Ask yourself: Is he or she:

❖ Sleeping too much or too little? (Having trouble getting to sleep? Staying in bed all day?)

❖ Acting irritable and/or intolerant? (More so than usual?)

❖ Moving restlessly or more slowly than usual? (Fidgeting?)

❖ Lacking in energy and motivation? (Not leaving home?)

❖ Complaining more about physical aches and pains?

❖ Being more confused or forgetful?

❖ Eating less? (Is the refrigerator empty? Does it contain spoiled food?)

❖ Not bathing or shaving as often? (Is he/she wearing the same outfit every day?)

❖ Not taking care of the home? (Is trash piling up?)

❖ Stopping medications or taking them incorrectly?

❖ Withdrawing from others? (Failing to answer the phone or to return phone messages?)

❖ Crying too often or too much? (For no articulable reason?)

❖ Expressing recurrent thoughts of death or suicide?

No one depressed person is like another. Having said that, I would advise that if you answered yes to any of these questions, you should make an appointment for your parent with his or her primary-care physician. To ensure that the doctor receives an objective account of the symptoms, accompany your Mom or Pop and relate what you have observed. If you're on the ball, you will have made dated notes of your observations to which you can refer.

The doctor should conduct a history and a physical exam. If clinically indicated, he or she also should arrange for blood and urine tests to determine if a physical illness is causing your parent's depression. But don't let the doctor engage in test-overkill. Make him or her LISTEN and be on your guard.

Primary-care doctors reportedly fail to recognize major depressive episodes in up to 50 percent of their patients of all ages. (If the patient doesn't mention depression, the time-pressed PCP is not likely to bring it up.) They also mistake depression in older people for dementia, as well as fail to distinguish when an Alzheimer's patient is depressed.[23]

Yes, it may be difficult to differentiate in an older person those somatic (bodily) symptoms that are related to depression and those that are related to coexisting physical illness. Yes, elders often have chronic medical illnesses or pain syndromes and unexplained physical symptoms. But medical professionals are supposed to be able to make the necessary cause-and-effect distinctions.

Primary-care physicians can do much more than they currently do to uncover cases of depression, starting with asking more on-point questions and listening to their patients' responses. Questions such as "How are things at home?" or even "Have you been feeling sad/depressed/blue lately?" can elicit valuable information. Communication + empathy = results.[24]

Assuming your Mom's doctor diagnoses depression, she may be treated in primary care or referred to a psychiatrist. The duration and severity of her depression should determine the choice. Cognitive impairment, if a factor, also should be weighed.

PCPs commonly prescribe antidepressants, but they do not engage in structured psychotherapy (talking), which has been shown in studies to benefit more elders than once thought. They also do not conduct electroconvulsive therapy (ECT), which may be indicated for patients with severe depression resistant to other treatments or at risk of serious harm to themselves.

In choosing an antidepressant for your Mom, the PCP *should* consider her prescription drug history, both in terms of efficacy and adverse effects. The potential for an adverse interaction between the antidepressant and her preexisting medications also is important to evaluate. People 65 and older have a lower tolerance for unwanted effects of antidepressants and are more likely to have cardiovascular disease and other medical illnesses that might complicate their pharmacologic treatment. Brain levels of chemical messengers, such as serotonin, norepinephrine, and dopamine, usually decrease with age. For this reason, older people should take lower doses of antidepressants that regulate one or more of these transmitters.

I have not researched ECT, but one of my mini-medical school authorities, Dr. Steve Epstein, chair of Georgetown's psychiatry department, says it can be used safely and effectively in older people with intractable major depression. It is strictly last resort.[25]

Ironically, elders who kill themselves often have seen their primary-care doctors shortly before their deaths! While they are less likely than younger patients to consult mental-health specialists, people over

65 with psychiatric disorders tend to visit their primary-care doctors regularly.[26]

Count yourself lucky if you have a Mom or Pop who articulates her/his depressed mood and/or anhedonia and asks for help. I think it is more likely that your aged parent will not talk about depression, instead stoically enduring it, rationalizing it as normal, or being so lethargic as to not want to discuss it. Cognitive impairment may complicate her or his awareness. Don't let a lack of perception complicate yours.

DELIRIUM: THE OVERLOOKED DISORDER

Of the three D's of cognitive impairment that I identified in Chapter Eight, delirium is the most overlooked and misdiagnosed. It is also one of the oldest disorders known to medicine, having been described 2,500 years ago by Hippocrates, who wrote about dementia, as well.

When my heavily medicated father saw my absent brother in his hospital room while he was convalescing from his 1998 rooftop fall, he was unquestionably delirious. Pain medication also rendered him delirious after he was discharged home.

I've witnessed more recent episodes of transient confusion by my parents and have reason to believe that these, too, may have been delirium, but I do not have a definitive diagnosis.

According to my research, delirium is common among older people during hospitalization, but 14 percent of all elders 85 and older living in the community also suffer from this attention-deficient and confusional state.[27] My friend Linda's remarkable 100-year-old grandmother knew she could no longer care for herself when she saw people in her kitchen who she knew were not there. Then living temporarily with her grandmother, Linda says the hallucinations "came on without warning."

Outside of the hospital, people typically suffer from delirium because of 1) infection, 2) neurological crisis, 3) drug-related effects, or 4) a metabolic breakdown.

Surely you've read about old people who have been "found down" in their homes, either alive and confused/incapacitated or dead, after days of being unable to summon help. Most likely, infection felled them, but they might have suffered a stroke, a seizure, or a subdural hematoma, the latter typically after a fall. Other explanations for their confusion, I've learned, include the taking of an opiate (which is what Dad did in 1998) or a sedative or a metabolic disturbance such as alcohol withdrawal, uremia, or a sodium disorder.[28]

CHARACTERISTICS OF DELIRIUM

Delirium is characterized by:

* **Inattention**–difficulty focusing, sustaining and shifting attention, maintaining conversation, following commands
* **Disorganized thinking**–disorganized or incoherent speech, rambling or irrelevant conversation, unclear or illogical flow of ideas
* **An altered level of consciousness**–clouding of consciousness with reduced clarity of awareness of the environment
* **Cognitive deficits**–typically global or multiple deficits, such as disorientation, memory deficits, language impairment
* **Perceptual disturbances**–illusions or hallucinations
* **Psychomotor disturbances**–either hyperactivity, marked by agitation and vigilance, or hypoactivity, marked by lethargy, or a mix of both
* **An altered sleep-wake cycle**–typically daytime drowsiness and nighttime insomnia, and
* **Emotional disturbances**–intermittent symptoms of fear, paranoia, anxiety, depression, irritability, apathy, anger, or euphoria[29]

The disorder has an acute (sudden) onset–usually over a period of hours or days–and a fluctuating course of symptoms, which come and go or increase and decrease in severity over a 24-hour period, along with lucid intervals. In contrast, dementia is a chronic confusional state with no lucid intervals.[30]

Delirium has three clinical subtypes.[31] Experts agree that the psychomotor behavior of delirious people can be 1) hyperactive, 2) hypoactive, or 3) mixed hyperactive-hypoactive. Hypoactive delirium has a silent or passive presentation, devoid of the hyperactive restlessness, delusions, and agitation that we–and, unfortunately, healthcare professionals—automatically associate with this condition.[32]

According to delirium expert Dr. Sharon K. Inouye, who is director of the Aging Brain Center at Hebrew Senior Life's Institute for Aging Research in Boston, physicians and nurses frequently fail to recognize delirium because it fluctuates and symptomatically overlaps with dementia. Also, they often lack a formal cognitive assessment of a delirious patient; underappreciate delirium's clinical consequences; and fail to consider the diagnosis important.[33]

Too frequently, ageism leads medical professionals to assume, *ipso facto*, that confused older patients have dementia. Once again, preconceptions and biases (CDRs) determine what they see and, thus, diagnose.

Studies suggest that healthcare workers, even nurses who observe patients throughout the day for a period of days, miss more than half of all delirium cases.[34]

HOSPITAL VULNERABILITY + INSULT

Hospital delirium differs markedly in cause from found-down delirium. According to Inouye, hospital delirium is a multifactorial syndrome that results from the "interaction of vulnerability on the part of the patient [with] hospital-related insults."

Hence, patient vulnerability + hospital insult = delirium.

Some predisposing factors that may render an elder vulnerable, says Inouye, are dehydration, *cognitive impairment*, alcohol abuse, severe illness, neurologic disease, immobility, and visual or hearing impairments. Common insult-causing factors that precipitate delirium include:

* Drugs, especially sedatives and narcotics
* Surgical and medical procedures
* Intercurrent illnesses, which occur during the course of another illness and include infections, iatrogenic complications, shock, and dehydration
* Emotional stress, sometimes brought on by sensory deprivation or sensory overload and/or by social isolation
* Use of Foley catheters and other medical (and physical) restraints
* Prolonged sleep deprivation[35]

The hip-fracture patient, in particular, is exposed to a number of insults: first, the accident (such as a fall), then pain, relocation, clinical and radio-physical examinations, anesthesia, and surgery. Perioperative (occurring during surgery) and postoperative conditions may cause him or her further insult. Delirium is associated with long waits for an operation, anemia, urinary tract and wound infections, urinary retention, fever, feeding problems, and immobility.

The combination of an elder's vulnerability with *just* the simple business-as-usual of hospital care can be cognitively devastating. According to Inouye, delirium annually "complicates" hospital stays for at least 20 percent of patients 65 and over. The incidence among them varies by clinical situation as follows:

- ❖ 10 to 30 percent in emergency departments
- ❖ 14 to 24 percent at the time of hospital admission
- ❖ 15 to 53 percent after surgery
- ❖ 70 to 87 percent in intensive care (thanks to isolation/noise/lighting/a variety of stressors imposed on critically ill patients)[36]

Although an ancient disorder, delirium became much more prominent in the 1950s and 1960s with the emergence of hospital intensive care. In this context, it has been called the "new madness of medical progress," as well as ICU psychosis.[37]

Up to 60 percent of patients in nursing homes or post-acute care settings also experience delirium. (Remember the dementia link.)

I always thought that my mother's bed-in strike at the Sentara Nursing Center "hellhole" was a display of delirium. Having studied this disorder and considered its links to dementia and depression, I now believe she may have been delirious (clinically hypoactive) in Sentara Norfolk General and at home, during my father's hip-fracture convalescence, before her hospitalization. What Dad labeled "decompensation" may have been delirium.

Delirium is a *huge* problem among elders. When illness is compounded by delirium, a person's chances of dying from that illness increase significantly.

ANTICIPATING DELIRIUM

A diagnosis of delirium can be made clinically, without technological aids, on the basis of 1) a history from family members, caregivers, and other in-the-know third parties; 2) a physical examination; and 3) bedside observations. If your parent is going to be hospitalized, I urge you to assist medical professionals by evaluating his or her vulnerability. Think of the predisposing factors as *predictive* risk factors that you can monitor and then minimize the risk by ensuring that interventions occur.

For example, if immobility is an issue, make sure that your parent walks often and engages in regular range-of-motion exercises. Evaluate with the healthcare team the use and necessity of a Foley catheter or other physical restraints. Whenever it is safe to do so, encourage your parent to walk, with assistance, to his or her bathroom, rather than to rely on a catheter or bedpan.

To enhance your Mom's or Pop's sense of cognitive connectiveness, be sure he has needed eyeglasses and portable amplifying devices, if hearing loss is a problem. Then keep track of these aids, so they don't "go missing."

Your parent may feel isolated in a hospital room. Orienting influences from home, such as calendars, clocks, and photographs, may help to ease his unrest, as may the presence of comforting family members. But leave the hot-button relatives at home.

I could go on with preventive measures, but you catch my drift. There is much that you can do to safeguard your Mom's or Pop's hospital environment and treatment if you fear delirium. Above all, strive to cut down on the hospital noise and enhance your Pop's chance for restful sleep.[38]

And, finally, if you observe a sudden disturbing change in your Pop's cognition, perceptions, and/or emotions, speak up! Hyperactive delirious patients run the risk of hip fractures or cardiovascular complications, according to Inouye. Those who are delusional or hallucinating may do violence to themselves or others. Hypoactive patients may become dehydrated or malnourished or suffer from that old bed-rest scourge of pressure sores.[39]

Remember, delirium is a *sudden* decline in attention and cognition. Dementia is not sudden—at least, not Alzheimer's disease dementia—but depression can be.

Besides my father, the only other older person I know who became undeniably delirious in a hospital was my friend Beth's 84-year-old father-in-law, who "freaked out," she said, after knee-replacement surgery. His precipitating factors were textbook.

During this crisis, Beth emailed me: "He's in pain and very anxious and seems to be going in and out of lucidity. He wants to pull all the tubes out and is very upset about still having a Foley catheter. My mother-in-law, who is sleeping in his room, went home for an hour today, and he freaked out because he did not remember that she told him she was leaving briefly."

The situation deteriorated when an attempt was made to transfer the poor man to another hospital. He became so "disoriented and combative in the ambulance," Beth said, "that he hit his head and cut his hands when the EMTs tried to restrain him. Huh? Two burly EMTs got into an alteration with my 84-year-old father-in-law?"

Yes, they did, and the police had to intervene.

Although he was initially agitated in his new room, Beth's father-in-law improved in the much calmer environment of a smaller private hospital. His family wisely reduced his stress by eliminating bright lights, noise, and other environmental irritants.

Before the surgery, Beth said, her father-in-law had shown no signs of dementia, but he does suffer from Parkinson's disease, which, as I noted in Chapter Eight, can cause memory deficits. This gentleman turned out to be vulnerable to hospital insults that restrained him, starting with his surgery. At no time during his hospitalization did any medical personnel identify his distress as delirium, leaving the family in a prolonged state of painful confusion.

By the time Beth's father-in-law went home, he had regained his former self. He seemed fine. Studies show, however, that delirium is independently associated with subsequent functional disability, dementia, admission to long-term care facilities, and death. Up to 90 percent of all terminally ill patients experience delirium in their last weeks of life.[40]

Chapter Twelve

The Aging
BODY

Normal Physiological Changes

When a doctor poses that maddening question, "What do you expect at your age?," to your Mom or Pop, or to *you*, you will be able to respond confidently—and defeat the implied ageism—if you know what you *can* expect. Age-related physiological changes happen to everyone, regardless of how successfully he or she has aged. The real question for the advocate, the caregiver, and the diligent patient is: What are they?

In this chapter, I give you an overview of normal aging. While I strive to be practically selective, offering what I consider to be physiological highlights, which, of necessity, include some anatomical facts, you nonetheless may be overwhelmed by my system-to-system presentation. If so, I suggest you use this chapter as you would a website about normal aging. Apply your research skimming skills. If your parent has a digestive problem, flip to that section and, when you have time, backtrack to my discussion about the heart, the lungs, and the brain. Cardiovascular and neurological aging became especially important for me to understand as I sought to help my ailing father.

As you undoubtedly have observed, no part of the human body better reflects the changes that occur over a lifetime than your skin, but I'm not going to start with your outer covering. Instead, I'll look first at your core or essence: your brain. All of the other systems of your body function to protect your brain. It is your control center. When it is dead, so are you. Indeed, you are your brain.

Your brain sends signals to your body through your nervous and endocrine systems, which are interconnected, but distinct. Impulses from your nervous system travel rapidly—in milliseconds—by electrochemical means, while the endocrine system releases chemicals (hormones) that act upon their targets in speeds varying from seconds to hours.

Let's take a closer look at the all-powerful nervous system and how age affects it.

The Nervous System

Your nervous system has central and peripheral components and is involved in some way in nearly every one of your body's functions, both voluntary and involuntary. Chief among its operations are:

* Receiving and interpreting sensory input
* Initiating responses to sensory input, including memory storage
* Maintaining homeostasis
* Controlling mental activity
* Controlling muscles and glands

The working unit of the nervous system is the **neuron** or nerve cell, which I previously mentioned in Chapter Eight. Each neuron has a cell body with a nucleus; an **axon**, also called a **nerve fiber**, which takes an electrical impulse away from the cell body; and one or more appendage-like **dendrites**, which bring electrochemical impulses from other nerve cells to the cell body.

Nerves are projections of neurons. They are made up of bundles of nerve fibers (axons) that transmit information between the central nervous system (CNS) and the peripheral nervous system (PNS).

Your CNS consists of your brain, which is jello-like and water-filled; your brain stem, and your spinal cord.[1] Your PNS encompasses all of the nerves and ganglia outside of the CNS, including the 31 pairs of spinal nerves that branch off of your spinal cord and the 12 pairs of cranial nerves in your skull. The PNS has two functional divisions: the **sensory (afferent)** division and the **motor (efferent)** division. The motor division subdivides further into the **somatic nervous system** and the **autonomic nervous system**.

Neurons, which are categorized as sensory or motor, are found in the brain, the spinal cord, and the peripheral nerves, whereas nerves exist only in the periphery. Ganglia, as I explained in discussing shingles, are structures that contain a number of neurons linked by synapses, which are junctions where neurons pass signals to other neurons or to muscle or gland cells.

Sensory neurons transmit **action potentials** (loosely, excitations) from the body's sensory receptors in the periphery to the spinal cord and thence to the brain, where they are interpreted. Sensory impulses are said to ascend and, therefore, to be **afferent** in relation to the CNS. Sensory receptors monitor external and internal stimuli through touch, taste, smell, sound, temperature, blood pressure, and body position.

Motor neurons work in the reverse, transmitting action potentials from the CNS toward the periphery, for example, allowing you to flex your bicep or curl your big toe. Their impulses descend and are **efferent** (away).

Nerves are not so neatly typed. Some of the cranial nerves, for example—the olfactory (smell), optic (vision), and vestibulocochlear (hearing and balance) nerves—are sensory only; some are exclusively somatic motor, such as the hypoglossal nerve that controls the tongue muscles; and the rest have mixed sensory, somatic motor, or parasympathetic functions.

The Autonomic Nervous System

Your autonomic nervous system (ANS) is vitally important and worth exploring further. The ANS regulates all **involuntary** nerve-controlled actions in the heart muscle, the smooth muscle, and the glands. In contrast, the somatic system influences the skeletal muscles, which are muscles attached to your bones, such as your biceps and quadriceps. The fibers of skeletal muscle are striated (streaked), whereas the fibers of **smooth muscle** are not. Smooth muscle can be found in the walls of your internal organs, such as your bladder, and your blood vessels.

Your autonomic nervous system consists of the mutually antagonistic **sympathetic** and **parasympathetic nervous systems** and the **enteric nervous system**, which is associated with the digestive tract. The ANS is unique in its two-neuron **efferent** pathway. The preganglionic autonomic neuron must synapse onto a postganglionic neuron before it can innervate (stimulate) the target or so-called effector tissues, such as those in the heart. (Think of ganglia as relay stations where nerves communicate with each other.)

Your sympathetic nervous system triggers the speed-up part of this automatic-response system, while the parasympathetic nervous system controls the opposing slow-down part. They oppose each other in a complementary way.

Surely you have experienced the "fight-or-flight" response to danger or stress. When you are confronted with a fearful or intensely anxious situation, your sympathetic nervous system reacts (i.e., your brain sends impulses), stimulating the release of two hormones, **epinephrine,** another name for adrenaline, and **norepinephrine,** from the medulla (the inner core) of your adrenal glands, which sit atop your kidneys. Your adrenals secrete these hormones into your bloodstream, thereby inducing what you know as an "adrenaline rush," the effects of which include increased muscle strength, stronger heart contractions and respiration, and elevated energy.

This adrenal secretion is 80 percent epinephrine and 20 percent norepinephrine. During fight-or-flight, your brain also triggers the release of norepinephrine at the end of postsynaptic autonomic neurons, so that it can more directly reach effector organs and other cells in the body. In this stimulation, **norepinephrine** acts as a **neurotransmitter**, not as an adrenal hormone, serving to mediate nerve signals that will boost your heart rate, blood pressure, and respiration, release glucose into your blood, inhibit your digestion, and otherwise get you ready to respond.

Norepinephrine is the key neurotransmitter of the sympathetic nervous system.

Your parasympathetic nervous system calms the physiological responses that epinephrine and norepinephrine incite by mediating rest and recovery. **Acetylcholine**, which I mentioned in relation to Alzheimer's disease drugs, is the preganglionic neurotransmitter for both divisions of the ANS, as well as the postganglionic neurotransmitter of the parasympathetic neurons. Acetylcholine exerts its effect on muscle cells at synapses called neuromuscular junctions.

The **vagus nerve** (cranial nerve X), which my father was able to stimulate in order to stop his irregular heartbeat, is command central for your parasympathetic functioning and also acts as a gateway between your sympathetic and parasympathetic nervous systems. It innervates the heart, lungs, liver, and stomach, among other organs.

Lost Neurons and the PNS

With aging, we lose a substantial number of neurons, but how this loss affects functioning is not always discernible.

You can expect older people to lose some **tactile sensitivity (touch)** because of a decline in their dermal sensory receptors. If your Mom or Pop cooks on an electric stove, beware the scorching burner inadvertently left on low heat.

Elders also experience a normal decline in sensory cranial nerve function. This *could* mean impaired smell, taste, vision, and/or hearing; but the impairment does not occur simply because of neuronal loss or dysfunction. It is multifactorial and could reflect cognitive deterioration or other change. As I previously mentioned, Alzheimer's patients typically cannot smell even the most pungent odors.

Motor neurons undergo a significant decline with age, hampering **locomotor function**. But just as with sensory changes, other factors that have nothing to do with age-related neuronal loss may come into play. In the case of an older person's altered gait and foot stride, for example, muscle strength, coordination, and visual acuity may be involved.

As many as half of the lower motor neurons in the lumbar region of the spinal cord may be lost by age 60. But, according to my "Merck Manual of Geriatrics," aging affects spinal-cord *function* primarily through "indirect" changes, such as "degenerative disease of the spine and intervertebral disks with compression of the spinal cord and entrapment of the nerve roots."[2] In other words, the loss of neurons does not translate to neurological dysfunction.

The neurologic examination of an older person can be complicated: "Normal aging," explain neurologists in *Brocklehurst*, "may be associated with the loss of normal neurologic signs or the exaggeration of others. It may be associated with the appearance of findings considered abnormal in younger patients or the reappearance of physical signs usually seen in infancy and early stages of development.

"The geriatric neurologic examination is also influenced by involvement of other systems (e.g., rheumatologic disease), the frequent co-occurrence of multiple conditions in a single patient, and the presentation of non-neurologic disorders (e.g., myocardial infarction, urinary tract infection, fecal impaction) as neurologic signs (gait difficulty and confusion)."[3]

Diagnosing a neurological condition in an older person, as I would learn firsthand with my father, can be challenging.

Lost Neurons and the Brain

The number of neurons lost in the brain with aging varies from next to none in some areas and from 10 to 60 percent in others, including the **hippocampus** and areas of the vital **cerebral cortex**. Not all older people experience hippocampal shrinkage, but those who do typically perform less well on some memory tasks. (As you'll recall, AD's ravaging of neurons occurs first in the hippocampus and later in the cerebral cortex.)

The brains of people with **Parkinson's disease**, which is characterized by tremor, muscular rigidity, and impaired motor control, show a *marked* loss of neurons in the **substantia nigra**, a layer of large pigmented nerve cells that produce **dopamine**, another essential neurotransmitter.[4]

In Chapter Eight, I looked in detail at normal cognitive aging. A normally aging person's intellectual performance tends to be maintained until at least age 80, after which it may take your Mom or Pop longer to perform intellectual tasks.[5] Typically, older adults favor a slower, more deliberate approach to decision-making and other thinking.

With normal aging, the pigment **lipofuscin**, which is essentially a lipid, accumulates in neurons, and **amyloid**, a starchlike substance that results from protein breakdown, accumulates in cerebral blood vessels. There is no convincing evidence that increased deposits of lipofuscin compromise neuronal function in normal brains or that the usual buildup of amyloid plaques affects cognition, but a proliferation of amyloid plaques in autopsied brain tissue is a telltale sign of Alzheimer's disease.

Other notable age changes in the brain include:

❖ From age 20 or 30 to age 90, the brain, which weighs about three pounds, loses about 10 percent of its weight. The amount is uncertain because postmortem changes occur in the brain's fluid compartments that can reduce its overall weight. (You can't weigh a living brain!)

❖ After age 60, cerebrospinal fluid, which bathes and cushions the brain and spinal cord, begins to increase. Between ages 20 and 50, the normal brain occupies more than 90 percent of the cranial cavity. Thereafter, the brain-to-cranium volume significantly decreases as the CSF volume proportionately increases.[6]

Any clinical effects from these weight and volume reductions, says *Merck,* are difficult to determine because they may not correlate with intelligence. In other words, we know these anatomic changes occur, but we don't necessarily know what effect they have on functioning.

Cerebral blood flow normally decreases with age by about 20 percent, but apparently without adverse consequences.[7]

THE ENDOCRINE SYSTEM

Like the nervous system, the endocrine system is a principal physiological regulator, helping to control body temperature, basal metabolic rate, growth rate, protein metabolism, stress responses, reproductive function, and other fundamentals.[8]

Your body's **endocrine glands**, such as the adrenals, produce and secrete hormones into your bloodstream. Hormones then bind to receptor molecules on the cells of their target tissues. Control over the release of most hormones begins in your brain with your **hypothalamus**, which also regulates your autonomic nervous system.

Your hypothalamus influences your **pituitary gland**, which is located at the base of your brain, to release nine different hormones that have stimulatory effects on lower endocrine glands, including the **thyroid**, **adrenal**, and **gonadal** glands. These lower glands, in turn, produce their own hormones and may perform additional functions. The gonads, for example, produce the sex hormones, such as estrogen and testosterone, with which you are probably most familiar.[9]

Within the endocrine system, but outside of the hypothalamus-pituitary axis, the pancreas secretes the critical hormones **insulin** and **glucagon**, which regulate blood levels of the monosaccharide sugar, **glucose**.

Chemically speaking, hormones are either proteins, peptides, and amino-acid derivatives, on the one hand, or lipids, on the other. Steroid hormones, produced mostly by the adrenal cortex and the gonads (ovaries and testes), are lipids.

The Pauses

Normal aging is marked by a variety of hormone-reduction or deficiency states also known as pauses. The affected hormones and their pauses are:

1)   Human growth hormone, in somato*pause*.[10]

Somatopause, induced by the body's dropoff in human growth hormone, causes a reduction of protein synthesis and a decline in immune function and contributes to the age-related loss of lean muscle, expansion of adipose-tissue mass, and thinning of skin. Its exact neuroendocrine mechanism remains unclear.[11] Research suggests that it is more likely caused by an age-dependent decline in the hypothalamic regulation of HGH secretion than aging changes in the pituitary gland. It has been shown that older people with poor physical fitness and/or more fat secrete even less HGH than those who maintain fitness and a trim body weight.[12]

HGH that contains the real hormone, not the substitute ingredients of over-the-counter pills, is available only with a prescription and administered only by injection.

The current consensus from clinical studies of synthetic HGH seems to be that short-term use by older people increases their lean muscle mass and decreases their fat, but does not improve their function, such as their cardiovascular endurance and muscular strength. HGH supplements also have produced worrisome adverse effects, including peripheral edema, carpal tunnel syndrome, joint pain, and even diabetes and glucose intolerance.[13]

2)   Estrogen, in meno*pause*

Menopause marks the cessation of a woman's cyclic ovarian function. It is the first full year during which no menstrual periods occur. The mean age for its onset is 51.4 years old. After menopause, the cycling production of estradiol, the most potent estrogen produced by the ovaries, is replaced by a very low, constant level. The consequences of estrogen withdrawal are numerous, including "an increased risk of cardiovascular events, rapid loss of skeletal mass, vasomotor instability [hot flushes], psychological symptoms, and atrophy of estrogen responsive tissue," according to *Brocklehurst*. Cognition also may be adversely affected.[14]

3)   Testosterone, in andro*pause*

Men experience their own sex-hormone pause caused by a gradual, progressive decline in testosterone blood levels. Unlike the sharp drop in estrogen at menopause, however, **andropause** "is more variable, with unclear clinical consequences," *Brocklehurst* experts say.

Aging men with declining testosterone typically experience "increased fat mass, loss of muscle and bone mass, fatigue, depression, anemia, poor libido, erectile deficiency, insulin resistance, and higher cardiovascular risk." But this phenotype also may occur in older men with normal testosterone levels.[15]

4)   Dehydroepiandrosterone (DHEA) and its sulphate, DHEAS, in adreno*pause*

Secreted by the adrenal cortex (the outer part of the gland), DHEA and DHEAS are the body's most abundant steroid hormones; but their physiologic functions, says *Brocklehurst*, remain "unknown." After age 25, the body's circulating levels of DHEA, a metabolic precursor to testosterone, and its sulphate gradually decline, resulting in **adrenopause**. This is true whether you are male or female. By age 80, your DHEA/DHEAS blood levels are only 10 to 20 percent of what they once were.

Some studies have described an association between declining DHEA and DHEAS and cardiovascular disease, breast cancer, low bone mineral density, depression, type 2 diabetes, and Alzheimer's disease. But, to date, no causation has been established. Further, when older people have taken DHEA replacement in trials, no improvement in well-being or cognition has been found. Just like synthetic HGH, synthetic DHEA has not proved to be the hormonal fountain of youth.

Unlike DHEA, levels of the adrenal steroid hormone **cortisol** tend to rise in older people. Cortisol mobilizes the body's reserves in times of illness, physical injury, and emotional turmoil. You may have noticed that your parents experience a prolonged response to stress, needing more time to quell their agitation after an upsetting encounter.[16]

The Pancreas

The primary function of your pancreas is to secrete digestive enzymes into your gastrointestinal tract, which it does via **exocrine glands** that empty into ducts. Only 1 percent of this organ is engaged in the endocrine function of secreting hormones into the blood to maintain normal sugar levels.

Insulin principally targets cells in the liver, adipose tissue, muscles, and the appetite-control area (satiety) of the hypothalamus. Insulin regulates the uptake of glucose into these cells, where the sugar is stored and used later for energy.

Blood-glucose levels typically elevate with digestion of a meal. Insulin ensures that **hyperglycemia**, an abnormally high concentration of glucose in the blood, does not occur. When blood-glucose levels dip too low, the other pancreatic hormone, **glucagon**, acts to raise them. Together, they maintain stability.

With age, the prevalence of the insulin disorder, **type 2 diabetes mellitus**, increases, but diabetes is hardly normal. According to the Centers for Disease Control and Prevention, 30 percent of all people 65 and over have diabetes, with a type 2 diagnosis accounting for 90 to 95 percent of them.[17] Type 1 diabetes mellitus usually appears in childhood or adolescence and is caused by insufficient production of insulin.

Physicians today view type 2 diabetes as resulting from "multiple defects," including the following:

- ❖ Insufficient or defective insulin receptors on target cells (a condition called resistance)
- ❖ An impairment in insulin's response to, and stimulation of glucose
- ❖ An overproduction of glucose by the liver, and/or
- ❖ A deficiency in the pancreas's insulin output (like type 1)[18]

Aging definitely causes some decline in insulin secretion, and insulin resistance is more common in older people. Most elders do not develop type 2 diabetes, however, because their bodies compensate by adequately increasing insulin output. The peripheral and hepatic insulin resistance that occurs with type 2 diabetes relates more to poor diet, physical inactivity, increased abdominal fat mass, and decreased lean body mass. The first-stage treatment for this chronic disorder includes an exercise program and a nutritious, calorie-restricted diet.

Type 2 diabetes can lead to serious eye, kidney, nerve, and cardiovascular damage, including blindness, kidney dysfunction or failure, a loss of sensation, hypertension, and heart attack. It also impairs the body's ability to fight infection. If your parents' families have a history of diabetes, your Mom and Pop need to be especially mindful of their weight and nutrition.[19]

The Thyroid

According to *Brocklehurst,* the prevalence of thyroidal disease increases with age, but the physiologic changes to the thyroid caused by aging have yet to be determined.

The thyroid gland, which is the body's thermostat, has two lobes, located on either side of your trachea (windpipe) and connected by a band called the isthmus. One of the largest endocrine glands, the thyroid contains numerous follicles, which produce and store the two thyroid hormones, **thyroxine** (T_4) and **triiodothyronine** (T_3). In order to make these hormones, the gland needs iodine—which is why iodine is added to commercial table salt.

Thyroid hormones regulate the body's metabolic rate and also play a part in tissue growth and development, sympathetic-nervous-system response, and mental alertness. Thyroxine has a longer half-life in blood than triiodothyronine and is 20 times more plentiful. You often see the two hormones referenced singly as thyroid hormone.[20]

Thyroid-stimulating hormone (TSH), released by the pituitary gland, stimulates thyroid-hormone production. If too much TSH is released, the thyroid gland secretes too much hormone, a condition called **hyperthyroidism**. Conversely, if the pituitary does not release enough TSH, the thyroid will secrete too little hormone, resulting in **hypothyroidism**.

If your Mom or Pop suffers from thyroid dysfunction, it is most likely to be hypothyroidism, which is characterized by sluggishness, muscular weakness, a reduced ability to perform routine tasks, and weight gain. You may think of it as a metabolic slowdown. Conversely, hyperthyroidism results in extreme nervousness, agitation, chronic fatigue, and weight loss—a metabolic overdrive.[21]

Normal aging is accompanied by a slight decrease in pituitary TSH release. Because the thyroid hormones' clearance from the blood also decreases with age, however, the concentration of thyroxine does not change.[22]

THE MUSCULOSKELETAL SYSTEM

Profound changes occur in your musculoskeletal system with age. The four hormonal pauses facilitate some of them. All of these changes affect your health as well as your appearance.

Speaking about 25 years ago at a conference about the nutritional needs of older persons, Dr. Irwin H. Rosenberg of the Human Nutrition Research Center on Aging at Tufts University observed: "No decline with age is more dramatic or potentially more functionally significant than the decline in lean body mass."

This decline differs between the sexes, with women showing a "rather sharp decline roughly at the time of menopause," said Rosenberg, who postulated that "no single feature of age-related decline [may] more dramatically affect ambulation, mobility, calorie intake, and overall nutrient intake and status, independence, breathing, etc."[23]

Rosenberg coined the term **sarcopenia** for the age-related decrease in muscle mass and muscle strength. Sarcopenia reflects atrophic changes primarily in skeletal muscles, but these changes also occur in skin, bone, liver, kidney, and spleen. A deficiency in muscle negatively affects all of your body's systems.

Sarcopenia

Sarcopenia* occurs largely because of skeletal muscle-fiber loss and muscle-fiber atrophy and varies from muscle to muscle. Generally speaking, when muscle quantity falls, muscle quality deteriorates. Functionally speaking, this means weakness.[24] Deficient muscles can ruin an elder's quality of life *and* lead to his death.

According to sarcopenia experts Drs. Ronenn Roubenoff and

---

*Most of the clinical data on sarcopenia derives from the study of Caucasian elders. African Americans and other blacks are known to have greater skeletal and muscle mass than whites, but the extent to which racial and ethnic differences might affect the development of sarcopenia is not yet known.

Carmen Castaneda at Tufts, "The loss of lean body mass reduces function, and [a] loss of approximately 40% of lean body mass is fatal."[25]

A quarter of all protein synthesis in your body occurs in muscle. It is the major source of protein for antibody production, wound healing, and white-blood-cell production during illness. If sarcopenia depletes your Mom's or Pop's protein reserves, she or he will have fewer reserves to mobilize when sick.[26]

It's important to understand that sarcopenia is a process or an outcome, not a disease. Do not confuse it with muscle wasting, which happens when a person's food intake is so poor that he or she undergoes extreme involuntary weight loss. This occurs with starvation, advanced cancer, and AIDS.[27]

Muscle-mass loss incident to aging is greater in the lower body than in the upper body, and in the extremities, generally, rather than in the diaphragm, which is the primary breathing muscle, although respiration mechanics also diminish. Aerobic capacity declines because of a diminution of muscle *and* cardiopulmonary reserves.[28]

Multiple causes exist for sarcopenia. Besides hormone withdrawal, metabolic, neurological, immunological, and nutritional changes can contribute to an elder's muscle-mass decline. So can a sedentary lifestyle.[29]

Clinical research clearly shows that a use-it-or-lose-it muscle strategy can reduce and even reverse sarcopenia, particularly when the "use it" consists of weight training or another exercise of a resistance nature. Building muscle will not only help your Mom and Pop to maintain body mass, strength, and endurance, it will help them to prevent injury to their joints and to maintain their flexibility and balance, which, in turn, will lower their risk of falling. Even frail 90-year-old nursing home residents can build and rebuild muscle mass and improve their functioning with strength training.[30]

Adipose Tissue Expansion

While lean muscle mass shrinks with aging, the body's mass of adipose tissue expands. People's fat tends to redistribute with age to the abdominal region.[31] This unfortunate shift happens irrespective of your Mom's or Pop's physical exercise, although maintaining an active lifestyle can reduce the amount of fat deposited.

Generally speaking, human body weight increases gradually from early adulthood until the 40s or 50s and then remains stable until age 65 or 70. Middle-aged people put on the most poundage. Women often gain weight when they transition from pre- to post-menopause, but after age 60, the body weight of both women and men usually slowly decreases. Sarcopenia contributes to this decline.[32]

If the gradual weight loss associated with aging does not stop, an elder may deteriorate into frailty, a syndrome that is defined by the presence of at least two of the following: balance impairment, slow gait, weight loss, undernutrition, sarcopenia, and osteopenia. Frail elders tend to be anorectic (lacking in appetite), weak, chronically exhausted, and inactive. They have impaired homoeostatic reserves and lack the capacity to withstand much stress. Fortunately, frailty is not a foregone conclusion; it can be prevented as well as reversed.[33]

The combination of low muscle mass and *high* fat mass, known as sarcopenic obesity, is also dangerous, in the absence of physical activity.[34] As you learned in Chapter Six, very little water exists in fat. The more fat you have, the lower your water reserves will be.[35]

Loss of Collagen and Elastin

You already know that age-related **bone thinning** accelerates in women after menopause and in men, after age 70. The loss of bone mass predisposes elders to fractures, kyphosis (the upper-back hump), and other conditions.

According to the CDC, **osteoarthritis (OA)** of the knees and hips is the most common cause of arthritis-related disability in the United States, and arthritis of all types is the No. 1 cause of disability among Americans of all ages. Back or spine problems reportedly rank No. 2, followed by "heart trouble."[36]

OA results from ulceration and destruction of joint cartilage, changes that eventually produce the painful bone-on-bone state that characterized my mother's worn-out knees. The cushion between the bones essentially wears away. Not surprisingly, obesity is a major risk factor for osteoarthritis. The more weight knee joints have to bear, the more damage they may undergo. Women may suffer more from OA than men because they have broader hips that put more stress on their knees.[37]

Collagen and **elastin**, two important constituents of bone and other body parts, also degrade with age and affect functioning. Their degradation has widespread implications.

Collagen is a fibrous protein. My father, who studied collagen and what were called connective-tissue diseases in the 1960s, once explained it to me as follows: *"Collagen makes up your connective tissues—your tendons, cartilage, ligaments, what have you—and holds together anything that is tied together, except the brain itself: the bone, the blood vessels, the heart, the lungs, the intestinal tract. If you didn't have collagen, you'd just fall apart. You'd be a little blob on the floor."*

You can't beat blob imagery for capturing functional essence. Collagen figures prominently in growth and also plays a role in the healing of wounds, scarring, and the pathogenesis of diseases, as well as aging.

As a person ages, more and more "cross links" form between adjacent collagen molecules, and they bind together "like rungs in a ladder," according to Dr. Al. Strands of cross-linked collagen polypeptides tend to be more fibrous and, thus, harder and less flexible.

The lens of the eye is one of the first structures to exhibit age-related changes as a result of increased collagen rigidity. Because of this rigidity, most people age 55 and older need reading glasses. But cross-linking also affects tissues in the heart, lungs, kidneys, and joints, greatly reducing their functional ability.

Elastin is a protein that, as you might deduce, accounts for elastic fibers in tissue. Wherever elasticity occurs, such as in the lungs, the bladder, the major arteries of the heart, and the skin, fibers containing elastin exist. Like collagen, elastin and elasticity decline with age.

THE INTEGUMENTARY SYSTEM (SKIN)

Your skin undergoes genetically determined **intrinsic aging**, aka chronological aging, as well as **extrinsic aging**, caused by environmental factors such as the sun's ultraviolet (UV) radiation, cigarette smoke, harsh weather, and even pollution.[38]

That's the bad news.

The good news is if you avoid environmental influences, especially UV exposure, you can generally preserve your skin's smooth and unblemished appearance (as my mother has).

Skin is part of the integumentary system—an integument being an outer covering—which also includes the hair, nails, and oil, sweat, and mammary glands. I will only look at the skin, which is the largest organ in the body.*

The skin consists of three main layers, which are, from the outside in: the **epidermis** (including the visible skin); the **dermis**; and the **subcutaneous tissue** (aka hypodermis). Intrinsic aging causes structural and functional changes in all of these layers.

Thinning of Skin, Lost Protection

Because of the abuse skin takes from the sun and other environmental elements, epidermal cells must be continuously replaced, a process that takes about 28 days in young skin. Between the ages of 30 to 80, the turnover rate of skin-cell replacement slows about 30 to 50 percent. This slower turnover causes thinning of the epidermis and diminishes the skin's repair and cell exfoliation. Wounds, thus, take longer to heal. The slowdown also contributes to the dull, rough skin surface that many elders have.

Melanocytes are epidermal cells that provide protective melanin pigment. With age, their number declines, as does the functional activity of the remaining melanocytes. This reduction leads to thinner, paler, and more translucent skin, as well as color changes such as mottled pigmentation and white spots. The decline of melanocytes also reduces your skin's protective capacity against UV radiation.

The dark spots or hyperpigmentation that you may see on older skin—especially in Florida—is caused by erratic melanocyte activity brought on by long-term sun exposure, not by a reduction of melanocytes.

The number of **Langerhans cells**, which are immunocompetent epidermal cells similar to melanocytes, also decreases—by nearly 50 percent in the very old. The loss of these cells compromises the skin's immune surveillance and leads to a higher risk of skin cancer. The longer sun exposure that older epidermal cells have because of slow turnover time also increases your Mom's or Pop's cancer risk.

There are three types of skin cancer: **malignant melanoma** (the worst); **squamous cell carcinoma** (which I have had); and **basal cell carcinoma** (fairly common). Because cancer is not inevitable with aging, I leave further details to your parent's dermatologist.

---

*Most of the available clinical data pertain to Caucasian skin, not black skin, which contains more protective melanin pigment.

A prominent change occurs with age at the junction between the dermis and the epidermis. The normally undulated membrane that separates these two layers flattens out, decreasing the transfer of nutrients between the layers and diminishing the renewal and healing of older skin.

During the aging process, the dermis can lose from 20 to 80 percent of its thickness. This is because of changes in collagen, elastin, and other protein biosynthesis.

Bruising and Wrinkles

As skin thins, **bruising** occurs more easily, and bruises heal more slowly. Also with age, the dermal microvasculature (blood vessels) becomes more fragile and subject to rupture. Not only do you lose vessels, thus reducing your skin's blood supply, but you lose the fatty subdermal layer that helps to protect vessels from injury. The loss of this padding leads to wrinkling and sagging of the skin and increases its susceptibility to trauma and bruising.

If your Mom or Pop takes an anticoagulant or aspirin, bleeding from capillary damage may take longer to stop and cause severe bruising. A diminished blood flow—perhaps caused by narrowed arteries—can further impair wound healing. If you see large, ghastly, discolored bruises on your Mom's arms or legs, don't panic. Given a plausible reason for the wound, allow it time to heal.

Because of the age-related decline in the density of the dermal blood supply, which provides oxygen and nutrients to the tissues and an efficient means by which to regulate body temperature, elders become more vulnerable to sunburn. This decreased density, coupled with a gradual loss of functioning sweat glands, predisposes your Mom and Pop to **heat stroke**.[39]

When many of us think of aged skin, we think of **wrinkles**, of which there are two types: Intrinsically aged wrinkles occur as a result of a reduction in muscle mass and skin thickness; cross-linking of collagen and elastin in the dermis; and dehydration in the epidermis. These are typically either "fine" wrinkles or expression lines. Extrinsically aged wrinkles, such as those on the face and chest, are deeper, coarser, and more numerous.[40]

Sun-induced **photoaging** is the chief perpetrator of your skin's extrinsic aging. Besides wrinkling, photoaging causes yellowing, irregular pigmentation, and the benign dermatologic lesions that we call "age" or "liver" spots, as well as other blemishes that multiply over time. Although most of the sun's damage to a person's skin occurs before age 65, geriatricians still advise elders to wear sunscreen. I wear it year-round.

Cigarette smoking also can severely age the skin, creating hard wrinkles and irregular splotches. This self-destructive habit can add 10 to 15 years to a smoker's facial appearance.

THE CARDIOVASCULAR SYSTEM

I have already told you a lot about the remarkable cardiovascular system. Every day, the average adult heart beats more than 100,000 times to pump the equivalent of 1,800 gallons of blood. With each contraction, about 70 milliliters of blood are ejected from both sides of the heart.[41]

Age renders this impressive organ less efficient, but it does not make it diseased.[42]

If you need a refresher on the atria and the ventricles, please refer back to Chapter Three. Aging affects the walls of your heart's four chambers, according to their layers, which, from the innermost out, are:

1) The **endocardium**, a simple endothelium* over a layer of connective tissues that allows blood to move easily through your heart

2) The **myocardium**, a thick middle layer that is composed of muscle and is responsible for your heart's contractions

3) The **epicardium**, a thin, serous membrane that forms the outer surface

With normal aging, the amount of fibrous tissue within the heart's myocardium increases, while the number of its **myocytes**–muscle cells–declines.

When cardiac myocytes reduce in number, the remaining cells react by increasing in size. They compensate. In similar fashion, fibrous tissue replaces the lost myocytes in order to contain the damage. This increase in fibrous tissue causes the myocardial layer

---

*An endothelium is a thin layer of flat epithelial cells, which form the membranous tissue that covers most internal and external surfaces of the body and its organs.

to thicken. Beginning around age 60, the number of **pacemaker cells** in the sinoatrial (SA) node, whose electrical impulses trigger the depolarization that initiates a heartbeat, also start to progressively decline.

Older hearts, therefore, have fewer active cells (myocytes, pacemaker cells) and **more fibroblasts**, which produce collagen in the heart's connective tissues. Increased collagen leads to increased collagen cross-linking and rigidity. When combined with changes in the mycocytes, this cross-linking promotes greater **myocardial stiffness** and a **decline in ventricular functioning**.

Fat and calcification may accumulate on the epicardial surface of the heart, and the endocardium may become fibrotic (scarred). The mitochondrial DNA in cardiac muscle cells undergoes damage, as well.

Bottom line: After performing well for many decades, the normal human heart has to start working harder to pump the same amount of blood through the body.

Stiffened Arteries

Your vast network of arteries also undergoes prominent aging. The walls of all of your large, blood-distributing arteries, including the aorta, its divisions, and main branches, **thicken** with age and become **less elastic** and more resistant to blood flow. These changes can promote hypertension.

As you know, the left ventricle propels blood out to the systemic circulation through the aorta, which subsequently branches into other important arteries, the first of which are the two coronary arteries. These arteries emerge from a short section called the **ascending aorta**, which passes in front of the right pulmonary artery. The aorta then curves in an arch between its ascending and descending portions.

To keep things simple, I will omit a lot of vascular anatomy. Suffice it to say that the **aortic arch** supplies the arteries through which blood flows to the head, neck, and arms, such as the two **carotid arteries**, which feed the brain. The **descending aorta** transports blood to the chest area and ends in the abdomen, where it divides into two smaller arteries that feed the legs and branch into other arteries. There is an extensive arterial network supplying blood to organs in the viscera.

Arterial blood eventually flows into **arterioles**, which are the smallest arteries that can be seen with the naked eye, before it reaches the **capillaries,** the site of the exchange of gases, nutrients, and metabolic waste. These substances transfer through a capillary's wall by diffusion, filtration, and osmosis. The **interstitial fluid**, which is fluid between the cells, allows them to pass to and from your tissues, as the blood moves from the arterial to venous capillaries.

Deoxygenated blood carrying waste flows from the venous end of the capillary bed into **venules (small veins)**, which increase in size to **veins**, as blood flows back to the heart. About 70 percent of your total blood volume is in your veins at any time.

The **superior vena cava** returns blood from your head, neck, arms, and chest—the superior or upper body—and the **inferior vena cava** returns blood from your lower limbs and your pelvic and abdominal viscera. Both of these large veins carry oxygen-poor blood to the right heart, thus completing the systemic loop. (The **coronary sinus** drains blood from most of the heart muscle, emptying it into the right atrium, as well.)

The IVC, with which you're familiar because of my mother's clot-protecting filter, goes through the **liver**, but it does not have any connections to this multi-purpose organ, which is also the largest gland in your body.

I mention this because another important circulation, known as the **(hepatic) portal circulation**, transports venous blood from your digestive organs to the liver through the **(hepatic) portal vein**. The liver, thus, has two blood supplies. In addition to the blood arriving from the portal vein for detoxification and nutrient absorption, the liver receives oxygenated blood, along with cholesterol and other substances that it needs to metabolize fats, carbohydrates, and proteins, through the **hepatic artery**.

Eventually, the portal vein divides into a capillary network that allows blood to exit the liver via the inferior vena cava, which travels to the right heart.

With age, the **liver's detoxifying ability diminishes**. The older liver also has reduced blood flow and does not regenerate as quickly after injury. Because of the liver's altered clearance, drugs, as well as toxins, remain in the older body longer. Elders, therefore, should take smaller doses of many drugs than younger people do. (The kidneys help in eliminating drugs and their breakdown products, but their efficiency, as you'll see, also declines with age.)

Like the walls of your heart's chambers, your arterial walls also have three layers. They are, from the innermost out:

1) The **intima**: a thin layer of connective tissue covered on the inner surface by endothelial cells
2) The **media**: smooth muscle bounded on its inner and outer surfaces by elastic connective tissue
3) The **adventitia**: a connective-tissue layer that contains the vasa vasorum (tiny blood vessels) that nourish the outer half of the arterial wall

Thickening of the aorta results from cellular changes mainly in the intima. The thickness of both the intima and media of the carotid arterial walls usually increases two- to three-fold between the ages of 20 and 90. Aging big arteries also elongate, dilate, and become tortuous (winding or twisting), further narrowing their lumens (openings).43 (Both of my parents would be diagnosed with tortuous aortas.)

While the total amount of collagen and elastin declines in arteries, the ratio of collagen to elastin increases. After its age-related loss, the remaining elastin, for reasons such as calcification and the formation of cross-links, becomes more rigid. (Before its reduction, elastin makes up about 90 percent of arterial elastic fibers.)

Response to Stiffened Arteries

Your heart responds to older stiffened arteries by raising systolic blood pressure, and, therefore, pulse pressure. Pulse wave velocity (PWV)–the speed with which the pressure radiates through the arteries–traditionally has been linked to structural changes in the blood vessels, including increased collagen, reduced elastin, elastin fractures, and calcification. It is a measure of arterial stiffness.

When the aorta and the pulmonary arteries stiffen, they do not easily expand and contract with a pressure change, and high arterial pressure usually results. Central-artery stiffness is thought to play a role in increasing the heart's **afterload** and in decreasing coronary artery flow. The afterload is the amount of *pressure* that the ventricles must work against in order to pump blood out.44

When arterial walls thicken and arteries stiffen, your likelihood of developing **atherosclerosis** increases. But these structural changes alone do not cause this serious vascular disease.

Atherosclerosis is a disorder in which cholesterol- and lipid-containing plaques accumulate in the walls of medium and large arteries. Increasingly, it has come to be regarded as a chronic *inflammation* of the arteries. (See Appendix Five, "The Scourge of Atherosclerosis.")[45] All of my sources advise that physical conditioning can lessen age-related vascular stiffening. So encourage your Mom and Pop to keep moving.

Although the walls of veins have the same three layers as arteries, they have less smooth muscle and connective tissue and, thus, are thinner and less rigid. Because they do not recoil, veins do not need elasticity.

(High) Blood Pressure

Hypertension is both a consequence of arterial damage or disease, as well as a risk factor for cardiovascular disease. According to my research, from 60 to 80 percent of all people age 80 and older have high blood pressure.

Christopher Wilcox, M.D., Ph.D., chief of nephrology and hypertension at Georgetown University, believes that 50 percent of all adults *age 50 and older* have hypertension, which he subjectively defines as "a level of blood pressure that increases the risk of stroke, renal or cardiovascular system diseases sufficiently to justify treatment."[46] Shryl Sistrunk, M.D., an associate professor of geriatric medicine at Georgetown, claims that 47 percent of all people *65 and older* have hypertension, which the majority control with medication. By age 80 and older, she says, 66 percent do.[47]

Despite—and whatever—its prevalence, hypertension is not inevitable with aging.

Physicians with older patients worry about **isolated systolic hypertension**, which is defined as two or more systolic-pressure readings of 140 mm Hg or greater on two or more visits, coupled with normotensive diastolic pressure. Increased systolic pressure is a greater risk factor for coronary artery disease than increased diastolic pressure.[48]

In general, systolic function is well-preserved in older people when they are at rest. The same is not true of **diastolic function** in the resting older heart. The rate of left ventricular filling in *early* diastole (the relaxation phase) progressively slows in people after age 20, so that by age 80, it is reduced, on average, by 50 percent.

A number of structural changes influence this slowing: Stiffness in the aorta increases the heart afterload, which compels the left ventricle to prolong contraction time at the expense of diastolic function. An increase in collagen deposits and alterations in elastin also combine to increase left ventricular stiffness, which reduces the chamber's compliance and thereby impairs its passive filling.

To compensate for **early diastolic slowing**, the left atrium contracts more forcefully, causing an increase in late or so-called *end* diastolic filling. Increased end diastolic filling pressure can cause **left atrial dilatation**, which can lead to atrial fibrillation and other arrhythmias in the aging heart. It also causes an enlargement of the left-ventricular wall, called **hypertrophy**.

Loss of the early diastolic contraction can result in a marked reduction in diastolic volume, which predisposes the aging heart to diastolic heart failure. This type of heart failure accounts for up to 50 percent of all heart failure in patients 65 and over.[49]

Heart failure, whether chronic or acute, usually occurs over time because of coronary artery disease or hypertension, which leaves the heart too weak or stiff to fill and pump efficiently. When failure occurs on the heart's left side, fluid may back up into the lungs. This is the status in congestive heart failure.

Decline in Cardiac Output

During exercise, older people often find themselves short of breath. Is their response to physical exertion normal aging? Nonagenarian sprinter Ida Keeling may not think so, but she is aging very successfully. To answer this question, you must look at **cardiac output**.

Cardiac output (CO) is defined as the volume of blood pumped by the left ventricle per minute while a person is at rest. It is calculated by multiplying heart rate, which is the number of heartbeats (contractions) per minute, by stroke volume, which is the volume of blood, in milliliters, that the ventricle pumps in one contraction.

A healthy, resting adult heart beats on average about 72 times per minute. The corresponding stroke volume would be about 70 mL per beat. Thus, the CO would be 70 multiplied by 72 or 5040 mL/min., which is the same as five liters per minute.

During exercise, your heart rate and stroke volume normally rise to meet the metabolic needs of your body, including the demand for increased oxygen. If exercise is vigorous, cardiac output can increase up to seven-fold, which, in the above calculation, would be 35 liters per minute. A decreased cardiac output, thus, would affect a person's response to exercise and contribute to decreased aerobic capacity.

Cardiac output tends to decline with age, but not precipitously. Although I have read reports that, by age 85, your Mom's or Pop's CO will have decreased by 30 to 60 percent, my mini-medical school geriatrics professors disagree. They say older hearts work harder, but generally maintain cardiac output.

Elsewhere I read that a 25- to 30-percent decline in CO is a "normal" average. This is largely because of an age-related change in heart rate, not because of a change in ventricular loading. Regardless of differences in fitness, older people generally have a lower maximum heart rate than young people during exercise, as well as when they are seated, but not when they lie down. Stroke volume remains unchanged or only slightly elevated in healthy older people.[50]

Also implicated in the change in cardiac output is a decline in the older heart's responsiveness to stimulation that triggers action by your **sympathetic nervous system**. Besides ramping up your heart rate, this system redistributes blood away from the less vital organs, i.e., those you're not using, to the working skeletal muscles, the brain, and the heart—as well as to the skin to dissipate heat.

Not only may an older heart require a greater amount of time to contract and relax, because of structural changes, it may not be able to respond as rapidly as a younger heart to the sympathetic nerve signals it receives during exercise. As we age, researchers theorize, the levels of norepinephrine and epinephrine circulating in our blood increase and thereby desensitize our hearts to their stimulation. A reduction in the older heart's pacemaker cells may contribute to its impaired response during exercise.[51]

Insufficient sympathetic nervous system activity also may account for the low blood pressure that older people can experience upon standing up too quickly—which I've previously identified as **orthostatic hypotension**—and the lightheadedness it causes.

Whether a decline in sympathetic nervous system response occurs with all older people is uncertain. Elders increasingly adopt a sedentary lifestyle, which affects their cardiac functioning and influences any conclusions that may be made on the basis of age alone. Clinical research unquestionably has shown that regular aerobic training can lessen the age-associated decline in cardiac output.

According to *Brocklehurst*: "Regular [aerobic] exercise attenuates the adverse effects of aging on the heart and vasculature and protects against the development of cardiovascular disease in older adults."[52]

The Hematologic System

I have mentioned blood often in this chapter, as well as in earlier chapters, but I have not yet looked at its components and how aging may affect them. The human body contains about five to six liters of blood, or about 1.5 gallons.

Plasma, a clear, yellowish fluid, makes up about 55 percent of your whole blood and is 95 percent water. Its remaining 5 percent contains clotting proteins, antibodies to fight infection, and electrolytes (sodium, calcium, magnesium, and potassium).

The other 45 percent of your blood's composition consists of red blood cells (RBCs), also called **erythrocytes**; white blood cells (WBCs), called **leukocytes**, of which there are multiple types; and **platelets**. Plasma fluid carries the erythrocytes, leukocytes, and platelets. It also transports nutrients, hormones, and proteins to the areas of your body that need them and helps to remove waste products from your cells.

Healthy people produce billions of white and red blood cells every hour of every day under normal conditions. In the event of infection, bleeding, or other stressors, new blood-cell growth increases. The blood-cell production process, called **hematopoiesis**, occurs mainly in your bone marrow, which is the spongy vascular center inside your bones. The RBC production process is called **erythropoiesis**.

Changes in Bone Marrow

According to *Merck*, "age-related hematologic changes derive mostly from changes in the bone marrow," including the replacement of active hematopoietic tissue with inactive adipose tissue, a significant reduction in the number of stem cells, * which are precursor cells, and a slowing of erythropoiesis, which results in a reduced incorporation of iron into the RBCs. Older bone marrow may have trouble keeping up

---

*In adults, stem cells act as a repair system for the body, replenishing tissues.

with chronic bleeding or other problems, but rarely are normal-aging changes clinically significant.53

Red blood cells contain **hemoglobin**, the iron-enriched protein that helps to transport oxygen in the blood, and last about 120 days. After squeezing repeatedly through small capillaries, RBCs undergo wear-and-tear that cannot be repaired. The spleen, an organ in the lymphatic system that filters the blood, removes damaged or old RBCs, and the bone marrow produces new cells.

Closely connected with the blood and the circulatory system, the **lymphatic system** consists of an extensive network of organs, nodes, ducts, and vessels that make and move **lymph,** a clear fluid containing a high number of **lymphocytes** (a type of leukocyte), from the tissues to the bloodstream. Lymphatic vessels branch throughout your body, in close proximity to blood vessels, and circulate around the interstitial tissues. As I previously mentioned, they drain excess fluid.

White blood cells protect your body from infection and cancer cells and significantly contribute to your inflammatory and allergic responses. They account for about 1 percent of your blood. After being produced in the marrow, they travel through blood and lymphatic vessels to organs such as the spleen, the tonsils, and the lymph nodes. Because some WBCs have life spans of only one to three days, your bone marrow is constantly producing them. The spleen also makes infection-fighting WBCs.

Platelets, which are made in your bone marrow and circulated in your bloodstream, assist in forming clots to stop the bleeding of a damaged blood vessel. They last about eight to 10 days.

Unexplained Anemia

When the rate of new RBC production equals the rate of old RBC destruction, there is no change in the oxygen-carrying capacity of the blood. The lab test to assess this capacity measures a person's **hematocrit,** which is the volume of RBCs in a blood sample. Hematocrit normally ranges between 42 and 54 percent in men and between 37 and 47 percent in women. With age, average values of hematocrit decrease slightly, but remain within these ranges. The concentration of hemoglobin in the blood also can be tested.54

Anemia, a common complaint in the older adult, is a deficiency in hematocrit or hemoglobin. It can have many causes and is not, contrary to popular thinking, a single disease. *Merck* defines anemia as "decreases in red blood cell or hemoglobin resulting from blood loss, impaired production of RBCs, or RBC destruction" and calls it a "sign" of an underlying benign or malignant (cancer) disease or a chronic illness.55

So-called iron-deficiency anemia occurs frequently in older people, but it is never normal. Do not let its familiarity fool you. Total body and bone marrow **stores of iron** increase, not decrease, with age.

A third of all cases of anemia in older people, apparently including my father's, are unexplained.56 I caution you to think of your Mom's or Pop's anemia as the tip of an iceberg of dysfunction or illness that an older person with lower physiological reserves can ill afford.

THE IMMUNE SYSTEM

Immunity is the ability that your body has to protect itself from invading pathogens, such as bacteria and viruses; harmful chemicals; and mutated (cancer) cells. Your immune "system" comprises all of the cells and organs that contribute to your body's immune response.

According to *Brocklehurst*, **normal aging compromises a person's immunity**, especially after age 70, but so do disease and other "pathophysiologic alterations": Older people "are more likely to have disease, conditions, or exposures that contribute to declining immune function."57

Immunity is viewed as existing in two complementary forms: 1) The **natural immunity**, also called innate, primary, and nonspecific, is your body's first line of defense. It provides rapid, but incomplete protection against disease and tumor threats, until your slower, more definitive, and versatile 2) **adaptive immunity** responds. Unlike your innate immunity, your adaptive immunity, which is also called acquired, secondary, and specific, requires sensitization or prior exposure before it kicks in.

You typically acquire an immunity to an offending microorganism by being infected by it and then recovering. Your body develops an immunological memory so that the next time it encounters the same invader it acts more swiftly and effectively to defeat it. (The historical observation that survivors of smallpox infections developed an immunity to this deadly viral disease led to the first-ever immunizing vaccine. Vaccines containing the live smallpox virus protected people who had not yet been infected.)

Adaptive immunity occurs as: 1) a humoral (blood)-mediated immune response (initiated by B lymphocytes); and 2) a cell-mediated immune response (initiated by T lymphocytes).

B lymphocytes, or **B cells**, are made and matured in bone marrow before going to your lymph nodes, spleen, and other lymphatic tissue. B lymphocytes differentiate into plasma cells that secrete **antibodies** designed to attack target substances (**antigens**) on bacteria or other foreign bodies **outside of the cells**.

T lymphocytes, or **T cells**, develop from stem cells in the bone marrow and go to the thymus gland, where they mature. T-cells destroy those microbes that hide **inside the cells**, most notably viruses.

Both B and T lymphocytes exist as "naïve" or new cells and as memory or stored cells. Memory B and T lymphocytes are primed and ready to go the next time the same or a similar strain of bacterium or virus invades your body.

Immune Senescence

The progressive immune deterioration that occurs with aging is most pronounced and most significant in the adaptive immunity, where both the quantity and quality of the lymphocytes, especially the T cells, decline.[58]

"Immune senescence," says *Merck*, "leads to an inappropriate, inefficient, and sometimes detrimental immune response."[59]

It is widely held that much of the increased susceptibility of older people to influenza and its complications is attributable to reduced antibody responsiveness and reduced influenza-specific-cell-mediated immunity. But how much is debatable.

Immune senescence can contribute to infection. A causal relationship definitely exists between an aged immune system and the reactivation of some infectious diseases, such as herpes zoster (shingles) and tuberculosis.

Chronic illnesses associated with older age, such as congestive heart failure, Alzheimer's disease, and diabetes mellitus, can adversely affect an elder's immune response, as can malnutrition, polypharmacy, stress, depression, and immobility. Some of these causes, obviously, can be reversed. Genetic and environmental factors also may play a role in immunity.

It is safe to say that the healthier and more physically fit your Mom and Pop are, the better their aged immune system will perform.

THE RESPIRATORY SYSTEM

Your heart and lungs work in tandem. While your heart pumps about 100,000 times per day, you breathe about 20,000 times, or about 14 times per minute.

Your respiratory cycle begins when you inhale oxygen-rich air through your mouth and nasal passages. This air flows successively through your pharynx (throat), larynx, and trachea, before passing into your lungs via large airways known as **bronchi**, which, like your pulmonary arteries, are designated as left and right.

Your respiratory and digestive systems are connected at the beginning of this journey, but separate after the pharynx. The **epiglottis**, a small piece of cartilage that folds over the **glottis**, which is part of the larynx, prevents food and liquid from entering the trachea during swallowing. Instead, they travel through the **esophagus**, which is located behind the trachea.

Diminished Function

According to *Merck,* aging definitely affects breathing, gas exchange, and other parameters of lung function, as well as the lungs' defense mechanisms—creating a condition much like mild emphysema—but "pure age-related changes do not lead to clinically significant airway obstruction or dyspnea [shortness of breath] in the nonsmoker."[60]

In assessing a patient's respiratory functioning, pulmonologists test lung **volumes** associated with different phases of the respiratory cycle and measure and evaluate lung **capacities**.

Aging affects your **forced vital capacity (FVC)**, but not your **total lung capacity (TLC)**. A chief fitness indicator, FVC is defined by pulmonologists as "the maximal volume of air breathed out during one forced exhalation after maximal inhalation." (Breathe in deeply; exhale forcefully.) TLC equals the total volume of air that your Mom's and Pop's lungs can hold.[61]

Because of changes in the lung soft tissue, FVC starts to decline steadily after the age of 25!

Your lungs are situated in your **thorax** or thoracic cavity, which is the space within the walls of your chest. The thorax is bounded above by the neck and below by the **diaphragm**. Each lung exists in a self-contained cavity, functioning independently of the other, which is why an entire lung can be surgically removed without killing the person who used it.

Once in the lungs, the inhaled air moves progressively through **smaller bronchi**, **bronchioles**, and **alveolar ducts**, finally reaching the microscopic **alveoli**, which look like clusters of tiny grapes. These thin-walled, capillary-covered air sacs serve as the primary site for gas exchange between the air and the bloodstream. Through **diffusion**, which is the movement of molecules from an area of high concentration to one of low concentration, oxygen and carbon dioxide cross (diffuse) between the alveoli and the capillary blood. In the alveoli, oxygen is high and carbon dioxide is low; in the blood vessels around the alveoli, the reverse is true.

You have about 300 million alveoli, which account for most of your air capacity and provide about 75 square meters of surface area—the size of a tennis court—for gas transport to and from your blood.[62]

Lost Elasticity, Other Deficits

When you inhale (inspire), your diaphragm contracts, thus lowering the thoracic floor, while muscles between your ribs contract to swing your ribs forward and upward. These actions help to expand your thorax.

When you exhale (expire), your breathing muscles relax, causing your thorax to contract to a smaller volume. This is accomplished chiefly by an elastic recoiling of your rib cage and lung tissue.

With age, lungs lose elastic recoil, and the small bronchioles tend to collapse, partially or completely, during exhalation. This collapse triggers air-flow obstruction and air trapping in the alveoli, causing a decrease in the rate of gas exchange. With age, the alveoli and alveolar ducts also enlarge, thereby reducing (up to 20 percent) the alveolar wall surface area. This reduction further hampers the exchange.[63]

Age-related skeletal changes also affect the older respiratory system. The older rib cage generally stiffens because of calcification of the cartilage between the ribs and the vertebrae. Calcification, as well as kyphosis, limit the mobility of the rib cage, making it difficult for the inhalation muscles to expand it.

The deleterious effects of normal aging on respiration can be hard to differentiate from the damage caused by a lifetime of breathing in **environmental pollutants**. Even if you're not a smoker or subject to second-hand tobacco smoking, you breathe in other pollutants, such as car-exhaust fumes and pesticides, that can harm your lungs.

According to *Brocklehurst*, early-life factors, such as premature birth, asthma, nutrition, and respiratory infections, as well as environmental insults, may further impinge on the lung function of a middle-aged or older person. "The mechanisms affecting respiratory function are likely to be multiple and cumulative."[64]

Predisposition to Pneumonia

Four respiratory diseases occur commonly in old age, but only one of them, **pneumonia**, can be considered a consequence of–or collateral damage from–normal aging.[65] The other three are **emphysema, chronic bronchitis,** and **lung cancer**.

Emphysema and chronic bronchitis are two of the diseases that physicians call **chronic obstructive pulmonary disease** or **COPD**. **Refractory (resistant) asthma** also may be diagnosed as COPD. Lung cancer and COPD are caused primarily, but not exclusively, by cigarette smoking or by *chronic* exposure to another form of unhealthy air, such as an asbestos-poisoned environment.

The term pneumonia refers to pulmonary infections characterized by fever, respiratory difficulty, and chest pain. Most pneumonias are bacterial, but some are viral; of the two types, the bacterial pneumonias tend to be the more severe. There is even a protozoan infection that results in a rare pneumonia suffered by people with severely compromised immune systems, such as AIDS patients.

Why are older people more susceptible to pneumonia?

According to *Brocklehurst*, aging leads to a breakdown of your lungs' **mucosal-membrane** barrier and to a reduction in **mucociliary clearance** so that disease-causing organisms can more readily invade the respiratory tract. Put simply, the mucus secreted in your breathing passages is not doing its job of protecting your lungs from invaders as effectively as it once did. Respiratory defense mechanisms, such as a forceful cough, also erode with age.

"Greater contact with pathogens and cumulative exposure to

environmental insults," *Brocklehurst* observes, also "increasingly challenge" the immune system in the aged lung.[66]

Offending microorganisms increasingly colonize in an older person's oropharynx, which is the area of the pharynx that includes the tonsils and soft palate. Such factors as repeated antibiotic therapies; endotracheal intubation; smoking; malnutrition; surgery; and therapies that lower gastric acidity and raise pH, also render elders more vulnerable to respiratory infection.

Most pneumonia in elders results from inhalation or aspiration. **Aspiration pneumonia** occurs when an elder aspirates (sucks or breathes) into his lungs contents that are laden with bacteria, notably *Haemophilus influenzae* and *Streptococcus pneumoniae*. This can happen when food "goes down the wrong pipe"–the trachea, rather than the esophagus. **Dysphagia**, a dysfunction in swallowing, is the chief mechanism responsible for aspiration pneumonia in older people.

Dysphagia is a major problem for stroke patients, but any elder who is debilitated by disease, using sedatives or narcotics, or undergoing therapy that impairs swallowing and the cough reflex is predisposed. Not surprisingly, aspiration pneumonia flourishes in nursing homes.[67]

Pneumonia is often the last event in a patient who has comorbid diseases, such as COPD, cancer, heart failure, diabetes, and dementia. Occurring after prolonged serious illness, this microbial infection has been called "the old man's friend," because it causes death and, thus, ends suffering. It also can be the advocate's enemy.

A pneumococcal polysaccharide vaccine can protect your Mom and Pop from most of the strains of the pneumococcus *bacteria* (but no viruses) that cause pneumonia.

THE URINARY SYSTEM

In Chapter Nine, I extensively explored the lower urinary tract in the context of my father's plumbing problems. The upper urinary tract, which consists of the kidneys and their ureters, is a wholly different realm. The UT is your filtering station.

The kidneys, which weigh about 4 to 8 ounces each, filter all of the materials in your blood–such as water, urea, salts, glucose, and toxic substances–and determine which materials will be **reabsorbed into the blood** for reuse by the body and which will be **secreted as waste** in the form of urine. In the process, the kidneys regulate the water and chemical composition of your blood and the content of interstitial fluid, maintaining homeostasis in your body's fluid compartments.

More than 450 gallons of blood pass every day through your two **renal arteries**, which branch off of the abdominal aorta and account for about 21 percent of your cardiac output. After filtration by the kidneys, the blood returns to your heart via the renal veins.

Age-Related UT Changes

According to *Brocklehurst,* the decline in kidney function caused by normal aging is "the most dramatic" aging-induced change of any organ or organ system in the body, with the possible exception of the respiratory system. Yet, despite dramatic physiologic alterations, textbook nephrologists still characterize renal aging as "variable between seemingly 'normal' individuals."[68]

Not only does heterogeneity rule, but it can be problematic to distinguish between normal aging and physiologic changes caused by disease.[69]

In general, renal function *substantially* diminishes with age. But—and this is a big but—older kidneys usually perform their tasks adequately enough, albeit at a **slower rate**. Difficulties arise when older kidneys must respond to physiologic and pathologic stresses. They do not easily tolerate disease or other disruption.

If the kidneys fail to perform their excretory and regulatory functions, nitrogenous waste products from protein breakdown can build up in the bloodstream and in the levels of water, electrolytes, or acid in the body, and alter normal processes. Older people more commonly suffer from acute and chronic kidney failure than younger people because their kidneys can't always keep up with the removal of toxic metabolites.

Misregulations

In discussing dehydration in Chapter Six, I mentioned some of the urinary-system "misregulations" that can accompany aging. One of them is the kidney's decreased ability to concentrate urine. *Brocklehurst* experts claim older people lose the ability to both concentrate and dilute urine "maximally."[70]

Other aging changes in renal anatomy and physiology take me

further into the esoteric kidney zone than I choose to venture. I will only scratch the surface here and try not to confuse too much.

The working unit of each kidney is the **nephron**, which consists of the renal corpuscle, the proximal and distal convoluted tubules, and the nephronic loop, aka the loop of Henle. (Just being precise!) Each kidney starts with about 1.3 million nephrons. The renal corpuscle and the tubules exist in your kidney's **cortex**, while the collecting duct, into which the distal tubules empty fluid, and the loop enter the **medulla.**

Older people have 30 to 40 percent fewer nephrons than they had when they were young. With age, the weight of each kidney also decreases by one to three ounces, and renal mass progressively declines. The loss of renal mass leads to a widening of the interstitial spaces between the tubules and an increase in interstitial connective tissue. Just like connective tissue everywhere, this means an increase in **fibrosis**.

Within each nephron's renal corpuscle is a ball-like cluster of capillaries called the **glomerulus**. The glomerular capillaries play a prominent role in fluid filtration and urine formation.

Of the total volume of plasma that flows through the glomeruli, about 19 percent passes through the nephrons' filtration network to become **filtrate**. The nephrons produce about 180 liters or 95 gallons of filtrate each day. Of this volume, only **1 percent or less** becomes **urine,** which primarily consists of water, but also contains organic waste products such as urea, uric acid, creatinine, and excess ions that are not readily reabsorbed. Most of the filtrate is reabsorbed.

With age, the number of glomeruli declines, thus reducing the effective filtering surface, but not its permeability. The number of sclerotic glomeruli also increases, proportionate to atherosclerosis elsewhere in the body. The walls of the large renal blood vessels undergo sclerotic changes, too.

The flow of renal blood progressively slows—by about 10 percent per decade after age 30. Thus, a typical flow of 1200 mL per minute at age 30 will be only 600 mL per minute at age 80. This decline occurs in the cortical blood; the medullary flow is preserved.

With aging, baseline levels of the kidney enzyme, **renin**, fall by about 30 to 50 percent, resulting in a reduction of plasma **aldosterone** levels and contributing to the development of fluid and electrolyte abnormalities.

Aldosterone is a steroid hormone that regulates salt and water and influences blood pressure. Its loss may contribute to an older person's advancing difficulty in maintaining homeostasis. Angiotensinogen II, the peptide that stimulates production and release of aldosterone from the adrenal cortex, also decreases.

GFR, Creatinine, and BUN

Physicians use the **glomerular filtration rate (GFR)** to assess kidney functioning, as well as tests of blood urea nitrogen (BUN) and serum **creatinine**.

The GFR estimates the volume of fluid filtered out of the blood plasma through these capillary clusters *per minute*.

It has long been thought that GFR inevitably declines with age, but this is not so. Longitudinal studies demonstrate that at least one-third of older people do not experience a decline, and some may even undergo an increase. Such a variance suggests that factors other than aging—among them, blood pressure—may be responsible for reduction in renal function.[71]

Urea is a nitrogenous end product of protein breakdown in the liver, which processes both the proteins that you eat as well as the proteins that your body makes. The waste product **creatinine** is principally produced by your muscles.

Because the blood levels of both creatinine and urea-produced **nitrogen** increase when their kidney-filtration clearance declines, they can be used to approximate GFR—and, thus, your Mom's or Pop's kidney functioning. (Your body's creatinine clearance also can be measured with a 24-hour collection of urine, but not as accurately as it can with a blood test.)

But there's a wrinkle: Even when an older person's GFR declines, his or her serum creatinine typically doesn't rise. This is because age-related declines in skeletal muscle mass (sarcopenia) tend to parallel those observed for GFR, causing overall creatinine *production* to fall as well. If the body produces less creatinine, there will be less creatinine in the blood, regardless of filtration clearance.

A BUN test may be done with a blood creatinine test, and the two values may be compared in a BUN-to-creatinine ratio, which can help a doctor check for problems, such as dehydration. The lab report of your Mom's or Pop's BUN and creatinine test results should provide a range of normal values. Keep in mind that not only do ranges differ from one laboratory to the next, but your parent's out-of-the-range value may be normal for him or her.[72] You should be concerned, however, with an abnormally high or otherwise aberrant value.

THE DIGESTIVE SYSTEM

I end my cursory examination of the aging body on an upbeat note. Fact: Aging has relatively little effect on the digestive system. Hooray!

The gastrointestinal tract has a large functional reserve capacity, and most new GI "complaints" in otherwise healthy older people, according to *Brocklehurst*, are caused by disease, not aging.[73]

Your digestive system processes the foods that you eat so your body can absorb the nutrients it needs to function and thrive. The system has an assembly-line tract made up of–in order of product delivery–the mouth, the pharynx, the esophagus, the stomach, the small intestine, the large intestine (colon), the rectum, and the anus. Each "stop" has a specialized function. Along the way exocrine glands, such as the salivary glands and glands in the pancreas and liver, aid in digestion and absorption.[74]

Let's walk the line.

From Ingestion to Elimination

According to *Brocklehurst*, up to 40 percent of healthy older people complain of dry mouth, known as **xerostomia**. Baseline salivary flow "probably" decreases with age, the textbook gastroenterologists say, but *stimulated* salivation remains unchanged in both healthy elders and those without teeth. Some medications, including antihypertensives, cause dry mouth; if your Pop complains of xerostomia, it may be because of his meds.

Older people also commonly experience **dysphagia**, which I mentioned in relation to aspiration pneumonia, but this problem does not occur with normal aging. You swallow because of a neuromuscular process that involves both voluntary and involuntary action. Hitches in the process can happen.

Studies from the 1960s introduced the concept of **presbyesophagus**, an age-associated failure of peristalsis in the esophagus, our next stop. Peristalsis consists of wavelike muscle contractions that propel food contents onward. More recently, research has shown that, although minor changes occur with age in motility of the esophagus, these changes do not result in abnormal motor function. Older people do, however, have a higher incidence of **reflux** symptoms than younger people. Reflux occurs when **gastric acid** from the stomach flows back into the esophagus.75

Similarly, it once was thought that aging caused a decline in the secretion of **gastric acid**, the chief agent of digestion in the stomach. Recent data indicate, however, that *Helicobacter pylori* (*H. pylori*) infections, not age, probably induce the histologic and acid secretory changes in older people's stomachs. *H. pylori* bacteria cause peptic ulcers and gastritis.

The **duodenum**, which is the initial section of the approximately 22-foot-long, tubular small intestine, receives the partially digested food, called **chyme**, from the stomach and continues the process of digestion. Assisted by secretions from the liver (which makes bile), the gallbladder (which stores bile), and the pancreas, the small intestine reduces some of the nutrient molecules to a size small enough to be absorbed through its walls by peristalsis, while the remainder of the digestive contents passes into the colon. Aging has little effect on either the small bowel's smooth-muscle contractility or its digestive function.

After leaving the small intestine, the residual chyme—largely water and undigestible fiber—enters the five-foot-long, tubular, and much wider **colon**, which is heavily colonized by normal bacteria. The colon reabsorbs most of the water and stores the remaining water and fiber as feces until defecation occurs. Feces pass through the **rectum**, which is the lower portion of the colon, before exiting the body through the **anus**.

It has been suggested that aging causes decreased motility of the smooth muscle in the large bowel wall, thus prolonging the time that feces are stored in the rectum and other portions of the colon and increasing the likelihood of constipation. This is not so.

I repeat: Aging does not cause constipation.

According to *Brocklehurst* experts, the "current thinking" is that colonic motility is largely unaffected by *healthy* aging: "Prolonged transit time in older people with constipation," they write, "is due to factors associated with aging (e.g., comorbidity, immobilization, drugs) rather than aging per se."

The older colon is definitely susceptible to cancer, however: The incidence of malignant **colorectal tumors** begins to increase at age 45 and reportedly doubles every five years thereafter. Colorectal cancer is second only to lung cancer in the leading causes of cancer death in the United States.

Besides age, predisposing factors for colorectal cancer include a family history of benign (polyps) or malignant colorectal tumors and preexisting inflammatory bowel disease. A diet high in animal fat and refined sugar and low in fiber has been suggested as another risk factor, but the diet-to-cancer causation has not been established.[76]

Beyond the colon, normal age-related changes in muscle mass and contractility may promote a decline in anal sphincter pressure that can lead to **fecal incontinence**, a condition more common in older women than men. Maximum sphincter squeeze pressure declines with age, as does rectal wall elasticity.

Potential Disaster

In his memoir, "Becoming a Doctor," Melvin Konner recalls a stern lecture from a superior about "the obscure presentation of certain abdominal crises in the elderly."

In a young person, Konner explains, there is no mistaking a "hot belly," which he defines as "a ruptured appendix or a twisted, infected loop of bowel."

Hot-belly "pain is usually excruciating," he continues, "and the 'chandelier' sign in response to pressing on the abdomen or to sudden release of the pressure—the patient screams and jumps up onto the chandelier—leaves little doubt as to the existence of a crisis. In the elderly, however, similarly dangerous and disruptive events in the abdomen can present without any severe pain or tenderness. Often the sensory nerves to the viscera are dulled by alcohol or diabetes or merely aging, and the result can be that only a mild nausea or sense of fullness signals an impending disaster."[77]

Two disaster-tripping digestive disorders commonly associated with, but *not* caused by, aging are diverticulosis and diverticulitis.

Diverticulosis is characterized by the development of diverticula—multiple pouches or small sacs—in the wall of the colon. These herniations often result from muscular spasms and increased intracolonic pressure associated with diets low in fiber and with straining to pass hard stool.

Diverticula most commonly occur in the **sigmoid colon**, which is the lower portion of the colon. When these pouches become inflamed, perhaps because of a fecal impaction, **diverticulitis** results. The danger is that the diverticulitis leads to infection and from there to a perforated bowel.

According to the National Institute of Diabetes and Digestive and Kidney Diseases, 10 to 25 percent of people with diverticulosis develop diverticulitis.[78]

Whereas most people with diverticulosis have no discomfort, people with diverticulitis usually have abdominal pain, which, depending on the patient, can be sudden and severe, or mild at first and then steadily worsening over several days. They also may experience cramping, nausea, vomiting, chills, fever, and/or a change in bowel habits, such as constipation.

My friend Beth lost her 79-year-old mother to disastrous consequences of diverticulitis, which went undiagnosed by her local county hospital's emergency department as well as her own primary-care physician.

On Tuesday, Beth's mother complained of constipation and slight abdominal pain, which she thought might be due to a fall she suffered that day at her gym. She speculated that she had fractured a vertebra and took pain medication for it.

By Sunday, she was dead.

The older woman had a gastroenterologist who had been treating her for six years for fecal incontinence and diverticulosis, but none of the physicians who examined her during her final week—including the ED team who kept her for a day—put two and two together; and Beth was out of the loop. Beth's mother went to the ED on a slow mid-November Wednesday accompanied only by her elderly, cognitively impaired husband.

Whether Beth's mother advised a history taker in the ED of her GI problems, which she considered humiliating, is not known. Beth did not obtain the medical records from that sad, wasted day. I'd wager, though, that no one bothered to think outside the box of a thoracic vertebral fracture—which the radiologist could not find. (Although it was there.)

An old woman walks into the ED, complaining of mild pain and constipation. What does she expect? An abdominal ultrasound?

Beth's mother saw her longtime primary-care physician on Friday.

This affable man certainly knew her GI history. He palpated her abdomen, found nothing significant, and sent her home with a different pain medication, Ultram® (tramadol), so she wouldn't endure any more presumably drug-induced constipation.

If diverticulitis leads to infection, an abscess may form in the colonic wall. Abscesses can be cleared with antibiotic treatment. Those that are resistant to drug therapy can be drained. Left unchecked, however, infected diverticula can develop perforations, and pus and bacteria-laden feces can spill into the normally sterile peritoneal cavity, causing **peritonitis,** a severe and life-threatening inflammation.

This is what happened to Beth's mother, whose acute pain fast worsened. On Saturday, when she arrived by ambulance at the county hospital, no one could overlook the massive infection in her abdomen. It was too late to save her.

Another friend of mine's mother endured a similar ordeal, but with a happier ending.

Genevieve's mother also went to a county hospital, alone, complaining of abdominal pain, but this older woman had no history of GI disorders. The local docs thought her problem was either gynecological or urological (LOL syndrome?) and treated her with an antibiotic.

Dissatisfied, Genevieve arranged to admit her mother to a larger hospital center. During her stay there, a university-affiliated specialist examined her and suggested that she see a gastroenterologist. Bingo!

Genevieve then "muscled and begged our way into [a university hospital] and a GI surgeon there," she emailed me. "He is absolutely top drawer and, for the first time, I think she is getting the medical care she needs."

Three weeks later, her mother had a successful resection of the damaged piece of her colon and reattachment of the severed ends in one procedure, rather than the usual two surgeries. Consequently, she did not have a temporary colostomy. Genevieve, a full-time practicing attorney, kept a 24/7 vigil in her mother's hospital room. As a reward, her mother recovered without "complications."

Chapter Thirteen

2012: The "Rescue"
COMES

With Pain and Atrial Fibrillation

I can best summarize the upshot of Dad's first appointment with Duke's Dr. Terse and his personable young resident, Dr. "PYR," by saying that my overwrought father gratefully hit the schmooze button, while I hit the dejection button. I was so burned out, I could scarcely speak on the drive home.

Every step of our trip from the Outer Banks to Durham had been an ordeal, as my anxious father second-guessed my driving and the route I took; my sense of direction; my hotel check-in and choice of rooms; the time of our checkout, you name it. As far as he was concerned, I was always late or lost, even though he knew, in what was left of his rational mind, I was neither, and he would be late or lost without me.

It wasn't like I was venturing into alien territory. I attended college and law school at the University of North Carolina in Chapel Hill, which is only 15 miles from Durham. Since receiving my law degree in 1981, I had traveled regularly to Chapel Hill, Durham, and Raleigh to visit friends. I also can read the heck out of a map.

At the hospital, which was undergoing construction (!! Mary had warned me), Dad's fussing extended to the parking (a trial run would've helped); his transportation to the urology clinic (I wheeled him a long way); and the excessive waiting time posted on a sign in front of the clinic reception desk.

Is there any reason to tell a patient that he or she will have to wait *two hours* to see his urologist?

It's doubtful a patient will slip away to do something more productive, and the news just might irritate the stuffing out of a family caregiver, especially if she busted a gut to get her nagging father there with time to spare.

I value communication when I'm in a hospital with my mother or father, but this wait-time notification widely missed the mark.

Fortunately, a nurse came much sooner than the posted time to escort Dad into an examining room. He started his schmoozing as soon as he saw the unusual name on her ID tag, and she graciously indulged him. Etiquette is something I find lacking in many doctors—a simple introduction, a "How are you today?"—so I'm always grateful when a healthcare professional understands the value of small talk. Dad visibly relaxed.

But then they forgot me. I sat in the waiting room for nearly four hours, wondering when this interminable day would end. No one thought to update me, including my father. Naturally, when a nurse came out to get me, I had exhausted all of my diversions and gone in search of a snack bar.

SPHINCTER HEMLOCK

When I saw my father again, he was over the moon impressed with Drs. Terse and PYR—"These guys are fantastic!"—and eager to schedule the implantation of his new artificial urinary sphincter, the same device he had rejected out of hand in Virginia Beach. He didn't even remember being told by Drs. Smith and Farrell that an AUS was an option. I felt my waning spirit sink. I was crushed.

"What happened to the sling possibility?" I sputtered.

Dad's incontinence was too severe, Dr. PYR said. The use of three pads per day is considered chronic severe incontinence; my father was using triple that number. (Thank you, Dr. Naylor.)

At the doctors' request, Dad had collected 24 hours of his urine-soaked pads and brought them with him to the clinic. The pads weighed 478 grams, which, in liquid terms, is about a pint, a full 16 ounces. Incontinent men who receive slings typically have 24-hour pad weights of 100 grams or less, roughly half a cup, or 4 ounces.[1]

Dr. PYR had performed the requisite urodynamics (tests of Dad's urinary-system functioning), and all indicators pointed to the sling being out. The resident launched into telling me about the sphincter, but I'm not sure how much of his explanation my weary mind absorbed. I adored my father and had promised I was in "it" for the long haul, but I couldn't help viewing the AUS as high-maintenance and, thus, a potential problem for me. The low-maintenance sling gave me an out. Allow me to explain.

The AUS is a simple device with three components: It has a doughnut-shaped *cuff* at one end; a *balloon* at the other end; and a *pump* in between. The cuff, which fits around the urethra where it meets the bladder, is connected to the balloon by fluid-filled plastic tubing. The fluid's pressure against the cuff keeps the urethra closed. In order to open up the cuff to relieve his bladder of urine, Dad would have to squeeze the pump, which would be implanted in his scrotum. The pump would force fluid away from the cuff and into the balloon for temporary storage. After urination, the fluid would flow back toward the cuff to close the urethra.

I know Dr. PYR told me all about this "gold standard" of care for male urinary incontinence, but all I heard was the part about Dad's scrotum.

"What happens," I asked, "if Dad can't open the sphincter?" If he can't prime the pump?

"What, do you think I'm going to get senile?" the giddy Schmoozer asked.

"I don't know, you could be incapacitated for some reason other than dementia. Like a serious illness."

"Then it would have to be opened up," PYR said matter-of-factly.

Come again? I gave an even blanker stare.

"He'd have to go to the emergency room."

Wonderful.

According to my notes, Dad was looking at three more trips to Duke: the first for an anesthesiology consult; the second for surgery, either outpatient or general, depending on his pre-surgical workup results; and the third for activation of the sphincter. Three interminably long and emotionally brutal trips.

Excuse me? *Activation*?

Yes, Dad's body would have to heal from the surgery, and the surgeons would have to ensure that the sphincter was properly in place before they would "activate" the device. For about six weeks, Dad would have a Foley catheter, or so I then mistakenly understood.

"Do you have any more questions?" Dr. PYR pleasantly asked.

"Yes," I thought. "Do I drink the hemlock now, or do I wait until after the surgery?" I felt nothing but despair.

This Q&A would turn out to be my only chance to speak with one of the surgeons before the surgery. Even if I'd known that, I still would have been stupefied. Tomorrow, after I'd processed this curve, and done some online research, I would have many questions for Dr. PYR, but all I could think about then was the scrotum pump.

I would have liked to have walked away that afternoon with a one- or two-page "what-you-can-expect" guide that would inform us about the steps in Dad's surgery. Something like an annotated timeline. But we received none. I later learned that, thanks to cooling my brain and heels all afternoon, I had the process wrong. There would be no separate trip for an anesthesiology consult before surgery—of course not—and there would be two appointments after surgery, not just one.

Dr. PYR went over the risks of the AUS. Besides problems with sphincter mechanics, post-surgery "complications" could ensue, the worst being infection, and Dad would have to return to Duke or go to the local ED. The balloon-and-cuff sphincter might have to be removed and replaced with another one. PYR might have said more, but that's as much as I got.

If my father is like other incontinent male octogenarians exhausted by hours of urodynamic testing, none of them is asking any questions when the surgeon is available to take them. If they're not Schmoozers, they're likely to be Snoozers, and they'll wake up feeling apprehensive later. Someone should be readily available to answer their questions by telephone, provided they're not annoyingly excessive. Duke had a "telehealth nurse" that I could call, but every time I tried in the weeks ahead, and I tried repeatedly, I got a busy signal.

Healthview, Duke's electronic portal for patients, was similarly useless. It enabled Dad to confirm his appointments and access his lab reports online, but it didn't get him any closer to talking with his doctors. Neither PYR nor Terse had given us an alternate number to call.

Dr. Terse's surgery days were Monday and Friday. Mary handled all of the scheduling, so I had to call her to set a date. Of course, Dad wanted the surgery to happen as soon as possible, but I was numb. I told him during the drive home that he shouldn't count on me. I was teetering at the abyss.

S.O.S.

It took me five days to come around. On Jan. 30, I sent an S.O.S. email to my siblings in which I said I wasn't "willing to rip my schedule all to shreds" for this continued ordeal, and, after 14 months of this urinary "nightmare," I was "burned out." I asked for volunteers to accompany Dad to Duke for the second and third appointments. I fell on my sword for the first.

As fate would have it, I had arranged with two friends to see an all-day theatrical production of Shakespeare's Henry IV and V plays on Saturday, Feb. 25, in Chapel Hill. Since I would be in the area anyway, I booked Dad's surgery for Feb. 24 and his pre-op appointments for the day before—but only after Dad agreed to hire a private-duty nurse on Saturday, so I could enjoy the Henrys without worry. Leslie volunteered to stay with Mom while we were gone, and Britt and Al waited reluctantly in the wings.

Britt actually suggested that these trips were suited to the "front lines"—meaning me—not the back-up troops, which she now was, thanks to a move from Alexandria to Florida. That my sister felt so unencumbered by family responsibilities that she moved hundreds of miles away meant she and I had tense times ahead. Being a plane trip away is not the same as being available at short notice.

Upon scheduling the surgery, I asked Mary about anesthesia, an issue that Leslie had brought up. Of course, we hoped Dad could have a spinal, but Mary didn't know, deferring to Dr. Terse and the anesthesiologist, whom we would not meet until the day of surgery. She also explained to me that Dad might not have a catheter between surgery and activation. He might be fully incontinent.

She shouldn't have said *might*. She should've said he *will* be incontinent. But she hedged, not wanting to trespass on M.D. territory. Thanks a lot. This "detail" was something that Dr. PYR should have made sure Dad and I understood.

A week later, I spent 45 minutes on the telephone with a representative from the Hilton hotel chain, arranging a three-night reservation of two adjacent or nearby rooms, next to an elevator on a lower floor in a Hampton Inn close to Duke. I confirmed that one of them had handicap accessibility and other safeguards. We also discussed the hotel's parking, its food services, its on-site handicap equipment, provision of a microwave and mini-fridge, everything I could think of to ensure that Dad would be comfortable and safe.

Not knowing what shape my father would be in after the surgery—more "what you can expect" info that I lacked—I planned to bring from home a walker, a wheelchair, and a portable commode. I wanted him to walk and me to wheel and haul the shortest distances possible.

After lining up the hotel rooms, I called a Durham-area nursing-care agency recommended by a friend whose elderly aunt had used it after she suffered a stroke. My phone contacts with the registered nurse in charge went very smoothly. I arranged for a minimum of eight hours' coverage, at $18.50 an hour, starting at noon Saturday, and left open the possibility that the CNA assigned would need to stay until 11 p.m., when I expected to return from my theater date.

The responsibilities enumerated in the CNA's contract were broad, including: assisting with all ADL; providing meals and snacks, as requested; encouraging fluids to prevent dehydration; assisting with all transfers and walking; keeping the living area clean and tidy; and emptying and cleaning the bedside commode. I also ensured that she would take Dad to Duke for emergency care, if necessary.

We left the Outer Banks around 7:30 a.m. on Thursday, Feb. 23, the second anniversary of Dad's hip fracture, for an afternoon of pre-op appointments. These exams went reasonably well; my schmoozing father was in good spirits. Mary had advised us to call the Ambulatory Surgery Center at 1 p.m. that day to find out when Dad should report for surgery. The call wasn't necessary. The pre-op nurses saved us the trouble. They also gave us detailed written instructions about Friday's itinerary. Yeah!

When we got to the hotel, however, the stress hit my fan. I might as well have talked with a phantom, for all the good my "coordination" with the Hilton did.

An unsympathetic desk clerk, who said she had no record of my reservations, assigned us to two rooms that were as far from an elevator as any two rooms could be. Not only that, they were at opposite ends of a long hallway. When the front-desk obstructionist wouldn't work with me on rectifying the situation . . . "Sorry, this is the best I can do," she said unapologetically. "We're full." . . . I asked to see the manager and gave her a proceed-until-apprehended earful. Suddenly two rooms next to an elevator opened up. Will wonders never cease. Who needs this petty nonsense?

PRECISION OPERATION

Fortunately, the sphincter surgery came off beautifully. Or so we thought.

Certainly, Duke had its outpatient surgical routine down.

We arrived at the Ambulatory Surgery Center at 9:15 a.m. and parked in an attached garage just outside the entrance. A nurse came to take Dad to pre-op well before 10 a.m.; the surgery started around noon; and I wheeled Dad out to the car at 3 p.m. Although there was some downtime, the kind of delay that we encountered with Dr. Naylor at Chowan County Hospital was unthinkable.

The clinic staff kept me informed and engaged in Dad's surgical process via an electronic monitor, much like the device you receive in a restaurant when you're waiting for a table. Because of this ingenuity, I never felt like I was alone and forgotten; instead, I felt involved.

Bravo. Very impressive.

The monitor first went off after Dad had been prepared for surgery. An OR nurse came out to take me to his pre-op waiting room, where he greeted me with the complaint: "Lousy prep for surgery. They wear you down before surgery." I saw Dr. Terse and his residents before the procedure and met the anesthesiologist, Dr. Mendelson, a very bright, warm, and vivacious woman who had University of Chicago connections and was interested in talking the talk with Dad. My father adored her.

When it came to deciding between a spinal or a general anesthesia, Dr. Mendelson flatly told Dad: "You want a spinal." Decision made. She was terrific.

I waited in one of several very comfortable lounges, reading, and received electronic notification that Dad's surgery was over much sooner than I expected. When I met with Dr. Terse in a small room down the hall from the lounges, he told me that all had gone well. It wasn't a Naylor-like boast; it was a report. He also confirmed that Dad was not catheterized. He would be incontinent. Damn.

Like Dr. Naylor, Terse had a stiffness to his manner, but it was more militaristic and formal than awkward or antisocial. I wasn't surprised later when I learned that he was in the U.S. Army Reserves. Terse didn't waste words or actions. He was spit-and-polish professional. He didn't smile warmly, but he did smile.

In the recovery room, Dad taxed the nurses' patience with his fretting, but once he was cleared to leave, he became a Teddy bear. During our exit, he hugged or blew kisses to all of them. Without me, he probably wouldn't have understood a word they said. I heard for him. I also read and collected the written home-care instructions that he signed. Still, his sentimental softness got to me.

At the hotel, I wheeled Dad to his room and got him situated. He needed sleep, but he was eager to get up and move about—especially to the bathroom, where he wanted to try "things" out. We had been warned that if he felt a sensation to urinate, but could not produce any urine, he was in trouble. Dad relaxed after he verified that the sphincter cuff had not interfered with his flow. Overall, he was none the worse for wear. He never used the walker or the portable commode I brought and even took an unassisted shower the night after his surgery.

The private-duty nurse I hired arrived 15 minutes late on Saturday. She also wandered about the hotel, even using the fitness room, despite my specific instructions that she should sit either in Dad's room or mine. She had expected to attend to a decrepit old man who needed help with his every move and bodily function, so when she met my able-bodied father, and he basically turned her loose, she enjoyed a holiday. I only found out about the fitness-room frolic because Dad let it slip.

My father dismissed the chatty aide hours before I returned, but she shouldn't have left. In doing so, she breached the contract I had with the agency, and I was the one who hired her, not Dad. She left a handwritten report of the day, but I have no idea how often she actually checked on Dad. Both of them were vague about that. Had he fallen on his own petard during the unattended period, he would've had a darn hard time getting up. And if he'd fractured a bone . . .

What's a daughter to do? It was better that I was annoyed than sorry.

We left early Sunday for home and gave into our exhaustion upon arrival. The next day Dad received an email from Duke informing him that his follow-up appointment would be Wed., March 28, when I planned to be in Washington. Dr. Terse's clinic appointments were only on Tuesday and Wednesday, and Dad "went ballistic," as I emailed Britt, when I suggested postponing his a week so I could go with him.

It would not be long, however, before he would have a good case for moving the followup to an earlier date.

Dr. Terse had implanted the sphincter successfully, but in the process, he had altered Dad's anatomy. Because of this alteration, my father was in terrible pain.

All I could say was: "Oy." What next?

EXTREME PAIN

When it comes to genital problems, I like to give people their privacy. I *can* be clinical, but I'd rather not talk with anyone, much less my father, about penile pain and inflammation. And yet, thanks to the surgery that cured his incontinence, Dad, who was not circumcised, now had unrelenting penile pain, and who else was going to ensure that he got relief but I?

I called Mary about this "complication." She would be my switchboard operator in what I came to regard as an infuriating game of telephone. At no time did she ever suggest that I talk to a physician assistant, who would be more accessible, and I had never met a PA in the clinic. A year later, I found out what nonsense that was.

My father (meaning I) could not reach Dr. Terse or his assistants directly; only Mary could. If Dad wanted a consultation, I had to call Mary who, in turn, would arrange for one of the junior M.D.s to call Dad during specific hours and then call me back to tell me when. After Feb. 24, the only time Dad communicated with Terse in person was during follow-up appointments, not on the phone or by email. He was an elite Unreachable.

Dr. Al identified his problem as balanitis, inflammation of the glans penis, caused by an unintended surgical "tuck" in the skin that shortened his length and tightened his foreskin. Its retraction was now painful. The first call-back physician Dad consulted was Dr. PYR, whose response was: "That's not possible." The great Dr. Terse could not have altered Dad's genitalia.

Well, of course, he did. Why would my father misrepresent what had happened? Call it an oversight or an accident, if you prefer, rather than a mistake, but do something.

Besides enduring pain, Dad was mopping up a pint of urine every day and trying to keep himself clean and infection-free. Within three weeks after the surgery, he again was so depressed that he was placing "You could lose your Papa" telephone calls to me, intimating that he was physiologically breaking down.

Terse had instructed Dad not to use the clamp, so he was spending much of his time in bed. He would call me during my work hours about a minor matter and then hang up when I didn't drop what I was doing and attend to him.

"I took the telephone cord out of the wall and now I can't get it back in. Can you come over?"

"Dad, you know how to put the cord in the jack. Just . . ."

CLICK.

"I can't get the TV remote control to work. Can you come over?

"I can't come right now. Have you checked the batteries?"

CLICK.

Although sympathetic, I was determined not to be run around by a deranged patient; but reaching a physician was a run-around that made me deranged. On one wretched Friday, I called Mary and told her I needed to book a doctor consult for Dad that day, if possible. He was miserable. She called back to tell me that Dr. Booker, an intern and the junior member of Terse's surgical team, would call Dad between 1 and 3 p.m. I then notified Dad and instructed him to stay awake and to keep the telephone next to him so he could hear it. I also suggested that Mom stick around.

Naturally, Dr. PYR (not Dr. Booker) called during a 45-second interlude when Mom walked down the driveway to the mailbox, and Dad nodded off. Upon reentering the house, Mom could hear the tail end of his voicemail, which did not include a return telephone number. Instead, he advised Dad to call Mary if he "still" wanted to talk with him. AAARRRGHHH! I was livid when I received word. There had to be a better way.

Again, I called Mary and went through this maddening telephone ritual, and this time it worked. Dad talked to Dr. Booker, who prescribed a steroid cream. This common-sense solution provided temporary relief for what had become a life-altering problem. Dr. Booker also suggested that Dad arrange to be seen in the clinic during the week before his planned followup. Like Dr. PYR, he didn't believe that Dr. Terse had made any inadvertent alterations. Ha! Instead, he thought there might be a problem with the artificial urinary sphincter itself. *Come on.*

This schedule change gave me a break. Leslie, who had been sending medical-supply products to ease Dad's discomfort, was visiting the Outer Banks that week with her family. I made an appointment for Dad to see Dr. Terse on Wednesday, March 21, and Les drove Dad to Duke. She pointedly chastised Dr. PYR for not helping our proud and dejected father deal better with his incontinence and, thus, facilitating his decline through neglect.

Dr. PYR replied: "They come to us incontinent."

That's ologist thinking for you. Not his problem.

"WHAT IF?"

During the followup, the resident examined Dad, affirmed Booker's decision to prescribe a steroid cream, and steadfastly refused to attribute Dad's pain to Dr. Terse's handiwork. For the latter, he put on his dazzling Duke blinders.

It reminded me of the time that I complained to a Johns Hopkins dermatologist that a previous Hopkins dermatologist had pressured me into removing a freckle on my forearm and left me with a scar that looked like one of those plastic stitch-marked scars you wear on Halloween. He said of his predecessor: "Johns Hopkins doesn't hire physicians that make mistakes like that." So I made it up?

At least Dr. PYR activated the sphincter on March 21, as we had hoped, thus obviating my return with Dad a week later.

You would think that after the sphincter's activation—a matter of squeezing the pump in the correct spot—my now-dry-all-of-the-time father would be relieved. Instead, he became obsessed with what-if, worst-case-scenario thinking, which he expressed to me because Mom didn't understand the sphincter system. What if, for example, he's in an auto accident, taken to a hospital emergency room, and catheterized without his knowledge? What damage could that cause?

Finally, he was well enough to ask questions . . . and he was badgering *me*!

I have no doubt that Drs. Terse, PYR, and Booker know from experience all of the questions that AUS patients are likely to ask. So why not send their weary patients home with an informative and simple-to-read factsheet that anticipates them? I'm talking about a concisely written, lawyer-approved handout that essentially says: Don't worry.

Another question that plagued my father: How easy would it be for him to deactivate his sphincter accidentally? A Duke factsheet with the answer, "It's difficult," would have gone a long way toward easing Dad's mind.

Instead, we received a multi-page "user's guide" published by the AUS manufacturer, American Medical Systems, Inc., which I don't think Dad ever understood. This guide listed the following four "commonly asked questions":

1) Can I ride a bicycle? (Dad probably hasn't ridden a bike in 75 years.)

2) Will the 800 [the AUS] affect sexual activity? (No comment.)

3) What about activities that put added pressure on the body? (Not a bad question, but the answer directs patients to talk with their doctors before engaging in sports and other activities.)

4) Can I have magnetic resonance imaging (MRI) or go through airport security? (This is the for-morons-only question.)

The user's guide definitely had good material in it, but this material would have carried more clout, and been easier to access, if it had been presented, and prioritized, by the Duke Urology Clinic. Patients don't want to hear from device manufacturers; they want to hear from their doctors.

I tried to reassure my father that local EMTs would not destroy his artificial sphincter or cause any other harm. To back up my claim, I sphincter-proofed him as best as I could.

I made multiple copies of the manufacturer's guide, sending one to each of my siblings, keeping one for myself, and putting another in a yellow folder on a book shelf near Mom and Dad's kitchen. I also prepared copies of the activation and deactivation sections of the guide to hand out to doctors and nurses in a hospital, if Dad should ever be admitted. And, as the coup de grace, I posted in my parents' garage instructions to emergency-medical personnel about how to deactivate the sphincter if Dad needed to be catheterized.

That darn sphincter wasn't going to beat me, not if I could help it.

CHECKING IN WITH MOM

Meanwhile, despite the Duke urological merry-go-round and Dad's travails, I did my best to keep a watchful eye on Mom, who was doing her best to hold onto her last vestige of independence.

In May 2012, my 88-year-old mother passed the tricky road-sign test required to renew her North Carolina driver's license. Many younger people fail to recognize road signs by their shape and/or symbols, absent explanatory words. Mom studied the N.C. Dept. of Motor Vehicles test booklet the night before and went by herself to the DMV office in Manteo, a half-hour's drive away. She took this challenge in stride.

In fact, she took all of her life in stride.

She still managed her hair appointment-swimming-short-errands driving orbit. She went out in the morning to buy a newspaper, as well as the occasional half-gallon of milk; ordered take-out food by phone and picked it up; and managed the drive-through at McDonald's. She shopped by herself at the local department store. Familiar territory, familiar tasks, yes. But memory and basic executive functions were involved.

On the downside, there were times when she forgot her standing hair appointment and had to be reminded to eat lunch and to change the blouse she'd been wearing for days. Dad complained that she asked him at 11 a.m. the same question she asked at 9 a.m.

Whenever I called Mom from out of town now, she always asked: "Where *are* you?" as if she couldn't imagine where I'd gotten to. She had stopped calling me on the road.

When I mentioned my writing, which I had countless times, Mom never failed to ask: "What book?" And then when I told her about it, she would say: "Is that what you're writing about?"

I even showed my first chapter to her, but she couldn't read it. Too many words. She asked: "Is that really what happened to me?" Later, when she wanted to be helpful and offered to read some more of my material, I reminded her that she already had. She had no recollection.

In 2012, Mom began forgetting peripheral people whom she had known for decades, such as the grandchildren of her friends. A wedding invitation from one of her great-nieces arrived, and she asked me: "Do you know who this is?"

It broke my heart when I mentioned Max, and she asked me if he was "the little white dog" in the framed photograph in her living room. Max, the Shih Tzu who visited her in the Durham nursing home, was her companion for nearly 15 years.

Since Max's death, I've arranged for Mom to adopt two senior rescue Shih Tzus, the first of whom died in 2011 of natural causes. A dog not only gives her pleasurable companionship, he gives her purposeful caregiving tasks to perform. I help with walks, feedings, and veterinary care. God bless dogs. They are such a comfort.

Although Mom's memory had deteriorated since that drive back from the dentist four years ago, she showed no evidence of aphasia, apraxia, or agnosia, but her executive functioning definitely had diminished. Because memory figures so prominently in this cognitive domain, I found the decline difficult to assess.

Where before Mom sought to mediate conflicts in the family, she now could not reason well enough to intervene beyond offering broad advice such as "Don't hold a grudge." She also was only aware of a conflict when it arose, not later. I learned that when I tried repeatedly to talk with her about a quarrel I had with Britt, and she never knew what I was talking about. "When did that happen?" she asked me each time. "Really?"

She passively "listened" during all substantive family discussions, her eyes often betraying a failure to comprehend. She was noticeably quieter and disengaged, and she laughed less.

She still made decisions, but they were on the order of what to have for dinner (a BIG question every day); when to go swimming; whether to watch one TV program or another. Dad also prodded and supported her.

Despite her impairment, Mom's empathetic nature still shone through, and people adored her. Neighbors, who met her when she was walking her dog, would tell me what a beautiful soul she is and how well she was doing "for her age." The rub is she used to be extraordinary.

Increasingly in the autumn of 2012, Dad called to report that Mom had fallen and not only could she not get up, he couldn't get her up, either. S.O.S. "We need you, Ann."

If my unsteady father tried to lift her, I feared that he, too, would go down, so I always rushed over. I didn't want any more fractured hips.

Mom first fell in the bathroom and bruised her shoulder and knee. Then she fell on her face (!) in the living room. Four days later, she stumbled in the dining room while she was putting wine glasses away and landed on her side. She could never explain why she fell. She said she didn't trip. As far as I could tell, loss of balance precipitated each incident, but I wondered if confusion, too, might have contributed.

Each time, I hoisted Mom onto a foot-high kitchen step-stool, and from there, she was able to stand. Each time, too, her injuries were not serious, although the shiner on her cheek after the face dive looked ghastly.

Increasingly, I was bringing up the need for in-home caregivers to help both of my parents. "No strangers!" each would reply, horrified at the prospect.

Sometimes when I visited, I would see new bloody sores or scabs on Dad's arms or knees and, upon my pressing him, he would confess to stumbling in or near the house. These falls were happening with such frequency that Dad started wearing longer-sleeved shirts so I couldn't see his injuries. He didn't want to fortify my in-home nursing-care argument with physical evidence.

Neither of my parents wanted to use a walker.

Why did I have to argue? I asked myself, when hot anger would well up inside me and bring lashing words to mind. Increasingly, I was losing my ability to be kind. Isn't part of being a responsible person planning for one's needs, one's infirmities in old age? I knew Mom and Dad could only skate on their denial for so long before the ice of reality (and, possibly, I) cracked.

And yet I understood that a reliance on caregivers represented an admission of dependency, a surrender of privacy and other qualities of life that were important to them. Like me, they were both introverts. They enjoyed being alone. They didn't want to *have* to talk with anyone, especially someone with whom they might have nothing in common. I tried to walk in their shoes, shoes that I might wear some day, but I was walking too closely behind them to be anything but distressed by their refusal.

NODULE UPDATE

In March 2012, I learned from Georgetown Mini-Medical School pulmonologist Charles A. Read that lung abnormalities with diameters of less than 3 centimeters are categorized as nodules; those larger than 3 cm. are masses. Solitary nodules, Read said, usually result from "bad infections," such as *histoplasmosis*.

In the Georgetown professor's experience, 70 percent of nodules measuring 1 cm. or more turn out to be benign scars, while the other 30 percent are cancer.[2] I further learned from the online Mayo Clinic that a nodule measuring 25 mm. (2.5 cm., or about an inch) or larger is more likely to be cancerous than a smaller nodule.[3] That gave me a working range with Dad's nodules of 1 cm. to 2.5 cm., if you catch my drift.

I also learned that, on *average*, smokers lose about 10 years of life.

Those who have habitually smoked cigarettes since early adulthood but stop before age 40 can gain back these years. Regardless of when you started and how many "pack-years" you smoked, if you kick the habit before age 40, you will achieve greater health benefits than if you quit at an older age. Younger lungs have a better chance of healing.[4]

But even with older damaged lungs, such as my father had at age 56, when he quit, studies indicate that as time after cessation increases, former smokers' *relative* risk of developing lung cancer, vis-à-vis people who never smoked, decreases. Nonetheless, they will always have "excess risk," because "of residual genetic damage that persists despite cessation of smoking," according to the WHO's International Agency for Research on Cancer (IARC).[5]

In the 2007 handbook, "Reversal of Risk After Quitting Smoking," the IARC analyzed all of the then-available data worldwide about the hazards of smoking and the benefits of stopping. Its bottom line: "There is persistent increased risk of lung cancer in former smokers compared to never smokers of the same age, even after a long duration of abstinence [such as 30 years]. Stopping smoking before middle age avoids much of the lifetime risk incurred by *continuing to smoke*. Stopping smoking in middle or old age confers substantially lower lung cancer risk *compared with continuing* smokers."[6] (My emphasis added.)

Regardless of what Dad's relative risk of lung cancer might have been, I think it's safe to say that he had outlived the majority of the never-smokers born in the United States the same year as he. Metastasized cancer from another body site, however, was a different story.

On May 29, before he signed off with Duke, Dad had another chest X-ray, ordered by Dr. Buchanan, and the results were not good. Dr. Exeter again did the honors.

The radiologist concluded that "some" change in the nodules had occurred, but, based on plain film alone, he couldn't document any size increase.

Of course he couldn't: This was just an X-ray.

Dr. Exeter suggested another CT scan.

Of course he did.

Hadn't we already been through this diagnostic process before? Remember the PET scan? Why Dr. Buchanan decided to schedule another chest X-ray, I do not know. My father followed his lead out of respect. Both seemed to me to be operating on automatic pilot, and Buchanan had no excuse. This was bullshit.

Buchanan offered to refer Dad to a pulmonologist in Elizabeth City, but he never mentioned an oncologist. Because I was not privy to the communications between Dr. Al and Dr. Buchanan, and I did not obtain Buchanan's medical records, I could not bash him with abandon. Even so, I adamantly felt that my father didn't need surveillance, he needed a primary-care physician who would stop testing and start advising.

In his film report, Dr. Exeter concluded: "Multiplicity of nodules is suspicious for metastatic disease."

"Suspicious." A new diagnostic word. The nodules had progressed from indeterminate to suspicious on the strength of their number. But was Dr. Exeter saying anything different than he had said before? Was there no other explanation than cancer?

I told Dad that once we signed off with Duke, we were scheduling an appointment with a pulmonologist in Norfolk. We weren't going to keep going round-and-round with Exeter and Buchanan in a dance of duplication and waste.

DUKE SIGNOFF

On June 20, Dad had his last checkup with Dr. Terse and Dr. PYR, whose residency at Duke would end in 10 days. Unfortunately, this visit would not be the end of Dad's pain or his exposure to urological loosey-goosiness.

Whenever I left town with Dad for the day, I had to ensure that Mom was "covered" with written instructions and check-in phone calls. She needed to be reminded to take her pills, eat lunch, and remove a frozen dinner from the freezer. Mom may not have understood her husband's ordeal, but she stayed strong. She cared for herself and her dog in his absence—and may even have enjoyed having a peaceful house for a change. Every one of my siblings called to check on her.

Dad saw the resident first. Dr. PYR talked with him about his foreskin-related pain, his prescription needs, his sphincter manipulation, and the device's performance. Dad raised the possibility of a circumcision to fix the anatomical alteration created by the AUS surgery, but he didn't press it. He felt awkward: How often do Duke urological surgeons perform circumcisions on 87-year-old men?

When Dr. Terse heard about Dad's pain, seemingly for the first time, the Teflon-coated urologist said, "LS," in a knowing aside to Dr. PYR. An *aside*. Meaning, in front of us, as if we were invisible.

LS, I found out later online, stands for lichen simplex, a skin condition characterized by small, highly irritating papules. Dr. Terse did not explain LS to my father, who most definitely did not have it. During his few minutes with Dad, the surgeon summarily accepted his own misdiagnosis and didn't say another word about his patient's pain. Dr. Al didn't push, so I didn't push, but Terse's attitude infuriated me.

Later, in the car, we discussed the brushoff Dad had received. "Basic care is beneath their dignity," he said.

What crap. My father had brought up his plight; he had complained. What more was he supposed to do? Get in the surgeon's face and demand that he respond? The message he and I both received was that Terse was done with him. Any "remedial" work would not be done at Duke.

The appointment was otherwise memorable because Dr. PYR made a move to examine my father, and Dad unhooked his belt buckle, before I could step out of the examining room or draw the all-important curtain.

Good Gawd. Was I invisible? Despite all that my father and I had been through together, I insisted on maintaining our respective privacy. I wanted to be clinical without being personal. A drawer-dropping exam of his genitalia struck me as very personal.

If you had told me then that in a year I would be watching another Duke urology resident perform a cystoscopy on my father, I would not have believed it. Incredibly, in a year, I would be thinking: Privacy, schimacy.

Father and daughter survived the drive home, and daughter vainly hoped for a respite. Some separateness.

But it was not to be. Nine days later, Dad's heart went haywire.

ATRIAL FIBRILLATION

You would think that urological surgeons at Duke would know something about the physiological toll of stress. A simple "How are you doing?" follow-up call from Dr. Terse's intern, if not the man himself, a week after Dad's last appointment might have made a big difference in his sense of well-being. Thirty seconds of empathy. He was an old guy who had been through an assault on his body and a lot of pain and anguish. Surgery is not a discrete act; it's a process, and recovery is a big part of it. Dad had traveled a long way. The sound of a doctor's voice—authoritative and confident—might have carried him to the finish line.

Instead, he awoke on Friday, June 29, with an irregular pulse: His heart was frequently skipping beats.

Twice before in his life, Dad had experienced a full-scale "attack" of AF, not just some irregular beats here or there. The first time, as you will recall, was during his Sentara Norfolk General hospitalization in 1998 when he spit out the digitalis that "can kill you." Each of the two AF episodes he had then lasted about eight hours.

The second attack occurred during the early months of 2005 when Dad was anxiously contemplating rotator-cuff surgery. At the same time, my older sister Leslie was experiencing massive blood loss from what turned out to be bleeding uterine fibroids.

Then 52, Les had stoically tolerated the bleeding as part and parcel of a hideous perimenopause until she became too ill to function. Later hospitalized in anticipation of a hysterectomy, my sister was still losing copious amounts of blood and being transfused. Dad was beside himself over her blood loss and the surgical team's lackadaisical response. Leslie had rated late-Friday-afternoon surgery, and it was still just Thursday morning.

What the hell? Dr. Al ran telephone interference with the hospital staff and insisted on a hematocrit, the test that shows the percentage of oxygen-carrying red blood cells in a person's blood. As I mentioned in the previous chapter, a normal hematocrit for a woman is 37 to 47 percent. Leslie's was 18 percent, dangerously low.

"She was slowly bleeding to death," my father recalled.

Shocked by her hematocrit, the surgeon ordered more blood and moved Leslie's hysterectomy up to first thing the next morning. While my sister fared well, my father took all of his anxiety out on his poor heart.

Between Feb. 3 and Feb. 13, 2005, he had five episodes of AF, each lasting from four-and-a-half to 12 hours. During this period, he saw Dr. Anthony, who documented Dad's AF with an ECG reading on Feb. 7 and put him on metoprolol (Toprol®), a beta blocker that slows the heart's rate.[7]

Bad idea: Dad's heart rate fell to just 40 beats per minute!

Beta blockers control heart rate, not heart rhythm. So Anthony switched Dad to flecainide (Tambocor®), an antiarrhythmic drug that stops atrial fibrillation and restores sinus rhythm.[8]

My father has what is called *paroxysmal* atrial fibrillation, which Johns Hopkins cardiologists, Drs. Hugh G. Calkins and Ronald Berger, describe as "a recurrent condition where the rapid heart rate and abnormal electrical signals spontaneously begin, typically last for a day or two, sometimes as long as a week, and then suddenly disappear as mysteriously as [they] began." Paroxysmal symptoms, they say, can range from "barely noticeable to severe."

Other types of atrial fibrillation are persistent AF, which lasts longer than a week, or is stopped short of that by a drug- or electrical-shock-induced restoration of normal rhythm, called a cardioversion; and longstanding persistent AF, which is continuous atrial fibrillation that lasts longer than a year.[9] I have seen a fourth category described as permanent AF, in which a medical decision has been made not to restore sinus rhythm.

The paramount concern with AF is not a sudden stoppage of the heart, as you might think, but a potentially fatal stroke. If cardiac blood slows, it is more apt to clot, just as venous blood does in the periphery. A clot can migrate to the brain. AF causes about 20 percent of all ischemic strokes.[10] (See Appendix Five for more about strokes.)

Thanks to an "Ah-HA!" turn of events, Dad never had surgery on his right shoulder to repair his rotator cuff. ("Do you know what a rotator cuff is?" Dr. Al would ask me, expressing skepticism that such a body part even exists.)

Hurt about 20 years before when he got knocked off of a tractor-lawn mower by a low-hanging tree limb, he had controlled his shoulder pain with steroid injections. By 2005, the pain was severe, and the injections, now being administered by an Elizabeth City orthopedic surgeon, weren't working. Uneasy about surgery, he decided to go see the orthopod for one more injection attempt.

"Nobody ever puts the needle right where my pain is, doc," he told the surgeon, indicating the spot. This time, the surgeon did. Voila! The pain stopped, and Dad never had pain again in that shoulder. Ever. True story.

When he returned home from the surgeon's office, the OR nurse was calling about his pre-op. He happily canceled the surgery.

AF Number 3

On June 29, 2012, the first day of my father's third-ever AF attack, Dr. Anthony was not available. Sadly, the dashing, "on-it" specialist who wore black lab scrubs was seriously ill with colon cancer and could no longer treat patients. Having no desire to go to the OBH's emergency room, Dad decided to drop by Anthony's office that morning to see if the cardiologist's fill-in or his staff could help him. While there, the fill-in's physician assistant felt Dad's pulse and informed him: "You need a pacemaker."

Not "You might need a pacemaker," or, better yet, "You definitely are in arrhythmia." No, this PA flatly informed Dad—who then told me—that he needed a pacemaker. I flipped. How does a person without a medical degree and a medical license come out with a bald statement like that? He should take lessons from Dr. Exeter on how to hedge. Or at least wait until after the doctor has talked to Dad and examined him.

Nonetheless, this advice struck a chord with me because my Uncle Pete, Dad's brother, has a pacemaker to control his heart rate. My grandmother, Dad's and Pete's mother, also had atrial fibrillation and other heart disease and died suddenly at age 68.

Pete's paroxysmal AF came on when he was about 60 and was more severe than my father's. His AF neither resolved on its own nor responded to medication: His heart had to be repeatedly shocked back into sinus rhythm. Eventually, my uncle underwent a cardiac ablation, a procedure in which a surgeon ablates (destroys) the heart tissue that is helping to cause the arrhythmia.[11] This, too, did not work, and the AF continued. Because Pete's heart rate was both irregular and too slow, he had a pacemaker implanted (just below the collarbone) to ensure a steady rate between 70 and 72 bpm.

I was preparing to leave on a labor-intensive weekend in the D.C. area when I heard the news about Dad needing a pacemaker. Still in sphincter meltdown, I was stunned. Are you *kidding* me?

Dad also told me that a nurse in Anthony's office had attempted to get an electrocardiographic recording of his heart's activity while he was lying down. The rate was normal! As soon as he sat up, it went wacky again. Acutely aware of the difference, Dad insisted that she try again while he was upright. Keep this in mind if your Mom or Pop knows her or his heart is in arrhythmia, and a technician or nurse denies it. That the patient had to instruct the nurse on ECG technique did not bolster my confidence in the Anthony-less cardiology practice.

But the quick-to-judge PA did one thing right that Friday morning: He wired a portable Holter monitor to Dad's chest in order to record his heart's electrical activity for the next 24 hours.

A Holter is a small battery-operated ECG device that can be carried in a pocket. Typically, patients keep a symptom diary during the test period. Afterward, a technician processes the Holter recording and prepares a report.

That weekend I planned to vacate a Baltimore studio I had been renting as a part-time getaway and move into Britt's Alexandria condo. My younger sister had defected—I mean relocated—to Florida about a year ago, and she had yet to sell her condo. I debated postponing my move until after Dad's AF had resolved, but I decided not to, and he didn't insist. I reasoned, hopefully, that, if necessary, Mom could call 911. The family could triage by phone. I needed to have a life, too. (An increasingly common refrain for me.)

Naturally, that decision kicked me in the butt, but not in the predictable way.

That night, while I was driving on Interstate 95 in Virginia, a massive, fast-moving, and other-worldly lightning and thunderstorm battered the area. To explain my stupidity in being caught in it, I cop to the pacemaker excuse. Even though I heard radio forecasts, I had been unfazed by the storm's approach. Around 11 p.m., nearly blinded by rain, I pulled off on an exit in Fredericksburg that I knew and took shelter in a protected hotel parking lot, crossing my fingers that my poor car would withstand the fierce winds.

I've hunkered down through many Outer Banks hurricanes, not having evacuated during a "mandatory evacuation" since the 1970s; but this storm's winds made a mockery of what meteorologists call hurricane-force. Through the relentless and hard-slanting rain, I watched as spectacularly brilliant lightning filled the night sky in a vast spider-web pattern. It was breathtaking.

It was also dangerous. When I returned to the highway, 95 had become a slow obstacle course of fallen tree trunks and other debris, which didn't stop idiot-drivers from proceeding at normal speeds. Soon their smashed vehicles added to the chaotic travel. It took me three hours to drive 50 miles. I arrived in Alexandria at 2 a.m., only to discover what I had feared even more than the intense wind: The electricity was out. With brutally high temperatures and stultifying humidity, this after-effect was even more challenging than the conditions on 95 had been.

I found it exceedingly difficult to sleep in Britt's condo. The building had settled, so that most of the windows wouldn't open—a problem she knew about, but had never addressed because she relied on air conditioning. The experience reminded me of my childhood when I got through hot, humid suburban-D.C. summer nights by wearing as little as possible and lying on top of the bed sheets. But in the dark ages before central air conditioning, we had windows that opened!

The next day, still without power, I learned that the other-worldly storm actually was an aggressive storm system that had originated in the Midwest and traveled more than 600 miles. It came with 70 mile-per-hour winds and an intriguing name: derecho.

Although the word describes the storm's straight-line path, it sounds like wreckage, and it caused plenty.

The derecho knocked out electricity in the greater Washington area, shutting down gas stations and other businesses and rendering all traffic-light-controlled intersections ridiculously hazardous. Without power, the urban areas that I drove through en route to Baltimore looked strangely desolate and abandoned, except for all of the idle people milling about! Starbucks, served by back-up generators, fared well that Saturday.

The electricity was out in my Baltimore apartment, but its ground-floor coolness kept me comfortable. I packed my car on Saturday, stayed overnight, then moved my things to Alexandria on Sunday and just kept driving. I refused to fry in Britt's condo another night. My early return to Carolina meant I could go with Dad to see Dr. Ramses at Eastern Virginia Medical School on Monday, July 2.

I had encouraged Dad to call Mom's internist at home—he had his cell number—instead of waiting until Monday to call Dr. Buchanan. Not only did I think that Dr. Ramses would work Dad into his schedule, which he kindly did, but I wanted to take advantage of EVMS ologists.

My slow zig-zag path through the derecho's destruction became an apt metaphor for my medical journey with Dad that summer. How much more wreckage would there be? And would we (I) have any power?

Chapter Fourteen

2012: A Runaway
TRAIN

With Too Many Station Stops

By Monday morning, July 2, Dad's atrial fibrillation had converted. His heart was beating normally again. Oddly, this seemed to me like good news-bad news. Dad was apparently out of danger, but now only the Holter reading would document, and thus characterize, his attack. An ECG done by a technician in Ramses's office later that day did not show an erratic heart rhythm.

Despite the conversion, Ramses gave Dad more than the usual 15 minutes of attention. I remained in the room while he gathered a thorough history and performed a basic physical. Like so many physicians today, even cardiologists, Dr. Ramses listened to Dad's heart and lungs through his clothing, a faux pas that Dr. Al never failed to point out to me. The sounds emanating from these organs are already barely audible. A layer of clothing only makes them harder to pick up through a stethoscope.

I usually don't obtain physicians' reports of Mom-'n'-Pop examinations that I observe, but this time, I did. I got Ramses's records for a six-month period that included the July 2 appointment as well as two subsequent appointments that I did not attend.

In his report, Ramses noted that his patient's "daughter thinks he has been going downhill over the last year." I certainly did. In just the months since his Duke surgery, Dad's loss in stamina had been profound, and he seemed increasingly confused. I knew he had been through an emotional ordeal, a lot of stress, and a lot of pain, and I appreciated that both could cause weakness. But I didn't think they could explain all of my father's symptoms.

As Ramses asked Dad questions about his general status, and

Dad minimized any problems—Stoicism? Not wanting to complain to a fellow M.D.?—I interjected what I considered to be relevant omissions. I tried to be selective and wished in hindsight that I had been more so. Although Ramses noted in his file that he spent 50 percent of the hourlong visit "in counseling & coordination of care," coordination of care really didn't occur.

I prodded Dad to tell the internist about the pulmonary nodules and the peripheral neuropathy and to elaborate on the chronic fatigue that he said was his primary concern—after his heart, of course. I was hoping to turn control of this multi-car healthcare train over to another conductor, but that never happened, in part because of Dad's careening and in part because Ramses neither prioritized nor analyzed Dad's problems: He merely cataloged them.

A catalog is not coordination. We needed focus. Although I recognized that Ramses was playing catchup, I wondered if he, too, was ageist and would let us down.

The internist's most significant contribution was the neurological exam he administered. The deficits Dad exhibited hit me hard.

I knew that my father's proprioception, his body's unconscious perception of movement and space—in a word, his balance—had eroded dramatically. He now teetered when he stood, and his gait was markedly ataxic. With such an uncoordinated walk, his legs, which had weakened without regular exercise, could easily go out from under him.

I also knew about the chronic numbness and tingling in both of his feet, and the progressive numbness, tingling, and tremors in each of his hands. But I did *not* know, as Ramses uncovered in his exam, that:

❖ Dad staggered to one side, losing his balance and risking a fall, when he stood with his feet together and closed his eyes. Dr. Al himself identified this phenomenon as "Romberg's sign," another indicator of a loss of proprioceptive control.

❖ He could not put one foot in front of the other in heel-to-toe fashion and walk; he was too unsteady.

❖ He had no vibratory sense in his calves and ankles. When Dr. Ramses placed a vibrating tuning fork on Dad's lower legs, he felt nothing. When the internist placed the fork on his wrist, he jumped.

Was Dad's nerve degeneration just really, really bad aging, or did he have a disease, a syndrome of some kind? If the latter, could it explain his fatigue, too? I still didn't trust the fallout from Ambien, flecainide, and other drugs Dad was taking. Could they explain any of his neurological symptoms? Or were they all related to degeneration?

MORE FRAGMENTATION

Ramses probed the possibility of Parkinson's disease, but the symptoms didn't fit. I considered this diagnosis far-fetched because my father could diagnose Parkinson's himself. I probably could, too.

The internist had no answers for us, just more tests for Dad to undergo and ologist appointments for him (i.e., me) to make. I soon learned how fragmentation–too many ologists–can break a sick older person's already weakened resolve. Hell, too many cooks in the healthcare kitchen can demoralize anyone, regardless of age and vigor.

It took Ramses's receptionist and me more than 30 minutes to schedule Dad's appointments with the cardiologist, pulmonologist, and neurologist whom he referred, and to arrange for an EVMS-interpreted CT scan of his lungs. I had to negotiate the physicians', my father's, and my own calendars, as well as the travel time to and from Norfolk, and the time of day. While I busied myself at the Internal Medicine front desk with this, a nurse came to wheel Dad to the pulmonary division, where he underwent lung-function testing. I wish they had waited for me. By the time I rejoined him, Dad had finished these tests and was exhausted, but pleased. He thought he had done well.

I later obtained a report of these arcane results and couldn't say otherwise–except there seemed to be a lot of asterisks next to numbers, signifying that they were outside the norm. Ramses never talked with Dad about his lung-function tests, nor did the pulmonologist he eventually consulted. Perhaps Ramses thought Dr. Al didn't need a discussion. He was wrong. No matter how brilliant my father was or had been, he was nearly 88 years old. He needed help. *We* needed help.

Generally speaking, when physicians don't explain test results to their patients, they lose their trust. They also deny them valuable information that belongs to them. Doctors shouldn't wait to be asked: They should just discuss them.

After the lung tests, Dad and I went to the lab so his blood could be drawn. Ramses had ordered a slew of blood tests, mostly designed to evaluate anemia, one of his cataloged assessments, but also including one for syphilis! Syphilitic myelopathy causes some of the same neurological symptoms that my father had, but I think Ramses was safe in taking Dad at his word when he said he'd never had syphilis. Talk about differential-diagnosis overkill.

Curiously, Ramses omitted a test for vitamin B-12, which Dr. Buchanan had been monitoring. A B-12 deficiency is associated with neuropathy and pernicious anemia, which is a severe anemia caused by a gastrointestinal failure to absorb B-12. When my father was at the NIH, he had treated a patient with pernicious anemia, which most often affects older people, so he knew its clinical signs and how closely his own symptoms correlated.

Despite the burden of multiple appointments, I was delighted that Dad was going to be checked out by presumptive experts. We were moving up through the cars of the healthcare-system locomotive. Or so I thought.

Wishful thinking.

My scheduling began to unravel the very next day when a pulmonology staff member called Dad and rescheduled with him, doing a nifty end-run around me. This woman had watched me struggle to book appointments and had worked personally with me on the pulmonologist's consult. Although Dad referred her to me for the final word, she didn't offer an acceptable substitute time. Instead she proposed to squeeze the pulmonology appointment in just ahead of the CT scan.

I balked. First of all, we wanted the scan results available before the appointment, and second of all, what she proposed would force Dad to hurry through his consult.

"You can't expect to have more than 15 minutes with the doctor," she told me when I objected.

The tyranny had spread.

"Then what's the point?" I asked this obstructionist. "Why would we want to go all the way to Norfolk for just 15 minutes?"

Ironically, her phone call and squeeze play gave Dad an opening: He indefinitely postponed the pulmonology appointment, then later canceled his neurology appointment, and refused to travel to EVMS for the CT scan.

He was overwhelmed, he said. Just skimming through the extensive paperwork that the neurologist's office had sent him to fill out defeated him. Why don't ologists *get* this and make a point of not encumbering their older patients? Like care fragmentation, medical paperwork is hazardous to elders' mental health.

"I can't deal with all of these doctors, Ann," Dad told me. "I'm worn down."

I understood.

Besides, he said, the only thing that mattered to him was his heart. His heart health was his priority.

The weekend bout with AF had left Dad worrying obsessively that his heart would stop before he could get medical care. I feared his cardiac neurosis would trigger an AF, so I backed off and reassured him that he could cancel whatever he wanted to cancel. He was the patient, not I, and I was concerned about his whole self, not just his parts.

On Thursday, July 5, Dad obtained his Holter monitor results from Anthony's replacement, Dr. Tridecker, as well as an electrocardiogram, which he could read without Tridecker's assistance. Dad told me that the tracing showed an absence of the P wave, which is typical with AF. He said there were "other irregularities" in the conduction of electrical impulses to his ventricles, but he didn't elaborate. If I needed to be more concerned, I reasoned, Dad would tell me.

A normal electrocardiogram of a heartbeat consists of a regularly spaced series of waves designated by the letters P, Q, R, S, and T, which indicate the order of the waves' appearance in the heart's depolarization-repolarization cycle.

Cardiac cells at rest are considered polarized. In order to beat, your heart undergoes rapid and repeated depolarization, electrical activity that stimulates its contractions; and repolarization, electrical activity that returns its cells and muscles to a non-electrical resting state. The P wave spreads from the SA node and represents atrial depolarization prior to contraction.[1]

Dr. Ramses referred Dad to Dr. Gotti, a cardiologist in Chesapeake, who, in turn, referred him to Dr. Eppi, an electrophysiologist in his practice group.

Electrophysiology is a subspecialty of cardiology and internal medicine that dates to the mid-1970s. It deals with diagnosing and treating the heart's electrical activities, especially rhythm disorders.

CARDIOLOGY CONSULTS

I went with Dad to see Dr. Gotti on Monday, July 23, 2012, but remained in the waiting room. Dad saw Dr. Eppi, who only had Friday hours, on Aug. 24. He went to this appointment alone. I obtained the reports that both specialists sent to Ramses, but, in general, I deferred to Dad on matters of the heart. In retrospect, I wish I had gone with him to the second appointment, not the first.

My father didn't like either Gotti or Eppi, so he was not inclined to take their advice. They didn't connect with him personally because, I suspect, they didn't do what Marcus Welby, M.D., would have done: get to know a little bit about him. He was strictly an ECG to them.

Dr. Gotti certainly wasn't much for small talk. I gleaned that much in the few detached minutes I spent with him. He didn't smile once.

My father remembers Gotti as "the guy who stole my Holter reading." The cardiologist had a photocopy made, but neglected to return the original. It got lost in the shuffle of our checkout with the receptionist, so Dad had to obtain another from Dr. Tridecker.

Based on the ECG performed in his office—they *all* do their own ECGs, no matter when the previous one was administered—Dr. Gotti suspected that Dad had an "underlying" atrial "flutter," which, like an atrial fibrillation, is a tachycardia in the atria. From what I gathered later, the basic difference between these two atrial conditions is that the electrical signal in a flutter moves in a regular and predictable circular motion, whereas the AF signal is disorganized and irregular. A flutter may or may not produce symptoms and can cause a fibrillation.[2]

In his report, Gotti could not say if Dad, who was "in regular rhythm in my office," was in a "sinus rhythm with first degree AV block vs. atrial flutter with 4:1 conduction." He referred Dad to Dr. Eppi to get the latter's opinion on whether he was a "potential candidate for flutter ablation."

My father had long known about the block at his atrioventricular node and scoffed at the flutter idea. I was clueless, however, and did some research on AV blocks.

I learned that the period of time between the onset of the P wave (the beginning of atrial contraction), and the so-called QRS complex, which represents three separate waves and marks the beginning of ventricular contraction, is called the P-R interval. Normally, the P-R interval ranges from 0.12 to 0.20 seconds. (You might see this range described as 120 to 200 milliseconds (msec.)) If there is a longer delay in the conduction of the electrical impulse from the atria to the ventricles, a block exists.

In a first-degree AV block, according to the National Heart Lung and Blood Institute, the electrical signals "are slowed" as they move between chambers, but each impulse still reaches the ventricles. There are no missed beats. An ECG will show a longer, flatter line between the P and R waves. This degree of block, of electrical-impulse delay, rarely causes symptoms and usually does not require treatment.

With the more severe second-degree AV block, of which two types exist, some of the heart's electrical signals do not reach the ventricles. A third-degree block is complete; no signals get to the lower chambers. The heart has to compensate with a backup system to create ventricular contraction. A complete block can cause cardiac arrest and sudden death.[3]

According to Dad, Dr. Gotti examined his Holter reading in great detail, noting, in particular, the space between heartbeats, and could see no reason to believe that a pacemaker would be helpful. When Dad confided his anxiety about sudden death, Gotti advised him not to worry unless the delay between heartbeats reached 10 seconds! That floored me. That's the best he could do?

In contrast, Dr. Eppi didn't care about his Holter reading, Dad said—or about his heart history, for that matter—and told him so. He did his own ECG reading, which would be Dad's fifth in three months, and informed the skeptical Dr. Al: "This is all I care about." He only wanted to know about his heart's status then, that day.

"Can you imagine?" my father later complained to me. "He didn't want to hear anything from me. This is medicine?"

Dr. Al couldn't see how the electrophysiologist could evaluate his AF without knowing about previous episodes. That's when Dr. Eppi lost his patient, and I lost access to an expert whom I potentially could consult and rely upon.

As for the all-important ECG in his office, Eppi reported that it showed "sinus rhythm with a left atrial abnormality, nonspecific T waves changes and a marked first degree AV block." The T wave represents ventricular repolarization (return to the resting state). A first-degree AV block is "marked" when the PR interval exceeds 0.30 seconds or 300 msec.

Dr. Eppi was noncommittal about whether Dad had a flutter

and concluded that, if he were to develop "more problems," the implantation of a "dual chamber pacemaker" should be considered.

A pacemaker resets a heart rate that is too slow to an appropriate pace so that blood and, therefore, oxygen continue to be delivered, as needed, throughout the body.

This small device contains a powerful battery, electronic circuits, and a computer memory that work together to generate pacing signals. Thin, insulated wires, also called leads, then carry these impulses to the heart. A dual-chamber pacemaker has a wire in two chambers, one pacing the right atrium and the other pacing the right ventricle. A single-chamber pacemaker has a lead to carry impulses to and from the right atrium or right ventricle.

People with atrial fibrillation may have a slow heart rate, but Dad did not. Dr. Gotti, you'll recall, had not taken up the pacemaker baton.

CHADS SCORING

Both cardiologists discussed antithrombotic therapy with my father. Dr. Gotti reported that, because of his (controlled) hypertension, age, and dilated left atrium, Dad was at high risk for a clot and should be taking warfarin (Coumadin). This jibes with the stroke-risk indexes I uncovered in my research.

One of the most popular and simple indexes to use is known by the acronym, $CHADS_2$, which abbreviates the following risk factors:

C: Congestive heart failure
H: Hypertension (above 140/90 mmHg.)
A: Age (75 or older)
D: Diabetes mellitus
S_2: Stroke (prior stroke or TIA)

To compute your Mom's or Pop's $CHADS_2$ score, assign one point to the first four risk factors and two points to the fifth, S_2, prior stroke or transient ischemic attack. According to Calkins and Berger, the Johns Hopkins cardiologist-electrophysiologists whom I earlier quoted, a score of zero or one suggests a low risk of a stroke; two to three points connote a moderate risk, and any score of four or higher is a high risk. (Other physicians may evaluate a score of one as a moderate risk and any score of two or higher, a high risk.)

Physicians do not recommend anticoagulation for a low-risk AF patient, except a daily baby aspirin, if the patient chooses. The standard medical recommendation for the moderate-risk patient is an oral anticoagulant or aspirin; and for the high-risk patient, an oral anticoagulant, typically either warfarin or dabigatran (Pradaxa®).[4]

My father's CHADS$_2$ score was two. An AF patient who has a score of two and does not choose to anticoagulate purportedly has an annual stroke risk of 4.0 percent, which means that, of 100 AF patients with a two score who don't anticoagulate, four will have a stroke.[5]

A more recently derived index, CHA$_2$DS$_2$-VASc, refines and extends CHADS$_2$ and reportedly has proved to be a better predictor of risk. CHA$_2$DS$_2$-VASc stands for:

C: Congestive heart failure or left ventricular systolic dysfunction (1 pt.)

H: Hypertension, either blood pressure consistently above 140/90 mmHg or treated hypertension on medication (1 pt.)

A$_2$: Age 75 years or older (2 pts.)

D: Diabetes mellitus (1 pt.)

S$_2$: Prior stroke or TIA or thromboembolism (2 pts.)

V: Vascular disease (1 pt.)

A: 65 to 74 years of age (1 pt.)

Sc: Sex category (female, 1 pt.)

Dad's CHA$_2$DS$_2$-VASc score was three, which corresponds to a high risk and an annual risk of stroke without anticoagulation of 4.7 percent. Just as with CHADS$_2$, any CHA$_2$DS$_2$-VASc score of two or more indicates the need for oral anticoagulation.[6]

Over the derecho weekend, my father had taken some of Mom's warfarin. Dr. Ramses recommended a daily aspirin, as did both Gotti and Eppi. Dad obliged.

Dr. Eppi further suggested that Dad add the calcium-channel blocker, dilitiazem (Cardizem®), which is an antihypertensive, to his daily prescription-drug regimen. Calcium-channel blockers slow the flow of calcium ions into the smooth muscle cells of the heart and blood vessels and thereby help to decrease the number of electrical impulses that go to the ventricles. These blockers and beta-blockers, such as the pulse-lowering metoprolol that Dr. Anthony prescribed for Dad in 2005, control heart rate, not rhythm. According to the Johns Hopkins electrophysiologists, calcium blockers are usually recommended for AF patients with underlying heart or lung disease.[7]

My father knew the scientific and commercial history of Cardizem and had no respect for "this crappy drug." Already on lisinopril, an angiotensin-converting-enzyme inhibitor, he didn't want to take two antihypertensives. He decided to continue with his current dose of flecainide, which does not affect blood pressure.

I think it's safe to say that Gotti's and Eppi's conflicting advice and their obvious lack of communication with each other; Gotti's flutter speculation; and Eppi's disinterest in Dad's cardiac history left my father feeling alienated and unimpressed.

When I asked Dad whom he would consult in the event of another AF attack, he said—you guessed it—Dr. Tridecker. Why? Because he could talk with him.

CT Scan No. 3

I had great hopes that the chest CT Dr. Ramses ordered, scan No. 3, would be done at Eastern Virginia Medical School, with a state-of-the-art scanner, and interpreted by the eyes and mind of someone other than Kitty Hawk's Dr. Exeter. I didn't stop to think that any new radiologist would be evaluating a new CT in the context of Exeter's interpretations. He/she would want to have the imaging history.

It ultimately didn't matter because my chronically fatigued father refused to travel to Norfolk. The scan went to default: Exeter.

Dr. Exeter began his 7/30/12 CT-scan report with a white lie. He said that Dad "refused the IV contrast material for today's study," when, in fact, Exeter refused to perform the imaging with contrast because Dad's creatinine and BUN levels hadn't been checked within the past three months. There was no patient refusal.

Later, Dr. Ramses said he preferred a CT scan without contrast.

Exeter found "at least 7 separate noncalcified nodules in the right lung," the largest being in the right upper lobe and measuring about a centimeter. This nodule, he wrote, "has shown progressive enlargement over the last two studies." If this were indeed the original "solitary" 5-mm. nodule, then it had doubled in about two years—assuming Exeter's measurements could be trusted.

Does it take two years for (some) cancerous tumors to double in size? You typically hear of more rapid growth with metastatic cancer, but I didn't know.

Georgetown pulmonology Professor Charles Read had said that 70 percent of nodules measuring 1 cm. or more turn out to be benign scars, while the other 30 percent are cancer. But he wasn't talking about a proliferation of growing nodules.

In the left lung, Dr. Exeter found "at least 7 separate noncalcified granulomas present," several of which "have increased in size with the largest one measuring a centimeter." Granulomas, not nodules. In about eight months, these granulomas apparently had grown between 1 mm. and 2 mm.

For the first time Exeter mentioned the calcification of all of the nodules. Why hadn't he done this before? Calcified nodules, I learned later, are more likely to have a benign cause, but their status also depends on where the calcification is within the nodule.

The "solid component"-"irregular density" that Exeter saw earlier had morphed into a "triangular band of soft tissue density with a single punctate calcification." It had not "significantly" changed in size or character.

Bottom line, the radiologist concluded: "The progression in size of the multiple nodules would suggest we are probably dealing with metastatic disease."

"Probably." Would you care to offer some odds?

Dad still had no respiratory symptoms.

I wanted to hospitalize my father and have him thoroughly checked out by a multi-disciplinary team of specialists working *together*: pulmonologist, cardiologist, neurologist, oncologist, whatever ologist. I wanted him to receive the patient-centered care that large academic centers like Johns Hopkins boast they can provide. Maybe Dr. Ramses could open a door. I still believed the system could help Dad (and me); but Dr. Al did not.

"The hospital could kill me!" he protested—which is true. He also didn't trust hospital personnel to know about or protect his artificial urinary sphincter: "What if they have to catheterize me?" he asked.

I wasn't going to argue with him. My father was nearly 88 years old. He could do what he wanted to do. But not knowing bugged me.

LOCAL PCP

Having been through the ologist appointment fiasco, and being alarmed by my father's fatigue, I insisted that he and Mom find a local primary-care doctor to whom they could go for diagnostic tests and referrals.

Although I recognized that I was contributing to the healthcare fragmentation that occurs with physician handoffs, and three PCPs (Drs. Buchanan and Ramses plus a new recruit) were at least one too many, I wanted to ensure that they could consult someone, other than an ED doctor, in a pinch. I knew that Dr. Eagan, a late-30s/early 40s internist who had trained at East Carolina University, was receiving high praise for the practice that she had opened at Kitty Hawk Regional, so they both arranged to see her.

On Aug. 9, 2012, Dr. Al had a grand old time talking with Dr. Eagan, a very attractive and vivacious woman who was in awe of him. Like my parents, she and her husband, an orthopedic surgeon, were a medical-doctor couple. That my parents had met and married more than 60 years ago made them a bit more unusual than Dr. Eagan and her spouse, and Eagan appreciated that. Upon hearing about this exchange, I held my breath that Dr. Eagan had more to offer than just her entertaining company. I needed some medical chops.

In her file report, Dr. Eagan described anxiety and insomnia as Dad's chief complaints, but the truth is they were just the complaints that she easily could address. In notes to himself, which he gave to the PCP, Dad cited the full menu of his complaints:

"Major: chronic fatigue; erratic systolic blood pressure; anxiety (especially since recent (6/29-7/1) episode of atrial fibrillation/ flutter, (confirmed by Holter)), non-recurrent on increased dosage of flecainide to 100 mg. TID.*

"Minor: Hand/foot (stocking/glove) paresthesias and penile pain secondary to balanitis, Rx by topical steroid."

On Aug. 22, Dad returned to Dr. Eagan, telling her that his stamina and endurance had decreased, and his muscle weakness had increased. He asked her for a referral to physical therapy, which she readily gave him. In a memo to himself of the same date, Dr. Al described "progressive muscular weakness, especially in legs (stumbling and ataxia)" and complained of nightmares while taking the melatonin

---

*TID means three times a day. It's an abbreviation of the Latin phrase, ter in die.

and diazepam (Valium®) that Eagan had prescribed for his extreme insomnia and anxiety.

Dad discontinued the melatonin, but not the Valium, an old drug that he knew well: He had treated flareups of back spasms for years with this muscle relaxant. I couldn't see how any good could come of my father taking Valium.

His worsening fatigue and weakness left me worried and wondering: Was he slowly succumbing to cancer, or did he have a serious neurological disorder, or both? Whatever was happening, the lightweight Dr. Eagan wasn't going to be able to help me.

PULMONOLOGY CONSULT

On Sept. 11, 2012, my father finally consulted an EVMS-affiliated pulmonologist, Dr. Dorrey, but I did not go with him.

No, that's not a mistake. I didn't go.

I wanted answers, but I had a greater priority: enlisting my siblings to shoulder more of the responsibility for our parents' healthcare. Sorry to say, I had grown resentful. I also increasingly felt that the caregiver needed to take better care of herself. Long drives aggravated my chronic back and leg pain, which I kept in check by not sitting for extended periods. (Hell for a writer.)

In my reflective and pain-free moments, I could appreciate the error of stepping aside, because only I provided continuity in Dad's alleged healthcare, but in the daily-life moment in which I had to act, I often felt anguish and yearned for relief. Why was every PCP and ologist a disappointment?

On Sept. 11, Dad had both a follow-up visit with Dr. Ramses and his postponed pulmonologist appointment. I asked Al, who was visiting the Outer Banks, to accompany him to Norfolk. Afterward, I received a debriefing from my brother and obtained all of the medical records.

According to Ramses's report, Al told him that both his "father and mother are doing reasonably well for their age." When I read that, my spirit sank. If Dad's son thinks he is doing well, and Dad himself doesn't press Ramses for help in deducing the cause of his fatigue or other symptoms, and, regardless of their origin, how they might be treated, why should the PCP do more than catalog his ills?

Why? Goddamnit, I rallied. Because he is the primary-care doctor. The conductor of the healthcare locomotive. I had told Ramses less than two months ago that Dad was going downhill, and I, unlike my brother, saw my father every day. I had known Ramses now for six years and had even seen him as a patient myself, so my credibility should have been established. I now questioned Ramses's credibility.

I also didn't appreciate that Ramses obviously wrote his summation of Dad's Sept. 11 visit after reading Dorrey's report and that he did not discuss the results of Drs. Gotti's and Eppi's exams with Dad. He also didn't talk with Dad about his neurological deficits.

Did he actually believe that my run-down father was on top of his healthcare?

All Ramses seemed to be good for was ordering lab tests and imaging studies. This was no followup. This was cr*p.

According to my father, the 40ish pulmonologist Dr. Dorrey spent 15 to 20 minutes looking at a DVD Dr. Exeter had prepared of the most recent CT scan. That's *all* he did. He didn't bother to examine Dad. He didn't even listen to his lungs. Was this a joke?

Dorrey said he thought the nodules were a metastasis from somewhere else, an opinion that knocked my brother, who had been out of the loop, *for* a loop.

Until you're in the white-lab-coat environment yourself, you sometimes can fool yourself into believing that what your Mom or Pop tells you on the phone has to be minor because, heck, she/he sounds fine. That's what my brother had done. My minimizing father would rather talk sports with his son than CT scans, and Al doesn't ask probing questions. When Dr. Dorrey came right out with the cancer word, he was stunned.

Dorrey specifically mentioned the colon and the prostate as primary-tumor sites—thus, earning him poor marks with Dr. Al, who thought both unlikely.

"Prostate cancer metastasizes to bone first," Dad had told me umpteen times. And he had no symptoms of colon cancer.

My father reportedly told Dr. Dorrey: "I'd be dead if I'd had a metastasis for two years." He had told my siblings and me this many times, too, and we'd been at a loss for how to respond. Ramses also had refrained from commenting when Dad said the same thing to him in July. If Dorrey had a response, he failed to record it, and neither Dad nor Al remembered one.

I also don't get this. Why consult a physician if he's not going to advise you?

Dr. Dorrey might have said: "No, Dr. Sjoerdsma, that's not true." Or, "You're absolutely right. It's quite unlikely. Let's explore other options." Or, "Frankly, I don't know." A patient doesn't see (and pay) a doctor for avoidance.

Dorrey offered to do a "needle biopsy"—my father's and brother's words—of one or more of Dad's nodules, which elicited another unfavorable reaction from the patient.

Always quick to consider what could go wrong with any invasive procedure, Dr. Al demurred. No one was sticking a needle in his lung, Dad told me later, piercing an artery, causing profuse bleeding, etc., etc.

Besides, even if the biopsy showed he had cancer, he wasn't going to undergo chemotherapy or radiation, and the nodules were too diffuse to be addressed surgically. He didn't want to die, but he had no interest in extreme measures that would make him sick and offer little therapeutic payoff. He may be "a walking museum of pathology," as he phrased it, but he still had no cough, no shortness of breath, no cancer-like symptoms except his damn fatigue.

Dad told the pulmonologist that he wasn't going to do anything further except cooperate with Dr. Buchanan's suggested monitoring. Absolutely no biopsy.

To this, Dr. Dorrey replied with magical words that redeemed him in my father's opinion: "Off the record, I wouldn't do anything either."

The clouds parted! The bluebirds sang! The ologist seemed to be showing care for my father. Dr. Dorrey didn't put this advice into the report I obtained, but my father heard it, as did my brother.

Then, no doubt mindful of his CYA posture, and, perhaps, his responsibility as a physician, Dorrey offered to arrange a thorough workup—CT scans of Dad's chest, abdomen, and pelvis; a colonoscopy; a prostate exam—and to "follow" his case, if he wanted.

"Sorry to disappoint you," the pulmonologist quoted Dad as saying, "but I do not want any more CT scans at least for a few months."

Had I been there, the one question I would have asked was: What, if anything, could these nodules be *besides* cancer?

But I wasn't there, and this question didn't occur to my brother.

While I supported my father in his decision to decline Dr. Dorrey's intervention, I did not buy his kitty-dander-disease diagnosis, which he still believed and did not mention to the pulmonologist. Contrary to what some of my friends later suggested, I could accept that Dad had cancer, if I had to. I could prepare myself for his death. But as long as he lived, and if I could, I wanted to improve the quality of his life. I wasn't in denial.

That Dorrey knew all of Exeter's interpretations before he formed his own conclusion was a great disappointment to me. I continued to believe that one radiologist should not have so much power.

I also was disappointed when I read the pulmonologist's opinion in his report to Dr. Ramses that "likely primaries could be from colon, kidneys, prostate, thyroid, breast, lung, etc."

Clearly, Dorrey didn't know cancer. I can catalog common cancers, too. For the record, he omitted stomach.

Dr. Dorrey further said that, because of the size and location of the nodules, a bronchoscopy "would not be able to get tissue samples," and a "TTNA likely will have low yield and lung biopsy would have highest yield."

In a bronchoscopy, a pulmonologist looks inside the lungs' airways, takes pictures with a small camera, and removes tissue with a thin flexible tube (a bronchoscope) inserted into the patient's lungs through his or her nose or mouth. In a transthoracic needle aspiration (TTNA), the pulmonologist uses a long needle inserted through the patient's chest wall between the ribs to obtain a biopsy.

It would seem the "needle biopsy" to which Dad objected promised only "low yield." Perhaps that's why Dorrey didn't push it. Presumably, a "lung biopsy" is open surgery to resect a tissue sample.

Summarizing the results of all of the physician examinations that Dad had undergone from July to September, including his own and Dr. Dorrey's, and carrying over some diagnoses from previous years, Dr. Ramses listed the following "assessments" in his September report:

- ❖ Gait abnormality
- ❖ Multiple pulmonary nodules
- ❖ Atrial fibrillation
- ❖ First-degree AV block
- ❖ Benign essential hypertension
- ❖ Pulmonary hypertension
- ❖ Benign prostatic hypertrophy [we told him about the AUS]
- ❖ Subclinical hypothyroidism
- ❖ Peripheral neuropathy
- ❖ Anemia [an ongoing worrisome problem]

And so?

If this is medicine, I don't get it.

Less than six months after he saw my father, Dr. Dorrey left his practice and the area. I actually thought to follow up with him, but couldn't.

DAD'S NEUROPATHY

In an Oct. 10, 2012 document that he titled "memo to self," my father made his own assessment list, which he titled "Major Present Neural Symptoms/Signs." It included:

1) Fatigue (languor/weakness)*
2) Numbness/tingling of hands (symmetrical)
3) Loss of proprioception (position sense)
4) Total loss of vibratory sense in lower legs, weak legs
5) Ataxia
6) Constipation

By November, it had been nine months since Dad had been able to play a round of golf. Evaluating all of the healthcare that he had received that year, I realized that none of it had enabled him to do what he wanted to do more than anything else. He couldn't even go to the driving range.

Would that always be so? Were this progressive neuropathy and fatigue, his "new normal"? What, if anything, could be done?

None of Dr. Ramses's write-ups of appointments he had with Dad in 2012–in July, September, and a third in December–gave a hint of a professional evaluation. He expressed no medical judgments, his reports reading like transcriptions of my father's dictation of his symptoms, neurological and otherwise. Besides Parkinson's disease and syphilis (ha!), which he had explored in July, Ramses had no diagnostic thoughts.

A test of Dad's serum B-12 level performed in October through Kitty Hawk Regional Medical Center showed a normal result: 748 picograms per milliliter (pg/mL), with 211-946 pg/mL representing the acceptable range. (A picogram is one-trillionth of a gram.)

Much to my chagrin, during the Dec. 5 checkup, Ramses allowed

---

*The parentheticals are Dad's, not mine.

my father to get away with a pathetic excuse that I couldn't fight: He wrote in his records: Dad "had appt. with neuro but did not go—got tired of filling out forms." This was acceptable to Ramses even though he noted: "Currently he is having overwhelming fatigue at times and some ongoing problems with gait."

It was true that five months ago, Dad had blown off a neurologist appointment. But, now he was having *overwhelming* fatigue and serious problems with ataxia. He had regressed. Is it too much to ask a PCP to arrange another consult with a neurologist who wouldn't insist on papering the old guy to death? I would have been so grateful if Ramses had assumed a Welbyesque approach and said: "Al, don't worry. I'll line you up with Dr. So-and-So, and we'll send your records ahead to him, so you don't have to be bothered"? In other words, if he had taken charge and actually coordinated my father's care.

Ramses easily could have controlled my controlling father by outlining a strategy and insisting that he adhere to it. Or, at least, he could have tried.

Instead, he just ordered another round of blood tests, a complete metabolic panel. He also prescribed an antidepressant, which Dad took for a few days before deciding he didn't like the way it made him feel.

Heart, lungs, nervous system, metastatic cancer . . . I don't believe Ramses viewed my father as a losing proposition or a hopeless cause, although many PCPs would. I think he actually cared about him, but he never talked about his status. If he was thinking terminal cancer, he never said it. Most egregiously, he failed to focus on how my father felt every day and how he lived, on his *quality* of life, which was profoundly diminished by the fatigue that no one could (or had yet to) explain.

I was increasingly frustrated. Forget the lab tests and the ologists, listen to the patient. Connect with him. A dose of humanity from a clinician would have made Dad feel better.

Sometime that fall I heard from Al that our father had something "major" to ask of me. He was still in severe post-sphincter surgery pain, so I figured it had to do with driving to Duke, a trip he knew I loathed. He didn't say a word to me until December, when he asked me to contact Duke about a post-Christmas appointment. Before we saw the distant Dr. Terse again, I suggested that he consult local urologist Dr. Carlson.

"He can't do anything for me, Ann," he protested.

"You never know, Dad," I insisted.

I was right, but nothing came easily with Dr. Carlson.

Dorsal Slit

My father saw Dr. Carlson in late December and returned with a new two-word term and a promise of salvation without Duke's intervention. Just as he had with the clamp, the old-school urologist was coming through. But first, he would go all loosey-goosey on us again. My nickname for him became The Gander.

The two new words were dorsal slit.

Dad could have a dorsal slit, which is a partial circumcision, performed by Carlson at the Outer Banks Hospital. The Gander would cut and remove some of his foreskin so its retraction would no longer be painful. Simple enough, yes?

Elated over this option, Dad scheduled his dorsal slit on Friday, Jan. 25, 2013, the first surgery date that the apparently in-demand Dr. Carlson had open. Naturally, I planned to go out of town on the 25th and was not pleased. But I wanted to accompany my father and be the designated post-op driver, so I postponed my trip until the following weekend. When I asked Dad what time we would need to arrive for his surgery, I received a reply that did not thrill me: We would not know until the day before, when Dr. Carlson's nurse or receptionist would call Dad and tell him.

I resolved to be flexible, but, on the Monday before his Friday surgery, I insisted on some organization and asked Dad a series of questions: How long will the dorsal slit take? What do you need to do to prepare for it? Can you take your usual medications the morning of the surgery? Will you have a local anesthesia and conscious sedation or just a local? How will you feel afterward? What pain medication will you need?

I wanted to know what to expect and how to plan.

Dr. Al didn't have the answers to all of my questions, including the critical time questions, so I prodded him into calling Dr. Carlson, with whom he hadn't spoken in a month. Despite his own worries, he had been reticent about getting in touch. When Dad did talk to the urologist, he framed his questions in the form of "My daughter wants to know . . .." Either he was protecting his physician's ego or he just disliked asking direct questions. I didn't care, as long as I knew how many hours to allot for the entire surgical process and what anesthesia

Dad would have. Leslie was bugging me again about the anesthesia.

Carlson told Dad that he would have a local "and maybe sedation." The surgeon would decide about sedation in pre-op. Not a fan of last-minute *anything* in healthcare, I was starting to feel doubts creep over me. Communications from Carlson's office the day before surgery only reinforced them.

On Thursday, Jan. 24, The Gander's assistant called Dad twice. Initially, she told him that he had the first surgery slot the next day at 9 a.m., and we needed to arrive at 8 a.m. Great! Then, she called back to say that an emergency case had arisen, and he would be the second surgery of the day. We didn't need to arrive until 10 a.m. OK, I could live with that. But then, at 7:30, the next morning, the day of the surgery, Dad received another call: He was the first case again and should come "ASAP."

All of this meant one thing to me: We were in La-La land. There were no surgical "openings"; there was just the ebb-and-flow of The Gander, who didn't care about how his on-again-off-again approach affected the feeble and anxious old guy he was about to circumcise! This is healthcare?

We arrived at the OBH at 9:10 a.m., which was our own "we're-not-rushing-for-you" ASAP time, and received superb service from volunteers. Thanks to them, the L-O-N-G outpatient registration with my hard-of-hearing, hard-on-schmoozing father went smoothly. I survived without losing my cool. As a volunteer and I wheeled Dad back to the pre-op area, I relaxed, blissfully unaware that I was minutes away from stepping in goose crap.

No-Go Crock

I actually was enjoying myself, chatting with exceptionally nice nurses and the equally nice volunteer when the scrub-attired Dr. Carlson arrived in a burst of frantic, self-important energy.

I extended my hand to the surgeon, who shook my elbow instead, à la Nobel Laureate Linus Pauling, so as not to pick up my microbes. Fair enough, but seeing as how there were a half-dozen sinks in the immediate vicinity, he might have done better just to wash his hands. I wouldn't have been offended. Lest I forget, however, Dr. Carlson was a virtuoso of standoffishness.

As soon as he let go of my elbow, and even before going into the curtained room where Dad lay on an examining table, wearing only a hospital gown and booties, he adamantly informed me that he was not going to operate if Dad had an active infection.

I was stunned. We were minutes away from surgery, and he was imposing a big contingency. All I could think was: You couldn't have brought this up *yesterday* while your assistant was jerking us around? You couldn't have examined Dad *yesterday* in your office? You couldn't have prevented this crock-of-shit-of-a-morning by thinking more than a minute ahead of your next move?

Shaking his head vigorously from side to side and acting more knowledgeable than he was, Dr. Carlson told me that if Dad had a skin fungal infection, the fungus could get into his bloodstream, travel to his artificial urinary sphincter, and disable it. He was not going to be responsible for damaging his sphincter. No, no, no, no, no. I will not operate, he emphasized, turning deaf ears to my flabbergasted sputters of protest.

If only I had that hypothetical Duke Urology Clinic factsheet that Dr. Terse's team never drafted, so I could hand it to Carlson and set him straight.

IF Dad had an infection? Well, of course, he had an infection. He had one in December when Carlson last examined him, and he had one during every examination before that one. Carlson treated Dad for infections. Carlson knew that Dad's altered situation had made it very difficult for him to keep clean.

All I could say was: "You need to explain this to Dad." And, by the way, I don't want to be in the room when you do. It turned out that I didn't have to be. Dad's voice carried far and wide. He did a good job of controlling the anger that I knew he felt: He just sounded supremely, wearily frustrated.

Over and over, he explained to The Gander that the sphincter was a "closed system," that it did not interact with the bloodstream, and that no risk of infection existed. Over and over, Dr. Carlson said he didn't care, he wasn't "taking a chance." Call Dr. Terse, Dad urged. Call Duke. Carlson was unmoved: Not going to happen.

I told everyone in the OR audience about the artificial sphincter and assured all that Dad had considerable medical expertise and knew what he was talking about. To bolster his authority, I dropped a few of my father's big-shot biographical details.

When scientific reasoning didn't work with Carlson, Dad tried another tact, proposing: "I'll assume the risk. I'll take my chances." The Gander still refused. No closed system; no assumption of the risks. That only left Dad to bitterly complain: Why didn't you bring this up earlier? Why didn't you examine me earlier this week?

Yes, why? Here he was, undressed and emotionally ready to go. Just getting to the hospital that morning had been a hardship for him. Surgery isn't a highly anticipated and longed-for date; it's a dreaded disruption, a stressful agitation. My father couldn't hide his disgust.

I believe the reason Dr. Carlson hadn't brought up infection and the sphincter earlier is that he hadn't thought about either until that morning, when, maybe, he'd done enough superficial research about AUSes on the Internet to back himself into a corner. He came out swinging a CYA bat.

Whatever predicated his decision, there was no changing The Gander's closed mind. He gave Dad a prescription for an anti-fungal ointment, showed him how to apply it (!), and advised him to call his office to schedule an examination next Thursday. If Dad passed an infection test then, Dr. Carlson promised he would operate on him first thing Friday morning. So much for having to wait a month for an opening.

Of course, I'd be out of town then. I had postponed my Jan. 25-28 trip to Feb. 1-4. I asked the OR nurse and the volunteer who had escorted us from the lobby if they would be on duty next Friday—they would—and if they could look out for Dad. They could.

Dad and I muttered our way out of the hospital—telling our story to the other helpful volunteers in the lobby who wondered what in the world had happened—and to the car. By the time I drove to Carlson's office, which was minutes away, and walked in, his nurse had heard about the urologist's refusal to operate and about my boasts. She had Googled my father. When I identified myself, she gushed: "Dr. Al is brilliant! I didn't know how brilliant he was. He was a pioneer. He never told us. He's famous!"

The next Thursday, when Carlson examined Dad, it didn't matter if my father had a skin infection or not. Now The Gander was asking Dad questions about his career, bending over backward to explain his incorrect reasoning about the sphincter, and deferring to him. True story. In this case, I didn't object to the deference. (And, for the record, he did not have an infection.)

I tried to line up a nurse friend of mine to accompany Dad to the hospital, but he insisted that Mom could be his designated driver, and they didn't need any reinforcement. I yielded to his stubbornness, but I was uneasy. While packing up Thursday afternoon for my Friday morning departure, I heard from Dad that the OR nurse had called him. She would arrange for volunteers to greet my parents in the parking lot and to wheel them both inside. She would look after them.

You gotta love the nurses, hospital support staff, and volunteers who really care and go the extra mile. They're invaluable. I was greatly relieved.

My parents arrived at the OBH at 8 a.m. and were met, as promised, by volunteers, who also managed the outpatient registration process, so Dad didn't have to go through it again. His surgery started at 9:45 a.m., and my parents left the hospital shortly after noon. Dad had a local, no sedative. He also drove home, contrary to Dr. Carlson's orders. Mom, he told me, "watched for red lights," sitting shotgun, like she was Bonnie to his Clyde. What can you do? Dad even stopped at the pharmacy to pick up a prescription. When I talked with them that afternoon, they sounded exhausted, but adrenaline-stoked.

In the ensuing weeks, my father would attend daily to his surgical wound and try to ameliorate the pain it caused. Unfortunately, the loosey-goosiness wasn't over yet.

ARCHIMEDES AT 88

A week later, on Friday, Feb. 8, at 11:15 a.m., my mother called to ask for my help in getting Dad out of the bathtub. At Dr. Carlson's suggestion, Dr. Al had soaked in a tub of warm water, and now he was stuck. His legs were so weak that he couldn't lift himself up. This mortifying predicament threatened to be a 911 moment.

I have some advice for all surgeons who would like their old, weak, fall-prone patients to avail themselves of the wound-healing power of hot water: Tell them to apply warm wash-cloth compresses to their wounds. Put them in a shower, if they have bars to hold onto and a chair to sit on. But don't ever put them in a bathtub unless you know they can get out.

Contrary to Dr. Carlson's belief, not all patients are created equally!!! There's more to a patient than his surgical site!!!

I arrived to find my father sitting in the upstairs bathtub with his back against the long wall, his useless legs dangling over the tub's

edge, and a towel strategically placed over said surgical site. Mom
suggested that we get on either side of him, grab an arm, and pull.
Seriously. My mother thought she and I could lift 200-plus pounds of
dead weight. I loved that she thought "can-do," but . . . not this time.

"Step aside, little lady," I told her. "I'm not going to the emergency
room if you fracture a vertebra."

Motivated by my strong desire NOT to call 911, I sized up the
logistics. The only way I could figure to get Dad out was to have him do
some of the work. He was too heavy for me to manage alone. After a few
minutes, I visualized a how-to.

I asked the captive bather to shift himself back into his soaking
position, with his head at the top of the tub and his feet near the drain.
I then got behind him and told him to put his feet on the wall under the
faucet and to push down, hard. At first, he pushed with his back, against
me, instead of with his legs and feet. Once he bore down on his feet,
however, I was able to use this shift in weight, and the relief it gave me,
to lift him onto the edge of the tub. From there, he transferred to a chair
and, eventually, with more help, he stood up.

I have told this story to my siblings and some of my friends, each
time demonstrating my technique, and nobody understands how I
got Dad out of the bathtub. As time passed, I couldn't figure it out
either. I *just did*. The dread I felt over calling 911 gave me super-human
strength. If only I possessed a super-human cure, for both of my
parents, especially my valiant mother.

COGNITIVE RESERVE

In February 2012, it seemed to me that Mom's cognitive impairment
had plateaued. Perhaps her cognitive reserve had delayed and would
continue to delay the inevitable. Maybe not all of the many words that
she had written on her mental blackboard would be erased. Certainly
she had an impressive reserve.

After my mother completed the second grade, local educators
identified young Fern as gifted, and she spent the next four years in
a special "Opportunity School," attended by only eight students. Not
only did she receive a superior educational foundation in the arts and
sciences, she received teachers' personal encouragement to take on
intellectually demanding tasks and to achieve higher-ability goals.

At home, her doting father, who was the town engineer, role-modeled an educated, accomplished person, as did her Aunt Grace and other extended family members. Her namesake mother studied at the University of Michigan for a year before choosing instead to work full-time.

Mom read voraciously like smart, curious kids do, danced, played tennis, wrote poetry, and knew no boundaries. As a teenager, she was featured in the Jackson, Mich., newspaper as the girl who collects and reads road maps. She went on to become valedictorian of her high-school class; to excel at the University of Michigan, studying zoology and acting in theater productions; attend medical school, showing talent for emergency medicine; train in psychiatry and have a fulfilling professional career; run a household, raise four children, and preserve and nourish her inner self.

She was a lifelong learner. Even now, when a subject came up on TV or in conversation that piqued her interest, she reached for an encyclopedia.

Eventually, Mom might progress from amnestic-MCI to dementia, as the Mayo Clinic's Dr. Petersen advises can occur, but I had reason to believe that any progression would be slow. In 2012, Mom still had Gertrude Stein's "there" there. Substance in the here and now. Trust me, I'm too much of a realist to lie to myself or to you.

I had given up on advocating for neuropsychological consultations, and I didn't talk about her memory loss anymore, as she had requested. If she lived in Baltimore or D.C., or within a half-hour of any teaching hospital, I would have persisted with testing. I had continued to read about MCI, AD, and other dementias, but nothing I read suggested a therapeutic breakthrough that could possibly benefit Mom.

I felt uneasy about my mother's future, but I didn't let her know that. I wanted her to be comfortable, and she seemed to be—certainly much more so than my father, who had confronted many physical infirmities in his late 80s and was well aware of each.

By this time I was doing what all of my friends who have lost their mothers had advised me to do: I was giving Mom lots of hugs and kisses. I also concentrated on how much she still could do. She was a joy, and she continued to surprise me.

Chapter Fifteen

2013: (Sub)Acute
WRECKAGE

Dad Loses Ground

While Dad waited for his dorsal slit, I ordered his medical records from the offices of Dr. Naylor and the Virginia Beach urologists to see what the Big Guy and his urological brethren had to say about Dad's BPH surgery. I was stunned when I read that during the *first* digital exam he performed, the bullish Dr. Naylor had felt a "suspicious nodule" on Dad's prostate. My father had never mentioned a prostatic nodule to anyone, not even after his PET scan revealed hypermetabolic activity in the gland.

On Nov. 3, 2009, Dad's PSA was 3.3. In a Sharpie-marker note at the bottom of the typed report about his appointment that day, Naylor wrote: "Re-examine in 4 weeks re: nodule."

For the followup Dec. 1, Naylor documented his previous diagnosis of "prostatic nodule with a PSA of 3.3" and recommended that Dad return in four months so he could "recheck his PSA and reexamine the prostate nodule."

Because of Dad's hip fracture, that followup occurred May 4, 2010. Afterward, Naylor again documented his diagnosis of a prostatic nodule and reported, "We repeated his PSA today." In the Sharpie writing below, the urologist instructed: "Please tell [Dad] PSA stable." It was 3.2.

Over the ensuing course of more than seven months and more than a half-dozen appointments, which included the GreenLight surgery, Dr. Naylor never did another digital exam on my father or ordered a PSA. He dropped the nodule from his diagnoses, without comment, and focused exclusively on Dad's BPH.

When I questioned my father about this nodule, he had no

recollection and was not concerned in the slightest.

"All men my age have prostate cancer," he said.

Yes, I know, but do all urologists expunge diagnoses of nodules from their records and fail to follow up? Was it possible that the nodule, and not BPH, had caused Dad's obstructive symptoms? That seemed far-fetched, but what did I know?

Naylor's practices struck me as more bad medicine, if not malpractice. By this time, my mission in life had become not allowing bad medicine, ageism, and/or other healthcare failings to defeat my parents.

"Prostate cancer metastasizes to bone first," Dr. Al informed me again, lest I think his lung nodules were a metastasis from a primary prostatic tumor.

With a PSA of 3.2, Dad definitely had been a candidate for watchful waiting, but Naylor had stopped watching. Physicians tend to take some intervening action when a PSA test result falls between a range of 2.5 to 4.0 ng/mL.

I reflected on Dad's urological treatment over the past three years. How many urologists had he consulted? How many had examined him? I counted two on the Outer Banks; two in Virginia Beach; and at least three at Duke. Heck, he was having urological surgery with Dr. Carlson in two weeks. Surely one of these ologists would have mentioned a nodule or a high PSA.

Dr. Buchanan had received copies of every report filed by Dr. Naylor. Had Dad's Elizabeth City PCP ever given him a digital? No, Dad said. A better question might be had Buchanan even read these reports? During his July 2012 appointment with Ramses, the Norfolk internist suggested a digital, but Dad declined. To my knowledge, Ramses subsequently had not pushed it.

How many urologists does it take to do one digital exam?

I felt stressed. I didn't have enough pairs of eyes or hands or enough hours in the day to protect Mom and Dad and also take care of myself.

Fortunately, the dorsal slit went well, and less than a week after our bathtub acrobatics, Dad's wound had healed. He had no pain. To build up his lower-body strength, he started walking laps in the house.

I shifted to a medical inquiry that I thought I could *somewhat* control.

LAPTOP DOCTORS

I decided Dad had no more excuses for avoiding a neurologist. Still too fatigued to travel to Norfolk, he agreed to see one of the two Elizabeth City-based neurologists that Dr. Buchanan routinely referred. Each had office hours on the Outer Banks every other week. I arranged for him to be seen in Kitty Hawk on Friday, Feb. 22, 2013.

It was a gamble. The Outer Banks had proved time and time again to be a medical wasteland, but what else could I do? Although I booked the appointment with Dr. Less well in advance, no one in her office sent the new-patient paperwork to my father, and I opted not to place a nudge call.

Every physician in private practice should have a website with new-patient registration forms and other information available for people to download. There's no excuse for not offering this courtesy and not informing a patient about it.

At 8 a.m. on the 22nd, I hurriedly completed the patient forms in the doctor's empty waiting room. Dad's hands trembled so much that he couldn't write.

Just as I had during the July visit with Dr. Ramses, I sat with my father in Dr. Less's examining room. Although he was her first patient of the day, she kept us waiting in that cold confined space for 40 minutes. I didn't expect a lot from her, considering where we were, but I'm always optimistic with new doctors until contrary evidence smacks me in the face. Her slap came quickly.

Early in their dialogue, Dr. Less referred to Dad facetiously as a "young person." Then she added insult to her closed-mindedness by interrupting my father while he was explaining his symptoms.

"Do you see this laptop?" she asked him, indicating the computer that seemed to be affixed to her ample waistline. "You can't talk faster than I can type into this laptop."

Wow.

You can't talk.

Here was a doctor who thought her keyboarding was more important than listening to her patient's concerns. And this was no neophyte physician weaned on technology. Dr. Less was 61 years old. I wondered what tool of patient avoidance she had used before her computer. Rudeness, most likely, because it seemed to come naturally to her.

In a 2009 *Academic Medicine* article, prominent gastroenterologist and then-Yale Medical School Professor Emeritus Howard Spiro regretfully observed how "diagnosis has turned from the ear to the eye."

"Doctors, who used to listen to their patients now look for disease on a screen or in a number," he elaborated. "'Laptop docs,' patients name them. Patients in person long ago disappeared from our [physician] conferences, but even worse for physician education, 'case' presentations now include a token history, physical findings, laboratory data, and *the images.* The patients remain unseen and unheard—no empathy for CAT scans!"[1]

Physicians and their critics have bemoaned the loss of humanism in medicine ever since the Scientific Revolution of the late 19th-early 20th century transformed the skill set of doctoring. Criticizing physicians as cold fish who don't truly care for their patients or even try to relate to them is old hat. Today, however, with technological dependency and a dramatically diverse U.S. population—in culture, ethnicity, language, and more identity traits—the empathy-compassion divide between doctor and patient has widened.

In recognition of this disconnection, the Association of American Medical Colleges has decided to recruit a new type of medical student, one who must have smarts beyond the organic chemistry lab. Starting in 2015, the AAMC's rigorous Medical College Admissions Test (MCAT) reportedly was to have sections designed to test aspiring medical students' knowledge of social sciences and psychology and their critical analysis and reasoning skills. Apparently the content of the MCAT would look more like that of the LSAT, the law-school admission exam.

Dr. Spiro trained at Harvard in what he described as "the mid-20th century," thus making him a contemporary of my parents. I Googled him and learned that he studied English in college, not the sciences, and was known for trying to bridge the gap between the humanities and clinical medicine. He died in 2012.[2]

In his article, Spiro wisely advised: "The eye is for accuracy, but the ear is for truth. The eye discerns diseases on screens or films, but the ear hears complaints of patients. Even more than examining the body, listening to our patients taps our sense of empathy. When we take the time to listen, we begin to do so."[3]

From what I've observed, laptop docs don't listen, reflect, and connect the dots, and they usually have little patience for patients' rambling, which may be important history. Some laptop docs manage to input while apparently listening and showing interest, but you can see in their eyes that they're distracted.

As a journalist, I know how challenging it is to listen to someone, take decipherable notes about what he or she is saying (in my case, verbatim quotes), and perpetuate the natural flow of a thoughtful conversation. You must be intellectually engaged in the moment. Quick and attentive. Interviewees will forgive long, even awkward pauses if you maintain eye contact and show that you heard and really understood what the person said.

Often during patient encounters, "the physician's back is turned because he or she is entering data into the computer," writes physician-author Dr. Abraham Verghese, Stanford professor for the Theory and Practice of Medicine, in a 2012 *New England Journal of Medicine* article about primary care. Verghese is a baby boomer about my age.

"I love technology," he continues, "but I think we're discovering that the physician-patient relationship is timeless. It cannot be abandoned because we have better tests and can do away with the human interface."[4]

I'm not wild about the word, interface, but I still say: Amen.

SUBACUTE CRAP

Dr. Less did a 10-minute neurological examination of my father–close your eyes and touch your nose with your forefinger; walk a straight line by putting one foot directly in front of the other (he still couldn't); can you feel this? that sort of thing–and, after remarking upon his many deficits, proffered a diagnosis: Subacute combined systems degeneration.

This sounded to me like "You're old and you're falling apart," but I wrote it down, anyway.

When I got home that afternoon, I Googled the term and couldn't find it, but I did find a similar condition: subacute combined degeneration of the spinal cord, or just subacute combined degeneration. I made a note to check it out thoroughly later.

Looking for disease "on a screen or in a number," Dr. Less ordered tests of Dad's B-12, creatinine, and magnesium levels, and an MRI of his lumbar spine. He had these *pro forma* tests done immediately.

Neither the bloodwork nor the spinal scan revealed anything unusual. In fact, Dad's serum B-12 level, which had been tested repeatedly, was high because he'd been taking vitamin supplements. If Dr. Less had figured on pinning Dad's neurological deficits on a B-12 deficiency, she would be disappointed.

As for the MRI, our radiology friend, Dr. Exeter, interpreted it and found bulging of the disks and other changes at every vertebral level from L1 to S1—but nothing dramatic, much less revelatory.

In a letter he wrote to Dad on March 5, 2013, he suggested that "the specific changes seen at L2-L3 can cause some of [your] symptoms," which he described in his report incorrectly as "chronic low back pain with leg numbness." Presumably, Dr. Less's laptop created that error.

Exeter also opined that "the focal left-sided protrusion of disc material [at L2-L3] is compressing the dural sac and causing some spinal stenosis. The asymmetrical bulging of the disc to the right of midline at L5-S1 could also cause some symptoms and needs to be correlated with the other clinical findings."

He was reaching, for a change, instead of hedging. Unfortunately, he was trying to explain an incorrect diagnosis.

Dad had a choice of following up with Dr. Less on the next Friday, when I had a conflict, or delaying two weeks. My father will never do something later when he can do it sooner. I didn't think the MRI shed any useful light, and I didn't expect anything from Dr. Less, so I didn't change my schedule. I also thought the neurologist might be more helpful to Dad if I were not in the room. I was wrong. It made no difference.

When I asked Dad how his appointment had gone, he told me Dr. Less had asked him to walk while she observed.

"You definitely need a cane to walk," she informed him.

No kidding.

She also told him "you can never get enough vitamin B-12" and recommended that he take supplements sublingually, meaning under the tongue, for better absorption.

She didn't say a word about his fatigue.

According to Dr. Al, doctor and doctor schmoozed. The Physician Shuffle. He enjoyed himself, but learned nothing.

Later, he rued: "I should have asked her how often she's seen my condition in other people my age." I doubt it would have mattered.

All Dr. Less had to offer was the next stop in her diagnostics checkout line: nerve-conduction velocity and electromyography studies, which her colleague, not she, would perform and, which, because of Dad's age, she considered a waste of time. Dad agreed.

An electromyograph is an instrument that records the electrical activity of a muscle. It produces a graphic record called an electromyogram, or EMG, which is used in diagnosing neuromuscular disorders.

"The studies will show dead nerves," Dr. Less told Dad. She said the same thing during his first appointment.

Diagnosis: Old age.

As we age, each of us loses a great many of the billions of neurons with which we start, but how this loss affects our motor, sensory, and other nerve-related functioning is not always clearcut. Nonetheless, I think a neurologist can do better than "dead nerves."

Dr. Less also could have made an effort to reach out to my father, a debilitated and anxious patient, an elder in need of a medical helping hand. She could've talked with him about his unsteadiness, his tingling feet and hands, his hand tremors, his loss of vibratory sensation, and his understandable despair over this decline. Just talking with a doctor has therapeutic value for a patient.

Dr. Less knew Dad had been a powerful person. Now his ataxia and weakness were so pronounced, he labored to walk down the driveway to the mailbox.

But Dr. Less didn't care about my father's suffering. She didn't even suggest that he get physical therapy.

On April 1, Dad finally quit taking Ambien. I had been trying to get him off of that damn hypnotic for the better part of a year. Unfortunately, he later resumed it as a quick fix for restless nights. I thought his hand trembling lessened during his abstinence, but I may have been kidding myself.

Dad had discontinued all of his other medications, even flecainide, at some time during the previous year, and had not noted an improvement in his energy level or his neurological symptoms. The B-12 had made no appreciable difference, either.

SCD

Nearly two months passed after my father's appointment with Dr. Less before I researched subacute combined degeneration of the spinal cord. Medical articles about this wordy condition exist in abundance. What I discovered was that Dr. Less wasn't being a conscientious physician. She was being a reckless gunslinger.

The majority medical wisdom seems to be that the term, subacute combined degeneration (SCD), was introduced in the United States in the late 1800s to describe a *myelopathy*, which is a disease of the spinal cord, "that develops over the course of a few weeks to a few months." One group of academic neurologists attributed coinage of the longer term, subacute combined degeneration of the spinal cord, to physicians who published an article by that name in a 1900 issue of the journal *Brain*. The related diagnosis of pernicious anemia apparently pre-dated both of these references.[5]

Myelin is the insulating sheath or layer around the axons of neurons, including those in the brain and spinal cord. Myelin sheaths, which are made up of protein and fatty substances, allow impulses to transmit quickly and efficiently. Demyelination, or myelopathy, describes damage or destruction of the sheaths, such as occurs with multiple sclerosis. This damage affects the entire nerve cell.

In the late 1950s an association between the myelopathy of SCD and a vitamin B-12 deficiency was made. Such a deficiency, which Dad did not have, is a *sine qua non*: SCD is described as a "rare neurological complication" of a B-12 deficiency.[6]

No B-12 deficiency, no subacute combined degeneration.

Besides, Dad's condition was better characterized as chronic rather than subacute. Nonetheless, his symptoms tracked those of SCD, which two Northwestern University medical specialists described as follows:

In SCD, "[n]umbness, weakness, and paresthesia [skin burning, prickling, or tingling] of the extremities primarily affects the lower extremities, is often symmetric, and progresses in a distal-to-proximal [bottom-up] manner. Later, this myelopathy progresses to unsteady gait, poor coordination, sensory deficits, and bowel or bladder dysfunction. At physical examination, signs of dorsal column involvement include loss of position and vibration sense and ataxia. Lateral column involvement includes spasticity, hyperreflexia, and a positive Babinski sign."[7]

Numbness, weakness, paresthesia of both legs that started in the feet, unsteady gait, poor coordination, loss of position and vibratory sense, ataxia . . . this was Dad.

Pathologically, the Northwestern professors said, the demyelination of SCD involves the dorsal columns predominantly in the lower cervical and upper thoracic regions of the spinal cord—not the lumbar region, which Dr. Less targeted for magnetic resonance imaging.

A "distinctive pattern of abnormal signal intensity . . . considered characteristic of subacute combined degeneration of the spinal cord" can be demonstrated in imaging of the cervical cord, from levels C2 to C5, and levels T1-T2, they write.[8]

The "combined" part of the disease refers to the fact that SCD affects the spinal cord, the brain, and the peripheral nerves. Experts believe that a lack of vitamin B-12 causes abnormal fatty acids to form around cells and nerves.

When Dr. Less speculated that Dad had "subacute combined systems degeneration," she was trying to dispose of him, not diagnose him: "Dead nerves," no hope, old age, go away.

People deserve answers from doctors, regardless of how long they've lived, if answers are indeed obtainable. Answers need not be cures. Thoughtful explanations suffice. Empathy is even better.

My father was fast losing ground. I had to do something.

"CONSULT" WITH DR. ROBERTS

On April 29, I outlined Dad's symptoms for Dr. Roberts in an email.

Nearly 11 years ago, on that interminable Friday night in Chesapeake when my mother lay moaning and breathing rapidly, her body bloated and her mind angrily confused, I called Dr. Roberts, the neurologist husband of a friend, for help. I now came full circle. I asked Roberts to think of Dad as a hypothetical patient, just as he had Mom. "What would you think" about a patient who had:

- ✓ A general feeling of weakness
- ✓ Chronic fatigue, excessive need for sleep
- ✓ Numbness, tingling, pins-and-needles sensations in both hands and feet
- ✓ Tremor in both hands
- ✓ Imbalance/loss of position sense (including Romberg's sign)
- ✓ Total loss of vibratory sense in his lower legs
- ✓ Ataxia/unsteady gait

He replied cautiously:

"The symptoms sound suggestive of a peripheral neuropathy and B-12 deficiency is certainly in the differential diagnosis. . . . [He then elaborated on B-12 testing and its replacement, before observing . . .]

"Peripheral neuropathy in an elderly patient is not uncommon and many times is cryptogenic in origin [of obscure or unknown origin]. Hopefully, his physicians have obtained bloodwork to assess for other causes . . . Unless a cause can be determined, one is left with symptomatic therapy, which is often physical therapy for gait training and lower extremity strengthening along with fall prevention. . . .

"The chronic fatigue is more problematic. Certainly patients experiencing daytime fatigue and somnolence considerations [sic] include depression, drugs, but also does the patient suffer from some type of sleep disturbance/sleep disorder which may be affecting his quality of sleep leading to daytime fatigue and somnolence. Hopefully his PCP has performed a thorough physical examination . . . Additional bloodwork as well as NCV/EMG [nerve conduction velocity testing and electromyography studies] could be used to assess for help confirming a peripheral neuropathy. . . . It may be worthwhile obtaining a second neurological opinion, perhaps at a university center?"

Dr. Ramses was in a university center. The previous year I had wanted to admit Dad to Norfolk Sentara General Hospital for evaluation by all relevant ologists, and he had objected that the hospital could kill him. His deteriorating condition troubled me *then*. I now looked at both of my wondrously intelligent and once-vibrant parents and saw Mom disappearing mentally, and Dad shriveling physically.

On the same day that I emailed Dr. Roberts, I wrote three words across the top of a page in my journal, in an attempt to analyze the anxiety and depression that were sucking the energy out of me. I wrote: STUCK . . . LOST . . . HURTING . . . and then I described why I felt stuck, what I had lost, and why I was hurting.

I didn't want to walk away, but I was consumed by anguish.

Among the "treatments" I outlined for myself was this one: "Adjustment in my thinking—letting go."

But that's not my style. I could never let go, and so I suffered periodically from mental distress and burnout. Soon the time between periods would shorten.

Another Miserable May

On Monday, May 13, 2013, Dad complained of a severe sore throat. On Tuesday, he had a cough. With each passing day, he became weaker. And then he started vomiting.

Dad had been without pain and able to walk with a cane for just three months.

I recalled that Mom's ehrlichiosis had begun with a "really bad headache." Now Dad was sick from no obvious cause, and my speculations ran rampant.

At the same time I coped with my own physical ills: two tick bites (I popped doxycycline as soon as I detected them and taped the ticks themselves to a calendar.); a smashed finger (I got it caught in a garage door!); and a sore throat and cold that knocked me down until Saturday.

At first we thought that Dad and I had contracted the same respiratory virus, but his vomiting dispelled that theory. Also, I didn't have a cough, and Mucinex® handled my symptoms. Dad's cough was intractable and nonproductive, meaning it was dry and didn't produce sputum. Mucinex didn't help him. Soon he was sleeping all day.

On Monday, May 20, I walked with my very weak father down his back-yard wooden walkway to the calm and shiny Currituck Sound. When he complained about his weakness, I said: "Well, at least you're using a cane. That's good."

The next day he couldn't walk without a walker. Worse, he couldn't get out of bed without assistance.

Britt was staying at Mom and Dad's house then. At 3 a.m. on Tuesday, May 21, she heard over a monitor next to her bed the sounds of Dad falling in the bathroom, and she rushed downstairs to help him. Within the next 24 hours, he fell two more times, crumpling to the floor from weakness.

On Wednesday, May 22—nine days into his illness—he vomited the Robitussin® he took for his persistent cough, as well as his dinner. Adding to his discomfort and the challenge of Britt's and my caregiving, he had bouts of fecal incontinence and trouble staying upright on the toilet.

I told Dad he needed to go to the local emergency room, that he was very sick, and Britt and I couldn't manage his care any more. He refused, being weary and frustrated with hospitals, and clinging to the belief that he could recover on his own. At my wit's end, I brainstormed another strategy that I thought he would approve. For the first time since my father had started seeing Dr. Buchanan, I called his office and talked my way into an emergency appointment with the internist at 10:15 the next morning. The nurse tried to pass me off to Buchanan's physician assistant, but I stood fast. Not that it turned out to matter that much.

On the designated day, at 7:45, I sat in the stressless chair in my living room, savoring a cup of coffee and trying to ready myself emotionally when a text from Britt came across my cell phone: "Call me when you get up." Crap.

Our father was now nearly dead weight. Britt couldn't handle dressing him alone, so I quickly pulled myself together and went to her aid. Between us, we got Dad into a pullover shirt, sweatpants, and sneakers, and wheeled him out of the house. If he hadn't been able to stand with our support and hold onto the porch railings, stepping down the front three stairs on his own, we would have had to call 911. There's no way Britt and I could have lowered the wheelchair with him in it. We would've ended up at the OBH.

PCP Pattern Recognition

Our hour-long drive to Elizabeth City was uneventful, and the crowded waiting room was comfortable enough, but as soon as I laid eyes on him, I knew Dr. Buchanan would be of no use to us. He had a look of resistance and detachment in his eyes. His stiff body language conveyed the same. Brusque and hurried, he did not reach out to us as a family in crisis. Instead, his posture was: What do you expect me to do?

Buchanan seemed not to believe that Dad needed a wheelchair and could not stand on his command. Although Dad's infirmity caught him by surprise, he wasn't that concerned. I wondered about their relationship. Buchanan clearly didn't like having two of his patient's daughters in the cramped examining room, answering his questions, but we couldn't trust Dad to recall the course of his illness.

In relating Dad's symptoms to Dr. Buchanan's nurse before the internist entered the room, I had used the term, fecal incontinence, and she had corrected me. "Diarrhea," she said. No, I replied, it wasn't diarrhea. How graphic do you want me to be? I know the difference. Buchanan did the same thing. They both sought to pigeonhole Dad's distress into pattern recognition: Nausea, diarrhea, vomiting, weakness = a GI virus. Fecal incontinence just didn't fit.

A discussion about his weakness elicited the B-12 theory from Dad, which Dr. Buchanan quickly and rightly discouraged. At least he remembered Dad's B-12 test results. The internist moved on next to pneumonia, more pattern recognition. I didn't think pneumonia was an issue, but I wasn't going to argue. His medical ego was too big.

I had strategized that Buchanan would be our entrée into nearby Albemarle Hospital, which I then considered to be superior to the OBH. I thought the PCP could exercise his admission privileges at Albemarle and save Britt, Dad, and me the time and aggravation of an emergency-department admission. Later, he could check in on Dad, ensuring some continuity of care.

But I was wrong and woefully ignorant. Dr. Buchanan's privileges had gone by the wayside when the hospital instituted its hospitalist system. After decades of practice, he could no longer admit and treat his patients in the hospital that was literally a stone's throw from his office. He let us know how unhappy he was about that.

Since 2002, when we first encountered Chesapeake hospitalist Dr. Amble, who seemed intent on killing my mother, the hospitalist model of primary care had swept the country. In 1997, there were 1,000 new-breed hospitalists nationwide. Five years later, the number had grown to 7,000. By 2011, about 30,000 hospitalists, spread out in every state in the nation, were practicing what had become known as inpatient medicine.[9]

The hospitalist trend grew out of managed care, the great cost-containment idea of the 1990s, and the emphasis that it placed on efficiency and cost reduction. Managed care put pressure on primary-care physicians to see more outpatients in their offices and on hospitals to shorten the length of stay for inpatients.[10]

Much has been written about the advantages and disadvantages and the gains and losses of the hospitalist approach, which is employed in academic centers, too, so that hospitalists are training house staff, and I will not belabor them. You can read the articles in my endnotes.[11] The way I see it, hospitalists are here to stay; they are a fact, and we all have to contend with the discontinuity of care that they bring to the healthcare process.

Every physician handoff—from PCP to ologist, sub-ologist, or sub-sub-ologist, and from ologist to ologist to all manner of subs, and back again—is a breakdown in patient care. Throw in the hospitalist, and you're back to square one, starting all over with a new PCP who has no familiarity with your Mom or Pop.

I'd like to meet the hospitalist who can take the handoff and race for the end zone without breaking stride. They all fumble, because all they have to go on are error-marred notes made by doctors in the ED or elsewhere in the healthcare chain, and they can't immediately know and prioritize your parent's needs. They're playing catchup and will do what they believe is necessary to feel comfortable about the decisions they make. Usually, that means unnecessary tests. CYA.

Dr. Buchanan offered to call ahead to the emergency department, and we gladly accepted. When I brought up my concern about catheterization and Dad's artificial urinary sphincter, he again acted surprised. He didn't know anything about an artificial sphincter, he said. Out of Buchanan's earshot, Dad insisted that he had told him, and I was sure he had. Another bad sign.

I gave Buchanan a copy of the AUS instructions that I had brought with me. I was on sphincter alert.

ANOTHER ER . . .

Around noon, Britt pushed our wheelchair-assisted father into the Albemarle Hospital Emergency Department while I went to park. Upon checking in, I received a pass and directions to a spacious and private room. The ED was quiet, so Dad received immediate attention.

I did not witness all of the nurse's history taking, but her notes, which I read later, accurately characterized the past two weeks of Dad's decline. In fact, her summation was superior to the young ED doctor's account, which incorrectly described Dad's chief complaint as shortness of breath. Dr. Buchanan had called the ED and expressed concern about pneumonia; hence, the SOB. But the nurse had it right with cough, weakness, fecal leakage, and general deterioration at the top of her list.

Dr. Jacey ordered "labs," including the usual "CBC with diff." and a urinalysis/culture (to check for infection), as well as a chest X-ray. Presumably because of his age and history of atrial fibrillation, she also ordered an ECG, even though Dad's blood pressure, pulse, respiration rate, and oxygen level (99 percent) were all strong, and he did not report an irregular heartbeat. Fair enough.

After she explained her plan of action to Britt and me, I mentioned the sphincter and offered her a copy of the AUS how-to. She declined the instructions, not seeing how the sphincter was relevant.

We whiled away 3½ hours as Dr. Jacey implemented her plan, and results began arriving. Whenever he was in the ED room, between tests, Dad got up to urinate. It seemed that no sooner had he laid down than we were calling for a male aide to help him up again.

Dad was receiving IV fluids, so his bladder was filling rapidly, but he didn't seem to be voiding nearly enough for all of his effort. He said he had an "urge sensation" that wouldn't subside.

Dad's chest X-ray was clear, no pneumonia. His labwork showed the now-usual low RBC, hemoglobin, and hematocrit, suggestive of anemia; an elevated BUN (29 mg/dL), which had occurred before; and something new: a sodium deficiency, the medical term for which is *hyponatremia.* Sodium is one of the body's electrolytes, which keep fluids in balance, and, therefore, your heart, brain, and other parts functioning as they should.

Body sodium normally ranges from 135 to 145 milliequivalents per liter (mEq/L). A milliequivalent is "one thousandth of a gram equivalent of a chemical element, an ion, a radical, or a compound," according to my medical dictionary. Cells need electrolytes, which ionize in fluids, to regulate the electric charge and flow of water molecules across their membranes. Dad's sodium level, evaluated from a urine sample, was just 122 mEq/L.

My father definitely had lost fluid when he vomited, and he had been taking a diuretic before he became ill, but to be sodium-deficient for those reasons alone seemed unlikely to me. Although Dr. Jacey said hyponatremia was likely "worsening his ataxia" and making him weaker, hyponatremia had not *caused* his illness. We were addressing effects, not causes. Jacey was practicing medicine-by-test. Was she also ageist?

I was going to push for an abdominal CT scan, but once I learned Dr. Jacey was admitting Dad for his hyponatremia, I let it go. I figured that the hospitalist could order one.

By 3:30 p.m., Dr. Al had a bed on the fifth floor of the hospital, which was a sight more worn and tacky than the emergency-department floor. Fortunately, the duty nurse was top-notch. In fact, she became our hero.

While writing some notes about Dad's status on the room chalkboard, she brought up the subject of toileting and catheterization, and I launched into my sphincter spiel. If she intended to catheterize Dad, I advised her, his artificial urinary sphincter would have to be deactivated. I also told her that he had been voiding frequently that day, and I was concerned that he might fall when he got out of the hospital bed to void again.

A lightbulb went off above her head, and she exited the room, returning with a machine that I recognized as a PVR ultrasound. She scanned Dad's bladder with the ultrasound and told him that it was filled with 1500 mL of urine. I didn't think a bladder could hold that much.

"No way," Dad said. "You're wrong."

"I'll do it again, then," she replied, without arguing.

No change. Dad's bladder was on the verge of bursting!

Here, at last, was a healthcare professional who knew something about artificial sphincters and had the smarts to put effects together with a possible cause. The nurse's father-in-law, she explained, had an AUS, and he had experienced a shutdown when the device malfunctioned.

I wanted to hire this brilliant nurse full-time, in place of the doctors, but, naturally, she would be off tomorrow and the next day and the day after that. We were just lucky to have her appear in Dad's room at all. She was a gift.

Not long afterward, Dr. Rodin, a very sympathetic nephrologist, dropped by to check on Dad and to tell us that a consulting urologist would be around soon to deactivate the sphincter, so Dad could be catheterized. The nephrologist was just filling in.

Dr. Rodin mentioned that he had seen Dad's chest X-ray and its interpretation: The lung nodules apparently had not changed since the last imaging. This was only an X-ray, but the fact that someone other than the omnipresent Dr. Exeter had read the image made me feel good.

My uptick was fleeting, however. It faded the moment the disheveled Dr. Rez arrived in the room.

ANOTHER ASS----

I have been known in my medical advocacy to get angry and, occasionally, to give voice to that anger, as I did when I threatened "to file a f–king complaint!" I believe anger, when it's properly channeled, can have a constructive role in conflict mediation. Meekness doesn't earn respect or get results. I was sorry, for example, that I didn't find my voice with Dr. Terse when he blew off my father with his preposterous "LS" aside.

Most of the time, though, I maintain a pleasant demeanor and trust my critical reasoning skills and powers of persuasion will prevail. There are those rare times, however, when I want to pound the smugness off of the face of an arrogant, condescending physician, with my fists, and Dr. Rez was such a physician.

What is it about urologists?

After brief introductions, during which Rez made it known to us how superior he was to any urologist Dad had consulted before—"I haven't seen one of these artificial sphincters in 30 years, not since my medical training. Don't use 'em."—I attempted to give him a copy of the AUS instructions I had brought so he would know how to deactivate it.

"I don't need that, honey," he said with a wave of his pudgy hand.

Honey? HONEY?

I saw red. Flaming red . . . hot, flaming red. For a millisecond, I thought: "Should I let him get away with that or should I take this asshole on?" In the next millisecond, I said:

"Please don't call me honey. I'm a very intelligent and well-educated person, and I have been with my father every step of the way in treating his incontinence. I've been with my father all day today, too. I know what I'm talking about."

"I call everyone honey," Rez replied, unabated. "I'm from the South. That's what we do down here. Everyone is honey—my wife, my daughters . . ."

"You may live in the South," I interrupted, "but you're not from the South."

New Jersey, he admitted, but he'd been in the South for decades, enough to have traded his Type-A, New-Yorker hardnose for down-home folksiness.

Yeah, when pigs fly.

"Regardless of where you're from," I said, my voice shaking a bit, "calling me honey is demeaning, and I don't appreciate it."

Whatever. Dr. Rez clearly didn't have time for feminists on their high horse.

A few minutes later, though, the asshole asked to see the instructions I had brought. He had attempted twice to deactivate the sphincter without them and failed.

Then acting as if he had known how to do it all along, Rez deactivated Dad's sphincter, said he would file a report on his "consultancy," and beat tracks.

I decided to catch up with him in the hallway and ask him some questions about the GreenLight surgery and Dr. Naylor.

"Your father wouldn't have been left incontinent if I'd done the surgery," he boasted. "I clean up after a lot of Naylor's patients." As for Dr. Carlson, he pronounced him "semi-retired," and, therefore, not a realistic option. I also asked him about Dad's small prostate size. He saw nothing unusual about it.

I never saw or dealt with Rez again, but I felt his vibe whenever I mentioned him to nurses during Dad's hospitalization. The knowing glances, the rolling eyes, the "Yes, I know Dr. Rez very well. He likes to have control of his patients."

One nurse, who was leaving in a week for a job in Northern Virginia and felt as if she had nothing to lose, told me how obnoxious and rude Rez was and how much nurses disliked him. She virtually high-fived me when I told her about my encounter.

Rez's notes for Dad's record had multiple errors in them, including a typo that made my father 68, not 88. "Urologic consultation [was] requested," he wrote, "since he is being hospitalized for hyponatremia and exacerbation of respiratory difficulty related to the rib fractures and a fall recently, apparently."

A doctor doesn't have to listen if he's just going to make things up.

Dr. Rez concluded that Dad's "high-volume retention [was] probably due to neurogenic causes given the sudden onset of neurologic deficits and particularly sphincter incontinence for stool."

Exactly which neurogenic causes and sudden deficits would those be? Rez didn't know Dad's history, and he hadn't examined him even perfunctorily. He spent all of 10 minutes in Dad's room, principally pissing me off.

On that day, from portal to portal, Britt and I put in 14 hours. We were wasted, and we were just beginning.

Hellhole Déjà Vu

The next morning, May 24, I tried to reach Dad on his hospital telephone, but he didn't pick up. I called the nurses' station for the floor and learned that he had been moved to another room (even more dreary) on a different floor. He didn't answer in that room, either. By the time I talked to my father, he was in all-out S.O.S. mode: He begged me to get him "out of this hellhole." I had heard that plea before.

Most of Dad's complaints concerned a CNA who had failed to attend to his needs: He had not received breakfast (he was sleeping, and she didn't save his tray), a bath, or a walk, and he had been unable to call out to speak with me. She had informed him erroneously that my number was long distance, and he couldn't call me directly.

I spoke to both the CNA and her supervisor to try to rectify the situation, but it wasn't until I arrived on the floor that I got results. The clueless CNA, who spoke much too softly for a hearing-impaired patient, claimed that Dad had declined food, drink, bath, any assistance. She had just left him lying in the bed, and the nurse in charge had looked the other way. I hustled up everything that Dad wanted and took him on a walk around the floor myself. A physical therapist had not evaluated him—another breakdown in care.

Later, I overheard the senior nurse reprimanding the young woman. The word family came up several times in her rebuke, leading me to believe that without my intervention, the CNA's neglect would not have troubled her. This aide simply did not know how to care for someone, especially an infirm old person. I would be very surprised if she still works in a healthcare setting today, even as bad as the system has become. Her eyes were as blank as a cable TV station without a signal.

Or should I blame management instead of labor? Both are culpable.

I asked the nurse to page the hospitalist, whom Dad had met and liked well enough. When Dr. Quinlan finally visited Dad's room, he didn't have much to say. He essentially functioned as a way-station attendant, punching Dad's ticket for three days and two nights. I started over with him, giving him a detailed history of Dad's recent illness and correcting the record that he was consulting.

According to his notes, which I obtained later, Dr. Quinlan treated Dad's hyponatremia as secondary to his diuretic use and "tubular dysfunction associated with bladder outlet obstruction." He encouraged me to get Dad to Duke as soon as possible for a sphincter checkup.

Dad's cough and respiratory distress, his nausea and vomiting, none of these symptoms made it into Dr. Quinlan's notes for the record. Apparently, he didn't read the ED nurse's report. All the hospitalist ever said in print about Dad's pre-admission status was that he had been admitted "for generalized fatigue over past several days and significant urinary retention," which wasn't true. Once his sodium level improved, Quinlan was ready to discharge my father, and Dad was champing at the bit to go. No exploration would be done at the Albemarle Hospital. What a worthless institution.

Amazingly, my father occupied a third room before his May 25 discharge, the hospital having decided to consolidate the space taken up by patients during the long Memorial Day weekend, when many nurses would be on leave. I can't see how playing musical rooms is good for the patients' welfare—which is supposedly the point of hospitalization—but at least Dad didn't have to change hospitalists.

The sphincter's malfunction puzzled me. Dr. Quinlan rubber-stamped Rez's opinion that Dad's urinary retention was "likely due to neurogenic causes," and that this retention caused his fecal incontinence, but I found that explanation improbable. The tests Dad underwent at Virginia Beach and at Duke should have revealed a dysfunctional bladder, if he had one. The fact he had peripheral neuropathy didn't mean he had a neurogenic bladder. In any case, no physician should diagnose a neurogenic bladder without first doing the appropriate tests.

After Britt and I got Dad home, he was still very weak. I was exhausted from having to explain to Quinlan and a changing cast of nurses what was (and had been) wrong with Dad and from having to protect him from hospital ineptitude. I was also demoralized at the thought of returning to the Duke Urology Clinic. While I recovered, Britt fixed all of Dad's meals, oversaw all of his transfers in and out of bed, held on to him when he walked on his walker, emptied his Foley bag, and did everything that a private nursing assistant would do.

Throughout May, I tried to convince Britt, who wasn't grounded by a job, to move to the Outer Banks for the summer, so she could help me to care for our parents, and I could catch a break. I hadn't worked in two months: Even if I'd had time, I was too depressed. Dad seemed to me to be going downhill, for reasons I couldn't specifically identify, and Mom couldn't be far behind. I even found a furnished house for Britt to rent, but my sister couldn't make a commitment.

It was a decision that she would regret.

SOMETHING HAS TO GIVE

On Wednesday, May 29, 2013, my father and I made an arduous eight-hour round trip to Duke to have Dr. Terse examine the condition of his AUS.

Dad was very weak, but, fortunately, he no longer had any GI upsets or abdominal pain. Neither one of us wanted to stay overnight in Durham, so we left the beach very early and took it easy en route, stopping frequently so Dad could stretch his legs and walk with his walker. I now had this trip encoded in my DNA. I not only knew the shortest route to take, I knew the Duke campus ingress and egress, the parking garage, the walkways, the elevators, the works.

A nursing aide came for Dad immediately after we signed in, and I accompanied them back into the clinic recesses. Ever since the first appointment, when I had rotted in the waiting room for hours, I had been accompanying my father everywhere.

After the nurse took Dad's vitals, we waited only a short while before Dr. Terse arrived. He thought it most likely that the sphincter had failed because of Dad's illness, not because of "operator error." Terse performed a cystoscopy on Dad, which I observed along with house staff, including two female residents. No longer did I draw the curtain. Now I was part of the healthcare team. All of us, including Dad, if he had known where to look, could see on a computer screen that the sphincter was OK. It was still intact. The catheterization had not destroyed it.

That was the good news.

The bad news was that, before the sphincter could be reactivated, Dad's urinary tract had to heal from the assault caused by the Foley. That meant—you guessed it—he would be incontinent for the next two weeks.

Boo!

The next day, Britt left for Florida. I was still hopeful that she would pull it together to return in a month and help me to salvage the summer. All I wanted was to be out of the healthcare trenches long enough to finish this book. A month? Two months? With every unproductive day that passed, I sank deeper into my emotional black hole.

Since his Elizabeth City hospitalization, Dad had improved, but he still suffered from weakness and general malaise. While Dad mopped up and counted the days until we returned to Duke, Mom waited on him hand and foot, except when I relieved her. I managed their groceries, bills, other household to-dos, and anything that came up. And, boy, did things come up. It became almost comical.

First, there was a leak in the hall bathroom toilet. Simple enough. I called the plumber. Then our adopted senior Shih Tzu, Tony, needed urgent care.

On Friday, June 7, I arrived at my parents' home at 5:30 p.m. and noticed immediately that Tony didn't come running to greet me. My father sometimes complained that I only visited him in order to "see the dog." Tony definitely was a great comfort to me, but that day, he didn't even glance my way. Upon closer examination, I found him to be lethargic and withdrawn, as if he had been injured. I had taken an energetic, confident, and affectionate dog to the groomer the day before; this canine wouldn't even lift his head.

My parents reported that during the past 24 hours, Tony hadn't mooched at the table during meals—a favorite activity—or touched the food in his dish. I shifted my problem-solving mind into gear: What had happened between the time that I saw Tony last and now that could've harmed him? That was easy: The groomer, that's what happened; so I called her.

After explaining Tony's altered demeanor and affect to her, I asked: "Did you use any new products on him? Anything that he might be allergic to?"

No. . . . No.

Realizing that I had been too specific, I opened up my questioning: "Did anything unusual happen to Tony while he was with you?"

"No," she replied.

This was like talking with a recalcitrant physician! She gave me nothing to go on.

Five minutes after our conversation ended, however, the telephone rang. I said to my parents: "That's the groomer."

Sure enough. She was "ashamed" and "embarrassed" to admit that she had lied to me. Tony had fallen off of the grooming table, a drop of about 4 feet, and she hadn't mentioned it before because he seemed OK. She apologized profusely and offered to pay for a veterinary examination.

The next day, Tony checked out fine at the vet's, except for a mild UTI, but he still wouldn't eat or drink. He remained in a Post-Traumatic Stress Disorder funk for more than a week, compelling me to take him to the vet twice for fluids; to force-feed him broth with a syringe; and to carry him outside and prop him up so that he could void. I was now caring for an elderly dog who had fallen! I had three patients.

On the Wednesday of Tony's PTSD week, Dad and I traveled to Duke to have his AUS reactivated. I knew Dr. Terse would be serving his Army Reserve time then, but I made the appointment anyway because sooner was always better for Dad, and I had been assured that someone would be available to treat him. Nonetheless, when I signed Dad in as Terse's patient, a whispered stir spread among the clinic staff. No one was sure what to do with us.

This turned out to be our best Duke appointment ever because it introduced us to the very smart, honest, empathetic, and all-around-fabulous Dr. Theresa Donovan, a resident who was leaving in three weeks for Hawaii to serve in the U.S. Army hospital there.

Dr. Donovan was excited about meeting a physician-scientist of Dad's caliber and had Googled him, which thrilled him to no end. She had boned up on his research and asked him questions about it. She couldn't have been more personable and engaging, a real pleasure. Dad was so enthralled by her that he didn't notice when she scoped him! Again, I stayed in the room and watched. All was well with Dad's lower urinary tract, and Dr. Donovan switched his sphincter on.

We went home relieved.

The next day, Thursday, June 13, 2013, a massive oak tree fell on my parents' house. Murphy had been lurking nearby.

Lightning Strikes

Medical advocate, nurse and caregiver (both human and canine), household fix-it person, grocery shopper, bill payer, prescription filler/pharmacy liaison, and now homeowner's policy claimant and tree-removal/roof-repair coordinator . . . I don't even know how to describe all of the tasks that I was doing for my parents.

Around 8:30 p.m. on June 13, Dad called to ask if I had heard a loud clap, like a tree falling, during that night's wicked lightning storm. No, I hadn't. "It was really loud," he said. "Not here," I told him.

The next night when I visited, I asked my folks if they had checked the back yard for any damage. Mom said she had looked outside and hadn't seen anything. Dad said he was too weak to make an independent assessment.

I think you could be on LSD, hallucinating about little green men on airplane wings, and still have seen the decades-old oak that fell on my parents' house. This enormous tree smashed portions of the back-yard chain-link fence and wooden walkway and crashed into two roofs, the top one protecting a bedroom, which now had a broken window, and the lower one on the garage. Open any door to the back yard, and leaves and branches would be in your face.

This Act-of-God "accident," caused by a lightning strike, made me angry. But I didn't rail at God or Nature. I was angry with Mom and Dad. They had chosen to live in a medical wasteland and in a natural environment that can be quite inhospitable to human beings. Their house was surrounded by big, old trees, some of them rotten. As much as they wanted to stay in their home, it wasn't safe.

I loved this 89-year-old and 88-year-old so much, but the drama was killing me.

I immediately called the insurance company and spoke to an agent for more than an hour, so that I would know what I had to do in the coming weeks. The next morning, Saturday, I called the two tree-removal companies in town. The owner of the smaller of the two came out, surveyed the damage, and gave me an estimate. The owner of the bigger company had taken the Father's Day weekend off.

The tree was securely lodged in place and didn't pose a danger to my folks or the house. The owner of Advanced Tree told me he would come back with his crew on Monday. In the meantime, I took photographs, contacted Dad's building contractor about covering the damaged roofs, and rearranged my schedule to accommodate all of the new business calls, meetings, and paperwork I had to manage. I would stay the course, getting Mom and Dad a nice financial settlement; new roofs, window, walkway, bedroom ceiling, etc.; and a clear yard. I further contracted with Advanced Tree to take down or cut back the branches of trees that were threateningly close to the house.

Dad couldn't help me with any of this business. While repairs were being done, he explained to workmen, with whom he always enjoyed talking, that he was ill, otherwise, he would be involved in what they were doing. He pointed to his side of the bed that he shared with Mom and said to one: "Right there. That's where I want to die."

Dad had told me years ago of his desire to die at home. He had expressed this intention in legal documents, as had Mom, and I had promised to honor their wishes. Still, I didn't like to think about it.

On June 18, amid the early cleanup, my father started a month's worth of in-home physical therapy with Coastal Rehab. He desperately needed to regain strength. I sat in on the first session with the therapist because I wanted to ensure that she received an accurate history of Dad's latest setback, but I did not observe his subsequent sessions.

By now, I knew the drill: range-of-motion exercises done in a supine or seated position, and walking as much as possible. Dad was motivated and doing laps around the house again with his walker. I spotted him in the evenings and also helped with dinners. Mom could still serve breakfast and lunch.

Britt returned on June 26, having dashed my hopes that she would spend the summer on the Outer Banks, but agreeing to pitch in for two weeks. After the tree fiasco, which closely followed the sphincter and Tony fiascos, I insisted on sibling help. With Britt assuming the caregiving, I could concentrate more on tasks for which I was better suited. It wasn't long, however, before Dad developed new symptoms.

Over the July 6-7 weekend, he suffered from what he diagnosed as severe heartburn and went through a succession of over-the-counter treatments: Tums, Tagamet, Prilosec. Nothing worked.

During the next week, Dad had nausea and a waning appetite, in addition to his heartburn. Although he continued to do his PT, he had no energy to join us for dinner. Instead, he lay on a nearby couch. My concern escalated, but I was determined to let Britt take the lead in assessing and attending him.

On July 11, the evening before my sister's departure, Britt and I had a heart-to-heart with Mom and Dad and again brought up the need for in-home caregivers. Dad was an invalid, Britt said. She had seen his disabilities for herself. This time, she and I pushed hard for help, but we couldn't push as hard as we wanted because of Mom's diminished capacity. We didn't want to alarm her.

I had lined up a male acquaintance who was prepared to take over the grocery shopping, the cooking, and many of our parents' ADL, but they wouldn't hear of it. That look of horror returned to their faces: "Strangers on the yard." Absolutely no strangers on the yard.

Instead, our anxious father wanted to talk about his burial: He had plots for Mom and him in his hometown of Lansing, Illinois, alongside his parents and grandparents, and plots in Southern Shores, which would be alongside his children, eventually. He also had definite ideas about his headstone. Such thoughts had been keeping him awake at night, he said, which made me feel so sad. Once Britt and I voiced our opinions, he made a decision and never mentioned any after-death arrangements again.

Was he dying? If so, I honestly didn't see it. I saw a very sick man, but I didn't see a dying man. I had learned how pessimistic Dad could be about his health, and how anxiety fueled that pessimism, and I no longer felt I could distinguish his neurotic judgment from his clear-eyed judgment. I saw a man who needed medical care, but had given up, understandably, on doctors. Dr. Buchanan and Albemarle Hospital had been useless. What was I going to do? Move my parents?

On Monday, July 15, at my father's request, I purchased Dramamine® and Zantac® for him. The next day, I bought Boost,® the nutritional drink, because he couldn't tolerate much food on his stomach, only soup and potpies.

While Dad slept during the day, I managed the tasks of my new multi-tasking job description. I called him every afternoon and checked on him every night. He continued to have nausea and a poor appetite, then started having pain in what he called his upper-gastric area, which to me meant esophagus and stomach. His symptoms were always worse during the night. Dr. Al now suspected GERD (gastroesophageal reflux disease), not heartburn.

During the week after Britt's departure, my mother ran herself ragged responding to Dad's requests, but they both still resisted hired help, and I was determined not to move in.

On Friday, July 19, the bottom fell out.

I emailed my siblings: "Our lives are never going to be the same again."

Chapter Sixteen

2013: Staying ALIVE

Mom and Dad Crash

I was seated at my parents' white kitchen table when I heard the crashing thud. It was about 9:40 p.m. I had arrived late that evening and was dismayed to see my mother looking so haggard and exhausted. Even so, when she excused herself to use the bathroom, I didn't think anything of it. Not until I heard the loud thud.

I ran into the bathroom and found Mom on the floor, pain crippling her lower body and distorting her soft face. Lying on her back, she managed to tell me that she had tripped on some panties she had washed and hung near the sink. I'm ashamed to admit that my first thought was about avoiding another trip to the emergency room. I so wanted to lift Mom up and have her be all right that I delayed an hour before I called 911. But no matter how I tried to hoist her, she cried out in agony: "My leg, my leg."

This was not going to be a bathtub magic trick. This was serious trouble. I made the call and became a crisis medical advocate again. I didn't leave the Outer Banks Hospital until 3:30 a.m. Saturday, by which time Mom was in a hospital-room bed, receiving intravenous morphine. I tried to process what would transpire over the weekend.

My mother had a fracture of her left distal femur, which is above the knee joint. This upside-down-funnel-shaped section of the large thigh bone had snapped like a twig, diagonally breaking through the middle into three fragments.

Impression: "Acute comminuted medially displaced fracture of the distal shaft of the left femur."

Mom would need emergency surgery and extended rehabilitation.

Meanwhile Dad was sick and wasting away at home.

One day at a time, I told myself repeatedly, reviving my mantra from the ehrlichiosis summer. Of course, then, my wonderful father was well and could help me. This was a two-fer, and I had no backup. I went to bed at 5:30 a.m.

"NERVOUS" SURGERY

A short four hours later, the telephone rang, waking me up. I could hear the voice recording on the answering machine in my office and decided it was a voice I should not ignore. Dr. Thompson, the orthopedic surgeon, left his cell-phone number for me to call. I did within minutes.

Thompson, who seemed to be a conscientious and empathetic professional, had scheduled Mom's surgery for 9 a.m. Sunday. What he said about the hardware he would use and where he would put it made sense to me when I heard his explanation, but when I talked with Dad later, I couldn't remember it all. What stuck with me was his admonition that Mom undergo surgery within 48 hours of her injury, in order for her to have the best chance at recovery, and his worry about blood loss during the procedure. I knew about the timing from my research on hip fractures, but I hadn't thought about bleeding, which is a concern for all surgical patients who are taking anticoagulants.

Thompson was going to "reverse the effect" of Mom's Coumadin with fresh frozen plasma, he said, long enough to repair the fracture, which, he emphasized, was of an old, osteoporotic bone. I had no illusions. Mom might not walk again, and, if she did, she probably would need a walker. Heck, she might not make it back from this calamity. Dr. Thompson had repaired more hips than distal femurs, but he had thought through how to fix this break, and I had a favorable first impression.

I tried not to notice that Thompson was the junior practitioner in the Outer Banks' only orthopedics practice, of which Dr. Faber, who repaired Dad's hip, was the senior. I knew he was the husband of Dr. Eagan, whom both of my parents had seen. When I Googled him later, I learned that he had graduated from Eastern Carolina University Medical School in 2004 and only finished his post-grad training in 2009.

I asked Thompson to call Dad. I needed my medical expert, even in his weakened condition, to evaluate what the surgeon said and to sign off on it. I was too tired to think.

Dad was holding his own, barely. I talked by phone with him and Mom—who vaguely remembered Dr. Thompson's pop-in visit that morning, but not what he said—then fed and walked Tony, did a few necessary errands, and slept the rest of the day. After another dog walk and check on Dad, I returned to the hospital to see Mom around 7:15 p.m. She knew she was having surgery in the morning and was resting without pain. I couldn't ask for more. After I left her, I visited with Dad and Tony again. Every day would be full like this for months to come.

I arrived at the hospital Sunday at 8:45 a.m., to find my poor mother agitated and in pain, thanks to a prescription screwup by the morning hospitalist, who was a local internist. I spoke with the OBH nurse, not the doctor, and calmed Mom. It was an inauspicious beginning.

Much later, I met a local florist whose elderly mother had been this same internist's patient when the older woman had to be hospitalized because of a dramatic physical decline.

When the florist spoke to the internist about the sudden change, he advised her: "You need to lower your expectations." Instead, she found a new doctor, who deduced that her mother was failing because Dr. Low Expectations had misprescribed her blood-pressure medications.

After Mom was taken to the OR, I retreated to the waiting room, where Dr. Thompson shortly joined me, and more unease settled over me.

Although pleasant and approachable, the young surgeon confided that he was "nervous" about the surgery because of Mom's age, osteoporosis, and Coumadin-altered blood.

He actually said nervous, a word that you don't want to hear from a surgeon. He didn't have to tell me my mother was high-risk. Heck, I didn't like the general anesthesia, the surgery, the rehab, any of it. But I had to play the hand dealt, and I needed support, not uncertainty, from my healthcare partners. The OR nurse was much more reassuring.

The procedure took about three hours, which I passed blissfully alone, reading. The next time I saw Thompson, he was a changed man. Mom had lost about 300 milliliters (10 ounces) of blood, he said, but she had done well, and he was pleased with the results.

I asked him to tell me again about the repair hardware, and he retrieved an X-ray of Mom's leg that showed a rod running through her femur, which connected the fragments, and two big screws, perpendicular at the distal end, that locked the rod in place. Dr.

Thompson had implanted another screw at the top of the femur, where he had inserted the rod. (The rod, called an intramedullary nail, went through the medullary, or innermost, cavity of the bone.)

I still didn't get it. The X-ray clearly depicted a femur that was displaced, with about an eighth of an inch of space between the two main bone fragments. Dr. Thompson acknowledged that he had not achieved total bone alignment, but he thought the less-than-complete alignment would hold up. Mom's first followup with him would be in two weeks. He advised me that she likely would need to keep weight off of her left leg for the next six weeks.

I stayed with Mom until 4 p.m. She was exhausted and aware of her surroundings, but not very alert. I had to start thinking about her rehabilitation. No weight for six weeks! How would she manage? Could we possibly care for her through home-health services?

There's no way I would allow her to be discharged to the Sentara nursing-home hellhole. That left me with only one other institutional alternative: the local SNF in Nags Head, which had such an atrocious reputation that I hadn't even considered it before. A female resident allegedly had been raped there by a stranger who walked into the facility. I also knew about deaths caused by nosocomial infections. Neglect by nurses was among the milder accusations leveled against "Harborside." People on the beach regarded it as a necessary evil. I needed time to process.

A TWO-FER WEEK

The next day, during the early morning hours, Dad awoke with excruciating abdominal pain, which he eased with Vicodin®, a drug that combines the narcotic, hydrocodone, with acetaminophen (Tylenol). He also drank some Boost and took additional medication to get back to sleep. He was now so sick that he was taking a hypnotic cocktail of Ambien, Valium, and Benadryl.

I saw Dad around 10:30 a.m. and insisted that he seek medical help.

Dad called Dr. Ramses, reaching him on vacation in California. Ramses advised increasing his Prilosec OTC dosage to twice what he had been taking (!), but also reinforced my suggestion that he see a local doctor. I called the nurse in Dr. Eagan's office and asked if she could work Dad in ASAP. She told us to come tomorrow morning.

On Tuesday, I took Dad to see Dr. Eagan. We waited in the hallway outside of her office for a long hour, during which time Dr. Al regaled other hallway dwellers with medical stories. He loved an audience, and the audience loved him. Once we got into Dr. Eagan's examining room, however, the great storyteller clammed up, minimizing his symptoms and claiming that the increased dosage of Prilosec had made him feel better.

What, I wondered, was the point of this wishful thinking? Anxiety?

Dr. Eagan went along with Dr. Al's GERD diagnosis, which frustrated the heck out of me. Who says he has GERD?

At least she did a hands-on exam. When she palpated Dad's abdomen, he recoiled in pain. She recorded in her notes: "pain with palpation over midepigastric area." (The epigastrium is an area of the central abdomen, and the abdomen is the area between the chest and the pelvis, or what we call the belly. It includes the stomach, which is an organ, not an area.)

Dr. Eagan suggested Dad try the laxative, MiraLax®, for his constipation and prepared to pass him off to a followup in a month, even though I told her that he had been ill since mid-May. I insisted that my father needed an endoscopy and a referral to a gastroenterologist. She went along with the scope, but referred Dad to a general surgeon who was "wonderful" and whom we "would love." Dad could see the surgeon much sooner than a local gastroenterologist, so I relented, but I didn't like it. I'd had a colonoscopy performed in Kitty Hawk by a creditable gastroenterologist: Why not him?

When I wasn't advocating for Dad, I was trying to figure out what would be in Mom's best interests. When I saw her on Monday afternoon, she had been in such an altered mental state that she scared me. She was absent. Vacant. I thought she might be in a painkiller haze or a delirium brought on by the surgery. Just as I had at the Sunshine Convalescent Center in Durham, I told her nurses that they weren't seeing the real person, and by Tuesday afternoon her affect had improved markedly, but she couldn't assist me in deciding her next move. She didn't understand what was going on.

After a day of wrestling with the idea of home nursing care and PT, which would be difficult even if Dad weren't there, I resigned myself to having Mom discharged to Harborside, which, in a break from its checkered past, was now known as Oakwood. The hospital caseworker said Oakwood's physical therapists were excellent, and my friends at Coastal Rehab agreed. The caseworker suggested that I go to Oakwood and tour the facility. I didn't have time for a tour, but I wanted to do a drive-by at least, so I drove to the nursing home, which is in the woods at the end of a residential street.

I almost cried. It was shockingly awful.

"How can I put my mother in this dump?" I despaired out loud, as I took in the dingy single-story red brick building that looked like an elementary school built in the 1960s and abandoned years ago. The part of the building that wasn't dingy brick was made of old wood painted a faded blue. You couldn't miss the hulking green dumpsters out front. Oakwood lacked a verandah, sidewalks, any grounds to speak of, and had nothing remotely charming about it, except the feral cats that roamed in the parking lot. Anxiety knotted my stomach.

"How can I?"

Because I have no choice.

OAKWOOD

On Wednesday, July 24, I spent eight hours with Mom, handling her discharge from OBH, which went smoothly enough, and her subsequent admission and introduction to Oakwood. The SNF's small front lounge had some nice features, including a piano and an aquarium, but overall, the place had a crummy, low-end feel about it.

By 11:30 a.m., I sat in the small cluttered office of a doughy man of about 65. Mr. Hill went through a stack of forms with me, repeating tired, one-size-fits-all phrases of explanation. He wasn't offensive, just blasé and perfunctory.

In two weeks, he explained—among other standard-procedure details—Mom and I and any other interested family members would have a care-plan meeting with representatives from the nursing, physical-therapy, dietary, and social-activity departments, to assess her progress. I had attended Mom's care-plan meetings at Sunshine, so I knew what to expect.

The nursing-home doctor, Dr. Steiger, who had a full-time family practice about 45 minutes away, would visit once or twice a week, Hill said. Mom might see her own private doctors, but all of their prescriptions would go through Steiger.

During the three months that I visited and interacted regularly with Oakwood staff, I never met Dr. Steiger or even saw him on the floor.

Oakwood was slowly getting a facelift. Three of the four residential hallways were open for use, but the fourth was closed for renovation. That meant Mom couldn't have a private room. She would be alone initially, which we preferred. Mr. Hill assured me that those residents who had been there longer than Mom would receive a roommate before she did.

The hallways of the facility were configured so that a nursing station served two of them, and a nurse, either an L.P.N. or an R.N., was on duty for each. I briefed as many people as I could about Mom's status while I helped her to get settled. I met Mom's R.N. and two CNAs for the day, as well as the wound nurse, who tended to Mom's incisions, one of which was weeping, and the thin skin on her swollen legs.

The tough-talking head of the physical therapy department dropped by and quickly set me straight about attending Mom's PT sessions.

"Against HIPAA," she said emphatically and authoritatively, citing the broad federal health-insurance act.

I have no interest in reading any of the Health Insurance Portability and Accountability Act of 1996, unless I absolutely have to. HIPAA, which is pronounced hippa, protects the privacy of a person's "identifiable health information," in any form or medium. The effective compliance date for HIPAA's Privacy Rule was in 2003, which, presumably, is why I had free access to the Sunshine physical-therapy gym in 2002. Even so, I bet if you asked other Oakwood residents who were in the gym when Mom was, they wouldn't mind my presence. People can waive privacy rights.

After what I'd been through in the past two months, I didn't want to argue with a hardnose. Mom would go to the gym in a wheelchair, without a family escort, and do strength exercises from her chair until Dr. Thompson allowed her to put weight on her left leg.

My mother's new residence measured about 12-by-20 feet. She had a twin bed next to the window, a nightstand, half of a dresser, a narrow clothes closet, and a big TV that needed servicing. With her wheelchair on the floor, the space was very cramped. One of the first requests I made of Mr. Hill was an armchair, so a visitor could sit at her bedside. I later appropriated a wooden desk chair from an empty room.

I did my best to make Mom's environment cozy with items from home: a lamp, a clock, a calendar, photos, as well as some personal effects. But I couldn't whitewash the truth: My mother was immobile and confused and at the mercy of her caregivers for everything, and those caregivers had to be very careful transferring her in and out of bed, and on and off the toilet. Each transfer would be a tough two-person job. I needed to be able to trust, depend, and get along with the nursing aides responsible for her.

Mom had a will strong enough to recover from this serious setback, but I wasn't sure if she had the mental awareness she needed. For the next two weeks, whenever I visited, she asked me:

Where am I?

You're in a nursing home in Nags Head, Mom, called Oakwood.

Why am I here?

You're here because you broke your leg, remember? And the people here are helping you to recover so you can walk again.

When can I leave?

As soon as you're well, Mom.

Am I here because Dad doesn't want me to come home?

She broke my heart time and time again.

After that first day, I spent four hours every night with Mom and developed a routine. I helped her with dinner and then wheeled her around Oakwood, so I knew that she was sitting up and getting some stimulation. Through my visits, I was able to meet all of the nurses and many of the CNAs. Everyone eventually knew "Miss Fern" had an involved family.

During our evening stroll, we wheeled to the front parlor area so Mom could visit two cockatiels in a cage, see the aquarium fish before the light went out in their tank, and watch "Jeopardy!" on the TV. One of the cockatiels, Wally, enjoyed being stroked. He represented the best that Oakwood had to offer: pet therapy. Small dogs wandered the hallways, too.

We were generally out of the room about an hour. I then helped Mom with her bedtime activities and lingered, just watching over her. She was not going to become a fracture statistic, not if I could help it.

THE BULLY PULPIT

The day after Mom checked into Oakwood, Thursday, July 25, I went with Dad to see the "wonderful" surgeon recommended by Dr. Eagan: Dr. Loudon turned out to be a bust.

Loudon, who was middle-aged and had gone to medical school as a second career, had a very loud, aggressive, and controlling manner. He overwhelmed my father, spending little time listening to him—or to me, whom he marginalized. Subject to such bullying treatment, my father again minimized his symptoms, saying he felt better.

Was Dad's denial anxiety? Fear? Cognitive impairment? Illness? All of my life I had counted on my father's brilliance and good judgment, but the steady rock was no longer steady. He even denied that he had lost at least 10 pounds in the past month.

Loudon performed a quickie physical examination, and it wasn't long before I saw where the surgeon was headed: Out the door. He treated us like an inconvenience.

The bully told Dad that he didn't want to do an endoscopy because of its invasiveness, and then he tried to convince Dad of that, so it would be his choice.

"You don't want me to do something invasive to you, do you?" Loudon virtually shouted at my hearing-impaired father.

"No," Dad agreed.

Oh, yeah, Dr. Eagan, we "love" your surgeon.

If an endoscopy is invasive, what do you call open-heart surgery, which is performed more often on elders than young people? Assault with a deadly weapon?

Dr. Loudon concluded this worthless appointment with a lecture about nutrition, exercise, and basic self-care. He talked to my father, an M.D., Ph.D., as if he were a child, instead of a very sick and anxious person who needed a real doctor's help. As a final insult, he wrote a prescription for Carafate®, a medication for intestinal ulcers, which he had no way of knowing Dad had or didn't have.

More crap.

What next? The OBH Emergency Department? Sentara Norfolk? Duke? Dad was deteriorating, but I couldn't do a lot to help him because of Mom. I was alone on a sinking ship. I saw Dad every morning for a few hours, and then again around 5 p.m., before I went to visit Mom. I also saw him at 10 p.m., after my nursing-home stint.

From Friday, July 26, until Monday, July 29, Dad tried the different meds he had: Prilosec, Carafate, MiraLax, and others. He mostly ate potpies and drank Boost and got around with a walker. He was not well, but he was not in acute pain. He described his stomach as feeling queasy, usually worse in the morning than evening, and also overnight. The MiraLax didn't help. On Monday he started having cramps.

It pained me to know that Dad was suffering so much. Was this the cancer?

Something had to give, and it did.

The Crash

Mercifully, my brother arrived the evening of July 29, so someone else could watch over Dad and, eventually, Mom—and walk Tony. The next day Dad said Carafate upset his stomach, and he could no longer drink Boost, his mainstay, because it tasted awful. Tuesday was a very bad night, with Dad getting up four times to void. Uh-oh. I asked Al to start documenting his illness.

On Wednesday, July 31, Al reported, Dad decided to discontinue Carafate and MiraLax and take only Prilosec, which he had been taking for a week even though he didn't have heartburn.

For breakfast, he ate a banana, half of a grapefruit, and half of a piece of cinnamon bread, and he drank half of a can of Pepsi. He said he was "aware of" his stomach—he could "feel it"—but he could "push it now and it's not painful."

"I don't feel too bad today," he told my brother. "Just a little weak."

For lunch he ate half of an egg salad sandwich, a chocolate chip cookie, and some cherries, and drank white and chocolate milk.

By evening, Dad began to lose control over his bowels, developing an urgency and then an incontinence like he had in May when Britt and I took him to see Dr. Buchanan. I asked him about his urination, about the sphincter's performance, and he said he had no problems. He drank a bottle of Boost at 10 p.m. and ate three scoops of ice cream at midnight. We were skating on thin ice.

At 5 a.m. on Thursday, Aug. 1, Dad drank more Boost. Upon awakening five hours later, he complained of severe abdominal pain and fecal incontinence. Al called to report that Dad had eaten half of an English muffin, half of a grapefruit, and a chocolate pudding cup and drunk some whole milk for breakfast, and then vomited all of it up in a clear brown liquid. He also was belching a lot.

Again, I desperately wanted to avoid the OBH Emergency Department, whose doctors were awful, 9.5 times out of ten. I knew my brother, who was a lieutenant in the Mom-'n'-Pop advocacy army, not a take-charge general, would not drive Dad there, and it would be up to me. Al took direction; he didn't chart it.

First, I sought help outside of the ED. I called Dr. Eagan—

she wasn't available—and even Dr. Loudon's office, whose nurses, I knew, couldn't help me, but I was processing my next move. I had an appointment in Chesapeake around 6 p.m. that I couldn't easily reschedule. By the time I returned, it was after 8 p.m. Dad had been unable to keep any solid food down all day, so I knew we had to go to the dreaded ED. Dad didn't argue.

"If you can't eat, you die," Dr. Al said.

At the OBH, we ran straight into an unpleasant battleaxe of a physician. I never use sexist terms, but this one fit—as a polite understatement. The battleaxe dispensed with introductions and reduced my thoughtful explanation of Dad's history to "an old man who can't eat." She also asked a question that I hate and don't think yields much of a return: "What brings you here today?" I think a far better opener is "What's been going on?" Ill health is rarely an event; it's a process.

Dr. More could have been Dr. Less's twin sister. She had ageist written all over her disagreeable face. Once again I was in the position of persuading a narrow-minded idiot that I wasn't an overreacting idiot. Dr. More didn't want to do anything for "LOM" or "SOG" disease, but she initiated the motions of bloodwork and an abdominal CT scan. You should've seen her face when the results came back. Her already slack jaw literally dropped, and her eyes betrayed disbelief.

My father had acute pancreatitis and prostate cancer, she said. I was stunned, too. Although I knew about the "suspicious nodule" that Dr. Naylor had diagnosed and then dropped from his reports, I figured if Dad had prostate cancer, one of his army of urologists would have noticed it. Dr. More told me the tumor was a 40-millimeter mass. An inch and a half! Although I stayed strong and outwardly calm, the size of the mass—no longer a nodule—hit me hard. My brother, whom I called, had the same reaction.

The pancreatitis diagnosis just confounded me. I knew of people who had been stricken with acute pancreatitis and died within a few days. How acute is acute? And how certain was the radiologist about this diagnosis? Surely Dad's distress was the same problem that he'd had in May when Albemarle Hospital's doctors attributed all of his ailments to a neurogenic bladder! (Incidentally, Dad was still anemic and hyponatremic.)

Dr. More ordered Zofran® (ondansetron), to thwart nausea and vomiting; Protonix®, a proton-pump inhibitor which, like Prilosec, reduces stomach acid, and IV fluids, and contacted the hospitalist on duty about admitting Dad.

Unfortunately, before he could be hospitalized, my father would have to be catheterized. This was a mandatory condition of admission. The hospitalist didn't want to risk harm befalling Dad or his artificial sphincter because the hospital staff was ignorant about such devices. Solution: Disable the device.

Remember, this is the same place where, three years before, the nurses didn't know how to operate a bladder scanner. Ordinarily, I would argue, because I knew catheterization endangered the AUS, but after an ultrasound (presumably used properly) showed a 598 mL post-void retention, I thought Dad's illness might have caused the implant to stop functioning again. Besides, where were we going to go for Dad's treatment if OBH refused to admit him? Albemarle Hospital? Norfolk?

The issue of who would deactivate the sphincter was quickly resolved when a fearless ED nurse named Summer took the instructions from me and quickly did the deed. Now *she* impressed me.

I stayed with Dad for nearly seven hours that night and got to bed at 3 a.m., grateful that I could turn over the parent watch to Al. That Friday I talked with Dad by telephone and learned that during his hospitalization, he would fast, in order to give his pancreas time to recover and his bowel time to rest, and receive pain medication, either Dilaudid or Vicodin, and fluids. His first meal would be broth and hot tea, and he would progress slowly from there to solid foods.

On Saturday, Aug. 3, I visited Dad for three hours and was able to talk in detail with the day's hospitalist, a nephrologist from Greenville, N.C., who told me that Dad's CT scan and an abdominal ultrasound had shown no evidence of disease in his abdomen, no gallstones, and no problem with his bile ducts. I also learned for the first time that his liver was scarred and cirrhotic, for no known reason.

From the hospital, I drove to Oakwood, where I discovered, much to my furor, that Mom had spent the entire day in bed, still dressed in her nightgown. No one had bothered to get her up. I tracked down all of the responsible parties I could find.

The previous day, in my absence, someone had removed some of Mom's equipment from her room so that "They messed up our [evening] system," she told Al. I instructed my tentative brother, who had added piano playing to Mom's nightly routine, to find the equipment and take it back. Proceed until apprehended. He did.

"Mischief" is often afoot in nursing homes on the weekends, when the physical-therapy department is closed, most of the full-time staff is off, and less "invested" part-timers often work. Regardless, all CNAs know that residents are to dress and get out of bed, *every* day, unless therapists inform them otherwise. Mom's aides should have transferred her to a chair to sit for as long as she could tolerate it. It was critical that she MOVE. Lest anyone try to say that Mom had refused to move, her roommate Judith, a very with-it lawyer mending from hip surgery, whom I quickly befriended, could set the record straight.

Judith's arrival in the room the day after Mom's admission exposed Mr. Hill's resident-roommate priority system for the lie it was. The dough man also conducted Judith's admission in the room while seated in the chair I had requested and while I was present! So much for HIPAA. I heard every word. Had Hill relinquished the chair when I arrived so I would have something to sit on, I might not have had a few choice words with him in the hallway. But I wasn't going to let any BS happen on my watch.

First thing Monday morning, I called to report the weekend neglect and to speak with an Oakwood physical therapist about Mom's rehab. I confirmed that she was to use both of her wheelchair's leg rests—which had been removed from her room—and to wear a boot on her left leg. The PT department posted a care plan in each patient's closet, but that didn't mean that the nursing aides checked it like they should.

On Sunday, Aug. 4, Dad confided to me that he had experienced some irregular heartbeats. Fortunately, the atrial fibrillation didn't last long, but I didn't like it. Fatigue, weakness, peripheral neuropathy, ataxia and other neurological deficits, pancreatitis, prostate cancer, AF . . . not good. Demoralizing, in fact.

Shortly before he left the OBH Monday, my father underwent the "invasive" upper-GI endoscopy that the "wonderful" Dr. Loudon was loath to put him through. It lasted all of 20 minutes. The surgeon informed me that he had seen nothing abnormal in Dad's esophagus, stomach, or small intestine except for mild gastritis. He did not have any ulcers. In fact, he said, "He's in great shape for a man his age." He then handed me a picture of the area scoped so I could see for myself.

The discharging hospitalist, an internist, told me that 95 percent of pancreatitis is caused by alcoholism or medications. Dad fell into the other 5 percent, but none of the most likely other causes—for example,

gallstones, infection, injury, pancreatic cancer, high blood calcium—
applied to him. So his pancreatitis was idiopathic. I couldn't help but
question if he really had it. The hospitalist also assured me that there
was no way the prostate tumor caused it.

How in the world had all of Dad's urologists missed that tumor?
Especially the Duke surgical team.

That morning I called Mary at the Duke Urology Clinic at 8:30 to
inquire about a referral from Dr. Terse to a prostate-cancer specialist.
I reasoned that we should coordinate with Terse because of the AUS,
and I told her so. She gave me a cold and unexpected brushoff.

"We don't handle cancer cases," she said, raising the gangplank. I
know, I replied. I'm concerned about the sphincter. "You need to talk
to a urologist who specializes in cancer."

"We don't do cancer," she said one too many times.

Frustrated, I asked her to transfer me to the Duke Cancer Center,
and I made an appointment later that week for Dad to see Dr. Judd
W. Moul, director of the Duke Prostate Cancer Center and an
internationally recognized prostate-cancer expert. Not long afterward,
I received a call back: We would be seeing Moul the next day, Aug. 6.
Perhaps Terse had intervened, after all.

After taking Dad home from the hospital around 2 p.m., and
helping him with his "new normal," which included contending with a
Foley catheter, I returned that night to spend four hours with him while
Al visited Mom. He was uptight and needed rest. Tomorrow would be
a long day.

DUKE SHOWDOWN, PART I

The Duke Cancer Center was like Emerald City in the Land
of Oz: a beautiful, sparkly new building with multiple clinics, each
of which had a large and luxurious waiting area and, presumably,
the same precision patient-checkin/exam/treatment process that we
encountered in the prostate-cancer clinic. I felt like Dorothy without
Toto. After driving 240 miles, and stopping often so Dad could stretch
his legs and walk with his walker around the car, and after pushing Dad
in his wheelchair from the jammed and distant parking garage to the
center, I had earned these amenities.

We waited only 10 minutes before being led to an examination
room where one of Dr. Moul's nurses took Dad's vitals and his

physician assistant obtained a detailed history. The PA had trouble keeping the facts straight, even though he seemed to listen intently. If I had doubts about the PA, and I did, I had none about Moul, in whom my father found a kindred spirit.

This urologist was delighted to hear about Dr. Al's association with Charlie Huggins, the original hormone king of prostate cancer. After Dad told him about his National Institutes of Health background, Moul shared his five-year experience at Walter Reed Army Medical Center, which had recently moved from Washington to Bethesda, across from the NIH, and they discovered medical acquaintances in common, despite the generational difference. Moul was my age.

Dad's PSA at the Outer Banks Hospital had been 22, a figure that didn't impress Moul, who was accustomed to "PSAs in the hundreds." He diagnosed Dad with cancer on the basis of a digital exam, alone, and said that the mass was small and would shrink with hormone therapy. When I brought up the lung nodules, the urologic oncologist said that they were unlikely to be a metastasis, but if they were, they, too, would shrink as a result of the treatment. In any case, Moul assured Dad: "You're not going to die from prostate cancer."

My father had a choice of receiving an injection of Lupron®, a testosterone-lowering drug that could be administered every six months, or degarelix (Firmagon®), a faster-acting testosterone inhibitor administered on a monthly basis. Each drug reduces the amount of testosterone released by the testes, but by different means. Dad chose the degarelix, which is injected into the stomach area, and scheduled a return appointment for September.

I asked both Dr. Moul and his PA about the artificial sphincter and how we should proceed. Both explained they do cancer, not incontinence, but the PA said he would get in touch with Dr. Terse, whom he didn't know. He later reported to us that Dad's PSA that day was 25.13.

The specialization of these urology specialists within the same medical complex seemed blindingly ridiculous to me. Medicine should be interactive, not insular. Knowing the risk of sphincter erosion, I probably should have insisted with Mary that Dad see Dr. Terse. I could have postponed the prostate-cancer appointment, but I was unnerved by the diagnosis and worried about the lung nodules, which I viewed as life-threatening.

I really am not a doctor.

I thought about stopping by the urology clinic and trying to arrange an on-the-fly cystoscopy after we finished in the prostate-cancer center, but it was 4 p.m., and Dad was exhausted. If I delayed our departure, Dad likely would arrive home in an immobile state. He lacked stamina and strength, and the time he spent sitting in the car and in the clinic already had taken a toll on him. If we stayed overnight in Durham, a hardship for which we had not prepared, I would have to reschedule his appointment tomorrow with the home-healthcare nurse who was coming to assess his needs AND he definitely would be immobile.

Besides all of this, Mom had her critical two-week followup with the orthopedic surgeon, Dr. Thompson, on Thursday, Aug. 8.

So Dad and I left. After he went to bed that night, he broke into night sweats, a temporary effect of the hormone drug.

The next day I learned for the first time that Dr. Terse had a physician assistant, because she called, leaving a frantic message that Dad had to be seen in the clinic *that* day. We exchanged messages, mine relating that Dad was too tired to travel, and I couldn't get him there.

When I finally spoke to PA Agatha Thursday, she urged us to go to the Duke Emergency Department that night, not having any idea that we were more than 200 miles away and couldn't possibly return so quickly. I told her about my first-thing-Monday-morning call to Mary and her brushoff. I also asked how it was that neither Dr. Terse nor anyone associated with him had mentioned her before. Here I was talking with her on her cell phone! Why hadn't I been given her name and number 20 months ago? Why? Because Dr. Terse didn't want patients to be in touch.

I volunteered to drive Dad to Duke on Friday, but Terse and his residents were in surgery all day and couldn't accommodate us. It wasn't until Tuesday, Aug. 13, that they worked him in.

In the intervening days, Dad became ill with upper-gastric pain again, and we received bad news about Mom. The alignment Dr. Thompson had achieved during surgery had not held up: The distal-femur fragments had come apart, so that the displacement looked much like the original fracture.

Britt arrived in town the day before and went with me to the orthopedic appointment. When she and I saw the new X-rays, we were aghast. Thompson was disappointed and genuinely apologetic, but short of a second surgery to repair the nonunion, which no one wanted, he had no treatment options for us. Perhaps time and natural healing would improve Mom's status. To support her leg better, he put it in a heavy-duty knee immobilizer that no one was to remove. We scheduled the next followup for Aug. 29.

Instead of driving Dad to Duke, I checked out the medical center's website to see if I could find an orthopedic expert who might be able to help Mom. Dr. Thompson seemed to be settling for low expectations, and I wanted to do all I could to ensure that Mom would walk again, preferably with a cane. Mom's roommate, Judith, recommended the highly sought-after orthopedic surgeon in Chesapeake who had operated on her, but I decided that his practice, although nearby, was too much of a cattle call: He did surgery on units or commodities, not people.

I also did a quick Internet study of open reduction internal fixation (O.R.I.F.), which is the surgical repair method that Thompson used to stabilize Mom's fractured bone. Open reduction refers to reducing or putting the broken bones back into place; and internal fixation is the hardware (screws, plates, pins, or rods) used to hold the bones together. I wanted to be able to speak, and use acronyms, knowledgably with whomever I contacted at Duke.

Eventually, I identified some surgeons who specialized in nonunions of repaired fractures and would have cold-called the Duke Department of Orthopaedic Surgery, if I hadn't had a friend whom I could call for a possible entreé. Shannon had worked at Duke Hospital in an executive business capacity and knew quite a few medical bigwigs. She contacted one of them, a physician whose son was a prominent orthopedic surgeon, and after a series of emails, I had a name: Dr. Robert Zura, director of orthopaedic trauma surgery. It didn't hurt that Shannon's contact knew Dad by reputation.

Although it never hurts to have a medical connection, you don't need a Shannon to get into Duke Medical Center or another top hospital. What you need is a physician's referral; so I also called Dr. Thompson and left a message for him about getting a second opinion at Duke.

On Aug. 9, Britt posted a photograph of Mom's latest leg X-ray on her closet door, and I spoke with the head of Oakwood's PT and the nurse du jour about the displacement. The hardnose and I were getting along quite well by now. Our interests had aligned, and she liked my sweet and accommodating mother a lot. She ordered nursing aides to transfer Mom henceforth on a wooden sliding board, so that neither of her feet ever touched the ground. This was a hardship for the aides, and Mom hated it, but the PT boss was determined to effectuate Dr. Thompson's new edict: Absolutely no weight bearing of any kind.

I now heard from the day nurse that another of Mom's incisions was weeping; her legs were enormously swollen (not surprisingly); and she had a nasty in-grown toenail. Then, Monday, Aug. 12, the wound nurse, with whom I also had an excellent relationship, called to say Mom was depressed and "wants to go home." After a weekend of sliding on the transfer board and hauling around the heavy knee brace, my already confused mother had melted down. She was miserable.

My emotional state wasn't that great, either, but I soldiered on and talked Mom out of her confusion. I gave her reasons to be hopeful.

That same week the PT chief or one of her associates removed the expensive knee immobilizer that Dr. Thompson had fitted and replaced it with a cheaper and lighter brace that, from the looks of it, didn't do much.

I added a new rule, beneath Murphy, in the healthcare rulebook. According to the Roseanne Rosannadanna rule of nursing homes, it's *always* something.

Duke Showdown, Part II

On the drive to Duke Tuesday, Aug. 13, I noticed for the first time *ever* that Dad was short of breath, so short of breath that his voice was barely audible. When I pointed this out, he said he had no awareness. He had lost so much of his vigor and will during the past three months that I didn't know how he was going to manage. *What good had three hospitals and umpteen doctors done him? How many doctors does it take to defeat an old man?* During this drive, I again stopped repeatedly, so Dad could get out and walk. He struggled.

After negotiating the highways, the parking garage, the hallways, the elevator, the patient check-in counter, the nurse's vitals, Agatha's questions, etc., etc., we found ourselves in an examining room at the Duke Urology Clinic, paralyzed by technology. The computer that was to display Dad's urinary tract while Dr. Terse scoped him was on the fritz. Every minute of this delay exacted a pound of energy from Dad's weak body. I don't remember how long the wait lasted, but I know we arrived at the clinic at 1:10 p.m. for a 1:45 p.m. appointment and didn't leave until 5:30 p.m. That's a lot of inertia.

When Terse finally did the cystoscopy, the imaging clearly showed that Dad's artificial sphincter had eroded: It was in pieces.

"Just what I was afraid of," Terse said, as disappointment rained over us. "It will have to be removed within the next few days."

I was already on edge because of the computer delay and because I had yet to hear anything remotely like an apology from Terse, just his head-shaking regret, "If only we'd known sooner," so I pounced.

"When? Tomorrow?" I asked, not liking his vague pronouncement about a "few days" or the Teflon surgeon himself very much. He had shown too much indifference when I explained Dad's latest setback. I could tell he didn't appreciate his vulnerable condition.

"No. I can't do it tomorrow," he replied, without offering an alternative time.

"Thursday?" I continued.

"No. I'll be in surgery all day."

"Friday, then?" I asked.

"No. I'm in surgery."

"Then when, Dr. Terse?" I pressed. "Wednesday, Thursday, Friday. That's the next few days."

"If only we'd known," he said one too many f–king times that afternoon. "We might have been able to save it."

That was it. A few days weren't actually a few days, and it was my fault that Terse hadn't seen Dad last week. Enough BS. I wasn't in healthcare. Duke wasn't paying my salary. How much is a patient's family supposed to do?

"I'm tired of hearing that," I said. "Let's tell the truth here."

Passionately I reviewed what had happened: I had called *first thing on the Monday morning* after Dad's cancer diagnosis and tried to reach Terse for a referral and an appointment and been *blown off* by Mary. Mary got rid of me, plain and simple. She didn't even bother to speak to anyone about my call. She knew Dad, and she knew me. We weren't cranks. Is it too much to ask that she try to be helpful?

"We've spoken to her about that," Terse said, in his sole admission of responsibility.

I kept rolling. Mary told me you don't do cancer. I *know* that. Even so, how did you miss the tumor?

"We're all so specialized," he said, or words to that effect. "We don't have anything to do with cancer." Uh-huh. And how is *that* good medicine? I wasn't thinking malpractice, but I got the sense that Terse thought I was.

Furthermore, why didn't I know about Agatha? I could've called her from the Outer Banks Hospital emergency room! Why didn't you tell us about her?

"Well, she was in the operating room" when Dad had his AUS surgery, he said lamely.

"I never met her."

And, another thing, I could've gotten Dad to Duke on Friday. Maybe the AUS would still have been intact four days ago. Couldn't *somebody* have scoped him?

I unloaded on this smiling iceberg, not rudely or disrespectfully, but unyieldingly.

After I finished, Terse excused himself and left the room. My dear father, whom I loved so much and was so worried about, immediately said: "You really gave him hell. I'm proud of you." His encouragement gave me strength to keep fighting. It gave me hope.

Terse returned to say that he had arranged to have Dad admitted to the hospital that night in anticipation of sphincter-removal surgery sometime tomorrow. If I hadn't been persistent, he would never have executed this 180.

Sensing an opportunity, I suggested that, during his hospitalization, Dad could be evaluated by a neurologist and other specialists, but my father discouraged me, and Terse, not having any stake or interest in his other problems, didn't support me. In fact, the urologist suggested that Dad could be discharged shortly after surgery, as if he were doing us a favor instead of saving the bed for a sicker ($$) patient. I explained again that Dad would be too weak and ill to travel until he had rested at least overnight.

For Dad's admission, we had to go to the main lobby of Duke Hospital, which, I discovered, hadn't changed much since Mom's 2002 hospitalization. I drove the car around to the parking garage I had used then and pushed Dad in from the garage through an underground tunnel I knew about, rather than drop him off in front. We needed some decompression time together. Inside the hospital, I easily found the admissions window, the cafeteria, and, much to my delight, a new Starbucks. Our wait passed pleasantly; and the admissions person had an upbeat attitude.

On the urology floor, though, I ran into testiness with Dad's first nurse, who was going off-duty in 15 minutes, at 7 p.m. She refused to allow Dad to stand without a physical-therapy evaluation, which wouldn't happen, she said, for another 15 hours.

"He's going to deteriorate," I said, explaining Dad's state.

"No one deteriorates in 15 hours," she replied.

"He will."

More crappola, having to do with the hospital's potential liability, not the patient's well-being. I'll sign a waiver, Dad said. Fortunately, the night nurses were not so rigid. Dad was up and walking, albeit slowly and for only a short distance, before I left to find a hotel room. Since Dr. Terse was working Dad into his schedule, we wouldn't know until tomorrow, at the last minute, when his surgery would occur. I told Dad I'd be back at 9 a.m.

On my drive into the hospital the next morning, I received a call on my cell phone from Dr. Thompson. He was more than happy to cooperate with a referral. He understood why I was seeking one and only wanted what was best for Mom. He would help in any way he could, starting with arranging for Mom's records and films to be picked up. His office did not digitize X-rays, so X-rays couldn't be emailed. He also wished Dad well.

This exchange gave me a lift. I still had to ask Britt to get the films; schedule an appointment with Dr. Zura; figure out how to transport Mom from Oakwood to Duke; contact nursing-home officials about the trip, and so forth, but I was on my way. Whenever Mom had a doctor's appointment, I had to arrange her transportation with the Oakwood van driver and sign Mom out of, and back into, the facility with the nurse du jour, as well as provide said nurse with the doctor's report. This appointment would require a tad more orchestration.

I would have the next four hours to brainstorm these details because the orderly didn't arrive to wheel Dad to the Duke Medicine Pavilion until 12:40 p.m. Ten minutes later, I arrived by foot in the pavilion's spacious and gleaming third-floor waiting area, where I checked in and received a monitor that would notify me when Dad was in pre-op and I could see him.

Newly opened in July, the Duke Medicine Pavilion was a spectacular state-of-the-art surgery and critical-care center, a sister Emerald City in Oz to the adjacent cancer center. A 608,000-square-foot, nine-leveled expansion that cost nearly $600 million, the steel-and-glass pavilion

had 18 operating rooms and many comforts and diversions for loved
ones of patients undergoing surgery, including a café, gift shops, a
chapel, and a patient resource center with computers. The pavilion's
floor-to-ceiling windows brought in warm natural light and, in many
cases, allowed views out onto green courtyards. What I liked most
about both the cancer center and the pavilion is that each reserved
space for quiet reflection and reading, far removed from televisions
and cell-phone conversations.

Unlike with the AUS implantation surgery, Dad was not given the
option of a spinal anesthesia; he received a general anesthesia with
a muscle relaxant. When he asked the young anesthesiologist what
anesthesia she would be using, she snapped: "General."

"Yes, I know, but what agents?" Dr. Al asked.

She wouldn't tell him, condescendingly informing him that he
wouldn't what she was talking about, if she did. Unbelievable. It wasn't
enough for this unfriendly and pretentious piece of work that Dad had
told her he was a doctor, she had to challenge him on his expertise.
After he provided his medical bona fides, she reluctantly told him
the drugs, which, of course, he knew. One of them was propofol,
which, according to Dr. Russell Wall, chairman of the Georgetown
anesthesiology department, is the most commonly used intravenous
anesthesia because of its quick onset and short duration.

Here, again, in this beautiful, awe-inspiring *patient-centered*
facility was that elitist Duke attitude that Terse copped so well. This
anesthesiologist was a far cry from Dr. Mendelson, who told Dad
everything about his anesthesia before he asked. Why would a doctor
withhold such information from a patient? So what if the patient
doesn't understand? The patient has a right to know.

Dad was unusually tense in pre-op, and we waited for quite a while
before Dr. Terse, who had trouble finding his way to the pavilion,
showed up. After he did, the surgery went well. I relaxed in a private
lounge, reading and calling all of my siblings, and joined Dad in
post-op. We never saw Dr. Terse again. One of his residents spoke
with me about the surgical followup: Dad would use a Foley catheter
for at least the next three weeks. If he wanted to undergo another
AUS implantation, he would have to live without a catheter, and be
incontinent, for three months while his lower urinary tract healed.

This was a dreadful blow. All in all, the day was exhausting.

HOMEWARD BOUND

The next morning Dr. Terse's residents deliberated with Dad and me about his discharge. Dad's blood-oxygen level had fallen below 90 percent; his sodium was low again; and they didn't want to release him. But, by this time, Dr. Al didn't care if he stopped breathing. He just wanted to go home.

Dad had reached his breaking point and told the residents that he would assume all legal responsibility for his discharge. They were good guys, but they were very young and inexperienced and didn't know how to persuade him. I, too, ran out of words to convince my father to stay.

I think Dad thought he might die in the hospital, which he was adamant about not allowing to happen, so I quit arguing with him, but I knew I was in deep s---. He couldn't even sit up. Just getting him into a wheelchair and then into my car at the hospital front entrance, *with* hospital-staff help, was an ordeal.

An hour into the drive home, I stopped so Dad could get out and walk around the car. He managed to stand up next to the car door with his walker, but he couldn't move. As the driving time passed, he slumped forward in his car seat, unable to hold his weight up. Yes, this was deep s---, been-there/done-that deep s---, and I have to tell you, because I want to be honest, I was angry. My father was asking too much of me. En route, he told me passionately: "Ann, I don't know what I would do without you. I love you so much." To which I replied: "You should be in the hospital, Dad." I wish I could edit that conversation: "I love you so much, too, Dad."

Later, he asked me to "just get me to my birthday," which was 13 days away. I insisted that he wasn't dying, and he had to hang in there and think more positively. I asked him to help me to help him. We needed to be a team. In retrospect, I wonder if he'd been having some irregular heartbeats that he hadn't told me about.

About an hour from Southern Shores, I called Britt to ask her to arrange for the Dare County transport service to meet us upon our arrival. There was no way that she and I could get Dad into the house. He would need to be strapped into a special chair and carried by some strong paramedics into his bedroom, and that's exactly what happened. The next day, Karen, the dynamo physical therapist from Coastal Rehab, came out to evaluate Dad. She managed to get him out of bed and sitting in his wheelchair.

While brainstorming how to care for Dad, I called the only assisted-living facility on the Outer Banks, a reputedly swanky place—I never saw it—and ran head-first into more healthcare crap.

The woman who answered the telephone was one of those close-mouthed (passive-aggressive?) employees, like Mary, who don't volunteer information. They make you ask every question, even though they know the questions you're going to ask. They even withhold information if you don't phrase the question properly. You have to pull teeth. You know who they are. God forbid they should be helpful.

I once saw a Johns Hopkins front-desk receptionist turn away a woman and her elderly father-in-law, who insisted that they were in the correct outpatient clinic, because in asking the receptionist whether they indeed were, the woman used the word, X-ray, instead of ultrasound.

"We don't do X-rays here," the receptionist said, instead of inquiring helpfully: "What type of test are you having?"

The two left and came back. Of course, they were in the right place.

The Duke Urology Clinic had such an employee at its reception desk, a sour woman who would ignore people at the front counter whenever she was stationed at the back counter, about seven feet away, even though she was the only employee out front and she heard patients talking with their families about how they should check in. She never greeted anyone; never said, "May I help you?" or "I'll help you over here"; never tried to un-befuddle befuddled people.

I'd fire all such petty power-mongers, antisocial nitwits, or clueless incompetents on the healthcare frontlines. They do great harm to already vulnerable people, as well as reflect badly on their employers.

Among the teeth I pulled from the Outer Banks assisted-living obstructionist was that a one-bedroom apartment, occupied by two people, would cost $8,000 per month, plus a move-in fee of $3,000. When I asked about in-house nursing services and physical therapy, she laughed at me.

"This is *assisted* living," she said in response to each question.

Finally, she informed me that residents have to be able to ambulate and transfer on their own, without assistance, to qualify for admission. She might have told me this threshold requirement at the outset of our conversation, but then she wouldn't have had any fun jerking me around.

If your Mom or Pop moves into assisted living, make sure they and you know what assistance they can expect and beware the facilities that don't offer much, unless you enjoy moving furniture and boxes a lot. Think like a lawyer and read the fine print.

Chapter Seventeen

2013: Failing to
THRIVE

"Ticky-Tack" Doctoring

My brilliant and imposing father was now an immobile 200-pound lump of bones and tissue that still had a sharp brain, when anxiety didn't cloud it. I felt very sad, but determinedly purposeful. I was going to bring him back.

Karen left on Friday with the promise to return on Monday to talk with us about a physical-therapy plan, if indeed she thought she could help Dad at home. Dad was taking the narcotic painkiller, oxycodone,* which Terse had prescribed, along with an antibiotic and a bladder relaxant, and, by Saturday, Aug. 17, he was very concerned about his bowels. He may have wanted to die at home, but he didn't want to die as the result of a bowel impaction and perforation.

Without informing me, Britt helped Dad to take the powerful colonic that the OBH nursing aide, Pam, had suggested, and his GI tract became a fecal faucet that couldn't be turned off. Because he couldn't get out of bed and walk on his own, Britt was rushing to help Dad get to a bedside commode and then changing his underwear, sheets, bed pads, all that was soiled, and cleaning up. Dad continued to have orthostatic hypotension, too, which meant he could pass out upon standing, fall, and break a bone.

I sized up this dreadful situation and decided that we couldn't care for our father at home and also look out daily for Mom, whom I needed to transport to Duke soon. We—*I*, after Britt returned to Florida—were going to burn out. So I came up with a plan. We could have Dad

---

*The most common brand name for oxycodone is OxyContin. Oxycodone also comes in combination products that contain acetaminophen (which is Tylenol), ibuprofen, or aspirin. Percocet®, for example, contains oxycodone and acetaminophen. Percodan® contains oxycodone and aspirin.

hospitalized at Sentara Norfolk General Hospital for at least three days, the Medicare prerequisite for coverage of 100 days of nursing-home care, and then discharged to Oakwood, where our parents could be together, and Dad could get physical therapy five days a week, instead of the maximum three that Karen could provide at home. Previously, we had discussed moving them both to Durham, but now Dad was in extremis.

On Sunday, Aug. 18, I called Dr. Ramses on his cell phone and arranged for my father to be admitted to Sentara Norfolk General on Tuesday. Dad would acquiesce in this plan only if Karen agreed, so before she saw him on Monday, I called the physical therapist to make sure that she would. I didn't twist her arm, but I feel bad now remembering this deceit. I thought I was acting in my father's best interests, as well as Britt's and my own, but later events caused me to second-guess, and even regret, my decision.

All you can ever do, though, is to judge the facts as you know them to be in the given moment. And then be compassionate.

Unfortunately, I was under the impression that Ramses, with whom I could communicate well, would supervise Dad's medical care, even though, as he explained, his "partner" would be the attending physician, and Ramses would only drop by.

But no supervision occurred, and that partner, Dr. Hedwig, turned out to be a physician who, if not from hell himself, certainly put Dad and me through it. Later at Oakwood, Dad contracted a "never event" infection that I had never heard of, but suddenly was reading about in newspapers. Ignorance is not bliss.

The next three months were a horror show.

KICKED TO THE CURB

Just getting our father into my car to be transported 75 miles to Norfolk was a task that Britt and I could not manage. He had no strength and could not stand. If Keith, the friend whom I had lined up in May to be our parents' caregiver, had not shown up to do yardwork, we would've had to call the county transport service again.

A big, sweet-natured man who looked like a Sumo wrestler, Keith handled both Dad and his wheelchair and transferred him into my car with a bear-hug lift. With that hug, Dr. Al bonded with Keith–"This guy is great!"–but we were a long way from "getting there."

For the next 90 minutes, my father lay uncomfortably contorted on the back seat of my 2005 Lexus. The scene in the semi-circular driveway in front of the hospital building where we were told to report for admission was even worse: No one working for the hospital offered to help me. A valet parking attendant, who tried hard to move me along, actually insisted that I close the back door of my car because the sight of my seriously ill father was disturbing children passing by.

Was this a hospital or a playground?

Reluctantly leaving Dad alone, I dashed into the hospital to find a wheelchair and some strong orderlies, and succeeded in my mission, but the orderlies dragged their feet. We waited and waited, while the parking attendants hovered and fretted, until a very kind young doctor stopped to assist. With her watching over Dad, I was able to go back into the hospital and hustle up my strongmen. The valet gratefully snatched my car keys as soon as the muscle arrived.

We didn't wait long for Dad's name to be called and the admissions paperwork to be completed (30 minutes, max), after which he was transported to the hospital room where he would live at least until the weekend. Despite his undignified arrival and obvious suffering, Dr. Al was in good spirits. He loved being around people, especially young people working in medicine.

In preparing to argue Dad's case for hospitalization to Dr. Ramses, I had written down some notes about his status, including: "Low O2/SOB; low sodium; fecal incontinence; weakness/immobility; chronic fatigue; chronic constipation; recent surgery for sphincter removal, taking antibiotic to thwart infection." Next to these words, I wrote: "GI, neurology, IM," IM signifying internal medicine. I also told Ramses about the pancreatitis and prostate cancer diagnoses, but I did not intend to pursue the cancer question unless the opportunity arose. I felt confident in Dr. Moul's treatment, and I knew Dad would not permit a lung-nodule biopsy.

Of course, Dr. Ramses never conveyed the content of this conversation to Dr. Hedwig. That would be much too organized and lawyer-like. To be a physician is to have no accountability for communication because, hey, "I'm too busy and don't have the time" and, besides, "I practice *medicine*." Apparently, there's no money in healthcare budgets to hire assistants to fill the communication gaps.

I never even saw Ramses. He popped in, for about 15 minutes, on Dad's first evening, precisely when I left the room to move my car from valet parking to a garage. He never visited again. So, as with every medical handoff, we started over. Had I known that Ramses would let us down, I would have persuaded my father to go back to Duke, which, despite Dr. Terse, had the superior medical staff.

An earnest young EVMS intern and senior resident stopped by Dad's room not long after his admission. They seemed personable, respectful, and bright.

When Dr. Roo, the senior house staffer, asked Dad the "what brought you here?" question, which he framed in terms of his concerns and objectives, Dad brought up his fatigue, weakness, immobility, and ataxia. I amplified this answer with more of his neurological symptoms and mentioned his shortness of breath and recent surgery at Duke, as well as the fecal incontinence.

Drs. Roo and Nar, the first-year resident (aka intern), performed what I considered to be a thorough systemic workup. Dr. Al enjoyed telling them about his Romberg's sign (loss of proprioception while standing with his eyes closed) and showing them the Dupuytren's contracture in his right hand that caused his pinky finger to be permanently bent.

In Dupuytren's contracture, which develops slowly over years, the palmar fascia within the hand becomes abnormally thick because of a change in the collagen. The pinky and/or ring finger may curl and lose function, and the ability to grip may diminish. Dupuytren's contracture primarily affects people of Scandinavian or Northern European ancestry, like my Dutch/Frisian father, and is known as the Viking disease. The contracture can be surgically corrected, but the correction doesn't last.[1]

Had Roo been left on his own or had a different attending than Dr. Hedwig, with whom, I later concluded, the resident was unjustifiably impressed, he might have given Dad better care. He seemed to have good patient instincts. He also was wide-awake, as was Dr. Nar, whenever he stopped by to see Dad. The last time I had been in Sentara Norfolk, I saw house staffers yawning excessively. (See Appendix Three, "The Paradox of the Better-Rested Resident.")

Unfortunately, the physician in charge was an egotistical showboater who played to a house staff that reinforced his showboating with undiscriminating hero worship. Even before Dad and I met him on Wednesday, Aug. 21, Roo was singing Hedwig's praises as an internist who had a neurological Midas touch and a specialty in geriatrics. Too bad he didn't live up to his hype.

CHEST PAIN AND POLYPHARMACY

I stayed late at the hospital on Tuesday and didn't return Wednesday until 12:30 p.m., so I missed Hedwig's morning rounds. Dad had chest pain during the night and underwent tests; an ECG apparently ruled out a cardiac source. He also had pain upon awakening and had a chest CT scan, after first being X-rayed at the bedside by an AP (anterior-posterior) portable chest radiograph. He now had a Holter monitor attached to him and was receiving oxygen.

Nothing in the tests seemed to explain Dad's acute chest pain, which was near his sternum (breastbone). Of the Holter results, he told me only that he was in sinus rhythm. That's all that concerned him. I found out after this hospitalization, when I read the medical records sent by Dr. Ramses, that an ECG showed Dad's first-degree AV block and "nonspecific IVCD with LAD," which translates to an intraventricular conduction delay with left axis deviation.

I'm not going to touch the LAD part of this assessment. It's over my head. The IVCD part apparently means that the electrical activation of Dad's ventricles by the atria had slowed, thereby widening the QRS complex, which marks the beginning of ventricular contraction.

My father had been worried about a prolonged delay between his heartbeats and sudden death, and the emotionally distant Dr. Gotti had advised him not to worry unless that delay reached 10 seconds. Was Dad now counting seconds?

Dr. Hedwig stopped by again on Wednesday afternoon, and I witnessed his standoffish response to my father's friendly attempts to get to know him. The glib, detached, and bow-tied internist was not inclined to talk medicine with Dad, and I got the impression that he didn't cotton to the admiration that Drs. Roo and Nar and his medical students expressed for Dr. Al. During Dad's hospitalization, I often felt that Hedwig prematurely terminated his visits with him. He always seemed to be in a hurry.

Hedwig speculated that Dad's chest pain might be pleurisy or heartburn (that sounded familiar), but he said nothing about the ECG. When Hedwig was able to reproduce Dad's pain by pressing on his sternum, he diagnosed him with costochondritis, which is an inflammation of the cartilage that connects ribs to the sternum. Dr. Al accepted this simple explanation. Just in case, Hedwig ordered a whole-body bone scan to rule out metastatic prostate cancer in his back.

This scan seemed ridiculously excessive to me. Dr. Moul had described Dad's prostatic tumor as small and the lung nodules as unlikely to be metastases from it. (The nodules now measured up to 12 mm., which is larger than a centimeter, but much smaller than the three centimeters that Georgetown pulmonologist Charles A. Read defined as a mass.) My father went along with the imaging and, despite the radiation exposure, I didn't think it would hurt to know if he had any cancer in his bones. He did not.

At least that is what I was told. Much later, I read in the medical records that the interpreting radiologist thought the "uptake" of the "radio-pharmaceutical," which Dad received intravenously three hours before the scan, "in the anterior left 6 rib, anterior left iliac crest and left ischium [is] suspicious for metastatic bone disease." There was that word again: suspicious. Would it have been suspicious if the radiologist had not known that Dad had prostate cancer? (The iliac crest and ischium are parts of the hip.)

At no time did Hedwig suggest a cardiology consult. If he and Dr. Al discussed his cardiovascular status beyond a mention of his orthostatic hypotension and known AF, I was not in the room to hear the discussion, and I was present quite often. Sentara Norfolk is known for its highly regarded heart center.

They also did not talk about the illnesses—i.e., his recent history—that Dad had suffered since mid-May. But they certainly talked about drugs. Hedwig zealously put the "polypharmacy" brand on my debilitated father, for whom he expressed no sympathy.

Acting quite appalled by Dad's "abuse," Hedwig eliminated his bedtime cocktail of Ambien, Valium, Benadryl, and meprobamate, and replaced it with the antidepressant, trazodone, which, like many antidepressants, has a sedating effect. (Meprobamate is a mild anti-anxiety drug that was popular in the 1960s, when it was known better by its brand name, Miltown®. President Kennedy took it.)

"I won't be able to sleep, Doc," Dad told him.

But Hedwig didn't care about how Dad slept. His chief concern was the impression he made on his house staff. As authority for the drug withdrawal, he grandiosely cited the American Geriatrics Society's (AGS's) "Beers list" of drugs that are contraindicated in the older population, not any expertise in clinical pharmacology, which Dad had in spades.

The Beers list was news to me. I have learned since that it is not a list, per se, but an evaluation of medications and medication classes by criteria that are designed to assess the appropriateness of their use by older adults, generally, and by elders with certain diseases and syndromes, specifically. According to its 2012 Beers Criteria Update Expert Panel, the AGS did not intend its recommendations "to supersede clinical judgment or an individual patient's values and *needs*."[2]

Of course not. Medicine is never about black-and-white rules, except when doctors choose to invoke some.

At the time, I supported Hedwig's decision, because I wanted an ally in my own effort to change my father's nighttime drug regimen. Nonetheless, I wasn't very keen on Hedwig's cold-turkey approach; the sudden withdrawal seemed like a major pharmacological jolt to inflict on a sick 88-year-old man. Surely, a tapering-off would be better.

I also didn't think there was any harm in Dad's taking meprobamate at the dosage prescribed by Ramses. Hedwig did not address drug dosage, just drug "appropriateness." I doubt he knew enough about meprobamate, a tranquilizer that has a short-term effect and is non-habit-forming (in Dad's and my experience), to evaluate its appropriateness. For years I've taken a small dose whenever anxiety has kept me awake at night.

I was much more concerned about trazodone. All antidepressants have adverse effects of some kind, and Dad had not tolerated Cymbalta well. I found out later that trazodone is a serotonin and norepinephrine reuptake inhibitor, just like Cymbalta.

The internist also discontinued Dad's antihypertensive, lisinopril, because he was experiencing hypotension; the bladder relaxant that Dr. Terse had prescribed; and the diarrhea inhibitor, lomotil, which Dr. Eagan had prescribed.

On Wednesday, I tried to work with Hedwig, rather than against him, even though I found him to be unpleasant and rigid. By Thursday, I had concluded that he was using Dad as a case study for his worshippers and couldn't care less about his welfare. He was sarcastic, too. Sarcasm in a doctor is a red flag. Beware.

Deep-Sea Fishing

Hedwig zeroed in on Dad's neurological problems. He thought his symptoms suggested a cerebellar source, meaning the underlying defect or disorder originated in the cerebellum, which regulates complex voluntary muscular movement, posture, and balance.

Hedwig hypothesized that Dad's nerves had degenerated because of demyelination—destruction of the myelin sheaths of nerve fibers—not axonal deterioration, and told us some diseases within his differential diagnosis. They included Guillain-Barré syndrome, which I had investigated and considered out of the question; and chronic idiopathic demyelinating polyneuropathy (CIDP), a condition unknown to me whose description by Hedwig did not apply to Dad's history. He even mentioned a copper deficiency, which I also had come across in my research. (I advised Dad to eat cashews.)

Hedwig's differential was the equivalent of the lawyer's kitchen-sink complaint. I knew from experience that horses sometimes turned out to be zebras, but I still preferred critical analysis to fishing expeditions. As Dad would say in imitation of the great Swedish physiologist Anton Julius (Ajax) Carlson, under whom he studied at the University of Chicago: *"Vas is the evidence?"*

It didn't seem to me that Hedwig knew or cared about the evidence. He was fishing in remote waters, and he planned to cast (order) as many tests as he could.

That afternoon, Aug. 21, I stayed by Dad's side, watching out for him, except for when I slipped out to my car to participate by cell phone in Mom's 3 p.m. two-week care-plan meeting.

It was a beastly hot August day, and the meeting lasted 45 sweaty minutes, but I—not Britt, who was in an Oakwood conference room with the various departmental supervisors—determined its length, as I struggled to hear what was being said and asked questions. Everyone was pleased with Mom's progress except the dietician, who reported that she ate only 58 percent of what was on her meal trays and didn't drink enough fluids.

Oakwood's kitchen fare was not one of its strengths, but, nonetheless, we discussed some foods that Mom might eat, if they were served to her more often. Getting Mom to drink water, however, was like getting a cat to swim: She just didn't do it—not unless you stood over her and said, "If you don't drink more fluids, you're going to get dehydrated." Britt suggested giving her milkshakes, an idea that seemed inspired, but didn't take off later because Mom had lost her taste for them. (Oakwood's milkshakes also didn't measure up with McDonald's.)

The physical-therapy manager reported that Mom was working hard, with "a great attitude," and had increased her upper-body strength. After this PT assessment, I brought up the Duke consultation. The top administrator present advised Britt and me that the SNF's transportation department could arrange for a private ambulance, and one of its CNAs could accompany Mom. Duke was definitely doable. Hooray!

Back in Dad's room that evening, an examination by an actual neurologist caused my opinion of Hedwig and his diagnostic approach to plummet further.

Sentara neurology consultant Dr. Ahmet started by taking a detailed history, which neither the ageist Dr. Less nor Hedwig's team had done. Ahmet also didn't need a laptop attached to his abdomen to remember the facts correctly later. He listened intently. His questions consistently led to thoughtful follow-up questions.

Ahmet thoroughly assessed Dad's mental status (his alertness, attention, orientation, concentration, speech, language, and memory); his cranial nerve functioning (sight, hearing, facial symmetry and sensation, tongue and soft palate); the muscle functioning in his arms, hips, knees, ankles, feet, and toes; the sensation in his arms, hands, legs, and feet; the tendon reflexes in his arms, knees, and ankles; his muscle coordination, as evidenced by such exercises as finger-to-nose touching and heel-to-shin flexing; and his muscle tone.

The Sentara neurologist noted the decreased sensation that Dad had in both feet and both legs, up to his knees, and in both of his hands up to his wrists, as well as the mild tremors he had in his hands. Dad had a trace of a deep-tendon reflex in his knees (the tuning-fork test), but none in his ankles. Ahmet couldn't evaluate Dad's gait or station because he couldn't stand unassisted, but Dr. Al told him about his longstanding Romberg's sign and his ataxia.

After all of this, Ahmet pronounced judgment: He had seen no signs of cerebellar dysfunction. Dad, he said, had a chronic idiopathic axonal (not demyelinating) peripheral polyneuropathy, "poly" as in a generalized disorder originating from "all over" the spinal cord, he told me, not just the "posterior column."

Having heard that word, idiopathic, a lot lately, I asked Ahmet to hazard a few guesses as to the polyneuropathy's cause. Dad was not diabetic, but his glucose levels had been consistently above the normal range for several years. Any relation? Ahmet attributed the nerve degeneration to aging—which I thought was a cop-out answer. This severe polyneuropathy wasn't normal. There had to be another reason for why Dad was aging so badly. No one in his family had been similarly stricken in their oldest old years.

Ahmet told Dad that nothing could be done medically or surgically about his polyneuropathy. He might be able to forestall its progression with physical therapy, as he had been doing, and balance therapy, but it would not improve. Henceforth, he would need to walk with a walker, so he wouldn't fall. He also told us that the polyneuropathy would not cause Dad's chronic fatigue. (What then? Cancer? Heart disease?)

"Dr. Less was right when she said dead nerves," Dr. Al said after Ahmet left.

"Come on," I replied. "I could've told you what she said, and I didn't go to medical school."

The Hedwig team had recommended an electromyogram and nerve conduction studies, whose usefulness Dr. Al questioned, but Ahmet went along with the group consensus. He thought Dad (and I) should know the extent and severity of his polyneuropathy and myopathy (muscle abnormalities), but thanks to Hedwig, Ahmet never got the chance to inform us.

THE HEDWIG EFFECT

The beginning of the end of our relationship with Dr. Hedwig and of the futility of this hospitalization occurred the morning of the next day, Aug. 22, when he suggested during rounds that Dad undergo a lumbar puncture to collect some cerebral spinal fluid for examination. CSF, as you will recall, serves as a protective cushion for your brain and spinal cord.

I was surprised by this. Dr. Ahmet had said with great confidence and certainty that Dad's polyneuropathy was due to an axonal deterioration, but Hedwig was still pursuing a demyelinating disease. I questioned him, not insultingly, but with some doubt. I admit, though, that the haughty way in which he had lectured Dad about polypharmacy, and Dad's ensuing restless night, had made me angry, so I wasn't smiling.

Affronted by my objection, Hedwig let me have it—in a defensive torrent of sarcasm that started with this priceless line:

"So [Ahmet's] the great specialist who's never wrong, and I'm just a ticky-tack doctor . . ."

I'll never forget that turn of phrase.

Hedwig turned on me as if I were an opponent he was trying to vanquish, instead of a worried daughter who did not want to put her poor father through an unnecessary procedure. I wish I could reproduce Hedwig's cutting remarks verbatim, but besides the ticky-tack crack, all I clearly remember is his comparison of Ahmet to Mike Tyson and himself to Woody Allen.

Sometimes, he said, Woody Allen wins the round. The hammering heavyweight falls to the cerebral lightweight.

"I like Woody Allen," I said, lamely. Jesus, who wants Mike Tyson making diagnoses?

In 2009 Britt underwent a lumbar puncture in the course of extensive hospital testing to determine what was causing her to have widespread pain and numbness in her extremities, her trunk, and even her face. Afterward, she developed a severe spinal headache that would not resolve on its own. The "headache"—a misnomer that Britt described as "crushing pressure in your head, as if you are deep-sea diving, and the water pressure is squeezing your brain"—eased when she lay down, but she couldn't get up without feeling nauseous and dizzy. She was in wretched condition.

To try to relieve her head pain, which was caused by a leakage of CSF, Britt's doctor ordered an epidural blood patch. This treatment involves injecting a small amount of the patient's blood into the space over the puncture hole to form a clot. Britt decided against intravenous caffeine, another common treatment for a spinal headache, because of all of the potential adverse effects. Delivered directly into your bloodstream, caffeine constricts blood vessels in your head.

Unfortunately, my sister fell into the 10 percent of patients for whom the patch does not work. She suffered head pain for weeks and also developed "paroxysmal positional vertigo" from lying flat for so long.

Like daughter, like father?

I mentioned the risk of a severe headache and Britt's experience to Dr. Hedwig, and he scoffed. That wouldn't happen, he said. He was an expert at performing a lumbar puncture—which, as you might imagine, took me back to Mom's ehrlichiosis crisis—and had never had a patient suffer a headache. What's more, he could do the CSF tap at the bedside with minimal disturbance to Dad.

Much later, I would learn that about 40 percent of people who undergo a lumbar puncture develop head pain. Had I seen that figure, I would have been more adamant about not permitting Dad to have one, but on this day, with Hedwig on the attack, I didn't have data, just anecdotal evidence and a bad feeling.3

After my exchange with Dr. Hedwig, he and his team of about five—residents and medical students—left Dad's hospital room, and I retreated to a quiet hallway to call my sister Leslie, who was flying up that night to relieve me. While I was briefing Les on the latest clinical developments and hotel arrangements, Hedwig and his loyal followers passed by. I'm tempted to call them toadies, but they truly believed in his genius. Sycophants, perhaps?

By the time I returned to Dad's room, Hedwig was well into the lumbar puncture after apparently obtaining Dad's consent.

No one will ever be able to convince me that he didn't deliberately act behind my back, expediting the procedure before I could return and exploiting Dad's vulnerability. Seeing my father, weak and disabled, sitting on the side of the bed, his face turned toward a wall and away from all onlookers, and his pasty white back, as well as the band of his diapers, exposed, while Hedwig pompously elucidated his technique for his wide-eyed minions, saddened and disgusted me.

I thought the entire episode was despicable, but I kept quiet.

Later that day, when Ahmet visited, and I told him what had happened, he just shook his head and said: "I can't stop them from doing what they're going to do." That's a heck of a commentary on medical teamwork, isn't it?

Ahmet advised us that another neurologist would be overseeing the EMG (electromyogram) and administering the nerve conduction test to Dad that afternoon, and Ahmet would drop by tomorrow to talk with us about the results and answer any questions we may have. I had to make sure that Leslie knew to insist upon this consultation.

In an EMG, which I've had myself, a technician inserts needles into your muscles and compares the amount of electrical activity present in your muscles when they are at rest with the activity present when they contract in response to the needles. An EMG can expose nerve and muscle disorders. Nerve conduction (velocity) studies measure the degree of damage in larger nerve fibers, thus revealing whether symptoms are caused by demyelination or by axonal degeneration. Neurologists use electrical probes to stimulate nerve fibers into producing their own impulses and then place electrodes along the nerves' pathways to measure the speed of the impulses along the axons.4

Neither of these procedures is a walk in the park. Compounding Dad's ordeal was the long walk that we took to get to the distant part of the hospital where he underwent the tests. An orderly transported my weary father by wheelchair, but it still wore him out.

The second Sentara neurologist saw the lumbar-puncture mark on Dad's back and asked about it. When I told him its source, he rolled his eyes disgustedly. Thus, the pugilistic specialists were unanimous in disagreeing with Woody.

I asked this neurologist about the possibility of damage in Dad's autonomic nervous system, which regulates involuntary action, such as that in the GI tract and bladder. He said he could test Dad's ANS functioning in his outpatient clinic; I would have to make such an appointment later.

During the painful tests performed that day, I hurt along with my father, but I believed, perhaps foolhardily, that we were on the cusp of finally getting solid advice and knowledge about his neurological condition. Ahmet would pull it all together for us (for Leslie and Dad) tomorrow. I would've liked to have been there, but I was hitting the wall and needed to go home to recharge for a night. Surely my older sister, a nurse, could pinch-hit for me. She could stand her ground.

Wrong.

After Hedwig got word that, as he wrote in the record, the lumbar puncture "showed no elevated proteins to support the diagnosis of CIDP," and the "EMG did not show any demyelination, but rather supported axonal degeneration with a sensorimotor polyneuropathy along with some carpel tunnel"—and Dad refused consent to any more fishing-expedition tests ("Antibodies looking for paraneoplastic cerebellar degeneration were order[ed]" and canceled.)—he couldn't move fast enough to discharge him. I left the hospital at 7 p.m. Thursday; when I reached Leslie at 9 a.m. Friday in Dad's room, the discharge was in the works. Although he had seen me caring for Dad every day, *all* day, Dr. Hedwig did not give me a courtesy call.

Perhaps Woody Allen didn't like being pummeled by Mike Tyson, questioned by a patient's daughter, and/or second-guessed (rejected?) by a patient. On Thursday, Dad refused Hedwig's offer of a lung-nodule biopsy, which, like the spinal tap, he said he could perform at the bedside without causing any harm.

I didn't tell Hedwig Dr. Dorrey's opinion that a transthoracic needle aspiration promised only "low yield," because I didn't have the facts to support it. I would've liked a biopsy, or an oncology consult, but I wasn't going to overrule Dad or try to persuade Hedwig to call in another specialist. Dr. Al declined a brain CT scan, too.

All Hedwig had to do to treat my father was to back off of the tests—and his ego—and discuss Dad's health and diminished life with him. All he had to do was to show concern for my father's well-being. But he lacked empathy. In that sense, he was a ticky-tack doctor.

I talked with Leslie at length on the morning of Friday, Aug. 23, but I couldn't persuade her to insist on receiving the EMG/NCS results and consulting with Ahmet before signing off on the discharge. She wouldn't even ask for the neurologist.

"When they want you to go, you have to go," she said, caving into Hedwig's pressure and lecturing me about discharges. Leslie also worried about getting back to the hotel in time for her extended-hour checkout and not being charged for another night. Small potatoes that I could manage later, I told her, but she wouldn't budge.

Never assume that people in healthcare and/or medicine, nurses or doctors, are advocates. While I understood that, being a new arrival, Leslie lacked a head of steam, I thought her failure to attempt a followup with Ahmet was disappointing.

When I spoke to Ramses later that day and explained that we hadn't received the final neurological report, he told me that the EMG and NCS showed "severe" nerve degeneration. End of story. The full written report, which I received by fax on Aug. 28, consisted of three paragraphs that didn't say much more than that. Perhaps Ahmet wouldn't have, either. It wasn't until six months later, during an appointment that I arranged, that Ramses told me Dad's polyneuropathy would not cause his severe weakness.

Why hadn't Dad's primary-care physician and friend explained this to me in August? Again, he failed to follow through. In the meantime, I assumed a link and spent hours researching idiopathic neuropathies.

What I dubbed the Hedwig effect followed my father to Oakwood, where I had arranged for my parents to share a room as soon as one was available.

Ironically, despite his zealousness about polypharmacy, and perhaps because of his haste to expel Dad, Hedwig made questionable prescription decisions at discharge. Leslie did not peruse the discharge paperwork with him or the nurse on duty, and mistakes were made. The sad truth is that the handoff from me to Leslie and Britt, who handled Dad's admission to Oakwood, contributed to his nightmare. The even sadder truth is that, because of the way healthcare functions today, handoffs between family members *really* matter.

My father and I were not out of touch for long, however. He was quick to call me from his new environs, voicing extreme and loud discontent.

Albert Sjoerdsma, M.D., Ph.D., had never been in a nursing home before, and he hated it now. He didn't think he should have to subjugate his will and self-determination to the will and control of others who didn't know (or might not know) how to care for him as well as he could care for himself. He objected to what was standard operating procedure in a skilled nursing facility, where the idea is that the staff looks out for you because you can't look out for yourself.

Bullshit, said Dr. Al.

Dad was especially incensed that he couldn't keep his medications in his room and take them when he wanted to take them. I explained that nurses would round with medications in the morning and evening about the same times every day, provided they weren't delayed by "emergencies" elsewhere.

Unfortunately, Dad started with a weekend nurse, whom I called Yogi because she was slower than the average bear. Yogi took her sweet time dispensing meds and started at the opposite end of the hallway from Dad's room. Any medications that Dad had on him would be confiscated, so he had to go with the SNF's flow until he (we) could convince the SNF head nurse to go with his.

By Sunday, Aug. 25, when I visited him, my unhappy father was decidedly unwell, coughing, breathing in a labored fashion, and generally acting out of it. What the heck? Was he delirious? Sick? Had he contracted something in the hospital? Over the next two weeks, he went rapidly downhill, sometimes declining to participate in physical therapy—which was the reason he was there!—and transforming from Dr. Frankenstein into his monster, as the nurses, who did not know his history, and I struggled to understand what was going on.

After Leslie and Britt left on Monday, Aug. 26, I was on my own until Al Jr. returned on Friday, Sept. 6. By Sept. 11, when I thought I might have figured out what was happening with Dad, he was a near-psychotic wreck.

NEW BONE GROWTH

Meanwhile, despite the constant fussing of her new roommate (Dad, that is), my sweet, confused, and unbelievably resilient mother was making strides.

On Aug. 29, after I finally succeeded in getting orders from Dr. Steiger for labwork, so I could find out, at minimum, if Dad had an infection, and other actions of mine got a part-time CNA fired—a red-letter day!—Mom saw Dr. Thompson for her last followup. (Again, I arranged Mom's transport, signed her in and out of Oakwood, brought the doctor's orders back to Oakwood, etc., etc. I pretty much lived at Oakwood, or handled my parents' lives there, 24/7.)

Although the fracture nonunion had not improved, the latest X-ray showed new bone growth around Mom's distal femur that supported the broken bone.

There was "no further slippage," said Dr. Thompson, and I could see that was true. The surgeon upgraded his rehab order to "TTWB," which meant touch-toes weight-bearing. When she touched her toes to the ground, Mom put about 20 percent of her weight on her left leg. Thompson also ordered the removal of the knee immobilizer—the useless one that had replaced the expensive one—and the commencement of knee strengthening and range-of-motion exercises.

This was all great news, but . . . I had already expended quite a lot of time and effort to book a Sept. 3 appointment with Dr. Zura at Duke and to plan the trip, and I was not going to cancel it. I wanted to know what an expert on fracture nonunions would say.

I planned to drive to Durham on Sept. 2 and stay overnight. Mom would leave at 5:30 a.m. the next day and travel by private ambulance. Because of her movement restrictions, she would have to lie supine on a stretcher the entire distance, which was a hardship. A nursing aide named Barbara, who took care of both of my parents, but favored Mom, and, therefore, alienated Dad—Roseanne Rosannadanna, remember—would get her up and dressed and accompany her.

According to Dad, Barbara *always* got Mom up, dressed, and ready for breakfast first, leaving him in bed, grumbling and, as likely as not, unprepared for physical therapy when the therapist arrived to escort him to the gym. This infuriated him.

I didn't meet Barbara until the Duke trip, so I couldn't objectively evaluate this complaint. But when he also complained early on about aides taking 20 minutes to respond to his call button, which he didn't use excessively, I knew for a fact that his beef was genuine. I had witnessed such ennui with Mom and other residents when she and I strolled slowly around the facility. Whenever I noticed the call-button light outside of a resident's room illuminated for more than 10 minutes, I would seek out an aide.

One Saturday night at Oakwood, before Dad's admission, I heard a young male resident angrily accosting a nurse, at great length, about the inhumane treatment that residents received from nurses and nursing aides. His chief complaint was their failure to respond, for sometimes as long as an hour, he said. I remember him screaming, "Jesus Christ, somebody could die, for all you care!" The nurse hid from sight behind the door of a room next to the nurses' station, saying repeatedly, "I'm not going to talk with you if you disrespect me like this," but I knew who it was.

On another Saturday night, there was no one on the floor for a full 40 minutes because of overlapping and extended dinner breaks. When a CNA finally returned, she said to me: "We have to eat, too." Yes, but not at the same time, and not for longer than the 30 minutes allowed.

The part-timer who was terminated aroused my ire because she not only failed to calm Dad when he was in a confused and agitated state and help him to get back into bed, she stood by with one of her buddies and laughingly said: "He's a mess." This woman had no idea who my father was or what ailed him. He wasn't an individual to her; he was a nonentity, a mess. But I knew she was one of the malingerers that Dad justifiably had complained about, so I rebuked her.

She wasn't going to put up with criticism from a family member, so we had more words. I was civil, but sharp. By this time, stress was flowing in my veins, not blood. I knew aides had not been properly assisting Mom with her transfers, as well as ignoring Dad. The Oakwood director, Shirley, heard about my confrontation and asked to see me privately. She confided that the CNA was an agency hire who was on probation because of previous problems. She also encouraged me to come to see her if I had any other concerns, and I took her up on the offer twice more.

During my subsequent "Dad's adjustment to Oakwood" meetings with Shirley, she expressed sympathy for his complaints about lost independence and told me that federal regulations of SNFs were moving in the direction of increased resident autonomy and choice. She also worked with me on setting up a structured schedule for Dad, so my father, whose cognitive wits set him apart from other nursing-home residents, would not feel out of control.

While in Durham, I saw for myself how Barbara fawned over Mom, hugging and kissing her, so I started dropping by my parents' room in the morning to check on the status quo. I observed the same doting there and suggested to Barbara that she work with Dad first every other day, but she didn't vary her routine.

In one of my meetings with Shirley, I mentioned the preference that Barbara showed Mom, and the aide stopped coming to their room. I never saw her again.

I could have filled out a slew of incident reports at Oakwood, but I never complained in writing about neglect, and I tried to keep my verbal "requests" of staff to a minimum so as not to appear too demanding or elitist. I worried that Mom and Dad could be harmed by *Just who do they think they are?* backlash. I wanted them both to make it out alive.

Instead, I wrote up "You made my day" reports that complimented stand-out nurses and CNAs on their concern and helpfulness.

MOM'S HEALING

Mom's ambulance transport to Dr. Zura's orthopaedic trauma surgery clinic, and her time with him and his team, came off beautifully. Everyone was exceptionally nice, attentive, and efficient, especially the nurses. Mom had no idea where she was or what she was doing there, but she nonetheless made an important decision that I believe furthered her recovery.

After he'd had a chance to look at new X-rays taken by his technician that morning and the X-rays from Dr. Thompson's office that I'd sent, Dr. Zura talked with me about Thompson's O.R.I.F. and about what, if anything, could or should be done to correct the misalignment.

He was very diplomatic when I questioned him about Thompson's handiwork. He didn't criticize the Outer Banks surgeon, nor did I. He simply said that he would have repaired the fracture differently and told me what hardware he would have used and where he would have placed it. He also told me what he would do in a second corrective surgery, but he didn't recommend one for all of the same reasons that the first surgery was risky—plus the fracture appeared to be stable. I agreed.

Mom spoke during this consultation only when Zura asked her a direct question. I don't think he figured out that she lacked comprehension, although I did tell the nurses that she had cognitive impairment.

I asked the Duke orthopod, who was quite authoritative and commanding, if there was anything that could be done for Mom besides surgery and physical therapy, and this was when our conversation got interesting. After being candid about his financial interest in the product, he advised us about the availability of an at-home ultrasound system that Mom could use 20 minutes a day to stimulate bone healing. Acknowledging that clinical-trial results with the device had been mixed, he said he'd had good results in patients who had nonunion fractures similar to Mom's.

A device that stimulates bone healing through ultrasound. . . hmmm. Being my father's skeptical daughter, my first thought was: What kind of hocus-pocus is this?

But my second thought was: What do you know about ultrasound, anyway, Sjoerdsma?

What I knew was that ultrasonic sound could be used to visualize the condition of Mom's leg veins, the fullness of Dad's bladder, or the development of a fetus, but I didn't know much about using ultrasound for therapy. Later, when I saw the Exogen® bone-healing equipment and learned how to use it, I found it hard to believe that it generated ultrasound of any intensity, much less ultrasound of an intensity to stimulate bone cells and promote new growth.

Aside from effectiveness, cost was a big consideration. Medicare wouldn't cover the Exogen's expense, which a technician, who called the Durham-based manufacturer, Bioventus, while we waited, said would be about $3500. (Zura said "thousands," because physicians like to stay clear of messy money matters, which, I believe, is a major reason why healthcare costs have run amok—yet another lack of accountability.)

I thought Mom's supplemental insurance might pick up the cost (which proved, much later, to be the case). While still at Duke and deliberating, I called Dad to get his opinion, and he deferred to Zura's expertise and Mom's desire.

Yes, yes, yes. Mom voted yes, and she was as animated and as engaged as I'd seen her in months. She adamantly wanted to try the ultrasound. Just the thought of this non-invasive therapy lifted her spirits.

So, too, did Dr. Zura's new order that she put as much weight as she wanted on her leg and work on knee range-of-motion and strengthening exercises, as Thompson had recommended. Mom had been wanting to walk, but Thompson had hesitated in allowing her to do so. Not Zura. He freed her to walk as much and as often as she wanted, writing in his instructions:

"The longer she is in the bed the less likely she is to obtain good functional return to walking. We would recommend bearing weight as tolerated with the assistance of a walker, with the understanding that the fracture may move or shorten, but that the risk of fracture movement is less concerning than the risk to her health from staying in bed (pneumonia, blood clots)."

Zura's liberation of Mom from the wheelchair and all other ambulation restrictions proved to be a watershed moment for her. She never looked back, just persistently ahead with renewed determination and vigor. She amazed and delighted everyone at Oakwood, and soon I began planning for her discharge home.

Chapter Eighteen

2013: Never
EVENTS

Killing Him Slowly

M y father lived in Oakwood from Aug. 23 until Oct. 26—two weeks past Mom's departure date. On Thursday, Oct. 24, while I was on a short break in Alexandria, he called to plead with me to get him out.

"I'm going to die here!" he cried, and I couldn't argue with him. He clearly had plateaued in his physical therapy, and the nursing home itself now posed a danger to his health. Nursing homes, like hospitals, can kill slowly.

During his two months of confinement at Oakwood, Dad was "sent out" to the OBH Emergency Department three times and hospitalized for three days in the Albemarle Hospital Intensive Care Unit in Elizabeth City. He also contracted a life-threatening nosocomial infection. I got so I anticipated the 3 a.m. distress call from either the nurse on duty or my father and always picked up the telephone on the first ring. Instead of getting back on his feet with therapy five days a week, as I had imagined would happen, Dad—to use his word—decompensated.

More than once, I wished I had arranged home healthcare in August and watched over my father myself. But, 3½ years of continuous medical advocacy and caregiving had taken their toll: I surrendered to burnout.

Within a week after the consultation with Dr. Zura, my mother was walking with a walker. Meanwhile, Dad was undergoing monsterization. Increasingly, he missed PT because he was exhausted, anxious, abusive, and/or paranoid (*everybody* had it in for him)—in short, a bad actor. His moods swung like a clock pendulum, and he viewed all but a few staff members with suspicion. He also was having sudden problems with his vision so that he couldn't see to read with his customary eyeglasses. Another blow.

Discharged from Sentara Norfolk with an order for bedside oxygen, he wore the nasal tubing (called a cannula) connected to its supply only intermittently. Many times when he was supposedly receiving supplemental oxygen, the prongs at the end of the cannula were outside of his nostrils! They didn't stay in place. Whenever his O2 was above 90, Dad refused to wear the cannula at all.

I never thought my father was dying, in an imminent sense, but I couldn't deny that he was declining. Inexplicably so. And doctors only seemed to make his situation worse.

THE HEDWIG AFTER-EFFECT

Because of Mom's early-September appointment at Duke, I postponed Dad's return for his second degarelix injection until Wednesday, Sept. 11. I paired his prostate-cancer clinic visit with his month-follow-up appointment in the urology clinic.

Concerned that Dad had worn the same Foley catheter for four weeks, I wanted it to be replaced soon. Oakwood's director of nursing, with whom I had a good rapport, had informed me that her nurses could not remove and replace the Foley without a doctor's order. Because Dr. Terse's PA, Agatha, said he wouldn't order a new Foley without examining Dad first, and Dr. Steiger wouldn't order one without Terse's OK, I battled idiocy on two fronts.

Later I consolidated Dad's two Duke appointments by arranging with Dr. Moul's PA for a nurse from the cancer clinic to give him his injection in Urology. The day before we were to leave, however, Dad called to say that he was too tired to travel, and I had no choice but to call the Duke PAs and cancel my best-laid plans. Considering how he was deteriorating, I couldn't see how Dad was ever going to be well enough to go to Durham, so I reluctantly booked an appointment on Sept. 17 with Dr. Carlson, the bathtub urologist.

I should have figured out sooner what was going on with my father's bad behavior, but I didn't, in part because, with me, he behaved better. He was usually anxious—nothing new there; he struggled with being sick and out of control—but he was not argumentative or brutish.

It wasn't until 9 p.m. on Sept. 11 that I had a head-slapping epiphany. While reading the day's *Washington Post*, I happened upon an article headlined "Painkillers to Get New Warning Labels," about the dangers of opiates and opiate addiction and action by the FDA to address them.[1] I immediately called Dad and told him, "You have to stop taking oxycodone. I think it's screwing up your head, and you're addicted to it."

Dr. Al had told me many years ago that when a person exhibits a sudden change in mental affect or a sudden onset of symptoms that can't be explained logically by illness, one should think of drugs. What, if any, new medications is the person taking?

The answer for Dad was painfully obvious, but I had missed it.

On Aug. 14, Dr. Terse had prescribed oxycodone for post-surgical pain, and Dr. Hedwig had continued this prescription for another month upon Dad's Aug. 23 discharge to Oakwood. (Apparently, oxycodone isn't on the Beers list of drugs to avoid.) Thus, for four weeks, my father had been able to take 5 mg. of oxycodone every four hours "as needed," without physician oversight, and he still had another two weeks to go.

Since Hedwig eliminated his sleep cocktail, Dad had been taking oxycodone nightly "as needed" for sleep, not pain, but the Oakwood nurses didn't know that, and none bothered to question his use as he became more hostile and irrational. On the night of my epiphany, I recalled for Dad how he had "lost it" in the hospital and at home after his rooftop fall. He didn't have a good track record with opiates.

Dr. Al agreed that oxycodone could be distorting his thinking and his personality, and he determined to quit it, *immediately*. He also was experiencing persistent diarrhea, and we discussed his resumption of lomotil treatment.

Five milligrams may not seem like a large dose, but every person's tolerance to a given drug is different; and older people, as I explained in Chapter Twelve, do not metabolize drugs as quickly as younger people do. When I later checked the nurses' medication logs, I was shocked at how often Dad was taking his 5-mg. dose of oxycodone. If Dr. Steiger was monitoring his drug use, he was doing a damn poor job of it.

But I doubt Steiger bothered to look. As I mentioned earlier, nursing-home doctors are phantoms; voices on the other end of a telephone; prescription writers. I laugh whenever other physicians refer to them as if they actually take care of patients. SNFs need their own version of a hospitalist: an M.D. with geriatrics training on site, even if only part-time.

That night, Dad had nightmares about being abandoned by the family and becoming lost in a local supermarket parking lot.

He called me at 3:30 a.m. "I don't know how I got here and why," he said. "I must have used the red car."

"Dad, you're in the nursing home," I replied.

"I know. I've got to go to the bathroom," he said. "Bye." Click.

The next morning, Friday, Sept. 13, Dad and I spoke by telephone, and he told me the details of his vivid dreams. Was he suffering from withdrawal? Dad's first care-plan meeting was scheduled that morning, so I would soon see for myself.

Al and I arrived early for the 11 a.m. meeting and made eye contact with some very solemn faces while we waited in the conference room for Dad to arrive. Clearly, we could not expect feel-good reports from the Oakwood supervisors. No one would talk about Dad until he was present, but after he showed up, no one could.

Our father was stridently uncooperative, angry, accusatory, and paranoid. His impaired mind didn't understand the purpose of the meeting, and he didn't trust anybody in the room, including Al and me. *Who the hell were we to be talking about him? What were we plotting behind his back?* He rejected all of us, in a tirade of abuse, and left.

I didn't know who this impersonator was. He looked like Dad, but he bore no resemblance otherwise to the generous, funny, and loving guy who had nurtured and supported me for decades. This man had lost all reasoning.

Since his admission, my father had slowly descended into incapacitation and irrationality. He had become a willful invalid, refusing to do things for himself that he could easily do, such as fluffing up his pillows or reaching for the light cord above his head. Today, though, my brother and I were witnessing a tragedy, not mere acting out; but Dad was so nasty that we felt like the victims. I thought the chief administrator might expel Dad from the SNF on the spot. Surely everyone believed that, if he didn't have dementia, he was mean-spirited beyond redemption.

After he left, each supervisor detailed Dad's quarrelsome attitude and behavior. He was especially volatile with the physical therapists!

Why hadn't any of these alleged healthcare providers contacted me? I felt ambushed.

I did my best to convince them of my drug-abuse theory: Dad had become addicted to oxycodone. But I was unnerved, as well as aghast. If oxycodone wasn't the root of his evil, what was? What was altering his mind? Was it Hedwig's trazodone? Nursing-home delirium?

After the group dispersed, Al and I went by our parents' room to visit Mom and to check on Dad. He was lying in bed, napping on and off, and jerking and flailing his arms about as if he were conducting an orchestra during a convulsion. The movements always stopped when he woke up and resumed when he drifted off to sleep again. Nurses told me that he had been having tremors, but these were not tremors.

During this fitful cycle, Dad was in and out of lucidity. It dawned on me while I talked with him in a lucid moment that he was hallucinating, and I conveyed this to his favorite nursing aide, Keshia, so she would keep a close eye on him.

Al and I left, pledging to return that evening. We had been back in our respective residences for about five minutes when I received a call from an Oakwood nurse informing me that Dad had been "sent out."

I was astonished: "What? Sent out where? . . . I just saw him. That can't be right."

Already concerned about his "tremors" and his cognitive dissonance, the nurse du jour had seen Dad slip out of bed and become worried that he might hurt himself. The 911 call had been made. My brother and I were off to the Outer Banks Hospital ED yet again.

ER Purgatory, September 13

By the time we arrived—separately, and about a half-hour behind Dad—the physician assigned to our addled father had summarily diagnosed him with a stroke and set in motion the usual overkill of expensive tests. Apparently accepting the nursing-home nurses' clueless account as fact, or at least as the best evidence available, he had headed down the wrong street.

I will never forget standing beside Dad's bed with this somber and unsociable doctor while he pointed out to my brother and me how our father's tired face drooped on the right side. One-sided face droop is a sign of stroke. He also thought Dad's speech was slurred—another stroke sign.

Didn't we think so?

Dr. Unsoc didn't even introduce himself—a pet peeve of mine, as you know. He walked in while Al and I were talking with Dad, trying to catch up with what had transpired in our absence, and pointed at the alleged droop.

Didn't we think so?

Heck, no, we didn't think so. But he did. Ergo, we had a potential conflict, a potential power struggle. You don't need a degree in clinical psychology to recognize when an unsmiling and laconic doctor has graduated from the close-minded school of medicine and might dismiss you if you don't see what he sees.

I swear I don't go out of my way to have run-ins with physicians over diagnoses; I would rather put my faith in physicians. But, here again, was an ageist doctor—or one with an eye on the bottom line—who had veered dramatically off-course, and I had to disagree with his opinion (i.e., his professional identity and ego) without seeming to disrespect it. Such diplomacy is hard work. It's stressful.

"Ahhh, not really," Al and I said, exchanging "Are you kidding me?" glances, before we backtracked: "Well, maybe, sort of."

My mind processed the scene: How much testing should I allow before I approached Dr. Unsoc—he certainly wasn't going to approach me—and spelled out my theory of oxycodone abuse and withdrawal? I knew Dr. Unsoc wouldn't take my word for it. He would need some data, but how much?

When technicians came to wheel Dad to Radiology for a brain CT scan, I told them he wouldn't go for it, but Dr. Al surprised me. He permitted the brain scan, along with the standard-procedure blood and urine tests and chest X-ray, diagnostics that seemed like far more than enough to me.

According to the medical literature, roughly 30 percent of all healthcare expenditure is wasted on "nonbeneficial measures." I would speculate that much of this waste occurs in emergency departments, where doctors take the shotgun approach of excessive testing.[2]

When my friend Lynn's 92-year-old mother fell—actually more like slid down to the floor—landing on her buttocks, but not hitting her head, the ED doctor who called Lynn said he was going to do a CT scan of her brain to make sure that she hadn't suffered a stroke. He said this was standard ED procedure for all elderly patients who fall.

"Why?" Lynn asked. "What difference does it make? You're not going to do anything, if she has." Her mother was already taking warfarin for atrial fibrillation.

"That's true," the doctor answered; treatment would not be affected, "but people usually like to know."

Lynn said if she hadn't talked with me about my experiences, she never would have questioned this test and its expense.

While Al and I waited for labwork and imaging results to come in, I sat with my father and finally got to the bottom of his repetitive dyskinesia—the jerky movements of his hands and arms, the convulsive conducting. He was falling in and out of sleep, and every time he awoke, I asked him: "What were you just doing? What did you see?" And before his conscious mind could override his subconscious mind, he told me.

One time he was picking up pieces of paper that had scattered. Another time, he was drawing back a curtain and looking behind it. Yet another time, he was stacking books. He sincerely believed all of these objects to be in the room and was reaching and grabbing for them. "You're hallucinating," I said. "There's no paper on the ground," no curtain, no books.

I waited until the brain scan came back negative for hemorrhaging, clotting, or any other problem before I made the long walk to Dr. Unsoc's computer terminal, where he had parked himself since his face-droop encounter with Al and me.

"Doctor so-and-so," I said softly, "excuse me, if I may interrupt . . . . I think I know what's going on with my father."

He didn't give me a look of approachability, but he did listen. And he bought my theory.

In his report of Dad's emergency admission, Dr. Unsoc wrote: ". . . Evidently there has been a slow decline over the past week. Daughter thinks this is medication related as he had similar rx to pain meds in the past. I have made adjustments to meds (opiates stopped and trazodone tapered for a week before stopping). Daughter is comfortable with him returning to [Oakwood]."

I never liked the trazodone prescription. Hedwig's antidepressant could be causing some of Dad's aberrant behavior, either alone or in interaction with another drug.

Dr. Unsoc changed his stroke diagnosis to "confusion." If I had not been there, I wonder how he would have proceeded.

Three days later, the diagnosis would be much more serious, but no less bewildering.

September 16

On Saturday, Sept. 14, my father slid out of bed—a near-fall—and fell in the bathroom, collapsing while he stood in front of his wheelchair at the sink. These mishaps occurred without notice by nurses, and without injury, and, thus, did not result in his being "sent out." Dad wanted to get out of bed and stand and walk as much as possible, so his muscles would not deteriorate, but he was undeniably unsteady.

I stayed with him for five hours that day, from 3 p.m. to 8 p.m. At the beginning of my visit, he begged: "Protect me, please." His helplessness cut me to my core, and I promised him that I would. By the end of my visit, however, Dad was excoriating me for mistreating and betraying him. Although I knew he was delusional, his words still stung. I left in tears after Al arrived and sobbed all the way home, swearing that I was "done" with sacrificing my well-being for my father's.

DONE! DONE! DONE! I wrote on a piece of paper that I taped to my bathroom mirror. Burnout was coming more often and more intensely for me. It wasn't fair that I was suffering so much.

That night, Al and Keshia walked with Dad in the hallway outside of his room, and the worst happened: He collapsed, hitting the floor. Yogi was on duty that weekend, and she ran to Dad faster than she'd probably run in 30 years. Fortunately, he wasn't hurt, but everyone was shook up, especially my brother.

Being "done," I took a much-needed Sunday off, while Al tried to watch a football game with Dad at Oakwood. Dad couldn't stay awake. Before his illness, watching a Washington Redskins game with my father had been one of my favorite pastimes. We had been doing it for years. Our football friendship dated back to the 1960s, when Dad first took me to Redskins home games, and I'd had the benefit of season tickets from the mid-'60s until well into the 2000s, when we finally gave them up.

On Monday, Sept. 16, I was still smarting from my father's chastisement when he called at 9:20 a.m. to check in. Unaware of how he'd hurt me, he seemed fine, and with it, but very tired. Despite his fatigue, he was eagerly anticipating physical therapy at 11 a.m. I was hopeful that he had turned the corner, and my trip with him to the optometrist that afternoon would be uneventful. No such luck.

Unbelievably, a nurse called me at 11:30 to say that Dad had been sent out!! Apparently he had been too weak to do PT, and a therapist had escorted him from the gym back to his room. Once there, all hell had broken loose. While seated on the toilet, Dad had passed out and vomited, or vomited and passed out—I was never quite sure—fallen, of course, and, according to the nurse in charge, "aspirated" vomit into his lungs. A blood-pressure drop to 80/40 had brought on the syncope (brief loss of consciousness). The nurse said she had reached down into Dad's throat to clear it of vomit.

Cripe.

This time when Al and I got to the OBH Emergency Department, we found our father in an extra-large room, hooked up to an electrocardiograph as well as the usual monitor for vital signs. The diagnosis at his admission was aspiration pneumonia, according to the physician assistant attending him; but just because he had vomited didn't mean that he had aspirated food particles into his bronchi. We would need more than a freaked-out nurse's word for that.

Dad's systolic pressure had risen from 80 to 110. He was receiving intravenous fluid and supplemental oxygen and was alert and out of respiratory distress. Considering the diarrhea he had been having, I thought he might have become dehydrated. I didn't visit him on Sunday, so I had no idea what his fluid intake had been during the past 36 hours. The weekend nurses may not have monitored it.

The PA informed Al and me that Dad was in and out of atrial fibrillation. Oh, god. Eventually we learned that his urine was clear of infection, according to a quickie test, but his white-blood-cell count was elevated. Because a chest X-ray showed "signs of aspiration" in his lungs, the attending ED physician, Dr. Vallee, who just "consulted" off-stage with the PA, decided to admit him and passed him off to the hospitalist on duty.

I never saw Dr. Vallee. He did not examine Dad nor did he prepare the report that went into Dad's medical records. He merely signed off on what the PA wrote. If you were to read the PA's report months later, as I did, you would have no idea what actually ensued unless you had been there. According to the record, Dad went "home."

V-Tach

The admitting hospitalist, Dr. Keating, knew Dad from his August hospitalization for pancreatitis. She had handled his discharge then and been very helpful to me. I since had learned that she was the visiting hospice doctor at Oakwood. I considered her to be a caring physician and was happy to see her.

Before Dr. Keating's arrival, I had answered all of the nurse's questions about Dad's medical and hospitalization record—again correcting errors that I'd corrected during his earlier OBH visits—and felt like I had an ally in her. Dr. Keating greeted us warmly and explained the reason for Dad's admission, i.e., the aspiration. She then placed her forearms on Dad's chest and leaned toward him, so that her face was close to his. She called him sweetheart, stroked his hair, and told him how sorry she was about his plight.

"We don't like to ask this," she continued, "but we have to . . .," and out came the Do-Not-Resuscitate question. What was Dad's preference?

I had my father's healthcare power of attorney, and the document was on file with the hospital. I knew Dad's wishes about resuscitation, and I intended to honor them. Dr. Keating's question struck me as grossly ill-timed and brought to mind the OBH's robotic former medical chief, Dr. Langard, who asked Mom the DNR question when she was in the ED for a compression fracture. Out of respect, though, I didn't interfere.

Dr. Al said, hell, no, he didn't want to be coded, no extreme measures, and he was emphatic about it. I planned to tell my new nurse friend as soon as Dr. Keating left to disregard what he said, but not more than a minute later, my father was in crisis.

A cry of "v-tach!" went up, and I watched transfixed as nurses came running into the room with big defibrillating paddles.

Was Dad in cardiac arrest? Were we going to see the paddles applied to his chest and his tired, old body bounced?

Dr. Tridecker, the Kitty Hawk cardiologist, happened to be in the ED and came thundering into Dad's room. I had never seen him before. Massively obese, he consumed space and oxygen and bellowed orders. Al and I stepped back toward a wall. Time stood still.

Was this *IT*?

Surprisingly, my precious father was calm. In fact, his facial expression suggested that he was having an out-of-body experience. He seemed to be observing the emergency around him, but not participating in it. I always took my cue from him, so I was calm, too, but I was keenly in the moment. I watched Dad, and I watched the ECG monitor.

V-tach, I quickly learned, meant ventricular tachycardia, which can lead to ventricular fibrillation, which in turn can cause heart stoppage and death. Defibrillation sends an electrical shock to the heart that can kick-start it into a normal rhythm.

As the resuscitation team gathered around him, their energy sky-high, but focused, Dad looked at everyone with soft, dreamy eyes. If he died now, I think he would have died painlessly. It would be devastating for Al and me if he did, but we would be comforted by his peacefulness. I didn't expect him to die, however, because he didn't "tell" me with his eyes that he was dying. They showed that he was still very much here.

Fortunately, the paddles were not needed. Dad's v-tach spontaneously stopped, and the tension eased. My brother remarked to me on the proximity of Dr. Keating's DNR inquiry to Dad's sudden tachycardia. We both agreed the crisis was no coincidence. Keating had precipitated it.

Tridecker decided that Dad's flecainide use had caused both his atrial fibrillation and his ventricular tachycardia and switched his medication on the spot to amiodarone, starting an IV infusion of this alternate anti-arrhythmic drug. Dr. Al was in no position to argue with the big man, and I had no basis to challenge him except for an uneasy sense that he was being rash. Because the OBH didn't have an ICU, Tridecker arranged to admit Dad that evening to the Albemarle Hospital, where he would oversee his care.

While the ED team made arrangements for Dad's ambulance transport, I told the nurse to override his DNR decision. He wasn't ready to die yet, and until he was, I wanted him resuscitated. She readily complied. She also complimented me on my coolness under pressure. It never occurred to me to be otherwise. I was there to help, not hinder. Al acted the same way.

The paramedics finally departed with our father at 7:15 p.m., by which time Al and I had been in the ED for seven-and-a-half hours. We now had an hour's drive to and from the Albemarle Hospital ahead of us. Adrenaline would carry us forward.

When we saw Dad that night in the quiet ICU—there were only two other patients—he seemed better, less pale and weak, but he had traded peaceful for hyper and neurotic. He talked incessantly and loudly. He continued to have a wet cough and some chills, but no chest pain or shortness of breath. He was still on oxygen.

Because of his diarrhea, Dad frequently needed help to get up and use the toilet. The nurse was a muscular former college football player whom Dad pegged for a fullback, and he was right. He got along fine with Dr. Al, despite Dad's many demands and his own inexperience. We pumped the nurse for tales of his heroics and watched some of the Monday night football game. This was not a typical ICU admission.

During our two-hour visit, Dad sheepishly mentioned that he'd "made a mistake earlier." I told him I had corrected it. I knew it was too soon for a DNR. Other than that, I wasn't sure about anything.

ALBEMARLE ICU

The next morning I called the Albemarle Hospital ICU to see how Dad had fared overnight and to find out what was in store for him. I talked with the same nurse three times throughout the day. Besides being concerned about his heart and his presumed aspiration pneumonia, I was interested in getting his Foley changed while I had a means to that end. I later called Dr. Carlson's office to cancel Dad's appointment with him.

This three-day hospitalization would be a difficult one for me to figure, and I never did, even aided by the medical records. Disorders of the heart have that effect on me, generally, but so do medical about-faces, as in "Oops, forget what we said yesterday."

On Tuesday, Sept. 17, Dr. Tridecker's physician assistant informed Al and me that Dad didn't have aspiration pneumonia after all. False alarm. Whatever the OBH radiologist had seen in Dad's left lower lobe was no longer there, and the "crackling noise" in his lung could no longer be heard. A sputum culture showed only normal respiratory flora, albeit a heavy supply. Nonetheless, Tridecker prescribed Keflex®, a broad-spectrum antibiotic, for 10 days.

I continued to think that Tridecker was ordering drugs too casually. Dad already was taking Augmentin, a combination antibiotic that contains amoxicillin, which Terse had prescribed and Hedwig had continued for 30 days. I had told the OBH nurse about Dad's Augmentin use, so it should have been in the record.

Dad also told me that an echocardiogram done that day had produced "crappy" pictures. The message that I received from the PA in the hospital—I did not speak with Dr. Tridecker—was that Dad was fine. Yes, he had atrial fibrillation and had experienced v-tach, but he was now in sinus rhythm. He had not suffered a myocardial infarction.

That day, I went to Oakwood to brief Shirley on Dad's status and to visit Mom. That night I drove to Elizabeth City and spent two hours with my father. He seemed much-improved, albeit very tired. His chief complaint was his immobility. Physical therapists did not visit the ICU.

The next morning Dad called me to complain again about his bedridden status. Knowing that once he transferred out of the ICU to a "stepped-down" medical floor, his care would be a crapshoot, I contacted his nurse du jour and asked her if she could arrange for a wheelchair and allow him to push himself around. She turned out to be a jewel, a true patient's nurse. Sarah spent the day attending to my father's every need and seemed to enjoy the personal attention he gave her, as much as he enjoyed her. I had left Dad's walker, and Sarah found a wheelchair, so he received a lot of exercise.

Sarah also arranged to remove and replace Dad's Duke catheter. Yay! I wouldn't have to think about this bacteria conduit for at least another month.

Because of her schedule, Sarah would spend only a day with Dad, but it was just as well. His ICU stay ended that evening when he transferred into the main "hellhole," a necessary step to discharging him. He called me as soon as he arrived in his new room, which he hated. He also was worried about his atrial fibrillation and Dr. Tridecker's discontinuance of the flecainide upon which he had relied for eight years. He didn't have faith in amiodarone. Of course, he wanted out *NOW*.

On Thursday, Sept. 19, I spoke with Tridecker's PA about Dad's discharge later that day and opted to take the easy way out. Instead of driving to Elizabeth City and overseeing the discharge, including perusing the paperwork—which I recommend that you *always* do for your Mom and Pop—I allowed the hospital to deal directly with the nursing home. An ambulance transported Dad to Oakwood, and Oakwood received the paperwork. Thus, it wasn't until much later that I learned the full extent of Dad's cardiac evaluation.

(When I first tried to obtain his medical records, I was blocked by the hospital's new records policy, which arose after it partnered with Sentara. No longer could I get records upon request by fax or regular mail; I had to appear in person. What BS.)

Thanks to Dr. Tridecker, Dad now had Ambien and Benadryl available for sleep. The cardiologist had not prescribed an anticoagulant, however, even though Dad was high-risk for both DVT and an AF-related stroke.

In light of Dad's falls, the nursing home decided to attach a monitor to his bed and his wheelchair so that if he got up on his own, a dreadful version of "You Are My Sunshine" played. This was tough on my independent-minded father, who couldn't stay still, but it was worse for poor Mom. Disabling the monitor was a difficult job that required a nurse's intervention. Naturally, I took it upon myself to rid Dad of this encumbrance when it seemed an unnecessary precaution. Proceed until apprehended.

I spent three hours with Dad at Oakwood that afternoon, grateful that I could see both of my parents at once and not have to leave town. But there would be no rest for the weary. At 4 a.m., Dad called to tell me that his heartbeat was irregular again. He wanted his flecainide.

KITTY HAWK FOLLOWUP

My father and I spent the afternoon of Friday, Sept. 20, together, and he fretted a lot. Besides taking him to a 3 p.m. appointment with Dr. Tridecker, I drove him all around Southern Shores and Kitty Hawk so he could enjoy being outside in the bright sunlight. He didn't care that much, but I did. It felt liberating.

I planned to drive up to Washington the next day with Al, so we could go the Redskins' home opener together on Sunday. Despite the team's loss, that trip, too, was liberating. My world had been very small—claustrophobic and confining—for much too long. My siblings all had an out. I did not. I was Ground Zero.

Dr. Tridecker allowed Dad to resume his flecainide, even though he thought the drug had caused Dad's fibrillations on Monday. From what I could glean, both flecainide and amiodarone posed boomerang effects: The "cure" could bring on the disorder.

Tridecker also prescribed the antihypertensive/calcium-channel blocker, Cardizem, which Dad previously had refused to take. The frequency of his irregular heartbeats now scared him into acquiescence.

Although friendly, Tridecker had such a loose, shoot-from-the-hip style that I lacked confidence in him. He is the cardiologist whose physician assistant told Dad, upon checking his pulse, that he needed a pacemaker, but I never again heard talk of a pacemaker. That bothered me. I also found it hard to get past the fact that Tridecker was so obese.

A cardiologist might carry a few extra pounds, 20 or even 30, maybe, but 75?

When I suggested to him that Dad's extreme anxiety might be contributing to his heart-rate irregularity, Dr. Tridecker immediately offered to prescribe Xanax®, even though he didn't know my father or his drug history well. Was Xanax, which is a benzodiazepine, like Valium, and a definite Beers no-no, an all-purpose go-to drug for him? Ambien, Benadryl, Xanax . . . Dr. Tridecker was loading up Dad's medicine chest.

I accepted the Xanax prescription, but decided to book Dad's appointment for next week with the new cardiologist in town, who was using Dr. Anthony's former offices on Monday, Tuesday, and Wednesday, while Tridecker had them on Thursday and Friday. The receptionist who scheduled the appointment knowingly told me I had made a good choice.

Indeed. In time, I searched Dr. Tridecker's background on the North Carolina Medical Board website and discovered that he had "issues" similar to the notorious Dr. Naylor's.

Twice since 1999 the N.C. board had suspended Tridecker's license for substance abuse. In the first instance, he had been drunk while on call at the Albemarle Hospital on a Friday night and had stupidly substituted a patient's blood for his own when the hospital demanded a sample for testing. While in his inebriated state, he had implanted a temporary pacemaker in a patient. He voluntarily had surrendered his medical license after this "lapse," but the board reinstated it in short order.

In the next series of charges, Tridecker committed a Naylor-like infraction and flunked a urine test. From October 2002 to February 2004, he wrote prescriptions for hydrocodone and *Xanax* to "Patient A," without actually examining or treating A. Then on Feb. 25, 2004, he provided a urine sample to the North Carolina Physicians Health Program, which is a confidential recovery program for doctors impaired by physical or mental illness, including alcoholism and drug dependency. (Lawyers have their own such programs.) The sample was positive for cocaine and hydrocodone.

Dr. Tridecker, now 54, had been a large-living, coked-up, 45-year-old cardiac surgeon. We had hit the jackpot.

Again, Tridecker voluntarily surrendered his license, which, as any good lawyer will tell you, is a cooperative act akin to showing remorse if you've committed a crime. The board suspended Tridecker's license "indefinitely," and he was without it for four years. Although his record had been clean since the 2008 reinstatement, I was glad to be rid of him. My impressions told me he was off-kilter.

The newly arrived Dr. Newton earned high marks during Dad's Tuesday, Sept. 24 followup when he listened intently to my description of his recent medical history, advised Dad to stop taking his pulse all of the time—he was in and out of AF, which made him very anxious—and suggested that the diarrhea he was experiencing could be *C. diff*.

Newton was fine with Dad taking 200 mg. or more of flecainide twice a day, which was twice his prescribed dosage. This pleased Dr. Al. But it was his C. diff speculation that set him apart. C. diff apparently had not occurred to Tridecker

C. diff, aka C. difficile, aka Clostridium difficile colitis is a bacterial infection in the gut that causes at least three, but most often far more, bouts of nasty diarrhea a day and a host of other symptoms, depending on its severity, including nausea, abdominal cramping and pain, fever, and inflammation and swelling of the colon.

In its worst form, the infection can lead to dehydration, kidney failure, and damage to the colon that can cause a rupture or a perforation, sepsis, and death. C. diff, which is shorthand for both the bacterium itself and the infection it causes, can kill anyone, but elders are more at risk than younger, healthier people.[3]

Newton nailed it.

Unfortunately, this speculative diagnosis would represent his high point. We were still in a medical wasteland.

THE RETURN OF DR. CARLSON

Wasteland or not, my days continued to be chock-full of M.D. consultations.

Britt returned for a visit in late September and helped me to transport Mom, by car, to Duke for her Oct. 1 follow-up appointment with Dr. Zura. The next day, I took Dad to his second appointment with Newton, who ordered more bloodwork.

As always, I observed Oakwood's strict off-site transport protocol and returned with doctor-signed paperwork and updated orders. I also hauled around a heavy wheelchair and tweaked my aching back.

Dad and I went to the Kitty Hawk Regional Medical Center lab on

Oct. 3; and on Oct. 4, I met with Keith and his wife, who was a nurse, about caregiving for my parents. Keith, you'll recall, bear-hugged my father into my car so I could drive him to Norfolk in August.

Oakwood's head physical therapist told me on Oct. 2 that Mom probably would be discharged at the end of the next week. To prepare for her return home, I had to identify, interview, hire, and schedule caregivers, preferably better ones than we'd had the last go-round. Mom also would need home healthcare, including physical therapy.

I couldn't have done this without Britt, not and still remain coherent—especially after Saturday, Oct. 5, when Dad received a definitive diagnosis of C. difficile.

We waited about two weeks for this analysis because the stool specimen that the nursing home sent out to the lab it used was lost by said lab, and the nurses whom I repeatedly questioned about the results wouldn't level with me.

Initially, they told me results would be back within 24 to 48 hours. After two days, I started asking about the delay. Eventually, they had to own up to the lab's error and obtain a second specimen. (The Roseanne Rosannadanna rule.) Meanwhile, we held off on the stool-sample lab order that Dr. Newton had given us, and Dad suffered with multiple bouts of watery diarrhea throughout the day. This was inexcusable. So was the infection itself. But Dr. Carlson beat out the nursing home for most-obnoxious honors.

On Monday, Oct. 7, I took poor Dad to see the local urologist for a 3 p.m. appointment. After parking, but before I went through the back-breaking wheelchair transport process, I checked in with Carlson's receptionist. The waiting room was overflowing with people, and there was no room for Dad's chair. I told her about his C.-diff infection and asked how long the wait would be—at least an hour or more, she said— and if Dad could lie down while he waited. He would never be able to sit for that long. I also worried that he would have to use the toilet, urgently.

The receptionist knew and loved Dr. Al and hated to tell me no. But there was no open bed or even an open room. I had no choice but to cancel the appointment and leave.

That little interlude, although annoying, paled in comparison to the big aggravating interlude that occurred the next day when I returned with Dad for a priority first appointment of the afternoon with the on-again-off-again dorsal slit doc.

Whereas Monday's weather had been gloriously warm and sunny, Tuesday's featured a driving rain, cool temperatures, and a nor'easter. That's the Outer Banks for you. I almost gave up on hauling the damn wheelchair out of the trunk. Instead, I cursed a blue streak and slammed the chair to the ground. Things only got worse when we saw the egotistical Carlson, who was so loathsome, I considered walking out. He earned a new alias: Dr. Menace.

Dr. Menace started by attacking Dr. Al for not waiting the previous day. When Dad and I explained that he lacked the stamina to sit up for an hour, Menace didn't believe it. He thought we were exaggerating Dad's disabilities and doubted the need for him to be in Oakwood! He even dared him to stand! He really raised my hackles when he challenged my assertion that Dad wasn't emotionally up to such a long wait.

"How do you know?" he demanded. "Do you have a degree in psychology? Are you a psychologist?"

I said no, but after years of taking care of my father, I knew his psychology fairly well. And f*&k you, too.

It was difficult enough to fill him in on the medical events of Dad's summer, especially the erosion and removal of the sphincter, but to have to defend myself from Menace's jabs was beyond the pale.

I told him that Dad had been diagnosed with chronic idiopathic axonal polyneuropathy, to which Menace replied: "Says who?"

"He was evaluated at Sentara Norfolk General."

"When? By whom? What's the name of the neurologist? Give me his phone number."

The "interview" went downhill from there. All we wanted was another hormone injection and an order for a new Foley. We wanted continuity, and he was pelting us with offensive questions.

In preparation for this appointment, I had arranged with Dr. Judd Moul's physician assistant to fax the latest Duke records to Carlson's office and had confirmed their arrival a week ago. Of course, Menace hadn't looked at a single page. Not only that, but he doubted the prostate-cancer diagnosis! ("Says who?")

Maybe he was trying to save face, because he repeatedly had failed to do a PSA test or to check Dad's prostate for nodules, but he only succeeded in facing off with me. It wasn't until I mentioned Dr. Moul that he retreated.

"Oh, ho! Well, I certainly know the great Judd Moul," he said, or words to that effect. "He's the one who teaches the seminars on cancer that I attend."

This exchange was exhausting, and it wasn't getting us anywhere. Then it actually got worse. Menace didn't want to ensure continuity with a seriously ill patient; he wanted to start all over.

"Doctor," he said aggressively to Dad, "I'll treat you, but only if you agree to do everything that I tell you to do." First, he wanted to remove Dad's Foley and leave him freely incontinent. Second, he wanted to scope him.

Dad refused. He was not going to lie in urine and diarrhea at Oakwood (while "You Are My Sunshine" accompanied his every move).

Menace, in turn, resisted Dad's resistance until my father finally broke down in tears. Only then did this alleged physician decide to read some of the paperwork that had been forwarded to him and some of the reports about Dad's OBH hospitalizations. I had always thought of him as arrogant and sub-par; now I knew he was just a stupid bastard.

And, still, the torture wasn't over.

Menace abruptly got up and instructed us to follow him down the hallway to the room where he kept his computer. By this time, Dad was barely able to stay upright in his wheelchair and was saying that he needed to lie down. I wheeled my fading father down the hallway, remarking to the nurse and receptionist: "Why doesn't he believe that Dad is exhausted and can't move? Why do we have to go through this?"

Menace read enough data online to realize that he had screwed up, or at least underestimated the extent of Dad's problems, but he didn't rescind his treatment plan, nor did he apologize. After enduring his company for more than an hour, we left. On the way out, I made an appointment for Dad to have a cystoscopy, which I had no intention of keeping, and an appointment at the Outer Banks Hospital for a Lupron injection. The OBH didn't administer degarelix, and Menace knew nothing about the drug.

Once we were back in the car, soaked by the driving rain, I turned to my beloved father, who could no longer keep his chin off his chest, and said: "I'm so goddamn mad. We are never seeing that asshole again. Never."

And we didn't. Less than a week later I called Carlson's office and told the nurse that Dad was done with him. If we had to drive to Norfolk for a lousy injection, we would. Carlson called back and spoke to Britt, not me. He now offered to help. Too late.

MOM'S DISCHARGE

I would've called Carlson earlier to dispose of him, but I wanted to decompress first and calmly examine Dad's options. I also was busy with Mom.

Dr. Zura hadn't recognized his patient, at her Oct. 1 followup, now that she was cleaned up, coiffed, dressed in street clothes, and sitting in a wheelchair. She didn't know him, either, but for other reasons. Britt and I decided that Mom—who griped during the four-hour drive about how long the trip was taking—would have further follow-up X-rays done locally, and we would send the results to Zura.

When I told the surgeon how Mom had flourished after he allowed her to put full weight on her leg and encouraged her to walk, he said: "I just did what the other guy didn't do." Interesting strategy.

Since learning of Mom's imminent discharge, I had been asking for caregiver referrals among my neighbors and other people in the community. Word of mouth is the best way to find someone who is reliable, trustworthy, competent, and compatible with your Mom or Pop. The owner of the local auto-body shop referred me to Sharon, who was not a CNA, but had cared for her mother in her final years and currently had a client in a late stage of multiple sclerosis.

Sharon deserved to be fired many times during her early months of Mom's caregiving—and even later—but I gave her a long rope. She had a good sense of humor, a tender heart, and a sincere desire to improve on her job performance. Most important, I could talk with Sharon. I used the same basic criterion that Dad had with his ologists.

Sharon became devoted to Mom, but there were many times when I thought: "What was she thinking?" Answer: "She wasn't." I had to do far more micromanaging than I wanted to do, but, on the flip side, Sharon followed my directives. She also was a dog lover and took good care of Tony, who was very important to Mom.

Because Sharon couldn't work 24/7, and I hadn't found a second caregiver through the community grapevine, Britt and I talked with The Sitters. Maybe, just maybe, the agency had improved! When its consulting nurse decided that Mom's ultrasound therapy constituted medical practice, and, therefore, Sitters aides could not administer it, we knew that it hadn't. The nurse's liability concerns were absurd. We eventually contracted with the Sitters for overnight help because we had no choice. Sharon handled daytime responsibilities.

The agency sent a personable nursing aide, but then nickeled and dimed us in its billing. The aide would show up at 8:45 p.m. for a 12-hour shift that started at 9 p.m. and clock in by telephone with her supervisor 15 minutes early. The Sitters were expensive, and we had no intention of paying for off-the-clock time. Ditto for when the aide stayed beyond her agreed-upon departure time. Who needs this nonsense?

The overnight assistance lasted only two weeks. Despite her impairments, Mom clung to her independence and objected to having someone sit in the living room while she slept. She could manage, she said, and she *did*.

After Mom's Oct. 11 discharge from Oakwood, Sharon, Britt, and/ or I continued the Exogen treatments for months until the product gel, which serves as a mediator of the ultrasound signal, ran out. That November, after a Georgetown Mini-Medical School lecture about orthopaedic surgery, I asked the professor his opinion of this ultrasound therapy. Professor Michael W. Kessler answered: "With nonunions, it absolutely stimulates bone healing."[4]

Just as Zura predicted she would, Mom regained the baseline status she had before her catastrophic fall. She eventually walked with only a cane and started doing physical therapy at the Coastal Rehab gym.

She never ceased to amaze me. While Dad was deteriorating, Mom was rising from the ashes yet again.

THE SCOURGE OF C. DIFFICILE

I had so much going on in early October 2013 that I didn't have the time or the energy to do my usual disease research. I read enough online about C. diff to get by. Interestingly, when I contacted Dr. Ramses, Dad's Norfolk PCP, to whom we now turned exclusively for advice—Buchanan had not been in touch after the Albemarle hospitalization—I found out that I knew as much as he did.

One fact was indisputable: Oakwood had infected Dad. This was a never event.

Unbeknownst to me, but known to every nurse, physical therapist, dietician, administrator, etc., who came in contact with my father, C. diff was rampant on my parents' hallway, whereas the other two hallways were C.-diff-free.

Dad had started out in a double room with a man on hallway 200, near Mom's original room. Had we known the infection status of residents on hallway 300, we would have vetoed Mom's and Dad's move to room 312, which the automatic-pilot Mr. Hill based on room availability, not on the health of, or—more to the point—the antibiotic use of the occupants.

Clostridium difficile is a spore-producing bacterium that exists throughout the natural environment, in soil and water, for example, as well as in some people's guts.

A C.-diff infection typically occurs in the intestines of a patient who has recently taken antibiotics to clear up another GI infection. Antibiotics can wipe out healthy flora (microorganisms) that live harmlessly in the digestive tract and help to protect the body from infection, leaving a patient vulnerable when he or she is exposed to Clostridium difficile, typically in a hospital or a nursing home. C. diff takes advantage of the gut being out of microbial balance; it grows opportunistically and releases toxins that attack the colon's lining. These toxins can be detected in a stool specimen.

According to the Mayo Clinic, the antibiotics that lead most often to C. difficile are fluoroquinolones, cephalosporins, clindamycin, and penicillins. Augmentin contains amoxicillin, which is a penicillin; and Keflex, the broad-spectrum antibiotic prescribed by Dr. Tridecker, is a cephalosporin.[5]

I was not happy about my father's antibiotic use, but I, sadly, had no knowledge of C. difficile, just a general sense that infections spread in SNFs. Ironically, *after* Dad's diagnosis, I began seeing newspaper articles everywhere about this bacterial nemesis: A noxious strain of C. difficile has emerged and is infecting people who have *not* taken antibiotics, but have recently visited a healthcare clinic. Annual death totals due to C. diff have skyrocketed.[6]

According to the CDC's most recent survey on hospital-acquired infections, Clostridium difficile was the most common pathogen identified among 481 pathogens in 183 acute-care hospitals in 10 states.* C. diff caused nearly 71 percent of all gastrointestinal infections suffered by patients and 12 percent of *all* hospital infections. *Staphylococcus aureus*, a major cause of pneumonia and surgical-site

---

*The 10 states surveyed were California, Colorado, Connecticut, Georgia, Maryland, Minnesota, New Mexico, New York, Oregon, and Tennessee

and bloodstream infections, came in second, accounting for nearly 11 percent of such infections.7

Clostridium difficile passes to humans by the fecal-oral route. People come in hand contact with contaminated human feces and then transmit the bacteria to their mouths when they don't wash their hands thoroughly. They also may spread the bacteria to food, surfaces, and objects that they touch. In institutions, C. difficile spreads between patients mainly by hand-to-hand contact: from infected Patient #1-to-nurse-to-vulnerable Patient #2, who puts his hand to his mouth.

It's possible that my father was infected within a week of his admission. That Oakwood had failed to ensure that its staff, especially its nurses, observed scrupulous infection-control measures, such as washing their hands and wearing protective clothing and gloves, made me angry.

After Dad was diagnosed and my parents' room was tagged for infection control, nurses still put their ungloved hands all over him. I walked in one time to find a nurse holding Dad's hand tenderly in her uncovered hand. To hell with comfort. This was life-and-death here.

I wanted to paper Dad's room with "Keep your bare hands off of him" signs, but I didn't want to presumptively insult anyone. Instead, I sought Keshia's help in caring for Dad. She had a special affection for him and always wore her protective gear.

Although it seems counter-intuitive, antibiotic therapy can cure C. difficile. For mild to moderate infections, physicians usually prescribe a 10-day course of oral Flagyl® (metronidazole), an antibiotic that the FDA has not approved for this use, but has been shown to be effective. Unfortunately, Flagyl often causes nausea and leaves a bitter taste. The potent antibiotic, vancomycin, is typically prescribed in more severe and recurrent cases, but as I would discover, only the oral form is effective against C. diff.

A course of Flagyl seemed appropriate to Dr. Steiger, the alleged nursing-home doctor, in Dad's mild-to-moderate case—or maybe that's what he ordered, perfunctorily, in *all* cases. Unfortunately, the drug made Dad vomit, so he took an antiemetic. After only seven days of Flagyl, his GI symptoms subsided, and the head nurse terminated the therapy. But C. diff is wickedly recurrent: Dad's relief lasted just two to three days.

I argued for resumption of the antibiotic before the results of another stool culture came back, and for a full 10-day course, regardless of symptoms, and Steiger agreed to sign off on that. But it didn't eliminate the infection.

Dad was now eating yogurt and taking probiotics in an effort to introduce healthy bacteria into his gastrointestinal tract that would outnumber and defeat the bad microbes.[8]

I recalled that the mother of an acquaintance of mine had died at Oakwood the previous summer from an infection, which she told me had not been properly treated by Dr. Steiger. At the time, I didn't know or recognize the name of the infection. When I saw her later, she confirmed it had been C. difficile.

MORE ER PURGATORY, OCTOBER 13

Sadly, C. diff was just one of Dad's problems. Two days after Mom's discharge, I received a 3:30 a.m. call from an Oakwood nurse. He had been sent out again.

I had visited with Dad Saturday night until 10:15. Scarcely five hours had passed. What the heck?! The nurse told me he had been on the toilet, stood up, and blacked out. Déjà vu.

I arrived in the OBH Emergency Department to find Dad resting and receiving IV fluids. The diagnosis agreed upon by Dr. Al and Dr. Vallee, who I found out much later had discharged Dad "home" a month ago when he actually went to the Albemarle Hospital ICU, was a "vagal episode." Dad had been having a "large bowel movement," according to the OBH records, stood up and lost consciousness when his systolic blood pressure dropped to 62! The blackout, he said, lasted about 30 seconds.

Drs. Al and Vallee were very casual about this episode. No big deal. For a change, the ED physician did not order an extensive workup. No bloodwork, no urinalysis, no chest X-ray, nothing. I couldn't figure out if Dr. Vallee was being eminently reasonable or eminently neglectful, and so I bluntly asked him: "You're not just diagnosing Old Person's Disease, are you?"

He assured me that he wasn't, but I wasn't convinced. I felt like he was giving Dad short shrift.

I had never heard of a vagal episode, but I knew generally about the vagus nerves' widespread functioning in the parasympathetic nervous system. It seemed odd to me that when a similar episode occurred to Dad in September, no one had used this term. They all talked about aspiration pneumonia.

According to the online Mayo Clinic, a vagal episode, aka vasovagal syncope, "occurs when your body overreacts to certain triggers, such as the sight of blood or extreme emotional distress. The . . . trigger causes a sudden drop in your heart rate and blood pressure. That leads to reduced blood flow to your brain, which results in a brief loss of consciousness."

Other common triggers include standing for long periods of time, being exposed to heat, having blood drawn, and, yes, straining during a bowel movement. (I don't know how much you strain when you have diarrhea, however.)

"Your heart rate slows, and the blood vessels in your legs widen," says the Mayo Clinic. "This allows blood to pool in your legs, which lowers your blood pressure."9

Vasovagal syncope is "usually harmless and requires no treatment," absent injury, the website explanation concludes. But "your doctor may recommend tests to rule out more serious causes of fainting, such as heart disorders."10

Dr. Vallee had no intention of wiring Dad to an electrocardiograph or doing any tests. He pronounced my father normal in every respect and couldn't be bothered to talk with me. Two days later, I took Dad to see Dr. Newton.

INTERSTITIAL LUNG DISEASE

Dr. Newton had scored with Dr. Al when he diagnosed C. diff, but he lost all brownie points when he made another speculative diagnosis: interstitial lung disease (ILD). That's what Newton thought Dad had in his lungs, not metastatic cancer.

I never obtained the cardiologist's medical records for my father, and I can't remember when he first mentioned this diagnosis—it was either Oct. 2 or, more likely, Oct. 15, after the vagal episode—but as soon as he did, Dr. Al wrote him off.

"No way," Dad said, and that was the end of our cardiology consults on the Outer Banks. Henceforth, whenever I suggested that Dad see Dr. Newton, he'd say: "Ann, he can't do anything for me. He thinks I have interstitial lung disease!"

I sat in the examining room with my father during his October appointments with Dr. Newton. The discussion about Dad's AF concerned whether or not he was in sinus rhythm at the time and whether the doctor approved Dad's doubling of his flecainide dosage—from 200 mg. to 400 mg. per day. He did. Nothing else was said about his heart's status. No mention was made of a pacemaker.

I did some quickie research on ILD and learned that it is as broadly defined as it sounds. In fact, ILD represents a variety of illnesses "with diverse causes, treatments, and prognoses," writes Jeffrey T. Chapman, a pulmonologist and ILD specialist with the Cleveland Clinic, not a "specific disease entity." The diagnosis applies to more than 100 separate disorders that can be grouped by "cause, disease associations, or pathology."

According to Chapman, the histologic abnormalities that characterize interstitial lung disease "generally involve the pulmonary interstitium," which is "the area between the capillaries and the alveolar space," rather than the alveolar spaces or the airways. The interstitium allows for efficient gas exchange.[11]

Dr. Newton suggested that Dad had toxin exposure-related ILD. (This, of course, is similar to the causation track that I had considered earlier.) Among all of the environmental, occupational, and avocational hazards that Chapman listed in an online article, however, I couldn't find one that applied to my father. He also had not taken any of the drugs that Chapman identified as associated with ILD, except amiodarone!

I thought Dad was probably right about ILD. But Dr. Al didn't know everything, so when Newton proposed prescribing steroid treatment, I was in favor of it, but only as a last resort and only after Dad was C. diff-free. Curing his everyday misery remained my primary focus.

When the Oakwood healthcare team finally got around to considering a course of vancomycin, it opted for liquid vancomycin, which Dad vomited. I knew vancomycin was given intravenously for serious infections, such as endocarditis, but I had never seen a liquid form of the drug.

Before I got Dad out of hallway 300 and into a safe, C. diff-free environment, I secured a prescription from Dr. Steiger for oral vancomycin. If it didn't cure him, I was prepared to consider a fecal transplant.

By now I knew that severe, intractable C.-diff infections could be treated by a transfer of stool from a healthy donor, usually a friend or relative, to the GI tract of a sick patient. After a donor's stool is diluted into liquid form, it is infused into a C.-diff patient typically by one of two methods, according to Ellen Meredith Stein, a gastroenterologist at Johns Hopkins: by a colonoscopy or, less commonly, by a nasoduodenal tube that runs through the patient's nose to his or her small and large intestines.

Both procedures are relatively safe and are a "godsend" for longtime C.-diff sufferers, writes Stein, especially the 15 to 26 percent for whom antibiotics are ineffective. Most patients feel better within days of the transplantation.[12]

Fecal therapy didn't thrill me, but you gotta do what you gotta do.

DAD'S TRANSITION

When I first proposed to my father that he not move home, but rather into a hotel or a family rental cottage, so Mom wouldn't be exposed to C. difficile, he balked. He didn't like the idea, and I didn't press it. Instead, I let him chew on it while I figured out where and how I could set up a temporary hospital room for him. I wanted to have my plan well-formulated before I approached him again.

I decided to quarantine Dad in the beach cottage, which, like most such houses, had been built on pilings. That was a major drawback: You had to climb two flights of stairs to reach the living space. But I knew that whenever Dad needed to leave for doctors' appointments, I could call upon the Dare County transport service to carry him in and out of the cottage. The stairs were an inconvenience, not a deal-breaker.

That I pulled off this way-station transfer—arranging it and his discharge less than 48 hours after his "I'm going to die here!" distress call—*and* made it attractive to Dad so that he consented, was a coup. As Britt would say, I was cooking with gas.

After Dad got settled in the fancy, and heavy, hospital bed that I'd arranged to haul (with my moving crew) from a neighbor's garage into the master bedroom of the cottage and surveyed how I had rearranged the furniture to accommodate his wheelchair and other equipment, set up a large television, and otherwise provided for his comfort and welfare, he was pleased. In fact, he got so attached to his new digs that he postponed his return home. And why not? He could see the ocean during the daytime and hear it roaring at night. He also had control and privacy.

The cottage plan only worked because Keith agreed to work as Dad's caregiver as many hours as were needed—24/7, bunking overnight—and Keith had the patience of a dozen Jobs. I also hired Keshia, first to do private duty in Oakwood during the days leading up to Dad's discharge, when I was busy with Mom, and later at the cottage. Ever since Leslie had told me in 2002 to be on the lookout for CNAs at Duke Hospital whom I could hire to assist Mom at the convalescent center, I had made a point of noticing the job that nursing aides did. If Keshia hadn't worked out, I had others in mind.

The only hitches to Dad's controlled environment came from outside it, specifically, from employees of Sentara Home Care, which was one of the two home-care services that I could choose. The other was run by the county. I chose Sentara because it had a contract with Coastal Rehab, where Karen worked. Karen was now seeing Mom regularly at home, and I wanted her to help Dad, too.

Soon after Dad's discharge, however, a Sentara supervisor contacted me and asked if its own physical therapist, Penny, could handle Dad's case instead of Karen. Not wanting to be uncooperative, I reluctantly agreed.

On Monday morning, Oct. 28, Penny called me to schedule an appointment and asked nursing questions that seemed inappropriate. I had been through the initial home healthcare interview enough times to know that the nurse arrived first, then the physical therapist. Penny seemed very aggressive. She turned out to be that and far worse.

Emily, the Sentara nurse, called after Penny, and she and I arranged to meet at the cottage before Penny arrived. Emily was of the slower-than-the-average-bear variety and wanted to do as little as possible. I didn't expect much from her except for Foley catheter changes. That Emily and Penny locked horns with each other—Emily was displeased by Penny's overreaching, to say the least—did not speak well for Sentara.

After far too much talk and no action, Oakwood's nursing director had finally persuaded Dr. Steiger to prescribe a new Foley for Dad, assuring him, as I had assured her, *repeatedly*, that he didn't need to see his urologist first. God, what an effort I expended to fight this idiocy! The Albemarle Hospital had already replaced one Foley since his surgery! Use your heads.

The problem was Dr. Terse. His PA Agatha told me that there was a particular post-op test that Terse wanted to do on Dad, and that without it, he wouldn't issue any further orders. She said the same thing to the nursing director, thus muddying the waters.

When I later talked with Agatha about transferring Dad's case to Dr. Carlson, however, she confided that this test wasn't really necessary. Then, when our relationship with Carlson blew up, she once again insisted on this unimportant roadblock. The bottom line: Terse dumped my father. He was a Teflon doctor; nothing stuck to him.

Penny had two sessions with Dad during his first week in the cottage, one of which I attended. Dad's main goal would be going up and down the front stairs on his own. When she failed to show on Tuesday, Nov. 5, for her third appointment, I called to ask her what was going on. She explained that she'd "spaced out" and forgotten Dad. Unbelievable. Now I either had to micromanage her or insist upon Karen.

Ironically, on *that* day, I capitalized on Penny's spacing out.

Although Dad wanted nothing more than to be rid of his C.-diff infection, he didn't trust vancomycin. He decided to take a three-day trial of the potent antibiotic, from Oct. 31 to Nov. 2. When the drug apparently caused him to be extremely fatigued and short of breath, he quit it.

I checked vancomycin on the NLM-NIH's MedlinePlus for drugs and reported that neither fatigue nor SOB was listed among the adverse effects. Of course, drugs have different effects on different people, so I couldn't rule out a drug reaction or interaction, but I thought it was unlikely. I wanted Dad to resume therapy, but I was overruled. Leslie visited that weekend and backed up Dad's termination.

My sister left on Monday, Nov. 4, the same day that my ED buddy, Al, arrived. By Tuesday, Dad's SOB had worsened. When I brought Penny back to Earth, I asked her if she had an oximeter that she could bring to Dad's PT session. She did. Penny's oximeter measured Dad's oxygen-saturation at 83-84 percent. That was much too low. I almost cracked.

A pulmonary embolus? Not *again*. Now in exclusive control of his medications, Dad confessed that he recently had stopped taking the baby aspirin.

Before I resigned to the inevitable, I called Dr. Newton's office to see if I could bring Dad in and let him manage his care. No way, Ann. How about a housecall? Not a chance. I was desperate to avoid the OBH, but I rallied and called 911 and followed the ambulance to the hospital.

Among all of Dad's visits to the emergency department in 2013, this one was far and away the best. Why? Because we met someone I thought was a genuine doctor. When I looked him up online a few months later, I learned that he had already left town. Figures.

BACK TO PURGATORY, NOVEMBER 5

The 30-something Dr. Authentic was a 2006 graduate of UCLA medical school who, during his post-grad training in emergency medicine, had spent a year of residency at Duke. That he was self-assured, competent, compassionate, and knowledgeable only added icing to the cake.

Authentic immediately suspected a clot or clots. When I told him Dr. Al's vancomycin theory, he pronounced it highly improbable and left to research the issue. He returned with a report that only one percent of all patients who take vancomycin suffer fatigue, weakness, or shortness of breath. Wow! *Data*. A doctor after my own heart. Authentic said the only way Dad was going to rid himself of C. diff was if he took a two-week course of oral vancomycin.

"How many cases of C. difficile have you seen?" Dr. Al asked, challenging the young ED doc's experience.

"Hundreds," he replied. "You won't be cured until you take vancomycin."

Dad took his word for it.

When a chest X-ray came back negative for any acute change since October, including emboli, Authentic didn't believe it. "But it's not my call to make," he said. He did make the call to order a chest CT scan, however, and this time the radiologist diagnosed bilateral pulmonary emboli. My father reeled from this sucker-punch.

Later that day Dr. Newton, who was in the ED, remarked to me about radiologists: "If you don't tell them what you're looking for, they won't find anything." How's that for a skills assessment? I think Dr. Jerome Groopman would agree. (Chapter Four.)

Dad needed to remain on oxygen and be transitioned from Lovenox to Coumadin therapy. That meant hospitalization. The on-duty hospitalist admitting him again would be Dr. Keating, whom I asked not to pose the DNR question–*please*. She agreed.

For the first time in the nearly dozen years that I'd been a medical advocate for my parents, a physician mentioned hospice to me. In a three-way hallway conversation that included Dr. Newton, Dr. Keating referred to Dad's "widespread cancer" and encouraged me to consider hospice care. Don't "treat" his disease(s); just minimize his suffering.

She was trying to be empathetic, but I disputed her characterization and told her what I knew about the history of Dad's lung nodules, including the inconclusive PET scan, and his recently diagnosed prostate cancer. If Dad had cancer in his lungs, I doubted it was metastatic prostate cancer. Besides, the presumed cancer was growing slowly—the nodules now measured up to 1.5 centimeters—and I didn't think it was time for a hospice decision. Dad had not indicated to me that he was in intolerable pain nor had he given up on life.

This conversation took a sharp turn when Dr. Newton brought up interstitial lung disease as an alternate diagnosis. Previously, the cardiologist had pointed out on Dad's CT scan what he considered evidence of the disease, but I couldn't see a thing, and Dr. Al still didn't buy it. Newton now proposed hospitalizing Dad in Sentara Norfolk Hospital and having a longtime pulmonologist friend of his do a thorough workup.

Dr. Keating had no problem with this plan and went off to make the phone call to Sentara. I wasn't sure a transfer was a good idea for anyone, but I didn't have time to think. I was standing in Dad's room, explaining to him what had been going on, when Dr. Keating handed me a cordless telephone and said, "He wants to speak with you." The "he" turned out to be Dr. Hedwig! You might as well have handed me a dead rat.

The ticky-tack doctor identified himself, in part by recalling the odious lumbar puncture that he had performed, and asked which daughter he was speaking with: "The blonde or the other one?" He then asked me an open-ended question about the current circumstances, and I started to explain them. When I used the phrase, "He would be admitted at Sentara for a thorough pulmonological evaluation . . .," Hedwig interrupted me: "Not if I don't authorize the admission," he said.

Bam! He had set me up just to knock me down. Here I was in a hospital emergency room where my father had nearly died just seven weeks ago, feeling emotionally and physically spent and trying to absorb Dr. Keating's "terminal" talk and the need for hospice, and Hedwig was giving me a hard time. I thought I might burst into tears.

Dad's alleged healthcare was killing both of us.

Hedwig continued: What was the point in giving a bed to an 89-year-old man who was only going to refuse treatment? Why should he clear the way for "futile treatment of an 89-year-old man?"

The word futile got to me. No one likes to hear her loved one reduced to a mere age in impersonal doctor-speak. But futile? That's a hot-button word. I stopped listening to him; walked to the nurses' station where Dr. Keating stood; and handed the telephone back to her. "I can't talk with him anymore," I said.

His Royal Highness Dr. Ticky-Tack couldn't spare one bed for one night.

Dad remained at the OBH overnight and was discharged with oxygen and a prescription for Coumadin. Dr. Keating said she was seeing too much bleeding associated with the new anticoagulants, such as Plavix®, which are touted as requiring less monitoring than Coumadin does. No matter. Dr. Al would never take a new drug if an old, well-known, and reliable drug were available. Like Mom, Dad would remain on Coumadin for the rest of his life.

My father would never have gone along with a pulmonary workup at Sentara Norfolk, especially if Hedwig were involved. He might have agreed to go to Sentara Leigh Hospital in Virginia Beach, if I'd pushed it, but he thought a pulmonary evaluation was pointless.

I mention Virginia Beach because it turned out Dr. Newton's colleague was in Virginia Beach, not Norfolk. Newton, who never followed up with us on this referral, didn't know the difference.

Penny failed to show for her noon appt. on Thursday, Nov. 7, and I decided I'd had enough of her. I arranged for Karen to take over on Nov. 12 and adjusted to this new lifestyle in which I now depended on "strangers on the yard" in two locations. For the next month, I scheduled and micromanaged three caregivers and quickly came to appreciate how fluid a concept "common sense" is. I wrote a lot of to-do lists and always explained the do's. I knew that Murphy lingered nearby.

ONCOLOGY CONSULT

While Dad was in the Outer Banks Hospital, Dr. Keating helped to arrange an appointment for him with a hospital-affiliated oncologist so he could get his hormone injections locally. I told her of the difficulty

I had been having, and she, like the Oakwood nursing director, knew Dr. Carlson well enough to understand why I wanted to avoid him.

The OBH sent a release to Duke, which faxed Dr. Moul's records directly to the oncologist, Dr. Lan, so I didn't have to act as a go-between, and Dr. Lan, unlike Dr. Carlson, read them! We were making slow progress.

At the initial appointment Nov. 11, Dr. Lan cheered both Dad and me when he advised that the nodules could not be metastases from the prostate or the colon, an organ that I considered suspicious. My father's paternal grandfather had died from rectal cancer at age 90, and he himself had had a polyp (a nonmalignant tissue growth) removed from his colon before age 80, when his Johns Hopkins gastroenterologist told him that he no longer needed colonoscopies. Dr. Lan also confirmed, as Dr. Al had been insisting, that prostate cancer spreads to the bone first and does not present in the lungs as these nodules did. Nor does lung cancer.

Lan could discern much more from Dad's imaging studies than any of the radiologists ever had, so why hadn't Dad seen an oncologist before now? Instead of butting heads with Dr. Al over a needle biopsy, why hadn't Hedwig (or Buchanan or Ramses) brought in an oncologist? I didn't get it.

Lan agreed with Dr. Al that if he wasn't going to treat the nodules, there was no point in a biopsy, although he would be happy to do one. He also offered Dad the option of radiation therapy, which was available at a local University of North Carolina-affiliated clinic. After we left the oncologist's office, I wheeled my father to an OBH lab where he received a Lupron injection. We would be back in three months.

Dr. Authentic was right about the two-week course of oral vancomycin. It cured Dad. I also tip my hat to Keith, who did yeoman's duty in monitoring Dad's bowel movements and cleaning up after him. I was occasionally hands-on, but I mainly read Keith's notes.

Dad gradually weaned himself off of supplemental oxygen, which Britt and I had ordered in tanks, and regained some strength. After decades of weighing more than 210 pounds, he was down to about 189.

"Just get me to Christmas," he now asked of me. First, I had to get him home.

Chapter Nineteen

My
ENDING

There's No Place Like Home

On Dec. 7, 2013, after six weeks of working with Karen to gain some strength and master the cottage stairs, my father went home. Together, with the aid of vancomycin and probiotics, Dad and Keith's round-the-clock care defeated Oakwood's hideous Clostridium-difficile infection.

Just as I had cooked with gas to create his temporary home, I now prepared his real home with accommodations. I knew he would need workspace that he could easily reach by wheelchair, so I set up different stations—for his meds, his mail, his financial affairs. Leslie and Britt arranged to have new carpeting installed that would lie flat beneath Dad's walker and wheelchair. Things seemed to be looking up.

As for Mom, I decided it was long past time for her to try Aricept®, the front-line Alzheimer's disease drug, even though I didn't believe her impairment was Alzheimer's. As far as I could tell, she didn't have any other therapeutic-drug options.

My mother remembered nothing—literally, nothing—about the past six months. She couldn't remember Oakwood, the facility, much less living there and what she did while she was there, nor could she remember how she had broken her leg or why Sharon applied the ultrasound therapy. She had no recall of Drs. Thompson and Zura, her surgery at the Outer Banks Hospital, her two trips to Duke Hospital, *nothing.*

Truth is, if you asked her more than a half-hour after she ate dinner what she had to eat, she couldn't remember that, either.

Dr. Ramses agreed to prescribe 5 mg. of Aricept daily, which Dr. Al still did not approve. Much to my delight, the drug helped Mom and caused her no adverse effects. Her thinking seemed sharper, and she laughed more. Some glimmers of her former self shone through her new duller façade. Even Dad noticed the change. Unfortunately, it didn't last. Just as I'd read and heard from friends whose parents took the cholinesterase inhibitor, the marked improvement lasted only two months.

At 11 a.m. on Thursday, Dec. 19, Karen called to report that Sentara had canceled its contract with Coastal Rehab, effective immediately. She couldn't even keep her 1 p.m. appointment that day with Dad. We were stuck with Penny, who would be on vacation the next week. Because Penny was Sentara's *only* physical therapist, no one would come in her place. Great home healthcare, huh? Merry Christmas!

Over the holidays, Al, Britt, and I walked with Dad and helped him with his strengthening exercises. Al took Dad to his hairdresser and bank, and we divvied up the caregivers' duties, so Sharon and Keith could have two weeks off. All things considered, we enjoyed a nice Christmas.

Dad watched a lot of "Home Alone," which ran continuously on one cable network, and never tired of the scenes when the kid gets the slip on Joe Pesci (a favorite of his) and Daniel Stern. He also discovered G.K. Chesterton and read passages from his novels to me. His vision troubles had cleared. After eight months of caring for my parents full-time, I decided that I would go back to work.

That decision would haunt me.

JANUARY 2014

Britt stayed on the Outer Banks until Jan. 9. Until she left, I continued my research into the cause of Dad's chronic idiopathic axonal polyneuropathy. I uncovered the best hypothesis in a 2004 article in the British neurology journal, *Brain*, about a CIAP clinical investigation that led London researchers to identify environmental toxins and hypertriglyceridaemia (high blood levels of triglycerides) as the causes most worthy of further study.

I liked the stuff about triglycerides, which are a type of fat, and told Dr. Al so. Very high triglycerides, according to the researchers, can result in pancreatitis. They also reported that glucose intolerance—or "pre-diabetes"—which I knew Dr. Buchanan had diagnosed in my father, after tests by Dr. Anthony showed "borderline" diabetes, is "not a significant risk factor" for CIAP.

Elsewhere, however, I read an article by Mayo Clinic investigators who observed that "abnormal glucose metabolism is twice as common among patients with CIAP than among the general population and [possibly] a risk factor for the condition."[1]

Dad, who debunked the diabetes branding, didn't dismiss the triglycerides hypothesis out of hand. Or maybe he was just humoring me.

"Could be," he said, but that's as far as we got because, once again, he was having urinary problems. The misery wrought by Big Guy Naylor seemed to be unending.

Urine was leaking around Dad's Foley, and the device was hurting him. Britt, who also saw blood around the tube, called Dad's new home-care nurse. Joan came out to check the catheter and found nothing amiss. Nonetheless, Dad continued to be in pain. I arranged for an appointment with a new urologist in Virginia Beach, and Britt and I took Dad there on the day of my sister's departure.

The young doctor did an interesting thing when he sat down in the examining room—after not introducing himself. He issued a disclaimer, essentially saying that he was a plumber and plumbing was all he knew, so don't ask him any non-plumbing questions, such as about prostate cancer. He gave Dad a cursory exam and prescribed a bladder-spasm drug for the urine leakage, but nothing for the pain.

"He didn't give me the time of day," Dr. Al complained later, and that was true. If I never see another urologist, it will be too soon.

The only encouraging words from Dr. New Urologist came in regard to Dad's ability to get a new artificial urinary sphincter. My father was a long way off from being healthy enough to undergo surgery, but he was thinking about it. Dr. Terse had advised that he would have to be incontinent, without a Foley, for three months, in order to heal. Dr. New-U said that would not be necessary. He could do the surgery whenever Dad felt up to it. Frankly, I'm not sure if his willingness was a plus or a minus.

For the next week, Dad's status was up and down, as he coped with what he called "penile pain." Eventually, the blood in his urine and around the catheter tube eased and, for a while, it seemed that he might regain some of the functioning he had lost. He was strong enough to climb 14 stairs to his second-floor office, with a spotter walking beside him, and he was optimistic enough to renew his magazine subscriptions for a year.

I now worked during the daytime and stopped by every night to check on my parents. I also spent Sundays with them. I rediscovered my soul-satisfying writer's groove and stopped waiting for the sky to fall. (But, on the downside, my teeth again bothered me, as I endured yet another root canal.)

On Jan. 14, Dad enlisted Keith's help in preparing an income-itemization statement to give to his accountant for my parents' 2013 tax return. He tried to draw me into this work, and I agreed to do a small part, but I declined to spend hours at the dining-room table poring over his financial statements. Keith had a college degree and a background in accounting. He could manage this chore.

Unfortunately, my father obsessed over his tax preparation, an annual task that he always discharged in January, and became increasingly irrational and volatile, a change that I attributed to extreme anxiety, not medication. I eventually relented, but whenever we talked about tax matters, we talked past each other, as if we were speaking different languages. Dad got angry with me, and I got frustrated with him. He never understood what I was saying, even when I was agreeing with him. I overheard him telling Britt on the telephone that "Ann and I don't get along any more. I just can't deal with her."

While my father and I clashed in the evening, Keith reported that during the daytime Dad was lucid and productive. They made progress at the dining table. Dad also participated wholeheartedly in his physical therapy, when Penny bothered to show.

Home physical therapists typically tell you approximately when they'll arrive for an appointment and then run late. Most will call, however, and let you know *how* late. Penny showed no concern for punctuality or courtesy. She also changed appointment dates and times at the drop of a hat.

In retrospect, I wish I had attended every one of Dad's PT sessions, so I would know exactly what was happening. Keith merely noted, "PT today," or "Penny canceled" in his daily log. I stayed away in part because I wanted Keith to step up, so I wouldn't have to manage so much, and I could work more. I also had a lot to handle: an emergency root canal; the dog's sudden illness; my parents' bills and various household concerns, etc., etc. And I wanted an occasional hour of a social life, too.

My father needed a personal assistant, as well as a private-duty nurse, a caregiver, and a live-in family advocate/coordinator to oversee all of the activities and decisions of his life. He was not "heavy, dead evolutionary weight," as Dr. Sandeep Jauhar callously had categorized people of advanced age. Many people still depended on Dad and sought him out for medical advice, *and* he had work to do.

Because Keith did not record detailed notes, I was caught unaware when my father called me at 9 p.m. on Tuesday, Jan. 21, shortly before I was to see him, to say that his catheter had stopped flowing, and we needed to go to the OBH Emergency Department.

I later learned that Dad had called Dr. Ramses that afternoon and requested a prescription for oxycodone, but he hadn't mentioned the catheter blockage, and Keith hadn't encouraged him to do so. (Maddening.) If he had, I probably would have headed to the ED earlier, rather than having to make a decision at the end of a long workday.

I decided not to call 911. I evaluated how much urine Dad likely had in retention, based upon when the urine bag was last emptied, and decided we could wait until the morning to have Joan remove the Foley. That was a selfish mistake.

When Keith arrived the next morning, he said he found pills strewn all over the floor next to Dad's bed, as he apparently had tried Valium, Benadryl, Ambien, meprobamate, and God knows what else, to sleep. Keith threw the pills out before I could examine them, so I had no idea what Dad actually consumed. (Wrong, again.) To say my father was confused was an understatement.

Joan finally replaced the Foley around 2 p.m., and Dad immediately improved. He called me, and I was relieved to hear him sounding cogent and to know that he was no longer in pain. I thought I had dodged a bullet. If I had, then what occurred later was a new bullet.

Keith reported in his log that during the evening Dad had vomited and become "disoriented." When I arrived, he was sleeping. The next day he vomited everything he ate for breakfast and lunch and mostly slept. He got up for dinner and kept down some chicken soup and crackers, but by the time I saw him, he was wildly out of it. For the first time, I was really scared.

"Survival Mode"

Curled up on his bed in a fetal position, my father said he was in "survival mode." He was excessively weak, fatigued, disoriented, and restless, and unable to speak clearly because his mouth was so dry it seemed to be pasted shut. I didn't understand this sudden decline other than, possibly, as a reaction to the catheter insult. He did not have a fever.

Dad's hunkering-down started Jan. 23 and lasted on and off for about a week. When I questioned him about what he was experiencing, he rebuked me, calling me a dictator and saying that he no longer loved me. I was not injured by his words, just bewildered.

Because Dad had trouble completing his sentences, I was often at a loss to understand him. Keith bought him Biotene®, an over-the-counter treatment for dry mouth, but it just made him vomit. He seemed to be in deep mental anguish, as well as physical erosion and pain. But, for some reason, he always rallied in the daytime, getting up, walking, eating, and doing some exercises—or so Keith reported, and Sharon didn't tell me otherwise.

On the morning of Jan. 26, Dad's heart started skipping beats, an irregularity that lasted several hours. He responded by taking more flecainide. How much, I didn't know. He was already consuming 400 mg. of the antiarrhythmic drug daily, an amount Dr. Newton had approved. After the emboli episode, I bought an oximeter at the local CVS and regularly tested Dad's oxygen saturation and pulse. While his heart beat erratically, his blood-oxygen level remained above 90, usually around 95.

My only conjectures, besides his AF, were an infection or a medication reaction, but I was confused by Dad's resurgence in the daytime. Keith continued to tell me that he had physical strength and a good appetite—when he wasn't sound asleep.

I called Dr. New Urologist's office and spoke with his physician assistant, who insisted that Dad would have to be seen before any advice could be given. Well, that wasn't going to happen. She also told me that a urine culture wouldn't be "urologically significant," which Dr. Al regarded as helpful. Without a doctor's order, Joan couldn't get a urine sample, and I couldn't find out if Dad actually had a UTI or another infection.

I was struggling.

Leslie visited for a weekend at the tail end of this survival fight and noticed sediment in Dad's urine. This led me to research causes of catheter blockage, and I came up with what I thought was the most plausible one in Dad's case: catheter encrustation, which occurs when mineral salts deposited on the internal and external surfaces of the catheter block the urinary flow.

Normally, urine is slightly acidic. When natural bacteria living on a catheter turn urine alkaline, mineral salts become crystals. In acidic urine, salts will dissolve.

Encrustation is reportedly very common, affecting 50 percent of all patients with indwelling urinary catheters. A buildup of crystals can be seen if the catheter tube is cut open upon removal. I asked Joan if she did this as a matter of course. She not only did not examine catheters for crystallization, she had never heard of encrustation.

A blockage can cause a urinary bypass or leakage around the catheter; painful urinary retention; and pain upon catheter removal. Removal itself, according to one medical source I read, can result in "urethral trauma," such as I theorized Dad might have.[2]

I prescribed water for Dad, and lots of it, and I asked Keith to measure his fluid intake and output. This therapy seemed to help. By early February, Dad definitely was stronger and more alert and rational. His mouth dryness eased, so he could speak clearly again. I felt hopeful and was surprised when my father told me for the first time that he was dying.

"From what?" I asked, ready to spring into action. Heart? Lungs? A systemic failure?

"My heart is going to stop," he said.

I took this to mean sudden death from a cardiac arrest, so I said, "Then let's go see Dr. Newton. Maybe he can help."

"He can't do anything for me, Ann," Dr. Al replied, again mentioning Newton's improbable diagnosis of interstitial lung disease.

"Then let's see someone else."

He wasn't interested. There was no one.

We talked a little about the nodules in his lungs. "So you don't believe in kitty dander disease anymore," I observed.

"No."

On Sunday, Feb. 9, 2014, I called Dr. Ramses at home and asked him to work Dad into his schedule that week. He agreed. I didn't understand Dad's survival-mode meltdown, and I needed some insight. I knew Dad was having AF episodes that he wasn't telling me about because he had quarreled with Keith over his flecainide dosage. I also could see that he was running out of the physiological "reserves" that I had read about. But as long as my father hadn't given up, I wasn't giving up either.

ANOTHER MEDICAL LETDOWN

I cannot overemphasize how disappointed I was by Dad's Feb. 12 appointment with Dr. Ramses. After telling Dad that he looked much better than he expected him to look—despite his weight having dropped to 180 pounds—the internist then spent far too much of our hour with him talking about a durable do-not-resuscitate order. He even completed and signed a copy of a Virginia durable DNR order, which would have no legal effect in North Carolina.3

Durable DNRs have force outside of a hospital. Signed by a physician and by a patient or by his or her legal representative, a durable DNR relieves emergency medical personnel from trying to prolong the life of someone who has suffered cardiac or respiratory arrest.

"What are you going to do if you arrive and find your father on the floor, struggling to breathe?" Ramses asked me. "Are you going to call 911?"

"No!" my father yelled. "No!"

Excuse me, but could we talk about his survival, please? I needed medical help in understanding what my father was going through. How could it be good for Dad or for me to dwell on his death instead? And did Ramses seriously think that Dad and I hadn't discussed DNR situations before?

When I brought up my father's survival-mode shutdown, Dr. Ramses had no opinion. He gave no advice. Blank. He primarily addressed Dad's health status by ordering tests, the most obscene among them being a full-body MRI to see if his prostate cancer had metastasized to his bones, and if cancer was the reason why he was so weak by day's end. This was an "r/o" or rule-out order.

I had never heard of anything so asinine. Dad had been fatigued and weak for years, in case the PCP had forgotten. Ramses also knew about the full-body bone scan that my father had in *his* hospital just six months ago, upon the order of the charming Dr. Hedwig; and I told him about Dr. Lan's assessment. The idea that Dad's skeleton was now riddled with cancer was preposterous; but if it was, the last thing the poor man needed was to undergo a full-f&*king-body MRI.

At Ramses's direction, the receptionist offered to book an MRI appointment that afternoon in Virginia Beach. I was aghast. Dad would be lucky to stay upright for blood and urine samples to be drawn in the lab just two floors above Dr. Ramses's office. He was fading fast. (Had Keith not been with us, no urine would have been obtained, because the technician didn't know how to get it from a Foley!)

Out of respect, I didn't oppose the MRI in front of Ramses. I told him that we would arrange one in Kitty Hawk. Once in the car, though, I exploded, as I had after Dad's last appointment with Dr. Carlson, exclaiming that there was no way he was going through such a bogus exercise. Surprisingly, my father disagreed.

"He's trying to find something that he can do," Dr. Al said, sympathetically. "I'll do it for him."

Doing something just to be doing something is common in medical practice. It's the authoritative person's search for a fix, any fix, be it ever so much waste. Physicians feel compelled to provide answers and to search for them through testing. For my money, however, all a physician ever has to do is listen, empathize, and take well-reasoned and logical actions, if any exist.

From my perspective, the only good takeaways of this visit were 1) a prescription for a smaller sized Foley (which I had to talk Ramses into writing, because catheters and catheter-related pain are nurses' responsibilities); and 2) a prescription for an antidepressant, Celexa® (citralopram). My father had resumed taking Xanax for his anxiety, but I was concerned about him developing a dependency. Finally, he was ready to take something for his mental distress.

"Are you depressed?" Ramses had asked.

"Of course, I'm depressed!" Dad replied.

On our drive back to the Outer Banks, we listened to Mozart and said very little. Within a few blocks of home, Dad turned to me and said, "I'm dying, honey." That hurt so much on such a deep level that I couldn't respond, not in front of Keith. I encouraged Dad to hang in and told him I would do the same. I wish I had said more. With Mom incapacitated, Dad only had me in whom to confide meaningfully. I didn't want him to feel alone.

After caregivers came into my parents' daily lives, I felt a loss of intimacy and was well aware when I could be overheard by an aide. I didn't like *having* to share private family details with the caregivers, even Keith, and I increasingly cut my visits with Mom and Dad short. Only when one of my siblings was visiting, and the caregivers had the day off, would I linger. I hadn't anticipated how intrusive I would regard their presence. This drive was just another example.

The next morning I called the Kitty Hawk Regional Medical Center's radiology department and reluctantly arranged for Dad to go there later for his MRI. I also called Penny and asked her to delay Dad's afternoon PT appointment.

For a change, incompetence (the essence of Murphy's Law) worked to our advantage. Regional's MRI machine was housed in an auxiliary trailer that could be accessed only by climbing several stairs or by wheeling up a ramp. That day, the ramp was out. After several attempts, Dad—assisted by Keith and me—gave up on the stairs. Had we known, as the radiology technician told us after this failed effort, that the full-body imaging would take upwards of three hours, we wouldn't have bothered to try.

Three hours? Did Dr. Ramses know this? Chances are, he didn't. I doubt that when he or most other PCPs write an order, they concern themselves with how it's executed. Not their department. If he did know, then his judgment was seriously flawed.

I emailed Ramses about the aborted MRI and received in return a report on Dad's labwork, which showed the usual: mild anemia and slight hypothyroidism. There were inflammatory cells in his urine, but the culture results had not come back yet. Fortunately, his BUN and creatinine levels looked good. We didn't have to worry about kidney failure. Ramses suggested 325 mg. of ferrous sulfate daily and prescribed Synthroid® (levothyroxine) for his thyroid.

Dad had been on the hypothyroidism merry-go-round with Dr. Buchanan before, so I didn't expect anything to come of the Synthroid therapy, or of the iron, for that matter. Ramses seemed to miss the point. I just hoped the Celexa, which is a selective serotonin reuptake inhibitor that takes 10 to 14 days to kick in, would relieve my father's despair.

After the radiology fiasco, I texted Penny that Dad had to cancel and asked if he could reschedule to Saturday. I knew Penny would be on vacation (again) the week of Feb. 17, and she had indicated that she might be able to stop by the house on Saturday.

She said she would get back to me. She never did.

On Friday, Feb. 15, Dad investigated Celexa in the "Physicians' Desk Reference" and didn't like what he read. He called me to say that he thought the drug might be dangerous, and I urged him to talk with Dr. Ramses, which he did. Ramses assured Dad that he had many years of experience with Celexa and considered it very safe, especially at the low dose (5 mg. or half of a 10-mg. pill) that Dad would be taking.

Over the next two days, however, Dad vomited so much that he called Ramses again. The internist advised him to quit the antidepressant and the iron, but continue the thyroid medication. He complied and later cut the Synthroid dose in half. The vomiting stopped, but now he was sleeping during the day, when he wasn't eating or exercising, and lying anxiously awake at night. Again, he reached for his favorite nighttime pills.

Vivid Dreams

Benadryl, meprobamate, Xanax . . . my father suffered at night. Coincident with these sleep meds, he started having "strange" and "vivid" dreams. When he told me about his dreams, I thought they seemed more like hallucinations, and I wondered about the drugs. On Wednesday, Feb. 19, he experienced irregular heartbeats again. Over the next two days, his energy diminished, but his appetite improved, until he again vomited. I was beside myself with worry.

I begged Al and Britt to come and stay with Dad, but they couldn't, or wouldn't, come at once. They booked plane fares for March. When Dad slipped to the floor on Thursday evening as he was transferring from the sofa to his wheelchair and couldn't get up, I felt sick and abandoned and wanted to let down and sob. Dad couldn't move, and I couldn't lift him. He needed Keith's bear hug. All I could think was that the past six months of physical therapy had been futile, and I was losing him.

That night Dad had vomited his dinner. The next morning he was also sick to his stomach. Why was he vomiting so much?

I had spent months trying to figure out how I could help my father regain his strength and a semblance of his former life, and I had failed.

During this stressful time, none of the physicians that I took Dad to see ever reached out to him or to me. Dr. Buchanan hadn't called since Dad's emergency appointment in May, and Dr. Eagan never followed up with us about the Loudon referral.

Dr. Terse disappeared as soon as he finished the surgery to remove the eroded sphincter. Dr. Ramses resisted giving me advice, or Dad prescriptions, until Feb. 12, because he hadn't examined my father since December 2013—conveniently forgetting that I had arranged Dad's hospitalization at Sentara Norfolk in August so Ramses *could* examine and treat him. And Dr. Newton didn't follow up his referral to his pulmonologist friend.

I beseeched Dad to stop taking such potent drugs during the night, but he refused, and we argued. He rallied over the weekend, though, and reached out to me on Sunday, Feb. 23. I visited for an extended time on Monday evening. He was extremely tired, but alert. He had decided to stop taking the multivitamin that Dr. Ramses recommended and to resume the Celexa. He had quit taking Xanax about 10 days ago.

That night Dad again had very "vivid" dreams. When I asked him about the drugs he had taken for sleep, he admitted that he had taken some Ambien. His pharmaceutical intake over 24 hours had been flecainide, Synthroid, Cardizem, Celexa, Ambien, and meprobamate.

I could imagine how this mixture could stir up nightmares or hallucinations and do him harm. I asked him to please try to sleep without medication and, if he couldn't, to take just one meprobamate. The next day Dad had his second visit with the oncologist, Dr. Lan, and I was eager for the doctor to see him. He agreed to my medication request.

Around noon on Tuesday, Feb. 25, Penny came for Dad's PT appointment. According to Keith, who filled me in afterward, Dad tried to walk with her, but he was too tired. Penny thought he was malingering, and she walked off, refusing to work with him ever again.

Sentara's only physical therapist had been away for more than a week, and her first response to my father's cry of distress was to reject him. I was livid. I asked Britt to call Sentara to complain, but we never filed an official grievance because we had to go up the chain of command. We couldn't just deal with the immediate supervisor. It was one more odious imposition.

After this scene, Dad called to ask me if I would cancel the oncology appointment. He was exhausted.

"I'm not going to die of prostate cancer," Dr. Al said.

The highly esteemed prostate-cancer authority Dr. Judd Moul had agreed, and I had no quarrel with this point. I mostly wanted Dad to see Dr. Lan so I could get a medical opinion. I wanted to ask Dr. Lan about Dad's survival-mode behavior. Maybe he could help me.

I canceled the appointment.

I saw Dad that afternoon and thought he seemed OK, just very weary and tired. That night, though, his breathing was shallow, so I put the oximeter on his finger. It registered 87-88, too low, but not scary low.

I told him the value and asked: "What should we do about it?"

"Drop dead!" he forcefully replied.

Still smarting from our disagreement about sleep meds, I was hurt.

"Are you telling me to drop dead?" I asked, softly.

"No," he said. "I'm going to drop dead."

"I don't want that to happen, Dad," I said.

The next morning, Keith helped me take one of my parents' cars in for mechanical service, so I got to see both of them while they were still in bed. My mother, who had limited awareness of my father's ailments, complained that he had kept her up all night with "his talking."

When he saw me, Dad asked if "the kids were here." I knew he was talking about my siblings, so I told him that they were not, "just me." He had seen all of them during the night, he said. He also said that he might've called Dr. Ramses.

"I don't think so, Dad," I replied. "I think you've been hallucinating."

His delirium, he said, was "strangely comforting."

While I was talking with Dad, my cranky mother turned down her covers to get up, revealing that she was wearing only a bra and underwear. What the ----! It was wintertime, for goodness sake. Mom had promised me the previous night that she would put on her nightgown after I left. According to Sharon, who had arrived for the day, Mom had slept the night before last in her sweatshirt! Clearly, I could no longer trust her to change on her own. I had to help her.

Around 3 p.m. that Wednesday, Dad called to tell me that the hallucinations scared him, and he was going to quit taking meprobamate and any other sleep aids. He asked me if I thought he should quit the Celexa, too. I again deferred to Dr. Ramses, recalling his confidence in the drug and the small dose.

That evening, I debated over whether I should visit my parents early, before Mom changed for bed, or later, so I could ensure that she put on her nightgown. I decided to work out at the gym first and arrived at 9 p.m. My father was already asleep, and Mom was watching television.

Dad's breathing seemed more labored than it had been, and he was coughing. When I asked Mom about these symptoms, she said that Dad coughed a lot, and he had been fine earlier. Sadly, this once-keenly aware and perceptive woman couldn't help me at all. In his logbook,

Keith had written that Dad had been "in and out of delusions" between 6 and 7 p.m., which made my heart sink. He meant hallucinations, of course. He didn't know the difference. Why hadn't he called me? I would've come immediately.

Dad had eaten dinner at 7 p.m. and gone to bed about an hour later. In a final note, Keith concluded that he showed improvement from the morning.

I thought about calling 911, but I knew my father wouldn't want to go to the hospital. His resistance and the what-ifs of hospitalization, such as the possibility of an endotracheal intubation—its horror was reinforced during the durable-DNR talk with Ramses—stopped me from calling. That, and the fact that he would end up at the Outer Banks Hospital, not at a hospital that I might be able to trust.

If we'd had oxygen in the house, I would've woken him up and suggested that he put the cannula on, but we had returned the tanks. That seemed so stupid now. I considered waking Dad up, anyway, to ask him how he felt, but I worried that if I did, he wouldn't be able to sleep later and would resort to drugs.

I stayed at my parents' home for 45 minutes, running the scenarios over in my mind. I could tell that Dad was not in respiratory failure, but beyond that, I was uncertain. Eventually I decided not to wake my long-suffering father and to check on him in the morning.

I never got the chance.

THE LONG GOODBYE

About 9 a.m. on Thursday, Feb. 27, 2014, Sharon called me:

"Dad's gone," she said.

"What do you mean?" I asked. "He's not in his bed?"

"No, Ann, he's gone. He's dead."

"Are you sure?" A ridiculous question, but it came immediately to my mind.

"Yes," she gently replied. "He's still warm, but I'm sure."

I didn't believe it. I couldn't believe it. It hurt too much to believe it. What would have happened if I had awakened him? Why hadn't I acted?

Although I knew that all a person can do is make a reasoned judgment in the moment, I couldn't stop berating myself. Was I in denial? Did I succumb to burnout?

I hung up the phone and tried to sort through what to do and when to do it. Less than a minute later, I called Sharon back and told her to call 911, but not to let anyone take Dad away. I didn't know anything about removing bodies from homes. I just wanted to see my precious father again, to touch his face, kiss his cheek, and tell him how sorry I was. I didn't want to let him go.

I then called each of my siblings and delivered the news.

The EMS team estimated Dad's time of death at 6:30 or 7 a.m. I could've been there before that time, but, as worried as I was, I just wasn't thinking *this is IT.*

A few weeks before I lived through the worst day of my life, my father, convinced that he was dying, had said about this book: "Now you have your ending."

"But I don't want that ending," I cried out.

Months later, terrible months of corrosive anger, directed toward myself and others, and deep, stomach-knotting grief, I understood that this book isn't an ending, it's a beginning; and my father will never be gone, although I feel his absence and miss him every day that passes. I also survive and prevail. Dr. Al gave me strength.

Dad tried so hard to hang in. He tried so hard not to die. I have comfort in knowing that he didn't want to continue living as the invalid he had become; that he died where he wanted to die, at home in bed next to Mom; and that he probably died quickly. Mom sleeps lightly and would have woken up if Dad had uttered anything. Even so, I don't believe he "died in his sleep." His right leg was hanging over the side of the bed, a fresh abrasion visible on his shin where it apparently banged against the portable commode.

My father suffered a lot in his final months, but contrary to what well-meaning friends said to me, I didn't believe he was in a "better place." How could he be? He was gone forever from the people he loved and those who loved him. My amazing father had always been so vigorous and dynamic and so embracing of life's challenges and pleasures. That he was no longer around didn't make sense: The void was so big that at times I felt like he had never existed.

I couldn't eat and quickly lost 10 pounds, but I managed to remain purposeful and focused. I had to take care of Mom and all of the business of my father's large life and death. Before I did, though, I had to know, if I could, what had happened to him.

Dad's concerns about Celexa nagged at me. On Monday, he had

taken 5 mg. of the antidepressant, and his oxygen saturation had dipped. The day after that, he took another 5 mg.-dose and hallucinated all night. The third dose, death. Coincidence?

I looked up the antidepressant online, and what I read made me heartsick and then angry. No doctor should ever prescribe Celexa to anyone who has atrial fibrillation or any other underlying heart problem, regardless of the dosage. Had I done a little research, I would have known that and told my father not to take it. Instead, I let Ramses, the same doctor who had ordered the ridiculous rule-out MRI, make the call. I also let Keith stand in for me. Now, just seven short weeks after I scaled back my advocacy and resumed working, my father was dead. I was inconsolable.

SEARCHING FOR ANSWERS

According to the online sources I read, Celexa can extend the length of the QT interval in the heartbeat. The longer the QT interval, the longer it takes for the heart to recharge between beats. A long QT interval can upset the timing of the heartbeat and trigger ventricular tachycardia, which can lead to sudden death.

MedlinePlus defines v-tach as a pulse rate of more than 100 beats per minute, with at least three irregular heartbeats in a row.[4]

As I previously explained, an electrocardiogram traces the waveforms—labeled P, Q, R, S, T, and U—that signify electrical activity during one heartbeat. For men, a normal QT interval, which begins with the QRS complex and goes to the end of the T wave, is about 450 milliseconds. At Sentara Norfolk General in August, Dad's QT interval had been 452 milliseconds.

Celexa-induced QT interval prolongation is reportedly dose-dependent. In August 2011, the FDA advised healthcare professionals and patients not to use the drug at doses greater than 40 mg. per day. Less than a year later, the FDA recommended that patients 60 and older take a maximum daily dose of only 20 mg.[5]

My father's 5-mg. dose was much less, but I didn't care. Heavily griefstricken, I became convinced that Celexa had triggered his death. According to reports I read about its other adverse effects, Celexa also could have caused Dad's shortness of breath and delirium. I hadn't forgotten that delirium often afflicts terminally ill people in their final weeks, but Dad's delirium always seemed drug-related to me. He wasn't terminally ill in the any-day-now sense that a cancer patient can be, although he had said that he was dying.

On the day that I lost my father, I spoke by telephone with the local medical examiner, advising him that Dad appeared to have suffered cardiac arrest. When I mentioned the labored breathing I had observed, he jumped to a pneumonia diagnosis, a pattern-recognition conclusion that I discouraged.

Because I was searching for answers and the ME was solicitous, I brought up the nodules in Dad's lungs. He turned out to be an oncologist by training and said the nodules were probably metastases from Dad's prostate, contrary to what Dr. Lan had led me to believe.

That the ME would so speculate without being familiar with my father's history made me question his professionalism, but I couldn't resist asking him about the antidepressant. I described the symptomatic events of the past three days and then queried: Did the low-dose Celexa kill my father?

"Probably not," he replied. Which meant it was possible.

I elected not to have Dad autopsied, either in full or in part. His heart was diseased, and it had stopped. An autopsy wouldn't tell the family any more than that. He could take the undiagnosed nodules to his grave.

The next day I spoke with Dr. Ramses who said that, although he had thought Dad looked good, and he expected to see him for followup in a few months, he was not surprised by the suddenness of his death. Death could move in swiftly with older patients. "Heart attack, arrhythmia, pneumonia, even a pulmonary embolus," he enumerated.

Ramses thought the small dosage of Celexa that Dad had taken couldn't possibly have had a detrimental effect. I mentioned a prolonged QT interval, but he didn't respond to this terminology. He wasn't a cardiovascular physiologist any more than I was, but he did have Dad's history, including reports from the Chesapeake heart specialists and records from his own hospital.

Dr. Lan agreed with Ramses about the low-dose Celexa. He was the third physician I consulted in the aftermath of Dad's death. Lan was very empathetic, but he surprised me when he said, as the ME had, that the lung nodules were metastases from Dad's prostate. I knew for a fact that he had expressed an opposing view in November because I had written down what he had said when he said it, and I had my notes to back me up.

Why he would commit an about-face, I didn't know. Ours was an arranged call, not a cold call. Lan had time to review Dad's records.

Both Dr. Ramses and Dr. Lan assured me that my father had died as peacefully as one can expect. He had lived intelligently and with self-awareness, and he had died in the same manner. Ramses comforted me by saying that I was "right" not to have called 911. Both reached out to me emotionally, for which I was grateful. In this sense, they were healers. If only they had given my father the same kind of healing.

Eventually, I contacted the most erudite and accomplished of my father's former cardiology-clinical pharmacology colleagues—his prize student at the NIH—about my drug concerns. He advised me that a daily 5-mg. dose of Celexa alone would not bring about a fatal ventricular fibrillation, even in an AF patient, but an interaction between Celexa and another drug might. If this in fact did occur with Dad, he thought the most likely offender would be the 400 mg. of flecainide that he was taking daily.

I felt stupid. A drug interaction hadn't occurred to me, but it should have. Dad and I both knew that flecainide was a risky drug and that antidepressants can be dangerous when combined with certain preexisting medications. But we were both off of our games. The small dose had given us false confidence.

According to the Cleveland Clinic, flecainide is a potent antiarrhythmic drug that has "a good safety profile" as long as the patient doesn't have coronary artery disease.[6] Did my father have CAD? I decided to read some of Dr. Anthony's reports, which Dad kept in his personal files, and figure that out, if I could, once and for all.

CORONARY ARTERY DISEASE?

In February 2007, Dr. Anthony noted for the first time that my father had coronary "calcification," which apparently had been detected on a CT scan. A 2007 lipid test reportedly showed borderline elevated triglycerides—which I had read about in the context of chronic idiopathic axonal polyneuropathy—and borderline HDL (good) cholesterol, as well as borderline diabetes. The next year Anthony again reported calcifications and said Dad was "at risk for coronary artery disease."

Hypertriglyceridaemia is associated with atherosclerosis, as well as pancreatitis. Anthony suggested that Dad take a cholesterol agent (a statin), but he never did. I am unaware of other lipid tests.

In 2008, Dr. Anthony reportedly discussed with Dad flecainide's contra-indication in a patient with CAD, and my father had "assumed the risk." Dr. Al swore by flecainide, viewing it as his salvation, and Anthony supported him in this medical opinion, writing on March 3, 2008: "[I]f we just stopped the flecainide . . . and we just leave him on a beta blocker, it is highly likely he would go back into atrial fibrillation."

A chest X-ray done in 2010 at the Outer Banks Hospital after his hip fracture reportedly showed that Dad had "atherosclerotic calcification of the aortic arch." Dr. Anthony repeatedly suggested thereafter that Dad undergo a thallium nuclear stress test, a radioactive-imaging test used to scan the heart, at rest and during exercise (the patient walks on a treadmill), to see how well the blood is flowing. Dr. Al considered this test, which takes hours, to be both dangerous and nonessential, and he always refused. (He also thought cardiologists rang up their bills with such stress tests, and he resented that.)

After Dr. Anthony became ill with cancer and could no longer treat my father, CAD, or the risk thereof, stopped being mentioned among Dad's diagnoses in the various cardiologist reports he received. The emphasis was always on his atrial fibrillation.

In August 2013, however, the cardiac assessment by Sentara Norfolk General included "aortic atherosclerosis." Except for the incident in the Norfolk hospital, I had never heard Dad complain about chest pain.

By 2014, Dad had been taking twice his recommended daily dosage of flecainide for months. An excessive amount, his former NIH associate now suggested. Ramses had been concerned about the dosage, too.

In September, you'll recall, Dr. Tridecker had speculated that flecainide brought on Dad's v-tach in the OBH Emergency Department and had switched him immediately to amiodarone, which also poses dire risks. Amiodarone remains in a person's system for three to six months. I knew this from my reading, and Ramses also told me so.

Regardless of my father's coronary-artery status, Ramses should never have prescribed Celexa for him. It was the wrong antidepressant for Dad, and the Norfolk PCP should have known this.[7]

MY POSTMORTEM

When I finally obtained all of Dad's recent medical records and reviewed them, along with the notes I had taken during his doctor appointments, here is what I could say with certainty about his cardiac health:

❖ My father had paroxysmal atrial fibrillation, which had increased in frequency, and a first-degree AV block.

At Albemarle Hospital in September 2013, the radiologist who prepared the "crappy" echocardiogram—"technically difficult study with suboptimal views, secondary to poor acoustical access"—saw Dad's AV block, as well as left ventricular hypertrophy (LVH), and a "mild to moderate impairment in his left ventricular systolic function." My father was aware of all of these deficiencies.

There was no way that I could evaluate the extent of his left-ventricular-wall enlargement, which I knew occurred with normal aging, or his impairment in systole. But Drs. Tridecker and Newton could, and, as his personal cardiologists, they should have.

If they had studied Dad's records—and I'm not saying they didn't—they would have seen a 2007 reference by Anthony to "mild LVH" and a 2009 note about a "faint systolic murmur," which I'm assuming meant an insufficiency in the mitral valve.

Tridecker and Newton definitely knew about Anthony's 2010 diagnosis of pulmonary hypertension because they either mentioned it during office examinations when I was present or at the OBH and/ or included it in their own recorded diagnoses. When high blood pressure builds in the pulmonary circulation, the right ventricle must work harder to pump blood to the lungs, thus, causing the heart muscle to weaken.

(According to Dr. Adam Myers, a Georgetown University cardiovascular physiologist and pharmacologist, when pulmonary hypertension coexists with long-standing systemic hypertension, which Dad had, it occurs because of left-heart failure.)

An AF-induced increase in heart rate also can increase the risk of cardiac hypertrophy and heart failure. AF, I now learned from simple Internet research, is associated with a three-fold increased risk of heart failure.[8] According to an online interview with cardiologists at the Cleveland Clinic, "different patients have different rates of progression" in their AF. While some patients may not progress beyond paroxysms of AF, as Dad had not for many years, "the natural history of atrial fib is [a] progressive increase in duration and frequency of episodes."

As the duration of the disease progresses, they said, "the ability to maintain sinus rhythm reduces . . . because of the remodeling of the atrium."[9] The atria change. Things get worse.

At Sentara Norfolk General in August, Dad's ECG impressions showed "sinus or ectopic atrial rhythm; first-degree AV block; and nonspecific IVCD with LAD."

An ectopic atrial rhythm originates near the atrioventricular node, so that the PR interval, which is measured from the beginning of the P wave to the beginning of the QRS complex, is short. The PR interval is the time it takes for an electrical impulse to reach the ventricles.

A normal PR interval ranges between 120 and 200 milliseconds; a blocked interval is 200+ milliseconds. In a first-degree AV block, such as Dad had, the PR interval is prolonged, but constant. At Norfolk, Dad's recorded PR interval had been 212 milliseconds. I never knew him to worry about his AV block.

Cardiologists diagnose a nonspecific intra-ventricular conduction delay with left axis deviation (IVCD with LAD) on an ECG when the duration of the QRS complex is greater than 120 milliseconds, and none of the known causes for a widening is present. Among the causes are left ventricular hypertrophy, which Dad had; hyperkalaemia, which is high blood potassium; and bundle-branch blocks, which are delays or obstructions in the electrical conduction on either side of the heart after a signal passes the AV node. I had never heard about bundle-branch blocks.

In the notes that Dr. Tridecker wrote during my father's Albemarle hospitalization, he expressed concern about "wide complex tachycardia" (WCT), which he apparently had seen on Dad's ECG after the ventricular tachycardia stopped.

My research suggests that nonspecific IVCD and WCT are related. WCT is defined as a resting heart rate of greater than 140 beats per minute, paired with a QRS complex of more than 120 milliseconds. It may be associated with myocardial infarction or ischemia (decrease in blood supply); hypoxia (low oxygen saturation); atrial fibrillation with aberrant conduction; medication toxicity (including antiarrhythmics); and electrolyte abnormalities (such as low potassium or low magnesium), among other disorders.

According to the Albemarle Hospital medical records, the OBH recorded wide complex tachycardia while Tridecker was there, but Albemarle did not.

RATE VS. RHYTHM CONTROL

For more than eight years, my father had relied exclusively upon medication to control his atrial fibrillation. Nearly all of the AF rhythm-control drugs, such as flecainide, carry a risk of ventricular proarrhythmic toxicity—the boomerang effect. Amiodarone also can cause pulmonary and hepatic toxicity, thyroid dysfunction, and bradycardia (slow heart rate).

The point of AF rhythm-control is to restore normal sinus rhythm. In contrast, heart-rate control is achieved principally by using an "ablate-and-pace" strategy or negative dromotropic drugs.

Ablate-and-pace, which my Uncle Pete had by default because the ablation he underwent didn't restore his heart's sinus rhythm, effectuates rate control through atrioventricular node ablation and pacemaker implantation. Dromotropic drugs affect the conduction speed in the AV node, which electrically connects the atrial and ventricular chambers. Dad was taking the negative dromotropic drug, Cardizem.

Substantial evidence associates antiarrhythmic medications, but not rate-control drugs, with risk, especially in elderly patients with tolerable symptoms.[10] Until recently, Dad's symptoms had been tolerable.

When I read the notes that Dr. Tridecker made during Dad's Sept. 16-17 Albemarle hospitalization, I bristled. He described Dad as a "difficult historian," which is doctor code for "he's old; ergo, his memory is impaired."

My father was rational and coherent and had no trouble relating his history. I believe Tridecker employed this phrase to C-his-ample-A. After all, he was the one who switched Dad from flecainide to the more dangerous amiodarone.

Beyond that, Tridecker had nothing to offer, nor did Dr. Newton, who didn't follow up with Dad or the OBH hospitalist, Dr. Keating, after the emboli diagnosis in November. Dr. Keating didn't contact Newton, either, to let him know that "Ticky-Tack" Hedwig had shot down Dad's admission.

Newton assumed that my father had rejected his idea of a

pulmonology consult. I could barely speak with him when he told me, during a checkup with my mother after Dad's death, how much his colleague in Virginia Beach had been looking forward to meeting him! (Newton also thought Mom had interstitial lung disease.)

I have learned that atrial fibrillation can cause both anxiety and shortness of breath. My father certainly had both after September 2013, especially anxiety. I never really thought about which came first, the anxiety or the arrhythmia. I just knew anxiety was bad for him. My father always ran in overdrive, and Drs. Tridecker and Newton concerned themselves little with his mental state.

I have read that "optimal" AF management requires an individualized approach, because each patient's symptoms, hemodynamic tolerance, and thromboembolic risk vary widely. That's only common sense and good medicine.

Bottom line: My father needed a good cardiologist to advise him, and he didn't have one.

I wish Dr. Al could interpret for me all of the data that I've now read about his heart's electrical activity. But even without him, I can surmise that the root cause of the sudden stoppage of his heart—which he himself had predicted—was his atrial fibrillation. V-tach to v-fib. He did not have a myocardial infarction.

The effect of Dad's ingestion of Celexa, either alone or in combination with flecainide, will trouble me until an expert assures me, "Ann, no way." But that won't happen because, as Dr. Al told me during Mom's ehrlichiosis crisis, "Medicine is not black and white."

I am troubled by the possibility that the antidepressant pushed my beloved father over the edge, but I am not consumed by the possibility, as I once was. Dad ingested Celexa, along with his 400 mg. of flecainide, for two days about two weeks before he died and experienced some gastrointestinal distress, but no adverse cardiopulmonary effects. He also told me before he took the drug that he was running out of time.

CANCER

I haven't forgotten that Dad may have had metastatic cancer. Finally, I had time to do some research into metastatic distribution patterns, about which I thought Drs. Exeter, Buchanan, and Ramses should know more than they seemed to know. I started with the Internet.

All primary tumors are capable of metastasizing to the lungs. That's a given. According to the National Cancer Institute, which I previously quoted, tumors of the breast, kidney, and thyroid, and melanomas commonly metastasize first to the lungs.

The Cancer Treatment Centers of America, which is a for-profit network of hospitals, says that adult cancers of the bladder, breast, colon, kidney, and prostate, and sarcomas metastasize to the lungs first. Sarcomas are tumors growing from bone, muscle, or connective tissue. The nonprofit Cancer Research UK cites cancers of the breast, bowel, kidney, testis, bladder, and bone, melanomas, and soft-tissue sarcomas as commonly metastasizing first to the lungs.

Breast, kidney, bladder, bowel . . . I turned next to the medical literature.

"[U]nderstanding the distribution patterns of distant metastases from primary tumors," writes a team of researchers from the M.D. Anderson Cancer Center in Houston, has been a therapeutic and intellectual challenge for more than 100 years. The two prevailing hypotheses to explain these patterns, these scientists say, are 1) the "mechanical or hemodynamic hypothesis" and 2) the "seed-and-soil hypothesis."

The mechanical hypothesis, which dates to the 1920s, concentrates on the "anatomic delivery system": The tumor spreads first into the lymphatic system or the body cavity and then metastasizes distantly through the venous circulatory system.

The only problem with this logical hypothesis is that there are exceptions to it. Venous blood drainage and other blood-flow patterns do not predict all distant metastatic sites. The seed-and-soil hypothesis, which was first proposed in a landmark 1889 *Lancet* article, would seem to fill in the gaps.

Nineteenth century English surgeon Stephen Paget described metastases from a primary tumor as a "plant that goes to seed." According to the M.D. Anderson team, Paget wrote that tumor "seeds are carried in all directions, but they can live and grow only if they fall on congenial soil."

A recent challenge to Paget's seed-and-soil theory based on molecular-assay technology now suggests that "tumor cells may be hard-wired early on and that organ-specific metastatic gene expression signatures that are superimposed on a poor-prognosis signature in the parent tumor also may account for the various patterns observed."[11] In other words, tumor metastasis is genetically determined.

The M.D. Anderson researchers sought a better understanding of metastasis in a large study analysis that they performed with known primary tumors registered at the cancer center from 1994-97. I read their 2006 article in the journal, *Cancer*.

The scientists obtained "clinical evaluation-based" data about the metastatic patterns of diagnosed distant-stage adenocarcinomas and then used these patterns to develop algorithms to predict the location of the primary tumors.

Adenocarcinomas are malignant tumors that originate in the epithelial cells of glandular tissue. The researchers limited their analysis to adult patients with histologically confirmed adenocarcinomas of the 11 most common primary sites: the breast, esophagus, lung, liver, stomach, pancreas, kidney, ovary, colon, rectum, and prostate.

Although I read about their methodology, I really have no clue how the M.D. Anderson researchers performed their biostatistical analysis to arrive at their conclusions. What I do know is that the most common metastatic sites among patients with these tumors were the liver (remember the portal vein), bone, and lung. Ninety percent of the patients with prostate primary tumors had bone metastases, while only 5 percent had metastases to the lung.

If I were to use this study of 4,399 patients to predict where my father's primary tumor was located, assuming his pulmonary nodules were metastasized adenocarcinomas, my best guess would be in the kidney or the colon.[12] But Dr. Lan had ruled out colon cancer, and Dad's kidney functioning two weeks before his death was fine.

In 2007, UCLA Medical Center pathologists used a more tried-and-true approach to discerning metastatic patterns: They examined archival data from 3,823 autopsies of cancer patients that were performed between 1914 and 1943 at five Massachusetts medical centers. They found that the most common metastatic targets among 32 different primary-tumor sites were, in order of frequency, 1-2) local and regional lymph nodes, 3) liver, 4) lung, and 5) bone.

UCLA Drs. Guy diSibio and Samuel W. French had access to "carefully documented" postmortem histologic analyses of all organ systems of these patients, none of whom underwent chemotherapy or radiation. The cancers that predominantly metastasized to the lung, but not necessarily first, were breast, kidney, skin, and thyroid.[13]

TUMOR SPECULATION

Obviously, I can't diagnose my father, but I have some satisfaction in knowing that retrospective tracking to an unknown primary tumor, based on metastatic patterns, has been, and could be, done. If autopsies of cancer patients were routinely performed, pathologists could develop "detailed observational templates that highlight expected metastatic patterns" of primary tumors, write Drs. diSibio and French. Pattern templates would be of great "clinical benefit in both diagnosis and treatment."[14]

According to diSibio and French, only one other autopsy study of a scope similar to theirs has been undertaken, and it was published in 1950. You and I both know how often autopsies are done today.

In the few notes that Dr. Authentic, the OBH emergency-medicine physician from UCLA, made in his report Nov. 5 before signing off to Dr. Keating, he said: Dad's "CT in Aug. showed suspicious lesions for mets in abd. [metastasis in abdomen]."

August was when my father was hospitalized for pancreatitis. The OBH hospitalist on his case had told me that a CT scan and abdominal ultrasound had shown no evidence of disease in his abdomen. The surgeon who performed Dad's endoscopy also saw nothing abnormal in his stomach or small intestine except for mild gastritis.

I was confused.

Did Dr. Authentic see something on the abdominal CT scan that no one else did? Where were these "suspicious lesions"?

A month later, in September, an Albemarle Hospital radiologist had seen no "acute abnormality" in the part of Dad's upper abdomen that was visible on a CT scan. This would be the epigastric area where Dad felt so much pain over the summer of 2013.

Fatigue and weakness, which my father experienced from the fall of 2011 until his death, are typical cancer symptoms. Starting in February 2013, Dad also complained of a persistent cough that he could never resolve completely. Then, in May 2013, he started to vomit on a regular basis. Treatment of his pancreatitis did not stop the vomiting. Despite Dr. Lan's opinion, could he have had a cancer in his lower gastrointestinal tract? He certainly didn't think so.

I'm just grasping at straws here, but I do appreciate that a cancer somewhere in his abdomen could explain some of the symptoms that he had in 2013 and his "survival mode" mere weeks before his death.

I do not believe, however, that the assumption made by *all* of the physicians who examined Dad during the last eight months of his life—except Dr. Newton—that the lung nodules were metastases of his early-stage prostate cancer should have been made. His history belied that conclusion. Absent a biopsy, these No-Think doctors apparently preferred an unsubstantiated assumption to a thoughtful investigation.

A logical, open-minded, and knowledgeable physician might be able to connect the dots of Dad's tests and records and reach some probable conclusions, if he or she took the time to do so. During the long months that I advocated for Dad, I never encountered such a physician.

After Dr. Naylor's prostate surgery left him incontinent, my father became morose and beaten down. He was no longer the hard-charging Difficult Patient. Although he rallied after he got the artificial sphincter, he never regained the energy he needed to take on his own healthcare Hydra.

I am not a doctor, and my Dad wasn't Hercules.

PHYSICIAN, HEAL THYSELF

When I look back on the events that occurred and the medical professionals whom I encountered in advocating for my parents during the past 12 years, I see too much thoughtlessness and ineptitude; distraction and detachment; insensitivity and unreliability; arrogance and egotism; irresponsibility and—most of all—indifference.

All of these failures result from or in a systemic lack of:

- ❖ Empathy
- ❖ Respect
- ❖ Compassion
- ❖ Communication
- ❖ Accountability

. . . for, with, and to the patient.

Every honest and caring person working in healthcare today—and they do exist, often in quiet frustration or disillusionment—knows where and why these problems occur and who or what causes them, just like all of the nurses at Albemarle Hospital knew how obnoxious Dr. Rez was. Fixing them is another matter. If I were to take a crack at reform, I would start with a simple proposition:

Physician, heal thyself.

I know the challenge to fix what's broken is daunting, and it often seems to physicians, chiefly because of healthcare economics (money, money, money) or the threat of litigation, that they can't even attempt to effect change, but they have to try—much harder than they do now. The burden of all of these failures should not continue to fall on patients and their families, especially older, more vulnerable patients who, having successfully endured or thrived and contributed to life, have earned your time, care, and attention and really need you.

Far from being dead evolutionary weight, older patients are heads of households, role models, mentors, educators, advisers, leaders, and survivors whose fates are intertwined with preceding and succeeding generations. When you treat an elder, you treat a family, a community, a society, and an era. Rather than regarding their care as pointless, you should consider it an honor.

Once upon a time, medicine was "based," writes Dr. Richard L. Byyny, executive director of Alpha Omega Alpha, the national medical honor society, "on a covenant of trust, a contract we in medicine have with patients and society."[15]

In the past 50 years, with the tremendous wave of scientific and technical advances, the rise of medical specialization, and the corporatization of healthcare, that trust has eroded because the medical profession has fundamentally failed to protect the doctor-patient relationship. Physicians have failed to get out in front of all of these changes and lead the way.

Physicians are the most respected (if not revered) and educated (at least on paper) professionals in our society, but when the healthcare world changed and Marcus Welby died, they failed to stand up for humanity and humanism. Even those who felt a deep commitment to professionalism allowed themselves to be defeated.

Physicians have one sacred duty, and it is to the patient. That means they have to care for the patient's welfare and well-being, not just his prostate, his peripheral nerves, or his heart. A patient is not just an age, a disease, a prognosis, or an anticipated life span. To treat him as less than human—as an acronym!—is to breach that sacred duty, and I don't care how much of a nuisance he is, or how stressed a doctor is.

I agree with Dr. Byyny that the defining principles of medical professionalism should be those enunciated by CANMEDS2000, an initiative that The Royal College of Physicians and Surgeons of Canada established to promote high standards of medical care in Canada and to define core competencies that all physicians need, to wit:

"Physicians should deliver the highest quality of care with integrity, honesty, and compassion and should be committed to the health and well being of individuals and society through ethical practice, professionally led regulation, and high personal standards of behavior."[16]

- ❖ Integrity, honesty, compassion, commitment.
- ❖ The well-being of *individuals* and society.
- ❖ Ethical practice, professionally led regulation, and high personal standards.

These are the ingredients for reform.

Even just observing the Golden Rule—treat others as you would have others treat you—instead of the CYA Rule, would go a long way toward healing what ails U.S. healthcare. If each patient situation were handled with Golden-Rule integrity and compassion, and appropriate checks and balances were in place to ensure high standards, chip-away reform could occur, and out of it, bigger reforms could come.

Where are the "Doctors Without Fear"—or those who are "Mad as Hell and We're Not Going to Take it Any Longer"?—who can found a movement to save medicine and restore sanity?

"Professionally led regulation" should start informally from within—at the insistence of physicians—not with formal complaints filed against them with state medical boards. Cancers should be excised before they metastasize and become too widespread to cure. That means self-scrutiny and workplace reviews to ensure the highest quality of care.

If physicians cannot discharge their duty to patients because, for example, they're blind and cold fish at the bedside (I think of the many distant doctors who formed my mother's ehrlichiosis trail), ticky-tack showboaters in the hospital (the narcissistic Dr. Hedwig), 15-minute turnstile pushers in a primary-care practice (the automatic-piloting Dr. Buchanan), or prideful blowhards (Big Guy and other problem urologists), then they must be neutralized by people whose sole mission it is to look out for patients' well-being.

The neutralizers could be outside consultants brought in to overhaul a system and ensure professional compliance; supervising physician-administrators and support staff who talk regularly with patients, make spot checks, and investigate complaints; and/or facilitators/coordinators who ensure that patients receive clear communications and continuity of care.

Proactive watchdogs and overseers must exist within the medical workplace, doing whatever it takes to ensure ethical, responsible, reliable, and respectful care. I'm not saying that such people don't already exist, especially in large facilities; I'm saying that they must.

BAD APPLES

I also believe that bad apples should be identified and plucked from the crop.

The medical profession is notoriously poor at policing itself—doctors tend to close ranks—and physicians, like lawyers, prize their autonomy and control and resent being told what to do. But it is far preferable to have a professional regulatory authority weeding out the bad apples and improving the orchard, than to have change driven by lawyers and litigation.

There are 70 state medical and osteopathic boards, and I have neither the time nor the resources to evaluate each one's effectiveness. I do know that when state medical boards such as North Carolina's discipline bad apples with slaps on their wrists and admonishments to "do better," they do not protect the public or strengthen the profession, as they profess to do. The bad apple is not the victim. The patient and the public trust are.

While I don't propose to brand disciplined physicians with lifetime scarlet letters, I do think the public has a right to know, through minimal effort, who has been disciplined, when, and why. State medical boards should have a link on their website homepages to an alphabetized-by-physician's-name registry of medical disciplinary case-file records and the actions taken, and physicians should be required to make disclosures to patients after their sanctions. Such exposure might even serve as a deterrent for future bad-apple acts.

I also believe there should be an online registry that informs patients and their families about surgeons' track records. Just how experienced is a surgeon, especially in a solo or small practice, in performing the procedure that he or she is discussing with you? How many such procedures has she performed? Those are difficult questions for a patient to ask, and surgeons have great financial incentive to lie or exaggerate.

The best surgeons will tell patients straight up, without being asked, how many surgeries they've done and their success rate. They may even offer to contact previous patients who have undergone a procedure and ask if they would be willing to talk about it with you. The best will seek to give you all that you need to know to make an informed decision and set your mind at ease. But it's not the best that the patient has to fear.

In one case-control study I read, researchers found that physicians who were disciplined by state medical-licensing boards for 1) unprofessional behavior (broadly defined to include substance abuse, negligence, sexual misconduct, fraud, etc.), 2) incompetence, and/or 3) other violations that constituted neither unprofessional behavior nor incompetence were three times as likely to have displayed unprofessional behavior in medical school than the controls were. Their "pattern" appeared early in their careers.

According to this study of post-1970s medical graduates from the University of Michigan, the Jefferson Medical College in Philadelphia, and UCSF, bad apples already exhibited in medical school: "irresponsibility, diminished capacity for self-improvement, poor initiative, impaired relationships with students, residents, and faculty, impaired relationships with nurses, and unprofessional behavior associated with being anxious, insecure, or nervous."

Hmmmm, maybe they just weren't cut out to be doctors.

Examples offered of "diminished capacity for self-improvement" included a "failure to accept constructive criticism" and "argumentativeness." Low MCAT (Medical College Admission Test) scores and low grades in the first two years of medical school were also significant predictors of later unprofessional behavior.[17]

I ponder the duty, if any, medical schools should have to future patients of those graduates who they know or have reason to believe will not conduct themselves professionally. I'll bet if you probed Dr. Naylor's and Dr. Tridecker's backgrounds, you'd find behavioral red flags. I doubt their professors would be surprised to learn of their later troubles.

Medical schools lay and develop the foundation for physicians' professionalism, humanism, and clinical skills through educational and training environments and experiences. I've read about how bright and altruistic young medical students get transformed during their matriculation into detached and disillusioned road kill. Not only are educators aware of the shortfalls among their graduates in integrity, character, and compassion—as well as in diagnostic and other clinical skills—they recognize their own complicity.

If I had a say in medical education, I would integrate into it as much problem-based learning, as possible, and I would compel medical students to ask "what if?" in changing scenarios. Brainstorm questions, not answers. Don't stop thinking and don't let technology do your thinking for you.

I also would introduce students to the real world of human life, not just life in clinics, so they would begin to appreciate its heterogeneity, if they don't already. I would arrange interviews for first-year students, who are the least jaded, with a cross-section of humanity, especially older adults who are healthy and belie ageist stereotypes.

I further would require prospective medical students to take literature courses. Yes, you have to read more than science textbooks if you want to treat patients. If you don't, sorry, you only get a Ph.D.

In an article about developing physicians, Drs. David T. Stern and Maxine Papadakis of the University of Michigan and UCSF, respectively, asked their medical-education peers to consider "whether we are cultivating in current students and residents the professional behaviors we would seek should we need medical care."[18]

Well?

TRANSFORMING PRIMARY CARE

In the past 20 years, 30 to 40 percent of doctors surveyed about their professional satisfaction reportedly said they would not choose medicine again as a career, and an even higher percentage would not encourage their children to do so. The dissatisfied typically cite as deterrents such factors as income, workload, and time consumed by administrative tasks, all of which are issues for the primary-care physician, whose income is not as much as the ologists' and whose workload and administrative time are excessive.[19]

The solution for the primary-care doctor, who is the No. 1 head of the healthcare Hydra, and his or her patients, is not to abandon medicine, but to abandon the primary-care practice model. The PCP's *modus operandi* needs to be revamped, so that it better meets patients' needs, first, which, in turn, will lead to meeting the PCP's needs, second.

New practice models have emerged, but too many take the easy capitalistic way out, making access to healthcare even more obviously contingent on patients' wealth. Driven by dwindling insurance reimbursements and the need to increase revenues, some PCPs have started concierge or retainer practices so that they can reduce the number of patients they see, but not lose income.

In a concierge practice—some of which are quite VIP and costly—patients buy guaranteed access to physicians, more personal time with them, top specialist referrals, and other advantages by paying monthly fees or an annual retainer. A retainer practice allows for increased access and longer appointment times, with the payment of fees, but offers fewer perks than the concierge practice does.

Concierge medicine makes the fulfillment of a physician's duty to a patient contingent on an extra fee being paid. It doesn't thrill me that the patient pays the physician to do what he/she should do anyway, without more money. I also don't know that concierge medicine fixes some of what ails traditional practices.

Consider Duke Signature Care, the Duke University Health System's concierge medicine that "encourages you to develop a richer, more meaningful relationship with your doctor." For an annual $2,000 retainer, you can buy into the following benefits:

- ❖ "Low patient-to-doctor ratios," enabling you to enjoy "more one-on-one time" with your PCP;

- ❖ "Unparalleled convenience," enabling you to arrange immediate or next-day appointments;

- ❖ "Expanded physician access," enabling you to reach your doctor by telephone after hours or while you're traveling;

- ❖ "Secure electronic medical records connection," enabling you to easily view lab results, request prescription refills, communicate with your doctor, and pay bills;

- ❖ "Specialty care referrals," enabling you to be seen by "specialists who are ranked among the nation's best";

- ❖ [A] "Comfortable environment," offering you "free, convenient parking and spacious, comfortable waiting rooms with complimentary wifi and coffee or tea"; and

❖ [A] "Skilled, compassionate team," enabling you to work and talk with the same group of "dedicated nursing, administrative, and clerical staff," who will "get to know you, and you them."[20]

So, does this mean that, when I arrive for my appointment, I can be assured that:

❖ My doctor has prepared for it by reading and re-familiarizing him or herself with my file/my history? Or, if he/she hasn't, a member of the "skilled, compassionate team" has briefed him?

❖ My doctor has read all of the ologists' reports, reflected upon them, calling the ologists themselves, if necessary, and is going to talk with me about their findings?

❖ My doctor will follow up with me after I've left his/her sight?

❖ My doctor will not prescribe any drugs that are counterindicated?

❖ My doctor will send (or post online in my electronic record, if I so request) a copy of the medical report of my appointment, so I won't have to contact the records clerk later? And he/she will have committed to writing an accurate and thorough account of my complaints and the dialogue we had about them?

What I would like a PCP to guarantee to a patient, especially an elder, is time spent in thoughtful preparation, continuity of care, and followup; safe and *informed* prescription-writing, so patients don't have to resort to the "PDR" to learn about the potential risks of medications (and daughters aren't left with regrets); accurate record-keeping; and actual medical advice, not just a litany of diagnoses.

Is concierge medicine conscientious or just convenient?

Primary-care reformer Dr. Thomas Bodenheimer of the UCSF School of Medicine proposes an alternate model that seems quite sensible to me, inasmuch as I believe that the PCP-patient relationship breaks down into readily discernible tasks, not all of which need to be performed by the doctor, but which must be overseen by the doctor or a responsible second in command.

Bodenheimer's "teamlet" (little team) model of primary care consists of a clinician and two health coaches, who are trained from among such people as medical assistants, community health workers, and licensed practical nurses. A teamlet clinical (patient) encounter involves four parts: a previsit by the coach; a visit by the clinician with the coach; a postvisit by the coach; and between-visit care by the coach. Depending on patient need, the clinician could be a nurse practitioner or a physician assistant instead of a physician.[21]

Bodenheimer aspires to replace the 15-minute physician visit with actual healthcare. I'd say this is a step in a better direction than the surcharge models.

Currently a sea change is under way in healthcare to convert and store patients' paper records as electronic files that can be easily accessed by patients and all of their physicians. Experts say we probably won't know for about 20 years how the electronic conversion will affect medical practice. According to Dr. Paul B. Rothman, the dean of the Johns Hopkins School of Medicine, that's how long the "transition in utilizing technology" will take.

"It's a cultural change," he says, and right now, "we're not in a good place."[22]

Call me a skeptic, but I don't think this change will reduce the number of errors being committed, much less eliminate No-Think and ageism.

If physicians show patients professionalism, patients will respond with trust and respect, and physicians just might enjoy their work more. What we need is a doctor-patient revolution that takes us back to the roots of good medicine without jacking up the costs. Payers and policymakers need to be on board, but physicians must conduct the runaway train.

PATIENT ADVOCACY

During one of my many visits to the Duke Urology Clinic, I spoke with a friendly and experienced nurse about the subject of my book.

"Oh, patient advocacy is so important," she said enthusiastically, "even here at Duke. I see situations all of the time when a patient needs an advocate."

There should be a line on a patient's hospital intake form for identification of his or her advocate. Your Mom and Pop *and* you need an advocate. Some hospitals offer on-site patient advocates, but these advocates work for the hospital, not necessarily for you. They can work to your advantage, however.

Just suggesting that she would arrange a meeting with a N.Y. hospital's patient advocate and her own attorney enabled my friend Louise to thwart the premature discharge of her seriously ill and pain-stricken 93-year-old mother, who had been neglected by doctors.

Louise, who lives in North Carolina, dealt first by telephone and then in person with a hospital case worker, who wanted to ship her mother out to a nursing home—any old nursing home, sight unseen by family—after doctors ascertained that the older woman's heart was stable. But her heart wasn't causing the pain in her hip, which no one had addressed.

Outside of hospitals, patient advocates can be found in for-profit (employer-based) and non-profit organizations, as well as in independent businesses. If you search "patient advocate" online, you'll find a number of resources, such as the Professional Patient Advocate Institute; Patient Advocates LLC, a Maine-based corporation; and the Boston-based non-profit Health Care for All. (Patient "navigators" usually assist cancer patients in the healthcare system.)

The patient-advocacy field has not evolved enough for a consumer to rely on an Internet referral, regardless of how much due diligence you do. I also am not keen on the way the field is shaping up.

Patient advocacy has emerged as a lay specialization within the healthcare industry. Advocates typically have a background in nursing, social work, counseling, physical therapy, health benefits, or gerontology. For my money, I want a well-rounded, out-going, and confident person who possesses the critical objectivity that comes from being and working *outside* of the system. I want a quick study who has leadership ability and a little lawyer in him or her, in the best sense of the lawyerly thinking process.

Right-stuff advocates are assertive, not aggressive; well-organized; big-picture- and task-oriented; medically knowledgeable or else able to do medical research and to understand what they read; logical and skeptical; and available at all hours. They are at ease with speaking up and aware of the risks and opportunities for healthcare error. They also are familiar with the special fears, concerns, wishes, and instructions of the person for whom they're advocating. They are trustworthy and deserving of respect.

And they know how to do homework.

People often ask me what I would do differently in my advocacy, if I had a chance for a do-over. That's a question that I tried to answer throughout this book.

I was always very aware of being in the moment and of not having the benefit of hindsight. I dealt with the facts as I knew them to be at the time. I also consciously tried to protect myself from emotional and physical exhaustion without harming my parents. I made a point of retreating—into exercise, reflection, a movie, sleep—so that I wouldn't burn out. The wearier I became, however, the more my decisions suffered. I never gave up, but I did give in on some occasions.

I regret that I opted to care for myself more and for my father less during the last week of his life. I was hurting. If I could've known on Sunday that he would die on Thursday, I would never have left his side. I still feel the pain of the choice I made. In hindsight, I'm also sorry that I didn't refuse to go to Edenton so Dad couldn't have surgery with the Big Guy.

During the summer of 2013, I desperately needed help, and none of my siblings would make a long-term commitment to help me, despite my pleas. They wouldn't or couldn't rearrange their lives as I had mine. (That's another book: siblings and shared responsibility for Mom and Pop.)

With Mom incapacitated by her broken leg and Dad seriously ill, I learned on the go how important it is to have a "double team." Even when only one parent is stricken, it helps to have backup. One advocate can rest and recharge while the other is on the frontlines. If I'd had a sibling helping me throughout that summer, I would have brought Dad home from Sentara Norfolk in August, rather than have him discharged to Oakwood. Then he wouldn't have become addicted to oxycodone nor would he have contracted the dreaded C. diff., which debilitated him in ways that I'll probably never understand.

I'm aware that, had Dad come home, he might not have lived as long as he did. His heart may have stopped in September. That's a chance that, in hindsight, I would take.

My father wanted to age "in place"—at home, as his father had, and as I would like. I think he believed that he would not be ill until his final illness and then he would go, quickly, with little need for medical intervention. He counted on following in my Grandpa's footsteps. Otherwise, it's hard to explain why he and Mom relocated to a medical wasteland. Dr. Al knew about the shortcomings of today's healthcare.

My advice to others who may believe as my father did: Don't move to the Outer Banks or any other remote location after age 70, unless you plan to move again—at a moment's notice—or you don't want to reach 80.

I plan to live my senior years near what is presumed to be a top-notch hospital, preferably a teaching hospital, if I can find one in a town or city that I can tolerate. (Winters in Rochester, Minn., and Boston are forbidding.) I also plan not to be hospitalized there, if I can help it. I'm going to age successfully. I have no daughter to advocate for me, but I know how to take care of myself. (See Appendix Six, "Taking Care of Yourself.")

If my health becomes an every-day issue that I can't manage, I'll have a Plan B, and I'll communicate it to my family and friends. I will try my best to preempt a crisis.

～

My mother turned 90 in 2014. She still lives comfortably in her home with her "little dog," thanks to my father's financial planning and the assistance of caregivers and family, and she will for the rest of her life. I promised her that, and my siblings are equally committed to that goal.

Because the trip to Durham for Mom's follow-up appointment with Dr. Zura exhausted her, I arranged for her next follow-up X-rays to be done at Kitty Hawk Regional Medical Center. Dr. Zura sent an order to Kitty Hawk Radiology, and, at my request, the local radiology department mailed a disk of the X-rays to the Duke surgeon. Zura and his team couldn't make heads or tails of what they received, however. His PA, with whom I spoke, was bewildered by the local department's failure to scan what Zura had ordered. As I recall, the angles were all wrong. An irrelevant interpretation by Dr. Exeter also accompanied the disk.

We decided not to bother with any more followups. The ultrasound therapy had been successful, and Mom was doing well walking with a cane.

My mother has neither heart disease nor cancer, but her lungs wheeze occasionally: An inhaler helps. Her memory loss is profound, and, yet, she still has Gertrude Stein's there *there*. I find her mental state hard to explain to people, especially those who readily apply the Alzheimer's label.

I recently recomputed Mom's score on the Functional Activities Questionnaire, which I shared in Chapter Eight. It is well past the threshold identified by the Mayo Clinic's Dr. Petersen for mild dementia. Mom no longer writes letters or reads books, but she still can manage many basic tasks alone, such as making a cup of coffee, playing a simple card game, and toileting. If she did not have arthritis in her shoulders and hands, she would be able to dress herself, without assistance, from the waist up. Pulling up pants is beyond her physical capability.

Mom no longer drives, but she still gets her hair done in a salon once a week and does physical therapy twice a week. She rarely calls me now, but she knows my telephone number. When I ask, she always recites it. We watch British mystery shows together—which I usually have to explain to her—and she still answers the occasional question on "Jeopardy!"

Mom lives in the moment, engaging in simple conversation and pleasures, and expressing curiosity in goings-on around her. She still looks things up in the encyclopedia.

She enjoys being with her children, even though she doesn't say much, and we enjoy her. Her smile brightens her countenance and fills our hearts with joy. She rarely complains.

My mother is a survivor. She embraces life, accepting the challenges that come, and perseveres. I can only marvel.

Appendix One

The Risks of
HOSPITALIZATION

In 1999, the Institute of Medicine (IOM), a nonprofit, non-governmental organization, dropped a bomb about hospital safety when it reported that at least 44,000 and as many as 98,000 hospitalized patients died annually because of medical error.[1]

The IOM's statistics came from two previously conducted studies, one analyzing 1992 data from Colorado and Utah (for 44,000), and the other analyzing 1984 hospital records in New York (98,000).[2] The former study relied upon the method of the latter, which was known as the Harvard Medical Practice Study.

That the high-end number of deaths exceeded the numbers attributable to all but the then-top four causes of death was appalling. You assumed more risk checking into a hospital than you did by traveling in an airplane or driving a car.[3]

The IOM's report was titled "To Err is Human: Building a Safer Health System" and became known simply as "To Err is Human," which has a pass-the-buck ring to me. Still cited often today, it upset the complacency of the media and the public about the quality of U.S. healthcare and forced members of the medical profession to acknowledge some harsh realities. It also spawned the professional field of patient safety.

The Institute defined a medical error, in part, as a preventable "adverse event." It further distinguished between an error of execution, which is "the failure of a planned action to be completed as intended," and an error of planning, which is "the use of a wrong plan to achieve an aim."

The IOM characterized an adverse event as an "injury caused by medical management." Thus, a medical error was a preventable injury caused by medical management.[4]

Regardless of whether such medical management constitutes legally actionable negligence or not, it is what you and I would call a screwup. The IOM's totals didn't even account for the *non-fatal* errors that prolong patients' hospitalizations and leave them worse off than they were upon admission.

Medical authorities disputed the IOM's figures then and still do, with some saying they were a gross exaggeration, and others branding them a gross underestimation.

Unquestionably, defining what constitutes an error; calculating errors within a specified context, such as a sampling of hospitals; and extrapolating to the nation the frequency of errors found in a small hospital sampling, are tricky feats.5 All error-study results necessarily depend on the nature, collection, and analysis of data, and it is the rare number that cannot be assailed. But even one error is too many.

Rather than identify and reject bad apples, and assign blame of any kind, the IOM condemned the whole medical orchard, the "culture," the "system." It concluded that the U.S. healthcare system, especially within hospitals, but also in private physicians' offices, is seriously flawed.

Many good-apple doctors disagreed, arguing that the careless and incompetent among them should be called out and disciplined. Although I agree with eliminating the bad apples, I think the IOM's report falls far short of an orchard-wide review.

INFECTIONS & DRUG REACTIONS

Consider some other numbers. In 2002, according to the U.S. Centers for Disease Control and Prevention, about 2 million U.S. hospital patients, or one in every 20, contracted nosocomial infections, and 80,000 to 100,000 of them died. (It is not possible to know which of these patient-deaths met the IOM's adverse-event-by-medical-management causation standard and which did not.)

I defined nosocomial infections in Chapter One as infections that are hospital-acquired. Infections that occur in a hospital also may be termed **iatrogenic**, an adjective that describes harm caused to a patient *because of* medical treatment; physician action, inaction, or advice; and the like, such as negligent surgery or improper care. Nosocomial infections are an example of iatrogenesis.

Four types of nosocomial infection account for 80 percent of the

CDC's total:

* Urinary tract infections, usually associated with a Foley catheter
* Infections of surgical sites or wounds (See Appendix Two)
* Bloodstream infections, associated often with the use of an intravascular device that is a different type of catheter, and
* Pneumonia, typically because of ventilator use[6]

The CDC reported that 80,000 U.S. patients annually developed infections because of intravascular catheters, and 30,000 of them died. These catheters are tubes placed in the neck, chest, or groin to administer medication and nutrients, drain fluids, or collect blood samples and may be used for weeks or longer.

Central venous catheter-related bloodstream infections, or so-called CRBSI, typically occur because of a failure by hospital personnel 1) to take adequate sanitary precautions when inserting the catheter or 2) to regularly assess a patient's continued need for the device and to remove it as soon as possible. The longer an intravascular catheter remains in place, the greater the risk for a CRBSI.[7]

A contemporaneous analysis by other U.S. researchers concluded that another 100,000 patients died annually because of adverse drug reactions, which typically occur because physicians 1) ignore patients' allergies, by neglecting to read the medical records that document their allergies; 2) fail to anticipate adverse effects that can be anticipated; or 3) fail to expect unexpected reactions. In other words, they don't individualize their patients, and, as my drug-czar father always said, "Doctors don't know drugs."

At least 1.5 million preventable adverse drug *events*, which are not considered reactions, also reportedly occurred in hospitals, long-term care facilities, and among outpatient Medicare recipients, combined.[8]

Errors in medication, a type of event, can occur at any step in the drug process, which commences with the drug being procured from the manufacturer and includes prescribing, dispensing, and administering the drug, and monitoring its effects, all of which involve hospital professionals. I have read that a hospital patient can expect to be subjected to more than one medication error per day.[9]

AFTER THE BOMB

In the aftermath of the IOM's bomb, U.S. hospitals initiated reforms, targeting, in particular, the prevention of infections. Some achieved great success in their zero-tolerance infection campaigns,[10] but overall, the U.S. Dept. of Health and Human Services reported that, after 10 years, "very little progress" had been made. With the exception of cases of surgery-related pneumonia, which dropped 12 percent, the occurrence rates of most infections surveyed actually worsened.[11]

According to Dr. Lucian L. Leape, a chief author of the Harvard Medical Practice Study and a national figure in the patient safety movement, studies conducted since "To Err is Human" show that "half of Americans [overall, not just hospitalized] fail to get effective treatments they need, at least a third receive treatments of little or no benefit, and 10 percent or more are significantly harmed by preventable mishaps."[12]

This is hardly a confidence-boosting assessment.[13]

Contemplating knee surgery in 2005, Dr. Donald M. Berwick, a former president of the Institute for Healthcare Improvement in Cambridge, Mass., put errors in perspective when he wondered: How can the healthcare system kill me? And then he counted some of the ways, writing:

"You can give me an infection during my surgery. You can mix up a blood transfusion. You can fail to prevent a pulmonary embolism. If I need a respirator for a while when I wake up, you can give me pneumonia. You can misplace a decimal point in the order for morphine. You can place the endotracheal tube by mistake in my esophagus (which, in the United States, happens on average in 8% of non-intensive care unit intubations) and not realize it until it is too late."

Everything on his list, Berwick said, not only happens, but can be prevented, maybe not down to a rate of zero percent, "but awfully close to zero."[14]

AN UPDATE

Nearly 15 years after "To Err is Human," John T. James, Ph.D., of Patient Safety America in Houston, reported that 440,000 deaths—up from the previously accepted total of 300,000—now occur in U.S.

hospitals each year because of preventable causes.

James reviewed selected hospital studies published from 2008 to 2011 and developed an evidence-based estimate of patient harm associated with hospitalization. If he is correct, then preventable hospital error causes one-sixth of all deaths nationwide and is the third leading cause of death in the United States.

James also concluded that between 4 million and 8 million patients annually suffer nonlethal but serious harm as a result of hospital errors.[15]

There is good news, however, from the CDC, which reported in 2012 that the number of infections acquired in hospitals each year had dropped. In its most recent healthcare-associated infection (HAI) survey, the agency found that "on any given day" about one in 25 hospital patients has at least one healthcare-associated infection. This is down from one in 20, as reported by its 2002 survey.[16]

For me, the bottom line remains: Hospital errors are a significant public-health hazard. You have to be aware.

1. Institute of Medicine, Committee on Quality of Health Care in America, *To Err is Human: Building a Safer Health System*, ed. Linda T. Kohn, Janet M. Corrigan, and Molla S. Donaldson (Washington, D.C.: National Academy Press, 1999), pp. 1, 26-28 [hereinafter cited as IOM, *To Err is Human*]. For information about the IOM, go to its website, www.iom.edu.

See also Julia A. Hallisy, *The Empowered Patient: Hundreds of Life-Saving Facts, Action Steps and Strategies You Need to Know* (San Francisco, CA: Bold Spirit Press 2008), p. 92; Gail Van Kanegan and Michael Boyette, *How to Survive Your Hospital Stay: The Complete Guide to Getting the Care You Need—And Avoiding the Problems You Don't* (New York: Fireside, 2003), pp. xv-xvi; and Rahul Parikh, "It's So Hard to Say I'm Sorry: The Financial and Personal Ramifications That Come When a Doctor Apologizes to a Patient," at http://www.slate.com/id/2234322/pagenum/all/. (Dr. Parikh is a pediatrician in San Francisco.)

2. Eric J. Thomas, et al, "Incidence and Types of Adverse Events and Negligent Care in Utah and Colorado," *Medical Care* 38 (2000): 261-71; Troyen A. Brennan, et al, "Incidence of Adverse Events and Negligence in Hospitalized Patients: Results of the Harvard Medical Practice Study I," *New England Journal of Medicine* 324 (1991): 370-76; and Lucian L. Leape, et al, "Incidence of Adverse Events and Negligence in Hospitalized Patients: Results of the Harvard Medical Practice Study II," *New England Journal of Medicine* 324 (1991): 377-84.

3. The top four causes were heart disease, malignant cancers, cerebrovascular disease (stroke), and chronic obstructive pulmonary diseases. See IOM, *To Err is Human,* p. 26; and U.S. Centers for Disease Control and Prevention (National Center for Health Statistics), *National Vital Statistics Reports* (1997 data), vol. 47, no. 19, June 30, 1999, p. 27.

4. IOM, *To Err is Human,* p. 28.

5. Lucian L. Leape and Donald M. Berwick, "Five Years After *To Err is Human*: What

Have We Learned?" *JAMA* 293 (2005): 2385; Clement J. McDonald, Michael Weiner, and Siu L. Hui, "Deaths Due to Medical Errors Are Exaggerated in Institute of Medicine Report," *JAMA* 284 (2000): 93-94; and Lucian L. Leape, "Institute of Medicine Medical Error Figures Are Not Exaggerated," *JAMA* 284 (2000): 95-97.

See also Robert J. Blendon, et al, "Views of Practicing Physicians and the Public on Medical Errors," *New England Journal of Medicine* 347 (2002): 1933-40; and Thomas H. Lee, "A Broader Concept of Medical Errors," *New England Journal of Medicine* 347 (2002): 1965-67.

6. R. Monina Klevens, et al., "Estimating Health Care-Associated Infections and Deaths in U.S. Hospitals, 2002," *Public Health Reports* 122 (2007): 160-66; and John P. Burke, "Infection Control—A Problem for Patient Safety," *New England Journal of Medicine* 348 (2003): 651.

7. Leonard A. Mermel, "Prevention of Intravascular Catheter-Related Infections," *Annals of Internal Medicine* 132 (2000): 394-97. Dr. Mermel lists recommended prevention strategies for intravascular catheter-related infections on p. 399.

In a major online survey, a majority of 2,075 responding infection-control workers cited the following factors as leading to CRBSI: insufficient time to train personnel on proper procedures; cumbersome paper-based systems for tracking patients; and neglect by ignorant and penny-foolish administrators. N.C. Aizenman, "Basic Practices Could Help Prevent Hospital Infections," *The Washington Post*, July 13, 2010, p. A3; and "Preventable Bloodstream Infections Still a Problem in Hospitals, Infection Prevention Group Finds," July 12, 2010 press release from the Association for Professionals in Infection Control and Epidemiology, obtainable at http://www.apic.org/AM/Template.cfm?Section=Home1.

8. Jason Lazarous, Bruce H. Poneranz, and Paul N. Corey, "Incidence of Adverse Drug Reactions in Hospitalized Patients:A Meta-analysis of Prospective Studies," *JAMA* 279 (April 15, 1998): 1200-05.

9. The Institute of Medicine, "Preventing Medication Errors," Report Brief, July 2006, at http://www.iom.edu/Reports/2006/Preventing-Medication-Errors-Quality-Chasm-Series.aspx. Considerable variation in the number of errors exists from one medical facility to the next.

10. In intervention studies conducted in intensive-care units, first at Johns Hopkins Hospital and then in 67 Michigan hospitals, prominent patient-safety advocate Peter Pronovost, M.D., Ph.D., of Johns Hopkins, showed that catheter-related bloodstream infections can be markedly reduced. Pronovost and his team achieved near-elimination of CRBSI in the Johns Hopkins ICU and a 66-percent reduction in 103 Michigan hospital ICUs statewide. Peter Pronovost, et al, "An Intervention to Decrease Catheter-Related Bloodstream Infections in the ICU," *New England Journal of Medicine* 355 (2006): 2725-32; and Sean M. Berenholtz, Peter J. Pronovost, et al, "Eliminating Catheter-Related Bloodstream Infections in the Intensive Care Unit," *Critical Care Medicine* 32 (2004): 2014-20.

11. The Associated Press, "Hospital Infection Rates Continue Alarming Rise," April 15, 2010, at http://www.msnbc.msn.com/id/36465334/ns/health-health_care/ns/health-health_care/; see also Manoj Jain, "Focus on Patient Safety Hasn't Succeeded," *The Washington Post*, Dec. 21, 2010, p. E5.

HHS's Agency for Healthcare Research and Quality (AHRQ) issues the National Healthcare Quality and Disparities Reports. According to HHS's 2009 health-care quality report to Congress:

• Rates of bloodstream infections after surgery increased by 8 percent;
• Urinary infections from the use of a catheter after surgery (painful, but treatable with antibiotics) increased by 3.6 percent;
• The overall incidence of a number of common infections due to medical care increased by 1.6 percent; and

• The number of bloodstream infections due to *central venous* catheters remained essentially the same.

See AHRQ at http://www.ahrq.gov/qual/nhq09.

12. Lucian L. Leape, "New World of Patient Safety: 23rd Annual Samuel Jason Mixter Lecture," *Archives of Surgery* 144 (2009): 394.

13. To help hospitals reduce the number of errors committed, the IOM re-conceptualized its analysis. It decided to categorize errors by the nature of the threat they pose to healthcare quality. Thus: 1) *Underuse* of care is a failure to provide medical intervention when intervention would likely produce a favorable outcome (needed treatment is not given); 2) *Overuse* of care occurs when intervention becomes common practice even though its benefits do not justify the potential harm or costs (the treatment is of no value); and 3) *Misuse* of care creates a preventable problem that eliminates the benefit of an intervention (a defect or mistake in treatment occurs). "What's the use?" you may well ask. Leape, "Five Years After To Err is Human," p. 2385; and Lee, "A Broader Concept of Medical Errors," p. 1966.

14. Donald M. Berwick, "My Right Knee," *Annals of Internal Medicine* 142 (2005): 122.

15. John T. James, "A New, Evidence-Based Estimate of Patient Harms Associated with Hospital Care," *Journal of Patient Safety* 9 (2013): 122-28. See also Tina Rosenberg, "To Make Hospitals Less Deadly, a Dose of Data," *The New York Times,* Dec. 4, 2013, at http://opinionator.blogs.nytimes.com/2013/12/04/to-make-hospitals-less-deadly-a-dose-of-data/.

16. The HAI survey is based on data compiled from 183 acute-care hospitals in 10 states: California, Colorado, Connecticut, Georgia, Maryland, Minnesota, New Mexico, New York, Oregon, and Tennessee. For a summary of the data, see U.S. Centers for Disease Control and Prevention, "Healthcare-Associated Infections (HAIs)," at http://www.cdc.gov/HAI/surveillance/index.html. For a full report, see Shelley S. Magill, Jonathan R. Edwards, et al, "Multistate Point-Prevalence Survey of Health Care-Associated Infections," *New England Journal of Medicine* 370 (2014): 1198-1208. A table showing the infection types and their distribution appears ibid, 1204. A list of reported causative pathogens, according to infection type, is ibid, 1205.

Appendix Two

Surgical
HAZARDS

In surgery, the three big errors are wrong patient, wrong procedure, and wrong site. Overworked, careless, and/or fatigued surgeons have been known to remove the wrong leg, the wrong breast, even the wrong kidney.

Such mistakes are dramatic and usually well-publicized, but, fortunately, rare. Far more common, according to celebrity surgeon Atul Gawande, of Harvard's Brigham and Women's Hospital in Boston, are the three big killers associated with surgery: infection, bleeding, and unsafe anesthesia.

In his book, "The Checklist Manifesto," Gawande argues that the use of a simple preoperative checklist by a surgical team would substantially reduce the incidence of postoperative "complications," which he defines as the three killers, "the unexpected," and death.[1]

The unexpected, writes Gawande, a well-published medical author who is a frequent contributor to *The New Yorker*, "stems from the fundamentally complex risks entailed by opening up a person's body and trying to tinker with it."[2]

I think his definition of complications, especially the inclusion of the catch-all "unexpected," is rather loose, but what rational person can argue with a checklist? I live by to-do lists.

After the IOM's "To Err Is Human" report, discipline-specific procedural checklists in hospitals proliferated. Gawande and other physicians began to tout the aviation industry and its use of safety checklists—e.g., an airplane equipment checklist before takeoff—as models for basic healthcare quality control.[3] Hospital checklists, they contended, would reduce reliance on memory, standardize processes, and improve access to information.

In an initiative funded by the World Health Organization, Gawande helped to draft a 19-item safe-surgery checklist that takes two minutes for a nurse to run through. Some of the items on the list include: Has the patient confirmed his/her identity? Has he or she confirmed the surgical site? The procedure? His/her consent? Is the site marked?

Other key questions: Is the anesthesia machine and medication check complete? Does the patient have any known allergies? Has the antibiotic prophylaxis (to guard against infection) been given within the past 60 minutes?

Tested in eight hospitals around the world, the WHO checklist reportedly resulted in an overall decline in the aforementioned complications of 36 percent and a decline in deaths of 47 percent.[4]

But just because an integrated team checklist and preoperative briefing build teamwork, communication, and discipline and reduce the number of postoperative adverse events[5] doesn't mean that surgeons will (or do) embrace such a process.[6]

Safety advocates politely attribute surgeons' resistance to change, such as checklist thinking, to their "culture."[7] Dr. Donald Berwick, the former president of the Institute for Healthcare Improvement, asks whether the operating-room "culture" is "open and fair," and whether "it value[s] input from anyone in the know?"[8]

Gawande himself coats his prose with arrogance on most pages of his book, which he subtitled: "How to Get Things Right."

When I would bring up with my father the personality profile of the stereotypical surgeon—egotistical, profane, disdainful, haughty—he always said: "Ann, surgeons do surgery."

In other words, what do you expect? To change the preoperative procedure is to change the nature of some beasts.

But the buck has to stop somewhere.

---

1. Atul Gawande, *The Checklist Manifesto: How to Get Things Right* (New York: Metropolitan Books, 2009), pp. 136-57. Gawande identifies the big killers associated with surgery on p. 101.

2. Ibid, 101.

3. L. Lingard, S. Espin, et al, "Getting Teams to Talk: Development and Pilot Implementation of a Checklist to Promote Interprofessional Communication in the OR," *Quality and Safety in Health Care* 14 (2005): 340; and J.F. Bion, T. Abrusci, and P. Hibbert, "Human Factors in the Management of the Critically Ill Patient," *British Journal of Anaesthesia* 105 (2010): 26-28. See also R.L. Helmreich, "On Error Management: Lessons from Aviation," *British Medical Journal* 320 (2000): 781-85.

4. Gawande, *The Checklist Manifesto*, pp. 153-56. The checklist testing is reported in Alex B. Haynes et al, "A Surgical Safety Checklist to Reduce Morbidity and Mortality in a Global Population," *New England Journal of Medicine* 360 (2009): 491-99.

5. Lingard, Espin, et al, "Getting Teams to Talk," pp. 340-46; Yael Einav, Daniel Gopher, et al, "Preoperative Briefing in the Operating Room: Shared Cognition, Teamwork, and Patient Safety," *Chest* 137 (2010): 443-49; and Martin A. Makary et al, "Operating Room Briefings and Wrong-Site Surgery," *American College of Surgeons* 204 (2007): 236-43.

6. Gawande, *The Checklist Manifesto*, pp. 156-57, 161-62.

7. Makary, et al, "Operating Room Briefings and Wrong-Site Surgery," p. 241.

8. Berwick, "My Right Knee," endnote 14, Appendix One, *supra,* p. 123.

Appendix Three

The Paradox of the
BETTER-RESTED RESIDENT

In July 2011, after more than two decades of debate, the private, nonprofit Accreditation Council for Graduate Medical Education (ACGME) mandated a reduction in the maximum shift for interns from 30 straight hours to 16.

Seeking to prevent medical errors caused by *all* residents' sleep deprivation, ACGME also limited second- and third-year residents to 28-hour shifts, during the last four hours of which they cannot take on new patients.[1]

At the same time, ACGME, which oversees residencies nationwide, reaffirmed its controversial 2003 directive that limited the average workweek for all residents to 80 hours, but left the structuring of shifts up to hospitals. The directive also established the 30-hour shift, itself a reduction from earlier days.[2]

Many older doctors perceived these cutbacks as coddling. The generation of physicians who trained in the 1990s typically worked a 120-hour week. The ACGME's detractors predicted that the quality of medical post-doc training would suffer as a result of the changes. Has it?

Physicians have long been expected to manage their fatigue and function at a superior level. The first residency, pioneered by the celebrated medical titan, Sir William Osler, at Johns Hopkins in the 1890s, involved an around-the-clock shift by young doctors (all men) who actually resided at the hospital. Their internship year was an especially rigorous rite of passage: They, literally, had no life outside of medicine.

Not much about the Osler paradigm changed, even as medicine and society itself changed, until 18-year-old Libby Zion arrived in distress at a Manhattan hospital emergency department in 1984 and died of cardiac arrest after being mishandled by exhausted and inexperienced house staff working a 36-hour shift. Zion's father, an attorney and writer for *The New York Times*, persuaded the New York County district attorney to launch a grand-jury investigation into her death.3 No charges were filed, but his advocacy prompted action. In 1989, New York passed rules that limited residents to 24-hour shifts and 80-hour workweeks; but N.Y. teaching hospitals ignored them.

Other states tried to do the same, only to be defeated by medical groups who argued that such cutbacks 1) resulted in "work compression," essentially doing the same amount of work in fewer hours; 2) deprived residents of valuable education and experience; and 3) actually increased the number of medical errors that occurred because a shorter workday increased the number of patient handoffs.

I don't think there's any doubt that fatigue degrades work performance, affecting judgment, mood, perception, and much more, regardless of how stellar an intellect you have. Overwork also may foster arrogance in residents and the belief that the world owes them for the misery they have been through. They may seek to move patients out earlier than they should be discharged and take their frustrations out on weaker (older, sicker) patients who cannot fend for themselves.

As patients, we want well-rested residents; but we also want well-trained doctors. Can't we have both?

In 2013, members of the Johns Hopkins medical faculty, which has led the opposition to ACGME's restrictions, reported on a study involving more than 1000 internal-medicine residents in which it concluded that residents' increased sleep during their on-call period was "associated" with "deterioration in educational opportunities, continuity of patient care, and perceived quality of care."4

I do not know the full extent of the education that residents receive, but I have seen them quizzed at the bedside by senior staff during conferences in my parent's hospital room. I believe these real-time exercises are highly valuable, and I would not want doctor rounds to be shortened simply because work hours have been reduced.

I also know the importance of continuous care and would not want to "break in" a changing cohort of residents, who have to be brought up to speed on my parent's case. That happens with musical hospitalists and nurses, each new one being a blank slate. I much prefer to have a resident in charge, even a sleepy one.

If the quality of patient care is suffering because of residents' scaled-back duty hours, and ACGME stands firm, then nonresidents will have to pick up the slack. While I can appreciate that duty-hour reductions challenge hospitals to come up with ways to compensate for, and finance their compensation of, the loss of relatively cheap labor, I don't believe that challenge can be an excuse for compromising care.

Fundamentally, I think that no matter how many hours a resident works, a patient's care is going to come down to the strengths and weaknesses, the attitudes and biases, and the *modus operandi* of the physician in charge and the hospital for which he or she works. In my experience, better residents work for better attendings at better hospitals. No surprise, there.

1. Self-reports by residents at Eastern Virginia Medical School between 2005 and 2011 suggest that the predecessors of Drs. Roo and Nar, who cared for my father in 2013, did not have to endure the rigors of their counterparts at Johns Hopkins or Harvard universities. EVMS resident reviews are at http:/www.scutwork.com/cgi-bin/links/review.cgi?ID=37.

2. Thomas J. Nasca, Susan H. Day, and E. Stephen Arnnis, Jr., "The New Recommendations on Duty Hours from the ACGME Task Force," *New England Journal of Medicine* 363 (2010): e3(1)-(6). See also Sandra G. Boodman, "More Work, But Less Time: To reduce errors and fatigue, medical interns work shorter hours. But has their training suffered?," *The Washington Post,* July 9, 2013, p. E1; and Jenny Gold, "New Rules On Medical Residents' Hours Spur Debate," National Public Radio, July 1, 2011, at http://www.npr.org/2011/07.01/137532829/new-rules-on-medical-residents-hours-spur-debate.

3. For an excellent summary of the Libby Zion case, see David A. Asch and Ruth M. Parker, "Sounding Board: The Libby Zion Case: One Step Forward or Two Steps Backward?" *New England Journal of Medicine* 318 (1988): 771-75, and the *New England Journal (NEJM)* commentaries that follow it: Timothy B. McCall, "The Impact of Long Working Hours on Resident Physicians," *NEJM* 318 (1988): 775-78; Norman G. Levinsky, "Compounding the Error," *NEJM* 318 (1988): 778-80; and Robert M. Glickman, "House-Staff Training–The Need for Careful Reform," *NEJM* 318 (1988): 780-82.

Dr. McCall concludes that "[h]ouse officers are overworked, sleep-deprived, and unduly stressed. The result is damage to their well-being, to medical education, to patient care, and to the entire profession. Changes in residency training are coming. Some in medicine oppose them. Perhaps, as has happened before in medicine, many opponents will later view the changes as desirable. Residents and patients certainly will." McCall, "The Impact of Long Working Hours on Resident Physicians," p. 778.

4. Sanjay V. Desai, Leonard Feldman, et al, "Effect of the 2011 vs. 2003 Duty Hour Regulation-Compliant Models on Sleep Duration, Trainee Education, and Continuity of Patient Care Among Internal Medicine House Staff," *JAMA Internal Medicine* 173 (2013): 649-54. See also Lara Goitein and Kenneth M. Ludmerer, Invited Commentary, "Resident Workload–Let's Treat the Disease, Not Just the Symptom," *JAMA Internal Medicine* 173 (2013): 654-55. Goitein and Ludmerer argue for a focus on workload, rather than work hours.

Appendix Four

The PSA-Test
CONTROVERSY

In May 2012, after reviewing available scientific evidence, the U.S. Preventive Services Task Force concluded that the "expected harms" of the prostate-specific antigen (PSA) test "are greater than [its] small potential benefit."[1]

The task force gave this blood test, as a *routine* screening practice for prostate cancer, the lowest grade it assigns: a "D," meaning no recommendation. A "C" grade would have been a recommendation that "depends on the patient's situation."[2]

The USPSTF is an independent panel of primary-care physicians and epidemiologists who are appointed, funded, and supported by the U.S. Dept. of Health and Human Services' Agency for Healthcare Research and Quality. In theory, it is impartial. I do not know its politics.

According to the panel, the PSA test helps to save the life of just one man in 1,000 and steers many more who would never die of prostate cancer toward unnecessary surgery and treatment.

"For every man whose life is saved by PSA testing," the task force said in a statement, "another one will develop a dangerous blood clot, two will have heart attacks, and 40 will become impotent or incontinent because of unnecessary treatment."[3]

The USPSTF's "D" grade principally affects healthy men between ages 50 and 70. According to Johns Hopkins urologist H. Ballentine Carter, for men age 70 and older, "the likelihood that routine PSA testing will be [at all] beneficial is extremely low."[4]

Many men over age 50 get a digital rectal exam and blood drawn for a PSA test during a regular checkup with their primary-care physician. Research suggests that PCPs too often routinely order PSA screening without assessing the patient's family history, race, age, life expectancy, overall health, and other patient-specific factors. (The incidence of prostate cancer among African-American men is greater than among men of other races.)

If the test suggests a problem—and false-positive results are common—they then "was[h] their hands of responsibility once the patient is referred to a specialist for prostate-cancer treatment," according to two Harvard primary-care doctors in a 2011 *New England Journal of Medicine* article.[5]

Once a patient is in the care of a urologist, his potential for over-treatment and, thus, exposure to harm, increases. Surgery, intensive radiation, and other interventions can cause temporary or permanent urinary incontinence, erectile dysfunction, bowel damage, and other debilitating consequences.

That men in the United States have a 17 percent chance of being diagnosed with prostate cancer during their lifetimes, but only a 3 percent chance of dying from it, suggests that conservative medical management may be appropriate for many.[6] And yet, most men diagnosed with low-risk prostate cancer choose to undergo active treatment such as surgery or radiation, regardless of their age and life expectancy and despite the risks. Anxiety and fear—and urging from their urologists—prevent them from opting for watchful waiting only.[7]

According to Richard J. Albin, Ph.D., the pathologist involved in the 1970 discovery of PSA, and Allan S. Brett, M.D., a University of South Carolina medical professor, PSA test "thresholds" for physician action fall in the range of 2.5 to 4.0 ng per milliliter.[8]

"Action" by physicians has tended to mean PSA retesting, sometimes several times a year; prostatic biopsies, sometimes repeated; and even the use of antibiotics to lower mildly elevated PSA blood levels in asymptomatic men with presumed prostatitis (inflammation of the prostate).[9] Depending on the doctor, "watchful waiting" can mean active surveillance, with regular testing, or simple observation, without testing. You should be aware that any time your Pop undergoes a biopsy, he risks infection, bleeding, pain, urinary problems, and other "complications."

Once a cancer diagnosis is made, a urologist stages the tumor(s) for purposes of prognosis. Besides DRE and PSA test results, he or she typically relies on a grading of the cancer's aggressiveness, which a pathologist calculates from the tumor patterns he or she detects in biopsied tissue. Because Minnesota Veterans Administration hospital pathologist Donald Gleason devised this cancer-grading scale in the

1960s, the calculation is known as a Gleason score.

"Low-risk" or "low-grade" prostate cancers are those in which no nodule, or only a small nodule, is felt during a DRE; the patient's Gleason score is 6 or lower; and his PSA blood level is below 10 ng/mL.[10]

If tissue and biochemical analysis suggests that the cancer has spread, physicians usually proceed with imaging tests, including CT, PET, and bone scans, to find out the extent and location of the cancer. Many doctors, however, will order a full battery of such imaging tests even in the absence of metastasis.

The American Society of Clinical Oncology strongly recommends that imaging not be used to stage low-risk cancers because of the costs to the patient and the healthcare system. Scans sometimes reveal abnormal-looking areas that prove, after expensive additional procedures and tests are performed, to be noncancerous. Meanwhile, patients endure needless worry and hours of wasted time. Imaging tests also expose patients to radiation and, thus, increase their risk of cancer.[11]

CHEERS AND JEERS

When the USPSTF withdrew its support of the nearly two-decade-old PSA test, physicians responded with both cheers and jeers.

The 19,000-member American Urological Association was reportedly "outraged" by the action. The Large Urology Group Practice Assn., which represents 1800 urologists nationwide—purportedly 20 percent of all practicing urologists—said it was "appalled" by the panel's "irresponsible and inexplicable" recommendation. But the decision pleased other physicians, including oncologists, who believe prostate cancer is both overdiagnosed and overtreated.

PSA testing has become "big, big money" for testing companies, physicians, and hospitals, said the chief medical officer of the American Cancer Society, who praised the task force for "taking a really hard line here."[12] According to PSA discoverer Richard Albin, the nation's annual bill for PSA screening is at least $3 billion, much of it paid by Medicare and the U.S. Veterans Admin. He has called the test's popularity "a hugely expensive public health disaster."[13]

Dr. Carter agrees that "An elevated PSA score can lead to a prostate biopsy that turns out to be unnecessary. Conditions other than cancer can cause PSA levels to rise, and about one in four men who have a positive PSA test turns out not to have prostate cancer. Further, when biopsies do reveal signs of prostate cancer, 30 to 50 percent of these cancers (depending on a man's age) won't be harmful—even if left untreated."

Nonetheless, Carter is reluctant to throw out the baby with the bath water, saying, "PSA screening is currently the best test available for early detection of prostate cancer."[14]

Geriatrician-epidemiologist Dr. Paulo H.M. Chaves, M.D., Ph.D., of the Johns Hopkins Center on Aging and Health, disagrees. He supports the USPSTF's recommendation. Chaves stresses that the PSA test is too often inaccurate; that all men of a "certain age" have cancerous cells in their prostates; and that prostate cancer progresses so slowly that men who have it typically die from another cause.[15] (He sounds like Dr. Al.)

My own view is that men should make informed individualized decisions about this screening test in consultation with physicians whom they trust to know them and to serve their best interests. They should ask their doctors about the benefits and costs of PSA testing. What does the clinical evidence show? As always, I recommend doing your own homework. You can start with my endnotes.[16]

---

1. Among the clinical studies the task force evaluated was a nationwide trial known as PIVOT, which stands for Prostate Cancer Intervention Versus Observation Trial.

From November 1994 through January 2002, PIVOT researchers followed 732 men who were diagnosed with localized prostate cancer (no metastasis) and randomly assigned to a radical prostatectomy or to observation. Each trial subject had to have a PSA value of less than 50 ng/mL and be 75 years old or younger, with a life expectancy of at least 10 years. The average age of the group was 67; the average PSA value was 7.8 ng/mL.

Among their findings, the researchers concluded that men with low-risk prostate tumors in the observation group were no more likely to die of prostate cancer than men with a similar risk in the prostatectomy group. Significantly, only 52 of the 354 deaths that did occur among the low-risk group were attributable to prostate cancer or its treatment. Among men with a PSA value greater than 10 ng/mL, however, radical prostatectomy was associated with reduced mortality from all causes.

Timothy J. Wilt, Michael K. Brawer, et al, "Radical Prostatectomy Versus Observation for Localized Prostate Cancer," *New England Journal of Medicine* 367 (2012): 203-13. See also H. Ballentine Carter, Johns Hopkins Medicine, "Prostate Cancer: To Treat or Not to Treat?," *Health After 50*, vol. 24, issue 12, January 2013, pp. 1-2.

2. USPSTF at http://www.uspreventiveservicestaskforce.org/prostatecancerscreening.htm.

3. Brian Vastag, "Panel: Prostate Test Shouldn't Be Routine," *The Washington Post,* May 22, 2012, p. A3. See generally USPSTF at http://www.uspreventiveservicestaskforce.org/prostatecancerscreening.htm.

4. H. Ballentine Carter, M.D., Johns Hopkins Medicine, "Should You Be Tested for Prostate Cancer?," *Health After 50,* vol. 23, issue 11, January 2012, p. 5. Carter advises men who choose to be screened to have their first PSA test at age 40. For men who get a PSA test at age 50, he recommends a follow-up testing schedule dependent on the results. His cut-off action threshold is 3 ng/mL or above. With a test of this level, he recommends that the patient "consult a urologist." Ibid.

See also Manoj Jain, "Are We Relying Too Much on Cancer Screening? False Positives Show Need to Adjust Patients' Expectations of Tests," *The Washington Post* , Nov. 1, 2011, p. E5. Jain, an infectious-disease specialist and adjunct assistant professor at the Rollins School of Public Health at Emory University in Atlanta, concludes that when he turns 50, he will skip the PSA test.

5. Mary F. McNaughton-Collins and Michael J. Barry, "One Man at a Time—Resolving the PSA Controversy," *New England Journal of Medicine* 365 (2011): 1953.

6. Wilt, Brawer, et al, "Radical Prostatectomy Versus Observation for Localized Prostate Cancer," p. 204.

7. Carter, "Prostate Cancer: To Treat or Not to Treat?," p. 1.

8. Allan S. Brett and Richard J. Albin, "Prostate-Cancer Screening—What the U.S. Preventive Services Task Force Left Out," *New England Journal of Medicine* 365 (2011): 1950.

9. Carter, "Should You Be Tested for Prostate Cancer?," pp. 4-5; and Carter, "Prostate Cancer: To Treat or Not to Treat?," p. 2.

10. Carter, "Prostate Cancer: To Treat or Not to Treat?," p. 2; and American Society of Clinical Oncology, "Hard Decisions About Cancer: 5 Tests and Treatments to Question," *Choosing Wisely,* at www.choosingwisely.org.

11. American Society of Clinical Oncology, "Hard Decisions About Cancer: 5 Tests and Treatments to Question," *Choosing Wisely,* at www.choosingwisely.org.

12. Vastag, "Panel: Prostate Test Shouldn't Be Routine," endnote 3, *supra*; American Urological Association, "AUA Speaks Out Against USPSTF Recommendations," available on the AUA website, http://www.auanet.org/content/homepage/homepage.cfm; and Large Urology Group Practice Association at http://lugpa.org/defaault.aspx. See also McNaughton-Collins and Barry, "One Man at a Time—Resolving the PSA Controversy," endnote 5, *supra,* pp. 1951-53.

13. Richard J. Albin, "The Great Prostate Mistake," *The New York Times,* March 9, 2010, at http://www.nytimes.com/2010/03/10/opinion/10Ablin.html.

14. Carter, "Should You Be Tested for Prostate Cancer?," p. 5.

15. Paulo H.M. Chaves, M.D., Ph.D., "Addressing the Well-Being of Older Adults: Millions and More at a Time," lecture in "Aging and Health," Johns Hopkins University Mini-Medical School, Oct. 20, 2011.

16. See James A. Colbert and Jonathan N. Adler, "Prostate Cancer Screening—Polling Results," *New England Journal of Medicine* 367 (2012): e25.

Appendix Five

The Scourge of
ATHEROSCLEROSIS

Although the exact cause of atherosclerosis is unknown, it unquestionably starts with damage or injury to the intimal layer of an artery, after which inflammation and biochemical changes occur in the cells. Evidence of the atherosclerotic process can be detected in a person within the first 10 years of life. Already, fat buildup is occurring.

As the Mayo Clinic explains: "[Platelets] often clump at the injury site to try to repair the artery, leading to inflammation. Over time, fatty deposits made of cholesterol and other cellular waste products also build up at the injury and harden."[1]

When fatty deposits grow and arterial walls thicken, cells within the wall layers die, leaving behind a fatty paste called atheroma. To contain this damage, fibroblasts form fibrous (hard) connective-tissue capsules around the atheroma. We refer to such capsules as fibrous or fatty **plaques**.[2]

Fatty plaques may completely or partially block arterial blood flow, or they may break free of the wall and enter the bloodstream as clots. Plaque-thickened arterial walls resist blood flow, increasing the afterload requirement so that the heart pumps harder. When it does, the systolic blood pressure rises, creating the risk of hypertension.

Upon encountering the force of increased blood pressure, inner layers of arterial walls weakened by plaque deposits and connective-tissue proliferation may balloon out into a bulge called an **aneurysm.** Aneurysms can form in *any* large artery, rupture, and cause severe internal bleeding. In a cerebral artery, this bleeding is a stroke. (See below.)

While we are all prone to atherosclerosis, also called arterial sclerosis, several prominent risk factors seem to accelerate its process. They include high blood pressure; high low-density lipoprotein (LDL) cholesterol; smoking and other nicotine sources; and type 2 diabetes.

Obesity, poor physical fitness, and stress further contribute to its progression.

According to cardiac surgeon and Georgetown University Professor David L. Pearle, atherosclerosis is a systemic disease.

"If it's present," he says, "it's going to be present in all of your body's arteries."[3] But consequences differ depending on which arteries are affected.

IN THE CORONARY ARTERIES

Coronary artery disease (CAD) exists whenever atherosclerotic plaques have narrowed or obstructed any of the heart's big arteries. When plaques prevent your Mom's or Pop's heart from getting the oxygen-rich blood it needs, she or he may experience chest pains called **angina pectoris.** Angina sufferers say the pain feels like "Someone is standing on my chest."

Angina can be a recurring problem, in which case it is considered stable, or a sudden, acute concern. If the pain is sudden, time is of the essence. Call 911 immediately. The angina may signal a **myocardial infarction (MI)**, commonly called a heart attack.

An **infarct** is an area of tissue that has died (necrotized) because its blood supply has been obstructed. Thus, an MI refers to the death of oxygen-deprived heart-muscle tissue. Once dead, these cells will not be replaced. If the heart survives, it will be weaker. Non-infarcted tissue will try to compensate for the loss.

A lesser known condition called **coronary microvascular disease** (MVD) results when atherosclerosis affects the heart's tiny arteries. Plaque doesn't cause blockages in these vessels, but patients with MVD, most of whom are women, are at an increased risk for a heart attack. They also suffer angina and other debilitating symptoms.[4]

CAD TREATMENT ALTERNATIVES

Many treatment options exist for coronary artery disease and stable angina, depending on their severity. They include lifestyle changes, such as an altered diet, a program of exercise, and a cessation of smoking, and a variety of medications.

According to Dr. Pearle, there are about 110 to 120 antihypertensive drugs on the market in the United States. Your Mom's and Pop's cardiologists also may prescribe drugs that inhibit blood-clotting, reduce arrhythmias, and lower blood-cholesterol levels. Coronary artery disease can be managed long-term.

The same luxury does not exist with unstable angina, which is a crisis.

Depending on the occlusion of arterial blood in the heart, says Pearle, there may be a window of only about 90 minutes between your Mom's or Pop's first sudden chest pains and surgery to save her or his life. The window for using clot-busting drugs, such as tissue plasminogen activator (tPA), which I mentioned in Chapter Three, is only 30 minutes.

For decades now, the gold-standard surgical procedures for preventing or halting a myocardial infarction have been the **angioplasty**, also known as percutaneous coronary intervention (PCI), and the **bypass**. Angioplasty and bypass can be used to repair renal arteries and restore blood flow to the kidneys, as well.

In an angioplasty, the surgeon uses tube-like catheters, including one that expands like a balloon, to open up a blocked or narrowed artery and inserts a mesh tube called a **stent** to keep the artery open. In a bypass, the surgeon transplants or "grafts" a blood vessel from another part of the body or uses a synthetic tube of some kind to route the blood around the problem vessel. Once an artery is bypassed, it no longer functions.

THE RENAL AND PERIPHERAL ARTERIES

The development and accumulation of fatty plaques in the renal arteries can reduce blood flow to the kidneys, increasing blood pressure and injuring tissue. Renal atherosclerosis can lead to progressive **kidney dysfunction** and **failure.**

Renal artery stenosis (RAS) is the narrowing of one or both of the arteries. Just like with CAD, RAS can be treated with lifestyle changes and medications. If this therapy proves insufficient, surgery may be done.

An atherosclerotic blockage in major arteries in the legs, arms, and/or pelvis leads to **peripheral artery disease (PAD)**, aka peripheral vascular disease, a disorder suffered by about 30 percent of older Americans. PAD, which is characterized by severe pain, skin ulcerations, lameness (claudication), and numbness in the extremities, elevates the risk of blood clots. (Note that DVT describes a clotting problem in the veins, not the arteries.)

THE CAROTID AND CEREBRAL ARTERIES

Atherosclerosis also may affect the two big carotid arteries that carry blood to the brain, as well as arteries within the brain itself. If plaque-thickened walls obstruct cerebral arterial blood flow, an **ischemic stroke** may occur. The rupture of an aneurysm, or a ballooning out, of a cerebral arterial wall, causes a **hemorrhagic (bleeding) stroke**.

Roughly 83 percent of all strokes are ischemic; and 17 percent are hemorrhagic. According to Victor C. Urrutia, an assistant professor of neurology and director of the Johns Hopkins Hospital Stroke Center, 20 percent of ischemic strokes are caused by atherosclerotic cerebrovascular disease and 20 percent are caused by blood clots.[6]

Classic stroke symptoms include slurred speech, paralysis or numbness on one side of the face or body, blurred vision, mental confusion, a severe out-of-the-blue headache (the worst of your life, says Dr. Urrutia), dizziness, and a loss of balance. Within four minutes of being deprived of oxygen and nutrients, brain cells begin to die.[5]

The effects of a stroke vary from person to person and depend on its type, severity, and location. A stroke may impair a person's movement and sensation, speech and language, vision, cognition (reasoning, memory), perception, emotional control, bowel and bladder control, and other vital body functions.

A **transient ischemic attack (TIA)**, or so-called mini-stroke, produces symptoms similar to a stroke, but usually only lasts a few minutes and causes no permanent damage. A TIA may be a warning of an impending stroke, however, and should not be ignored.

According to Urrutia and Georgetown neurologist and stroke expert, Dr. Alexander W. Dromerick, giving tPA intravenously to a stroke sufferer within four and a half hours of the onset of symptoms substantially reduces the likelihood of his or her long-term disability or death. But note: The attending physician has to be certain from a brain scan that the patient's stroke is ischemic, and not hemorrhagic, because tPA will aggravate cerebral bleeding. To be confident of access to, and the proper use of tPA, your Mom or Pop should go to a university-affiliated or other known stroke center.[7]

Stroke is the third leading cause of death in the United States.

Don't second-guess stroke symptoms. Call 911 immediately.

---

1. "Causes of Atherosclerosis," Mayo Clinic at http://www.mayoclinic.com/health/arteriosclerosis-atherosclerosis/DS00525/DSECTION=causes.

2. "The Physiology and Pathology of Aging," by David A. Sandmire, M.D., in *Gerontology for the Health Care Professional*, ed. Regula H. Robnett and Walter C. Chop (Sudbury, Mass.: Jones and Bartlett Publishers, 2nd ed., 2010), p. 83

3. David L. Pearle, M.D., lecture on "Cardiology," Georgetown University Mini-Medical School, March 20, 2012.

4. "What is Coronary Microvascular Disease?," National Heart Lung and Blood Institute, at http/www.nhlbi.nih.gov/health/health-topics/topics/cmd.

5. Dr. Alexander W. Dromerick, "Under Pressure: Understanding How High Blood Pressure Affects Your Health," presented by the Georgetown Center for Hypertension, Kidney & Vascular Research at the Georgetown University Medical Center, March 31, 2012.

6. Dr. Victor C. Urrutia, "Stroke Essentials," presented in Johns Hopkins Medicine's "A Woman's Journey" conference, Baltimore, Md., Nov. 17, 2012. Of the remaining 60 percent, Dr. Urrutia says 30 percent of strokes are cryptogenic, meaning their cause is not known, and 25 percent are lacunar, meaning another defect is responsible. He has a 5-percent margin of error.

7. Ibid, and endnote 5, *supra*.

Appendix Six

Taking Care of
YOURSELF

If today's longer lifetimes only mean more years of disease, dysfunction, and decline, then extended longevity is a poor goal. Fortunately, you and your parents can take steps to avoid this fate.

Geriatrician Diane Snustad of the University of Virginia has compiled a list of the Top 17 things that you can do to age well. No. 10 is actually a "don't," but it's a big enough "don't" to constitute a do. I pass them along below, from the bottom up, with my own remarks included in parentheses:

- ❖ 17. Get an attitude! (Be confident and think can-do.)

- ❖ 16. Laugh, be optimistic!

- ❖ 15. Avoid noise trauma.

- ❖ 14. Avoid sun damage.

- ❖ 13. Get vitamin D and calcium. (Fortify your bones.)

- ❖ 12. Take antioxidants. (Evidence on this is conflicting. Eat fruits and vegetables instead.)

- ❖ 11. Maintain good nutrition.

- ❖ 10. Don't smoke.

- ❖ 9. Avoid polypharmacy.

- ❖ 8. Work with your doctor. (Provided you have a competent and compassionate one.)

- ❖ 7. Limit your alcohol intake.

- ❖ 6. Have good genes. (Especially maternal genes.)

- ❖ 5. Be female. (Ha!)

❖ 4. Keep up social contacts. (See Chapter Ten about depression.)

❖ 3. Exercise the mind. (Learn new things. Also Chapter Ten.)

❖ 2. Exercise the body. (The only "magic pill" there is.)

And, the No. 1 thing to do to age well?

❖ AVOID AGEISM. Don't accept from your doctor: "What do you expect at your age?"

Endnotes

Note: I elected to abbreviate the *Journal of the American Medical Assn.* as *JAMA* because that is how people refer to it. I decided not to abbreviate *The New England Journal of Medicine*, for similar reasons, although I do omit the "The" to make *NEJM* citations a bit more wieldy.

CHAPTER TWO. BECOMING AN ADVOCATE, And a Pox on Dad's Head

1. For more details about ehrlichiosis, see http://www.cdc.gov/ncidod/dvrd/ehrlichia, the website of the Viral and Rickettsial Zoonoses Branch of the CDC's National Center for Infectious Diseases.

2. Johns Hopkins Medicine, "Urinary Tract Infections: What Both Men and Women Should Know," *Health After 50*, vol. 25, issue 15, February 2014, pp. 4-5. With a short course of antibiotics being standard treatment for an uncomplicated UTI, writes Edward E. Wallach, M.D., an obstetrician-gynecologist, doctors often presumptively diagnose, without waiting for the results of a urine culture, and, thus, over-treat.

3. Sheldon P. Blau and Elaine Fantle Shimberg, *How to Get Out of the Hospital Alive: A Guide to Patient Power* (New York: MacMillan, paper ed. 1998), pp. xv-xxvi.

4. Ibid, 208.

5. Sandeep Jauhar, *Intern: A Doctor's Initiation* (New York: Farrar, Straus and Giroux, paper ed. 2009), p. 198.

6. Ann G. Sjoerdsma, "Medical Miracle Frustrated: A Wonder Drug for Sleeping Sickness Is Not Available to Patients in Africa," *The Baltimore Sun,* Dec. 10, 2000, p. 1C.

7. According to Johns Hopkins, more than 90 percent of all adults in the United States have had chickenpox. Johns Hopkins Medicine, "Taking a Shot At Shingles," *Health After 50*, vol. 24, issue 7, August 2012, p. 8.

8. Immunization Action Coalition, "Shingles (Zoster): Questions and Answers," content reviewed by the U.S. Centers for Disease Control and Prevention, October 2011, at www.immunize.org/catg.d/p4221.pdf.

9. Hung Fu Tseng, Ning Smith, et al, "Herpes Zoster Vaccine in Older Adults and the Risk of Subsequent Herpes Zoster Disease," *JAMA* 305 (2011): 160; and "Herpes Zoster," in *The Merck Manual of Geriatrics*, ed., Mark H. Beers, M.D., and Robert Berkow, M.D. (Whitehouse Station, N.J.: Merck Research Laboratories, 3rd ed., 2000), p. 1259.

10. Ann Arvin, "Aging, Immunity, and the Varicella-Zoster Virus," *New England Journal of Medicine* 352 (2005): 2266.

The vesicles usually appear along the affected *dermatome*, which is the area of skin innervated by a single spinal nerve. Along the torso, dermatomes look like horizontal bands.

11. My description of the symptoms, natural course, and complications of herpes zoster is culled from the sources in the preceding four endnotes and from Richard Whitley, "A 70-Year-Old Woman With Shingles: Review of Herpes Zoster," *JAMA* 302(2009): 73-80; and John W. Gnann and Richard J. Whitley, "Herpes Zoster," *New England Journal of Medicine* 347 (2002): 340-46. The 40 percent statistic comes from *The Merck Manual of Geriatrics, 3rd ed.,* endnote 9, *supra*, p. 1259.

The National Institute of Neurological Disorders and Stroke gives an excellent overview in "Shingles: Hope Through Research," at http://www.ninds.nih.gov/disorders/shingles/detail_shingles.htm. Less comprehensive, but also informative is the Mayo Clinic's review at http://www.mayoclinic.com/health/shingles/DS00098.

Any time a rash erupts on the nose, cheek, or forehead, both patient and doctor must think about ophthalmic consequences. In herpes zoster *oticus*, the virus infects the geniculate ganglion of the facial nerve (the seventh cranial nerve), and vesicles erupt on, in, and around the ear as well as in the mouth. This type of shingles, called Ramsay Hunt Syndrome, can cause facial paralysis, intense earaches, vertigo, tinnitus (ringing in the ears), temporary or permanent hearing loss, and diminished taste.

For more about the possible consequences of herpes zoster virus, see Donald H. Gilden, B.K. Kleinschmidt-DeMasters, et al, "Neurologic Complications of the Reactivation of Varicella-Zoster Virus," *New England Journal of Medicine* 342 (2000): 635-45.

12. Zostavax is a live, attenuated vaccine, meaning its developers modified the live virus in a laboratory to produce a microorganism that can grow and stimulate immunity in the vaccine recipient *without* causing the illness. In 2006, the CDC recommended that all healthy ("immunocompetent") adults age 60 and older receive a dose of the vaccine, even if they already had shingles. See Immunization Action Coalition, "Shingles (Zoster): Questions and Answers," endnote 8, *supra.* In 2011, the FDA approved Zostavax's use in people 50 to 59 years old.

Studies have consistently shown the vaccine to be quite safe, with only mild reported adverse effects, such as pain or tenderness at the injection site. Thus far, the clinical-study data support the proposition that Zostavax lowers the incidence of herpes zoster among vaccinated immunocompetent people age 60 and older; but its effectiveness is far from emphatic and seemingly declines with the recipient's age. More time/vaccine use and field studies are necessary to properly evaluate its efficacy.

There is some suggestion that among vaccinated people who develop shingles, the duration, but not the severity, of their pain is shorter than it would be if they had not been vaccinated.

Ibid. See Tseng, Smith, et al, "Herpes Zoster Vaccine in Older Adults and the Risk of Subsequent Herpes Zoster Disease," pp.160-66; M.J. Levin, M.N. Oxman, et al, "Varicella-Zoster Virus-Specific Immune Responses in Elderly Recipients of a Herpes Zoster Vaccine," *Journal of Infectious Diseases* 197 (2008): 825-35; and M.N. Oxman and M.J. Levin, et al, "A Vaccine to Prevent Herpes Zoster and Postherpetic Neuralgia in Older Adults," *New England Journal of Medicine* 352 (2005): 2271-84.

See also Johns Hopkins Medicine, "Taking a Shot At Shingles," endnote 7, *supra*; and U.S. Food & Drug Admin., U.S. Dept. of HHS, "Vaccines, Blood & Biologics," at http://www.fda.gov/BiologicsBloodVaccines/Vaccines/QuestionsaboutVaccines/ucm070418.htm.

CHAPTER THREE. 2006: BRONCHITIS OR A MASSIVE BLOOD CLOT?
When Precautions and Primary Care Fail

1. Victor F. Tapson, "Medical Progress: Acute Pulmonary Embolism," *New England Journal of Medicine* 358 (2008): 1048.

2. Nils Kucher and Samuel Z. Goldhaber, "Management of Massive Pulmonary Embolism," *Circulation* 112 (2005): e28.

3. American Public Health Assn., "Deep-Vein Thrombosis: Advancing Awareness to Protect Patient Lives," white paper, pp. 1-3, Public Health Leadership Conference on Deep-Vein Thrombosis, Washington, D.C., Feb. 26, 2003 [hereinafter cited as APHA, "Deep-Vein Thrombosis"], available at www.apha.org; National Quality Forum, "National Voluntary Consensus Standards for Prevention and Care of Venous Thromboembolism: Policy, Preferred Practices and Performance Measures," available at http://www.qualityforum.org; and James D. Douketis, Clive Kearon, et al, "Risk of Fatal Pulmonary Embolism in Patients with Treated Venous Thromboembolism," *JAMA* 279 (1998): 458.

4. Jauhar, *Intern: A Doctor's Initiation*, p. 6.

5. Tapson, "Medical Progress: Acute Pulmonary Embolism," p. 1040; and Giancarlo Agnelli and Cecilia Becattini, "Current Concepts: Acute Pulmonary Embolism," *New England Journal of Medicine* 356 (2007): 266, 269.

6. Tapson, "Medical Progress: Acute Pulmonary Embolism," p. 1040; and Agnelli and Becattini, "Current Concepts: Acute Pulmonary Embolism," p. 266.

7. R.K. Mani, P. Pandey, et al, "Pulmonary Embolism After Total Knee Replacement Despite Thromboprophylaxis," *American Journal of Respiratory and Critical Care Medicine* 179 (2009): A3286.

8. Charles W. Francis, "Prophylaxis for Thromboembolism in Hospitalized Medical Patients," *New England Journal of Medicine* 356 (2007): 1438-44; and Dale W. Bratzler, Gary E. Raskob, et al, "Underuse of Venous Thromboembolism Prophylaxis for General Surgery Patients: Physician Practices in the Community Hospital Setting," *Archives of Internal Medicine* 158 (1998): 1909.

9. Agnelli and Becattini, "Current Concepts: Acute Pulmonary Embolism," p. 266; and C. Gregory Elliott, Samuel Z. Goldhaber, and Robert L. Jensen, "Delays in Diagnosis of Deep Vein Thrombosis and Pulmonary Embolism," *Chest* 128 (2005): 3372.

10. Francis, "Prophylaxis for Thromboembolism in Hospitalized Medical Patients," p. 1438; and Victor F. Tapson, Hervé Decousus, et al, "Venous Thromboembolism Prophylaxis in Acutely Ill Hospitalized Medical Patients: Findings From the International Medical Prevention Registry on Venous Thromboembolism," *Chest* 132 (2007): 937.

11. APHA, "Deep-Vein Thrombosis," pp. 1-3; Hsing-Ting Yu, Michelle L. Dylan, et al, "Hospitals' Compliance with Prophylaxis Guidelines for Venous Thromboembolism," *American Journal of Health System Pharmacy* 64 (2007): 69; John A. Heit, Alexander T. Cohen, and Frederick A. Anderson, Jr., "Estimated Annual Number of Incident and Recurrent, Non-Fatal and Fatal Venous Thromboembolism (VTE) Events in the U.S.," *Blood* 106 (2005): 267a; Tapson, "Medical Progress: Acute Pulmonary Embolism," p. 1037; and National Quality Forum, "National Voluntary Consensus Standards for Prevention and Care of Venous Thromboembolism." See also Kucher and Goldhaber, "Management of Massive Pulmonary Embolism," p. e28.

12. Tapson, "Medical Progress: Acute Pulmonary Embolism," p. 1048; and Elliott, Goldhaber, and Jensen, "Delays in Diagnosis of Deep Vein Thrombosis and Pulmonary Embolism," pp. 3372, 3374-5.

13. Kucher and Goldhaber, "Management of Massive Pulmonary Embolism," p. e28.

14. Tapson, Decousus, et al, "Venous Thromboembolism Prophylaxis in Acutely Ill Hospitalized Medical Patients," p. 937.

15. In 1995-96, the International Cooperative Pulmonary Embolism Registry (ICOPER) enabled analyses and comparisons of choices made in prophylaxis, diagnostic tests, and treatment regimens of 2,392 PE patients in seven countries. The International Medical Prevention Registry on Venous Thromboembolism (IMPROVE) is an ongoing observational study to assess clinical practices.

For information about ICOPER, see: Samuel Z. Goldhaber, Luigi Visani, and Marisa de Rosa, "Acute Pulmonary Embolism: Clinical Outcomes in the International Cooperative Pulmonary Embolism Registry," *The Lancet* 353 (1999): 1386-89; and Nils Kucher, Elisa Rossi, Marisa De Rosa, and Samuel Z. Goldhaber, "Massive Pulmonary Embolism," *Circulation* 113 (2006): 577-82. For IMPROVE, see: Tapson, Decousus, et al, "Venous Thromboembolism Prophylaxis in Acutely Ill Hospitalized Medical Patients," pp. 936-45.

16. Tapson, "Medical Progress: Acute Pulmonary Embolism," p. 1048; Bratzler, Raskob, et al, "Underuse of Venous Thromboembolism Prophylaxis for General Surgery Patients," p. 1911; APHA, "Deep-Vein Thrombosis," p. 4; Tapson and Decousus, et al, "Venous

Thromboembolism Prophylaxis in Acutely Ill Hospitalized Medical Patients," p. 943; and Yu, Dylan, et al, "Hospitals' Compliance with Prophylaxis Guidelines for Venous Thromboembolism," pp. 73-75.

17. APHA, "Deep-Vein Thrombosis," p. 5.

18. Tapson, Decousus, et al, "Venous Thromboembolism Prophylaxis in Acutely Ill Hospitalized Medical Patients," pp. 942-43. Of course, VTE patients who have a counter-indicative underlying medical condition, such as an active peptic ulcer or a blood disease, should not receive an anticoagulant.

19. Bratzler, Raskob, et al, "Underuse of Venous Thromboembolism Prophylaxis," p. 1911.

20. Kucher, Rossi, DeRosa, and Goldhaber, "Current Concepts: Massive Pulmonary Embolism," p. 581.

21. Bratzler, Raskob, et al, "Underuse of Venous Thromboembolism Prophylaxis," pp. 1909-11.

22. Ibid, 1911; APHA, "Deep-Vein Thrombosis," pp. 4-5; and Francis, "Prophylaxis for Thromboembolism in Hospitalized Medical Patients," pp. 1439-40.

23. Tapson, "Medical Progress: Acute Pulmonary Embolism," p. 1039.

24. Ibid.

25. Francis, "Prophylaxis for Thromboembolism in Hospitalized Medical Patients," p. 1439.

26. Jack Hirsh, Gordon Guyatt, et al, "Executive Summary: American College of Chest Physicians Evidence-Based Clinical Practice Guidelines (8th Edition)," *Chest* 133 (2008): 78S; and David Rosenberg, "Venous Thromboembolism Prophylaxis: Implementing a Program That Works," *CHESTSoundings*, Jan. 1, 2010, at http://www.chestnet.org.accp/chestsoundsings/venous-thromboembolism-prophylaxis-implementing-program-works.

27. Elliott, Goldhaber, and Jensen, "Delays in Diagnosis of Deep Vein Thrombosis and Pulmonary Embolism," p. 3375.

28. Timothy Hoff, *Practice Under Pressure: Primary Care Physicians and Their Medicine in the Twenty-first Century*, (New Brunswick, N.J. and London: Rutgers University Press, 2010), p. 6.

29. Peter R. Ebeling, "Osteoporosis in Men," *New England Journal of Medicine* 358 (2008): 1474-75.

30. For a description of a vertebroplasty, see the Mayo Clinic website at http://www.mayoclinic.org/vertebroplasty/vertebroplasty.html.

Although the U.S. Medicare program has not promulgated national coverage policies for vertebroplasties, local Medicare contractors in multiple jurisdictions have covered these procedures since at least 2001. Vertebroplasty rates nearly doubled from 2001 to 2005 and increased by 32.3 percent from 2001 to 2002 alone. This growth preceded the U.S. Food and Drug Administration's approval in December 2004 of the use of polymethylmethacrylate cement for vertebroplasty. See Darryl T. Gray, William Hollingworth, Nneka Onwudiwe, Richard A. Deyo, and Jeffrey G. Jarvik, "Research Letter: Thoracic and Lumbar Vertebroplasties Performed in U.S. Medicare Enrollees, 2001-2005," *JAMA* 298 (2007): 1760-61.

31. See Rachelle Buchbinder, et al, "A Randomized Trial of Vertebroplasty for Painful Osteoporotic Vertebral Fractures," *New England Journal of Medicine* 361 (2009): 557-68; David F. Kallmes, et al, "A Randomized Trial of Vertebroplasty for Osteoporotic Spinal Fractures," *New England Journal of Medicine* 361 (2009): 569-79; and James N. Weinstein, "Balancing Science and Informed Choice in Decisions About Vertebroplasty," *New England Journal of Medicine* 361 (2009): 619-21.

32. Nortin A. Hadler, M.D., "Health Screening Gone Wild: Predicting Heart Disease, Cancer, and Osteoporosis," lecture in seminar, "Efficiency in Health Care: Effectiveness

and Value," UNC Center for School Leadership Development, University of North Carolina-Chapel Hill, Chapel Hill, NC, April 13-14, 2012.

33. Judith Graham, "A Different Prescription on Aging: Treatment or Overtreatment," *The Washington Post*, Feb. 21, 2012, p. E4.

CHAPTER FOUR. DOCTORTHINK AND NO-THINK
Psyching Out Misdiagnoses

1. David E. Newman-Toker, "Twenty-Five Year Summary of U.S. Malpractice Claims for Diagnostic Errors 1986-2010," *BMJ [The British Medical Journal] Quality & Safety* 22 (2013): 672-80. This analysis reportedly covered 350,000 malpractice claims extracted from the National Practitioner Data Bank, which is maintained by the U.S. government, and identified 100,249 claims of diagnostic error. See also Sandra G. Boodman, "Missing the Mark," *The Washington Post*, May 7, 2013, p. E1; and David Brown, "Diagnostic Mistakes Top Cause of Claims: More Than a Third of Malpractice Payments Are Rooted in Such Errors," *The Washington Post*, April 23, 2013, p. A6.

2. From Sherwin B. Nuland, *How We Die: Reflection on Life's Final Chapter* (New York: Alfred A. Knopf, 1994), as quoted in Pat Croskerry, "A Universal Model of Diagnostic Reasoning," *Academic Medicine* 84 (2009): 1022. See also Mark Graber, "Diagnostic Errors in Medicine: A Case of Neglect," *Joint Commission Journal on Quality and Patient Safety* 31 (2005): 108.

3. Graber, "Diagnostic Errors in Medicine," pp. 109-10.

4. Arthur Garson Jr. and Carolyn L. Engelhard, *Health Care Half Truths: Too Many Myths, Not Enough Reality* (Lanham, Md./Boulder, Colo./New York: Rowman & Littlefield Publishers, Inc., 2007), p. 59.

Two excellent articles about "mindful," "self-aware," and "reflective" medical practice are Silvia Mamede, Henk G. Schmidt, and Remy Rikers, "Diagnostic Errors and Reflective Practice in Medicine," *Journal of Evaluation in Clinical Practice* 13 (2007): 138-45; and Francesc Borrell-Carrio and Ronald M. Epstein, "Preventing Errors in Clinical Practice: A Call for Self-Awareness," *Annals of Family Medicine* 2 (2004): 310-16. See also Gloria J. Kuhn, "Diagnostic Errors," *Academic Emergency Medicine* 9 (2002): 748; and Robert M. Hamm and John Zubialde, "Physicians' Expert Cognition and the Problem of Cognitive Biases," *Primary Care* 22 (1995): 190.

5. Richard C. Cabot, "Diagnostic Pitfalls Identified During A Study of Three Thousand Autopsies," *JAMA* 59 (1912): 2295-98; Graber, "Diagnostic Errors in Medicine," p. 106; and Stephen J. McPhee, "The Autopsy: An Antidote to Misdiagnosis," *Medicine (Baltimore)* 75 (1996): 41.

6. For diagnostic error rates, see Mark L. Graber, "The Incidence of Diagnostic Error in Medicine," *BMJ Safety & Quality* 22 (2013): ii22-ii27; Pat Croskerry, "A Universal Model of Diagnostic Reasoning," *Academic Medicine* 84 (2009): 1022; Gordon D. Schiff, Omar Hasan, et al, "Diagnostic Error in Medicine: Analysis of 583 Physician-Reported Errors," *Archives of Internal Medicine* 169 (2009): 1881; Kuhn, "Diagnostic Errors," p. 741; Georges Bordage, "Why Did I Miss the Diagnosis? Some Cognitive Explanations and Educational Implications," *Academic Medicine* 74 (Supp. 1999): S138; Wilhelm Kirch and Christine Schafii, "Misdiagnosis at a University Hospital in 4 Medical Eras," *Medicine* 75 (1996): 29 [The hospital is in Germany. See endnote 18, *infra*.]; Lawrence L. Pelletier Jr., Friedrich Klutzow, and Hugh Lancaster, "The Autopsy: Its Role in the Evaluation of Patient Care," *Journal of General Internal Medicine* 4 (1989): 300-01, 303; and Lee Goldman, Robert Sayson, et al, "The Value of the Autopsy in Three Medical Eras," *New England Journal of Medicine* 308 (1983): 1000-05.

7. About "burying mistakes": Schiff and Hasan, "Diagnostic Error in Medicine: Analysis of

583 Physician-Reported Errors," p. 1886. See also George D. Lundberg, "Editorial: Medical Students, Truth, and Autopsies," *JAMA* 250 (1983): 1199-1200.

Re the autopsy rate: Jianguo Xiao, Gerhard R.F. Krueger, et al, "The Impact of Declining Clinical Autopsy: Need for Revised Healthcare Policy," *The American Journal of the Medical Sciences* 337 (2009): 41; Graber, "Diagnostic Errors in Medicine," p. 109; Kaveh G. Shojania, Elizabeth C. Burton, et al, "Changes in Rates of Autopsy-Detected Diagnostic Errors Over Time: A Systematic Review," *JAMA* 289 (2003): 2849; and Stephen J. McPhee, "Maximizing the Benefits of Autopsy for Clinicians and Families: What Needs to be Done," *Archives of Pathology and Laboratory Medicine* 120 (1996): 744.

See endnote 16, *infra*, for citations about some of the reasons for the decline in the autopsy rate.

8. Edward W. Campion, Victoria A. Reder, Albert G. Mulley, and George E. Thibault, "Age and the Declining Rate of Autopsy," *Journal of the American Geriatrics Society* 34 (1986): 866. See also McPhee, "Maximizing the Benefits of Autopsy for Clinicians and Families," p. 744. Campion et al point out that autopsies allow monitoring of "complications" and iatrogenic events, which are harmful events caused by healthcare.

9. Xiao, et al, "The Impact of Declining Clinical Autopsy: Need for Revised Healthcare Policy," p. 44; Mark L. Graber, Nancy Franklin, and Ruthanna Gordon, "Diagnostic Error in Internal Medicine," *Archives in Internal Medicine* 165 (2005): 1498; Kuhn, "Diagnostic Errors," p. 745; Bordage, "Why Did I Miss the Diagnosis?," p. S138; and McPhee, "Maximizing the Benefits of Autopsy for Clinicians and Families," p. 744. See endnote 7, *supra*, for additional citations.

10. Goldman, Sayson, et al, "The Value of the Autopsy in Three Medical Eras," p. 1002. For another take, see Pelletier, et al, "The Autopsy: Its Role in the Evaluation of Patient Care," p. 303.

11. Shojania, Burton, et al, "Changes in Rates of Autopsy-Detected Diagnostic Errors Over Time: A Systematic Review," pp. 2849-55. For the full report, see Kaveh G. Shojania, Elizabeth C. Burton, et al, "The Autopsy as an Outcome and Performance Measure," Evidence Report/Technology Assessment No. 58, AHRQ Publication No. 03-E002, in the archives of the Agency for Healthcare Research and Quality, at www.ahrq.gov. This analysis, prepared for the U.S. Dept. of Health and Human Services, also concluded that only 25 percent of all cause-of-death statements in death certificates are correct.

12. Lucian L. Leape, Donald M. Berwick, and David W. Bates, "Counting Deaths Due to Medical Errors (letter)," *JAMA* 288 (2002): 2405. In their letter, Leape, Berwick, and Bates cite a *Lancet* article for the proposition that autopsy studies consistently find undiagnosed disease as the cause of death in 10 to 20 percent of patients, of whom *half* could have been treated successfully. *The Lancet* is published in London.

See also Shojania, Burton, et al, "Changes in Rates of Autopsy-Detected Diagnostic Errors Over Time: A Systematic Review," p. 2853; and David E. Newman-Toker and Peter J. Pronovost, "Diagnostic Errors—The Next Frontier for Patient Safety," *JAMA* 301 (2009): 1060.

13. Shojania, Burton, et al, "Changes in Rates of Autopsy-Detected Diagnostic Errors Over Time: A Systematic Review," p. 2853.

14. Schiff and Hasan, "Diagnostic Error in Medicine: Analysis of 583 Physician-Reported Errors," p. 1883; Graber, "Diagnostic Errors in Medicine," p. 107; Goldman, Sayson, et al, "The Value of the Autopsy in Three Medical Eras," p. 1002; Pelletier, et al, "The Autopsy: Its Role in the Evaluation of Patient Care," pp. 301-02; and Bordage, "Why Did I Miss the Diagnosis?," p. S138.

15. Campion, et al, "Age and the Declining Rate of Autopsy," pp. 866-67; and Judith C. Ahronheim, Alissa S. Bernholc, and William D. Clark, "Age Trends in Autopsy Rates: Striking

Decline in Later Life," *JAMA* 250 (1983): 1182-86. Campion et al speak directly to ageism on p. 867. For a word on overconfidence, see McPhee, "Maximizing the Benefits of Autopsy for Clinicians and Families," p. 744.

16. Pelletier, et al, "The Autopsy: Its Role in the Evaluation of Patient Care," pp. 302; Xiao, et al, "The Impact of Declining Clinical Autopsy: Need for Revised Healthcare Policy," pp. 41-43; and McPhee, "Maximizing the Benefits of Autopsy for Clinicians and Families," p. 744.

According to Stephen J. McPhee, of the University of California-San Francisco School of Medicine, some of the reasons that a doctor may not request an autopsy include a lack of training in how to seek autopsy permission; the perception that technologic advances have rendered the autopsy obsolete; a delay in receipt of the autopsy results; a fear of malpractice litigation and/or of unexpected findings that would cause professional discreditation; defective training of autopsy pathologists and/or frustrations at poorly performed autopsies; and cost-cutting pressures. McPhee, "Maximizing the Benefits of Autopsy for Clinicians and Families," pp. 744-46.

Interestingly, while some physicians fear that the postmortem exposure of diagnostic discrepancies may result in malpractice lawsuits, the UCSF-Stanford study (Shojania, Burton, et al, "Changes in Rates of Autopsy-Detected Diagnostic Errors Over Time: A Systematic Review," endnote 7, *supra*) showed that autopsies often inure to physicians' benefit because they uncover "no-fault" errors, for example, those made by patients. Xiao, et al, "The Impact of Declining Clinical Autopsy: Need for Revised Healthcare Policy," p. 44. See also McPhee, "Maximizing the Benefits of Autopsy for Clinicians and Families," p. 744.

17. Mary Furlong, M.D., Director of Education, Georgetown University Medical Center Department of Pathology, lecture on "Pathology," Georgetown University Mini-Medical School, Feb. 28, 2012.

18. For example, a study of 400 autopsies performed over four medical eras at the First Medical University Hospital in Kiel, Germany, documented a correct final diagnosis based on the H&P in 60 to 70 percent of the cases, compared with just 35 percent of those based on imaging techniques. Kirch and Schaffi, "Misdiagnosis at a University Hospital in 4 Medical Eras: Report on 400 Cases," pp. 29-40. See also Bordage, "Why Did I Miss the Diagnosis?," p. S138.

But, as Kuhn points out, an inaccurate and incomplete history can lead to the wrong diagnostic tests being ordered. Kuhn, "Diagnostic Errors," pp. 743, 745.

19. An estimated 80 to 85 percent of medical diagnoses are made correctly on the basis of a patient's history. Jauhar, *Intern: A Doctor's Initiation*, p. 289; and Konner, *Becoming a Doctor*, p. 130. (See endnote 5, Chapter Two, and endnote 1, Preface.)

20. See Jerome Groopman, *How Doctors Think* (Boston/New York: Houghton Mifflin Co./First Mariner Books, 2008 paper), p. 192.

21. Sandeep Jauhar, "The Demise of the Physical Exam," *New England Journal of Medicine* 354 (2006): 550. See also Goldman, Sayson, et al, "The Value of the Autopsy in Three Medical Eras," p. 1004.

22. Gail Van Kanegan and Michael Boyette, *How to Survive Your Hospital Stay: The Complete Guide to Getting the Care You Need—And Avoiding the Problems You Don't* (New York: Fireside, 2003), pp. 189-90.

Here's a related tidbit to contemplate: According to Johns Hopkins researchers, doctors miss 9 percent of all cerebrovascular events (strokes) when the patients' symptoms are mild or transient, and thus, vague and unparticularized. Newman-Toker and Pronovost, "Diagnostic Errors—The Next Frontier for Patient Safety," p. 1060. See also David E. Newman-Toker, Karen A. Robinson, and Jonathan A. Edlow, "Frontline Misdiagnosis of Cerebrovascular Events in the Era of Modern Neuroimaging: A Systematic Review," *Annals of Neurology* 64 (2008): S17-S18.

23. Groopman, *How Doctors Think*, pp. 178, 197-98.

24. Ibid, 178, 190-91.

25. Ibid, 180-81, 197-98.

26. Van Kanegan and Boyette, *How to Survive Your Hospital Stay*, pp. 182-83.

27. Geoffrey Norman, "Research in Clinical Reasoning: Past History and Current Trends," *Medical Education* 39 (2005): 418-20; Pat Croskerry, "Achieving Quality in Clinical Decision Making: Cognitive Strategies and Detection of Bias," *Academic Emergency Medicine* 9 (2002): 1200-01; Kevin W. Eva, "What Every Teacher Needs to Know About Clinical Reasoning," *Medical Education* 39 (2005): 103; S. Coderre, H. Mandin, et al, "Diagnostic Reasoning Strategies and Diagnostic Success," *Medical Education* 37 (2003): 695-97; and Pat Croskerry, "The Cognitive Imperative: Thinking About How We Think," *Academic Emergency Medicine* 7 (2000): 1224-25.

28. Norman, "Research in Clinical Reasoning: Past History and Current Trends," pp. 49-20; and Kuhn, "Diagnostic Errors," pp. 742-43.

29. H.G. Schmidt, G.R. Norman, and H.P.A. Boshuizen, "A Cognitive Perspective on Medical Expertise: Theory and Implications," *Academic Medicine* 65 (1990): 611-21 (illness script is defined on p. 613); and Norman, "Research in Clinical Reasoning: Past History and Current Trends," pp. 421-23.

30. Norman, "Research in Clinical Reasoning: Past History and Current Trends," p. 425.

31. See Kuhn, "Diagnostic Errors," pp. 741-42; and Robert M. Hamm and John Zubialde, "Physicians' Expert Cognition and the Problem of Cognitive Biases," *Primary Care* 22 (1995): 186-87.

32. Kuhn, "Diagnostic Errors," pp. 742-46; and Tavinder K. Ark, Lee R. Brooks, and Kevin W. Eva, "Giving Learners the Best of Both Worlds: Do Clinical Teachers Need to Guard Against Teaching Pattern Recognition to Novices?," *Academic Medicine* 81 (2006): 405. See also Judith L. Bowen, "Educational Strategies to Promote Clinical Diagnostic Reasoning," *New England Journal of Medicine* 355 (2006): 2218-24; and Hamm and Zubialde, "Physicians' Expert Cognition and the Problem of Cognitive Biases," p. 185-91.

33. See Bowen, "Educational Strategies to Promote Clinical Diagnostic Reasoning," pp. 2217-21.

According to Croskerry, novices typically engage in another diagnostic strategy: exhaustion. Medical students and other medical trainees will search painstakingly for "all medical facts about the patient," he writes, without giving immediate attention to any, and then sift through a mountain of data for the diagnosis. The exhaustive patient workup reflects the trainee's high degree of uncertainty. Of course, when the diagnosis is, in fact, esoteric, exhaustion may be the appropriate strategy. *Quality in Clinical Decision-making* 9 (2002): 1200.

34. Robert H. Miller and Daniel M. Bissell, *Med School Confidential: A Complete Guide to the Medical School Experience: By Students, for Students* (New York: St. Martin's Press/Thomas Dunne Books 2006), p. 152.

35. See Evidence-Based Medicine Working Group, "Evidence-Based Medicine: A New Approach to Teaching the Practice of Medicine," *JAMA* 268 (1992): 2420-25.

36. Groopman, *How Doctors Think*, pp. 5-6. See also Lucian L. Leape, Donald M. Berwick, and David W. Bates, "What Practices Will Most Improve Safety? Evidence-Based Medicine Meets Patient Safety," *JAMA* 288 (2002): 501-07; and Rose Hatala and Gordon Guyatt, "Evaluating the Teaching of Evidence-Based Medicine," *JAMA* 288 (2002): 1110-12.

37. Donald A. Redelmeier, "The Cognitive Psychology of Missed Diagnoses," *Annals of Internal Medicine* 142 (2005): 115. See also Bordage, "Why Did I Miss the Diagnosis?," p. S138.

38. Perri Klass, "The Patient Narrative," p. 48, in *Becoming a Doctor: From Student to Specialist, Doctor-Writers Share Their Experiences*, ed. Lee Gutkind (New York: W.W.

Norton & Co., 2010).

39. Ibid, 46-48. See David Watts, "Cure for the Common Cold," *New England Journal of Medicine* 367 (2012): 1184-85.

40. Ibid, pp. 118-19.

41. Graber, Franklin, and Gordon, "Diagnostic Error in Internal Medicine," p. 1494; Croskerry, "When Diagnoses Fail," pp. 79-80; and Mark Graber, Ruthanna Gordon, and Nancy Franklin, "Reducing Diagnostic Errors in Medicine: What's the Goal?" *Academic Medicine* 77 (2002): 982-86.

42. Graber, Franklin, and Gordon, "Diagnostic Error in Internal Medicine," pp. 1493-94; and Croskerry, "When Diagnoses Fail," pp. 79-80.

43. Croskerry, "Achieving Quality in Clinical Decision Making: Cognitive Strategies and Detection of Bias," pp. 1201-02. Croskerry espouses a hard-wired theory of CDRs, viewing them as the nature of the human beast. I believe that cognitive gaps or biases are learned and can be unlearned. You just have to pay attention. See Croskerry, "When Diagnoses Fail," pp. 79-87.

44. Lucian L. Leape, "New World of Patient Safety: 23rd Annual Samuel Jason Mixter Lecture," *Archives of Surgery* 144 (2009): 396.

45. Croskerry catalogs his CDRs in a number of articles, including Croskerry, "Achieving Quality in Clinical Decision Making," pp. 1186-99; Croskerry, "When Diagnoses Fail," p. 86; and Croskerry, "The Importance of Cognitive Errors in Diagnosis and Strategies to Minimize Them," pp. 777-78. Groopman presents actual doctor-patient case studies of cognitive errors throughout *How Doctors Think*. The explanations related to anchoring, availability, confirmation bias, premature closure, and search satisficing appear on pp. 65, 169-70, 185, 197.

Katherine Hall, a New Zealand medical professor, gives a competent overview of physician heuristics ("rules of thumb") and biases in K. H. Hall, "Reviewing Intuitive Decision-Making and Uncertainty: The Implications for Medical Education," *Medical Education* 36 (2002): 219-21; and Kuhn probes the anchoring and premature closure CDRs in "Diagnostic Errors," pp. 743-45.

Hamm and Zubialde cover cognitive errors and heuristic strategies as recognized in the mid-1990s in Hamm and Zubialde, "Physicians' Expert Cognition and the Problem of Cognitive Biases," p. 191-97. They also tackle the thorny question of how to address cognitive errors through medical education.

46. See the Croskerry citations in endnote 45; and Groopman, *How Doctors Think*, pp. 45, 72, 126-27, and 170-71.

47. Psychiatric patients' illness is "in their heads." See Delese Wear, Julie M. Aultman, et al, "Making Fun of Patients: Medical Students' Perceptions and Use of Derogatory and Cynical Humor in Clinical Settings," *Academic Medicine* 81 (2006): 457; B.A. Teachman and K.D. Brownell, "Implicit Anti-Fat Bias Among Health Professionals: Is Anyone Immune?," *International Journal of Obesity* 25 (2001): 1525-31; E.L. Harvey and A.J. Hill, "Health Professionals' Views of Overweight People and Smokers," *International Journal of Obesity* 25 (2001): 1253-61; and M.R. Hebl and J. Xu, "Weighing the Care: Physicians' Reactions to the Size of a Patient," 25 (2001): 1246-52.

48. Pat Croskerry, "Diagnostic Failure: A Cognitive and Affective Approach," *Advances in Patient Safety* 2: 241-54, available at http://www.ahrq.gov.

49. For quote, see Groopman, *How Doctors Think*, pp. 239-40. For doing what others do, see Hall, "Reviewing Intuitive Decision-Making and Uncertainty," p. 218.

50. Newman-Toker and Pronovost, "Diagnostic Errors–The Next Frontier for Patient Safety," p. 1060; Olga Kostopoulou, Brendan C. Delaney, and Craig W. Munro, "Diagnostic Difficulty and Error in Primary Care–A Systematic Review," *Family Practice* 25(2008): 400; and R.L. Phillips Jr., L.A. Bartholomew, et al, "Learning From Malpractice Claims About

Negligent, Adverse Events in Primary Care in the United States," *Quality and Safety in Health Care* 13 (2004): 121-26.

51. Pat Croskerry, "When Diagnoses Fail: New Insights, Old Thinking," *The Canadian Journal of Continuing Medical Education* 15 (Nov. 2003): 79. Diagnostic error expert Dr. Mark Graber believes that "for every error we detect, scores are missed." Graber, "Diagnostic Errors in Medicine," p. 107.

52. Croskerry, "The Importance of Cognitive Errors in Diagnosis," p. 776.

53. See David J. Dula, Nora L. Dula, et al, "The Effect of Working Serial Night Shifts on the Cognitive Functioning of Emergency Physicians," *Annals of Emergency Medicine* 38 (2001): 152-55; and Gloria Kuhn, "Circadian Rhythm, Shift Work, and Emergency Medicine," *Annals of Emergency Medicine* 37 (2001): 88-98.

54. Kuhn, "Diagnostic Errors," pp. 744, 748.

55. Konner, *Becoming a Doctor*, p. 343.

56. Physicians' failure to recognize the severity of a patient's illness is a common medical error. Schiff and Hasan, "Diagnostic Error in Medicine: Analysis of 583 Physician-Reported Errors," p. 1885; and Bordage, "Why Did I Miss the Diagnosis?," p. S138.

57. Allen Kachalia, Tejal K. Gandhi, et al, "Missed and Delayed Diagnoses in the Emergency Department: A Study of Closed Malpractice Claims From 4 Liability Insurers," *Annals of Emergency Medicine* 49 (2007): 200-02. These same researchers published a report on misdiagnoses in the outpatient setting at Tejal K. Gandhi, Allen Kachalia, et al, "Missed and Delayed Diagnoses in the Ambulatory Setting: A Study of Closed Malpractice Claims," *Annals of Internal Medicine* 145 (2006): 488-96l

58. Van Kanegan and Boyette, *How to Survive Your Hospital Stay*, pp. 164, 183-86.

CHAPTER FIVE. 2010: FALLS AND FRACTURES, Life Turned Upside-Down

1. Johns Hopkins Medicine, Drs. Hugh G. Calkins and Ronald Berger, "Atrial Fibrillation: The Latest Management Strategies," (New York: Health Medicine, LLC 2011), pp. 4, 6-7; and Mayo Clinic Staff, "Atrial Fibrillation: Causes," at http://www.mayoclinic.com/health/atrial-fibrillation/DS00291.

2. Johns Hopkins Medicine, "Atrial Fibrillation," pp. 4-5.

3. James E. Groves, "Taking Care of the Hateful Patient," *New England Journal of Medicine* 298 (1978): 887.

4. Edward R. Marcantonio, Jonathan M. Flacker, et al, "Reducing Delirium After Hip Fracture: A Randomized Trial," *Journal of the American Geriatrics Society* 49 (2001): 516.

5. For an easy-to-understand description of the types of hip fracture and their surgical treatment, see Encyclopedia of Nursing & Allied Health, "Hip Fractures Rehabilitation," at http://www.enotes.com/nursing-encyclopedia/hip-fractures-rehabilitation/. The Mayo Clinic website, www.mayoclinic.com, and WebMD, online, also explain hip fractures for laypeople.

6. Ibid, for hip-replacement surgery.

7. Morton C. Creditor, "Hazards of Hospitalization of the Elderly," *Annals of Internal Medicine* 118 (1993): 219, 221.

8. Scott Schnell, Susan M. Friedman, et al, "The 1-Year Mortality of Patients Treated in a Hip Fracture Program for Elders," *Geriatric Orthopaedic Surgery & Rehabilitation* 1 (2010): 6-7; and Laurence Z. Rubenstein, "Falls in Older People: Epidemiology, Risk Factors and Strategies for Prevention," *Age and Ageing* 35 (Supp. 2, 2006): ii37-ii41. See also American Geriatrics Society, British Geriatrics Society, and American Academy of Orthopaedic Surgeons Panel on Falls Prevention, "Guideline for the Prevention of Falls in Older Persons,"

Journal of the American Geriatrics Society 49 (2001): 664-72; the endnotes in Gretchen M. Orosz, Edward L. Hannan, et al, "Hip Fracture in the Older Patient: Reasons for Delay in Hospitalization and Timing of Surgical Repair," *Journal of the American Geriatrics Society* 50 (2002): 1336-40; and Helen Hoenig, Lisa V. Rubinstein, et al, "What is the Role of Timing in the Surgical and Rehabilitative Care of Community-Dwelling Older Persons With Acute Hip Fracture?," *Archives of Internal Medicine* 157 (1997): 513-20.

9. According to researchers at the University of Washington's Dept. of Rehabilitation Medicine, about half of older adults hospitalized for fall-related injuries are discharged to nursing homes. Anne Shumway-Cook, Marcia A. Ciol, et al, "Falls in the Medicare Population: Incidence, Associated Factors, and Impact on Health Care," *Physical Therapy* 89 (2009): 325. See also A Place for Mom, "Hip Fractures in the Elderly," at http://nursing-homes. aplaceformom.com/articles/hip-fractures-in-the-elderly/; and Encyclopedia of Nursing & Allied Health, "Hip Fractures Rehabilitation," *supra,* endnote 5.

10. Mayo Clinic Staff, "Heart Failure: Tests and Diagnosis," at http://www.mayoclinic. com/health/heart-failure/DS00061; Johns Hopkins Medicine, "Atrial Fibrillation," p. 19; and UCLA Health, "Surgery and Procedures: Electrocardiogram," at http://www.uclahealth. org/body.cfm?id=593 (click on the "Medical Tests" link, then on "Electrocardiograms" in the next window). The quote about the echocardiogram is from UCLA Health, "Echocardiogram: How the test is performed," at http://www.uclahealth.org/body.cfm?id=593 (click on "Medical Tests," then on "Echocardiograms.")

11. The medical staff at a Cleveland hospital in the late 1950s first identified activities of daily living as an index of self-care functionality among aged people recovering from hip fractures. These activities collectively came to be known as the Katz index, named for the chief physician, Sidney Katz. See Staff of The Benjamin Rose Hospital, "Multidisciplinary Studies of Illness in Aged Persons: II. A New Classification of Functional Status in Activities of Daily Living," *Journal of Chronic Disease* 9 (1959): 55-62. See also Sidney Katz, Amasa B. Ford, et al, "Studies of Illness in the Aged: The Index of ADL: A Standardized Measure of Biological and Psychosocial Function," *JAMA* 185 (1963): 914-23.

Certified-nurse-aide training programs vary from state to state, but all teach basic medical tasks, such as taking blood-pressure readings and pulses, and usually consist of laboratory classes and clinical experiences. A high-school diploma or GED, while highly desirable, is not always a prerequisite for admission to a program. To become state-certified, a CNA-program graduate must pass a competency examination. Twenty-one states, including Virginia and North Carolina, and the District of Columbia use the National Nurse Aide Assessment Program (NNAAP) exam. See NNAAP, National Council of State Boards of Nursing at https://www. ncsbn.org/1721.htm.

12. Stephen R. Lord, Hylton B. Menz, and Catherine Sherrington, "Home Environment Risk Factors for Falls in Older People and the Efficacy of Home Modifications," *Age and Ageing* 35 (suppl. 2, 2006): ii55-ii59. See also Rubenstein, "Falls in Older People: Epidemiology, Risk Factors and Strategies for Prevention," p. ii40.

13. Orosz, Hannan, et al, "Hip Fracture in the Older Patient: Reasons for Delay in Hospitalization and Timing of Surgical Repair," pp. 1336, 1339-40. See also Hoenig, Rubinstein, et al, "What is the Role of Timing in the Surgical and Rehabilitative Care of Community-Dwelling Older Persons With Acute Hip Fracture?," pp. 513-20; J.D. Zuckerman, M.L. Skovron, et al, "Postoperative Complications and Mortality Associated with Operative Delay in Older Patients Who Have a Fracture of the Hip," *Journal of Bone and Joint Surgery (American)* 77 (1995): 1551-56; and R.A. Incalzi, O. Capparella, et al, "Predicting In-Hospital Mortality After Hip Fracture in Elderly Patients," *Journal of Trauma* 36 (1994): 79-82.

14. The Johns Hopkins data come from a Johns Hopkins Health Alert, titled "Osteoporosis: The Sobering Facts About Hip Fracture" and published online in October 2011. See http://

www.johnshopkinshealthalerts.com.

15. CDC, "Costs of Falls Among Older Adults," at http://www.cdc.gov/HomeandRecreationalSafety/Falls/fallcost.html.

16. Adam Darowski, *Falls: The Facts*, (Oxford/New York: Oxford University Press, paper, 2008), pp. 13, 15.

17. CDC, endnote 15, *supra*.

18. See Lesley D. Gillespie, M. Clare Robertson, et al, "Interventions for Preventing Falls in Older People Living in the Community," published in *The Cochrane Library* 2009, issue 2, available at http://www.thecochranelibrary.com; and Mary E. Tinetti, "Preventing Falls in Elderly Persons," *New England Journal of Medicine* 348 (2003): 42.

19. CDC, "10 Leading Causes of Injury Deaths, United States 2007, All Races, Both Sexes" and "10 Leading Causes of Unintentional Injury Deaths, United States 2007, All Races, Both Sexes," available at the CDC's website, http://www.cdc.gov. To put the number of fall-related deaths into context, consider that the CDC reported that 496,095 people age 65 and over died in 2007 from heart disease, and 389,730 succumbed to cancer. (With a U.S. autopsy rate of only 5 percent, you can safely assume that many actually died from pulmonary emboli.)

20. CDC, "Costs of Falls Among Older Adults" and "Falls Among Older Adults: An Overview," available, respectively, at http://www.cdc.gov/HomeandRecreationalSafety/Falls/fallcost.html and http://www.cdc.gov/HomeandRecreationalSafety/Falls/adultfalls.html; and the white papers, "Fall Prevention Facts" and "Don't Let A Fall Be Your Last Trip: Who Is At Risk?," by the American Academy of Orthopaedic Surgeons, available, respectively, at http://orthoinfo.assos.org/topic.cfm?topic=A00101 and http://orthoinfo.assos.org/topic.cfm?topic=A00118.

See also Shumway-Cook, Ciol, et al, "Falls in the Medicare Population: Incidence, Associated Factors, and Impact on Health Care," pp. 324-32; Rebecca Boyd and Judy A. Stevens, "Falls and Fear of Falling: Burden, Beliefs and Behaviours," *Age and Ageing* 38 (2009): 423-27; and J.A. Stevens, P.S. Corso, et al, "The Costs of Fatal and Non-Fatal Falls Among Older Adults," *Injury Prevention* 12 (2006): 290-95.

For the incidence of wrist fractures in people ages 65 to 75, see Rubenstein, "Falls in Older People: Epidemiology, Risk Factors and Strategies for Prevention," p. ii37.

21. Darowski, *Falls: The Facts*, p. 1.

22. Ibid, 16.

23. For different analyses of risk factors, see Rubenstein, "Falls in Older People: Epidemiology, Risk Factors and Strategies for Prevention," pp. ii37-ii39; Stephen R. Lord, Hylton B. Menz, and Catherine Sherrington, "Home Environment Risk Factors for Falls in Older People and the Efficacy of Home Modifications," *Age and Ageing* 35 (Supp. 2, 2006): ii55-ii58; Tinetti, "Preventing Falls in Elderly Persons," pp. 43-46; and American Geriatrics Society, et al, "Guideline for the Prevention of Falls in Older Persons," pp. 664-65.

24. Darowski, *Falls: The Facts*, pp. 14-15; Rubenstein, "Falls in Older People," p. ii38-ii39; and American Geriatrics Society, et al, "Guideline for the Prevention of Falls in Older Persons," p. 664.

25. Darowski, *Falls: The Facts*, pp. 5-10.

26. Ibid, 6-7, 14.

27. Ibid, 14-15. See also the citations in endnote 8, *supra*, especially American Geriatrics Society, et al, "Guideline for the Prevention of Falls in Older Persons," pp. 664-65; and Tinetti, "Preventing Falls in Elderly Persons," p. 45.

CHAPTER SIX. 2010 cont.: CONFUSION, PAIN, AND DECLINE
When Bad Things Happen While Others Watch

1. Jauhar, *Intern: A Doctor's Initiation*, p. 219.

2. Sharon A. Levine, Jeremy Boal, and Peter A. Boling, "Clinician's Corner: Home Care," *JAMA* 290 (2003): 1203-04.

3. Andrew D. Weinberg and Kenneth L. Minaker, "Dehydration: Evaluation and Management in Older Adults," *JAMA* 274 (1995): 1552.

4. "Body Fluid Compartments," *Essentials of Anatomy & Physiology* ed. Rod R. Seeley, Trent D. Stephens, and Philip Tate (New York: The McGraw Hill Cos., 2007), pp. 526-27; and Dale A. Schoeller, "Changes in Total Body Water With Age," *American Journal of Clinical Nutrition* 50 (1989): 1176-78, 1181.

5. See The Mayo Clinic at http://www.mayoclinic.com/health/dehydration/DS00561.

6. Weinberg and Minaker, "Dehydration: Evaluation and Management in Older Adults," pp. 1552-53; and Joan L. Warren, Tamara Harris, and Caroline Phillips, "Dehydration in Older Adults," *JAMA* 275 (1996): 912.

7. Weinberg and Minaker, "Dehydration: Evaluation and Management in Older Adults," p. 1554.

8. Ibid, 1553.

9. Marzia Leacche, Daniel Unic, et al, "Modern Surgical Treatment of Massive Pulmonary Embolism: Results in 47 Consecutive Patients After Rapid Diagnosis and Aggressive Surgical Approach," *The Journal of Thoracic and Cardiovascular Surgery* 129 (2005): 1018-19; and James D. Douketis, Clive Kearon, et al, "Risk of Fatal Pulmonary Embolism in Patients With Treated Venous Thromboembolism," *JAMA* 279 (1998): 458, 460.

10. According to Dr. Michael A.E. Ramsay, the scale he devised scores sedation at six different levels:
1) Patient is anxious and agitated or restless, or both;
2) Patient is co-operative, oriented, and tranquil;
3) Patient responds to commands only;
(The above three levels apply when a patient is awake; levels 4-6 apply to the sleeping patient. The glabella is the smooth area between the eyebrows just above the nose.)
4) Patient exhibits brisk response to light glabellar tap or loud auditory stimulus;
5) Patient exhibits a sluggish response to light glabellar tap or loud auditory stimulus; and
6) Patient exhibits no response.
Virtually every critically ill patient admitted into the ICU is given sedation therapy, Ramsay says, to "allow the patient to tolerate the physical environment, and the unpleasant procedures and therapies that are necessary in the ICU; to facilitate nursing care and management, and reduce both anxiety and stress, so that post-traumatic stress disorder does not occur after discharge from the unit."
Michael A.E. Ramsay, "How to Use the Ramsay Score to Assess the Level of ICU Sedation," available at http://5jsnacc.umin.ac.jp.
Ramsay first described the research that resulted in his scale in M.A.E. Ramsay, T.M. Savege, et al, "Controlled Sedation with Alpaxalone-Alphadolone." *British Medical Journal* 2 (1974): 656-59.

11. Mayo Clinic, "Complete Blood Count (CBC)," at http://www.mayoclinic.org/tests-procedures/complete-blood-count/basics/definition/prc-20014088.

12. An excellent resource online about Medicare coverage is "ElderLawAnswers" at http://www.elderlawanswers.com. The U.S. government website is www.medicare.gov.

CHAPTER SEVEN. AGEISM & AGING, A Study of Fear and Heterogeneity

1. Robert N. Butler, "Age-Ism: Another Form of Bigotry," *The Gerontologist* 9 (1969): 243.
2. Robert N. Butler, "Ageism," p. 22, in *The Encyclopedia of Aging*, ed. George L. Maddox, et al (New York, NY: Springer Publishing Co. Inc., 1st ed., 1987); and Robert N. Butler, "Ageism," p. 41, in *The Encyclopedia of Aging*, ed. Richard Schulz, et al (New York: Springer Publishing Co. Inc., 4th ed., 2006), vol. 1. See also Todd D. Nelson, "Ageism: Prejudice Against Our Feared Future Self," *Journal of Social Issues* 61 (2005): 207-21; and T.D. Nelson, "Ageism and Discrimination," in *Encyclopedia of Gerontology: Age, Aging, and the Aged*, ed. James E. Birren (Amsterdam/Boston/Heidelberg/London/New York: Elsevier Inc./Academic Press, 2nd ed. 2010), vol. 1, pp. 57-63.
3. Laura Diachun, Lisa Van Bussel, et al, "'But I See Old People Everywhere': Dispelling the Myth That Eldercare Is Learned in Nongeriatric Clerkships," *Geriatric Medicine* 85 (2010): 1221. Florida State University's College of Medicine has one of the nine departments. See http://med.fsu.edu/index.cfm?page=geriatrics.about.
4. Robert N. Butler, *Why Survive? Being Old in America* (New York/Evanston, Ill./San Francisco/London: Harper & Row, 1975), p. xi.
5. Zaldy S. Tan, "A Doctor of None," pp. 133-34, in *Becoming a Doctor: From Student to Specialist, Doctor-Writers Share Their Experiences*, ed. Lee Gutkind (New York: W.W. Norton & Co., 2010).

The following articles address ageism within the medical-student and physician populations:

Clare Harries, Damien Forrest, et al, "Which Doctors Are Influenced by a Patient's Age? A Multi-Method Study of Angina Treatment in General Practice, Cardiology and Gerontology," *Quality and Safety in Health Care* 16 (2007): 23-27.

Delese Wear, Julie M. Aultman, et al, "Making Fun of Patients: Medical Students' Perceptions and Use of Derogatory and Cynical Humor in Clinical Settings," *Academic Medicine* 81 (2006): 454-62.

Amy J.C. Cuddy, Michael I. Norton, and Susan T. Fiske, "This Old Stereotype: The Pervasiveness and Persistence of the Elderly Stereotype," *Journal of Social Issues* 61 (2005): 279 (medical setting).

Monisha Pasupathi and Corinna E. Lockenhoff, "Ageist Behavior," pp. 205-10, in *Ageism: Stereotyping and Prejudice Against Older Persons*, ed. Todd D. Nelson, (Cambridge, Mass./London: MIT Press 2002).

Genevieve Noone Parsons, Sara B. Kinsman, et al, "Between Two Worlds: Medical Student Perceptions of Humor and Slang in the Hospital Setting," *Journal of General Internal Medicine* 16 (2001): 544-49.

Atul K. Madan, Shaghayegh Aliabadi-Wahle, and Derrick J. Beech, "Ageism in Medical Students' Treatment Recommendations: The Example of Breast-Conserving Procedures," *Academic Medicine* 76 (2001): 282-84.

Barbara E. Cammer Paris, Gabriel Gold, et al, "First Year Medical Student Attitudes Toward the Elderly: A Comparison of Years 1986, 1991 and 1994," *Gerontology & Geriatrics Education* 18 (1997): 13-22.

Carols A. Reyes-Ortiz, "Physicians Must Confront Ageism," *Academic Medicine* 72 (1997): 831.

Carlos A. Reyes-Ortiz and Thomas Mulligan, "A Progressive Geriatrics Curriculum," *Academic Medicine* 71 (1996): 1140.

David B. Reuben, Judith T. Fullerton, et al, "Attitudes of Beginning Medical Students Toward Older Persons: A Five-Campus Study," *Journal of the American Geriatrics Society* 43 (1995): 1430-36.

Rolando Berger, "Age and Reversible Lung Disease: Let's Grow Old, But Not Be Forgotten or Ignored!," *Chest* 108 (1995): 897-98. (Writes Berger: "Do we really pay the same attention to the 80-year-old woman complaining of stomach pain or dizziness for the first time as we do to the 40-year-old executive with the same symptoms?" Ibid, 897.)

Michele G. Greene, Ronald Adelman, et al, "Ageism in the Medical Encoutner: An Exploratory Study of the Doctor-Elderly Patient Relationship," *Language & Communication* 9 (1986): 113-24.

Dawn L. Warren, Albert Painter, and John Rudisill, "Effects of Geriatric Education on the Attitudes of Medical Students," *Journal of the American Geriatrics Society* (1983): 435-8.

R. Adelson, A. Nasti, et al, "Behavioral Ratings of Health Professionals' Interactions with the Geriatric Patient," *The Gerontologist* 22 (1982): 277-81.

Alan J. Maxwell and Nicole Sullivan, "Attitudes Toward the Geriatric Patient Among Family Practice Residents," *Journal of the American Geriatrics Society* 28 (1980): 341-45.

Donald L. Spence, Elliott M. Feigenbaum, et al, "Medical Student Attitudes Toward the Geriatric Patient," *Journal of the American Geriatrics Society* 16 (1968): 976-83.

Articles documenting the negative effects of medical education on students include:

Mohammadreza Hojat, Michael J. Vergare, et al, "The Devil is in the Third Year: A Longitudinal Study of Erosion of Empathy in Medical School," *Academic Medicine* 84 (2009): 1182-91.

Liselotte N. Dyrbye, Matthew R. Thomas, et al, "Personal Life Events and Medical Student Burnout: A Multicenter Study," *Academic Medicine* 81 (2006): 374-84.

Lisa M. Bellini and Judy A. Shea, "Mood Change and Empathy Decline Persist During Three Years of Internal Medicine Training," *Academic Medicine* 80 (2005): 164-67.

Wayne Woloschuk, Peter H. Harasym, and Walley Temple, "Attitude Change During Medical School: A Cohort Study," *Medical Education* 38 (2004): 522-534.

(Other relevant articles in this issue of *Medical Education* include John Spencer, "Decline in Empathy in Medical Education: How Can We Stop the Rot?" pp. 916-20; and Mohammadreza Hojat, et al, "An Empirical Study of Decline in Empathy in Medical School," pp. 934-41.)

Jack Coulehan and Peter C. Williams, "Vanquishing Virtue: The Impact of Medical Education," *Academic Medicine* 76 (2001): 598-605.

Donald G. Kassebaum and Ellen R. Cutler, "On the Culture of Student Abuse in Medical School," *Academic Medicine* 73 (1998): 1149-58.

John K. Testerman, Kelly R. Morton, et al, "The Natural History of Cynicism in Physicians," *Academic Medicine* 71 (1996 Supp.): S43-S45.

Henry K. Silver and Anita Duhl Glicken, "Medical Student Abuse: Incidence, Severity, and Significance," *JAMA* 263 (1990): 527-32.

T.M. Wolf, P.M. Balson, et al, "A Retrospective Study of Attitude Change During Medical Education," *Medical Education* 23 (1989): 19-23.

Loretta Kopelman, "Cynicism Among Medical Students," *JAMA* 250 (1983): 2006-10.

6. I.L. Nascher, "Geriatrics," *New York Medical Journal* 90 (1909): 358. See also Susan A. Gaylord and Mark E. Williams, "A Brief History of the Development of Geriatric Medicine," *Journal of the American Geriatrics Society* 42 (1994): 335-40.

7. Theodore R. Brooks, "Gerontologists or Geriatricians? That is the Question," *Journal of the National Medical Association* 84 (1992): 749-51.

8. Tan, "A Doctor of None," endnote 5, *supra,* pp. 133-34.

9. I read the paperback edition: Samuel Shem, *The House of God* (New York: Bantam Dell, 2003). Bergman/Shem's worldly wise character, the Fat Man, a no-bullshit resident whose stubby fingers don't touch bodies unless they have to, especially the bodies of gomers, explains the acronym on p. 29, saying in part: "[G]omers are not just dear old people. Gomers are human beings *who have lost what goes into being human beings*. They want to die, and we will

not let them. We're cruel to the gomers, by saving them, and they're cruel to us, by fighting tooth and nail against our trying to save them. They hurt us, we hurt them." (my emphasis added)

10. Google gomer, and you'll learn more than you ever wanted to know about this offensive term, for example, that a 2007 poll by The Student Doctor Network showed that 17.29 percent of its respondents (23 people) considered it "wrong" to use the term gomer, because it is disrespectful to patients, while the other 110 (82.71 percent) said internships are "tough": "You need to laugh to survive." See The Student Doctor Network Forums, "Is it wrong to use the term, 'GOMER,' amongst ourselves?" at http://forums.studentdoctor.net/showthread.php?t=376277.

11. Diane G. Snustad, M.D., "Aging: Know Old With Me," University of Virginia Mini-Medical School, April 22, 2010.

12. Parsons, Kinsman, et al, "Between Two Worlds: Medical Student Perceptions of Humor and Slang in the Hospital Setting," p. 546.

13. Jauhar, *Intern: A Doctor's Initiation*, p. 90.

Speaking of smell, check out the results of a 2012 study conducted at the Monell Chemical Senses Center in Philadelphia and reported by the journal *PloS ONE* as "The Smell of Age: Perception and Discrimination of Body Odors of Different Ages," at http://www.plosone.org/article/info%3Adoi%2F10.1371%2Fjournal.pone.0038110. I think a study like this, in which 41 20-to-30-year-olds smelled underarm pads, is why we have the word idiocy in our lexicon.

14. I first heard these age divisions explained by Professor Shryl Sistrunk, M.D., in a lecture on "Aging," in the Georgetown University Mini-Medical School, April 20, 2010. Two days later, I heard Professor Diane G. Snustad, M.D., cite the same categories in her lecture, "Aging: Know Old With Me," a part of the University of Virginia Mini-Medical School, April 22, 2010. I later heard the divisions applied by medical professors lecturing in the Johns Hopkins University Mini-Medical School on "Aging and Health" in the autumn of 2011.

See "A Profile of Older Americans: 2010; Health and Health Care," Administration on Aging, U.S. Dept. of Health & Human Services, at http://www.aoa.gov/aoaroot/aging_statistics/Profile/2010/14.aspx.

15. Thomas A. Glass, Ph.D., "Late Life Development: Basic Theories, Concepts and Findings," lecture in "Aging and Health," Johns Hopkins University Mini-Medical School, Oct. 6, 2011. Reinforcing her colleague's "peak" pronouncement, Michelle C. Carlson, Ph.D., associate director of the Johns Hopkins Center on Aging & Health, pinpointed the age at which our body systems start to decline at 22. Carlson, "Mending the Heart, Feeding the Brain," lecture in "Aging and Health," Johns Hopkins University Mini-Medical School, Nov. 10, 2011.

Medical doctor Denham Harman of the University of Nebraska College of Medicine charted the same chances for death as a function of age. Harman wrote that changes due to the Inborn Aging Process (IAP) "are largely responsible for the now almost exponential rise in the limiting chances for death after about the age of 28 years in the developed countries. Only 1-2% of a cohort die before this age." Denham Harman, "Free Radical Theory of Aging: An Update, Increasing the Functional Life Span," *Annals of the New York Academy of Sciences* 1067 (2006): 11.

For a thorough, yet brief overview of heterogeneity, see Jean-Pierre Michel, Julia L. Newton, and Thomas B.L. Kirkwood, "Medical Challenges of Improving the Quality of a Longer Life," *JAMA* 299 (2008): 688-90.

16. "Fastest Running Nonagenarian: 95-Year-Old Ida Keeling Sets World Record," at http://www.worldrecordsacademy.org/sports/fastest_running_nonagenarian_95-Year-Old_Ida_Keeling_sets_world_record_112130.html.

See also Steve Wieberg, "Age may be irrelevant in Okla. State crash/Octogenarian pilots common," *USA Today,* Nov. 23, 2011, p. 10C.

17. Brian T. Weinert and Poala S. Timiras, "Theories of Aging," *Journal of Applied Physiology* 95 (2003): 1706.

18. Snustad, "Aging: Know Old With Me," endnote 11, *supra.*

19. Leonard Hayflick, "Aging: The Reality. 'Anti-Aging' Is an Oxymoron," *The Journals of Gerontology Series A: Biological Sciences Medical Sciences* 59 (2004): 575.

20. The HeLa cells came from 30-year-old Henrietta Lacks, who died of cervical cancer mere months after Johns Hopkins scientists harvested HeLa. Johns Hopkins kept HeLa cells multiplying in a lab culture and widely distributed them for research. Ms. Lacks, a poor, black woman born in Virginia, consented to the tissue biopsy that her surgeon performed, but had no knowledge of what happened to her cells. See Rebecca Skloot, *The Immortal Life of Henrietta Lacks* (New York: Broadway Paperbacks, 2010).

21. See "Cellular Aging: Growth Factors and Cellular Senescence," *Encyclopedia of Gerontology: Age, Aging, and the Aged,* endnote 2, *supra*, p. 257.

22. Glass, endnote 15, *supra.*

23. Data taken from Emily M. Agree, Ph.D., "Population Aging and Population Health," lecture in "Aging and Health," Johns Hopkins University Mini-Medical School, Oct. 20, 2011. See also Leonard Hayflick, "New Approaches to Old Age," *Nature* 403 (2000): 365.

24. Glass cited 2006 data from the World Health Organization for these statistics. According to the WHO, Japanese women had a life expectancy at birth of 86.0 years, and French women had a life expectancy of 84.0 years; their male counterparts could expect to live, on average, 79.0 and 77.0 years, respectively.

25. Matteo Tosato, Valentina Zamboni, et al, "The Aging Process and Potential Interventions to Extend Life Expectancy," *Clinical Interventions in Aging* 2 (2007): 401; and Weinert and Timiras, "Theories of Aging," p. 1707.

The public outcry incited by muckraking journalist Upton Sinclair's book, "The Jungle," a fictionalized exposé of the unsanitary U.S. meat-packing industry at the turn of the 20th century, contributed in part to congressional passage of the 1906 Pure Food and Drug Act. This first-ever food-and-drug law was an antecedent to legislation that decades later created the U.S. Food & Drug Administration. Sinclair himself exceeded his life expectancy at birth, living to age 90.

26. Hayflick, "Aging: The Reality. 'Anti-Aging' Is an Oxymoron," p. 575; and Leonard Hayflick, "The Future of Ageing," *Nature* 408 (2000): 268 (cited in Tosato, Zamboni, et al, "The Aging Process and Potential Interventions to Extend Life Expectancy," p. 401). See also Harman, "Free Radical Theory of Aging: An Update," p. 11; and Steven Horrobin, "The Value of Life and the Value of Life Extension," *Annals of the New York Academy of Sciences* 1067 (2006): 94.

27. Snustad, "Aging: Know Old With Me," endnote 11, *supra.* See "Centenarians" in *Encyclopedia of Gerontology: Age, Aging, and the Aged,* p. 269.

28. Harman, "Free Radical Theory of Aging: An Update," p. 15.

29. Hayflick, "New Approaches to Old Age," p. 365. See citations for Harman and Horrobin in endnote 12, *supra.*

30. See "Jeanne Calment" at http://en.wikipedia.org/wiki/Calment; and "Centenarians," *Encyclopedia of Gerontology: Age, Aging, and the Aged,* p. 269.

At age 13 Calment supposedly met Vincent Van Gogh, whom she called "disagreeable" and "dirty," when the artist visited her uncle's fabric shop.

31. Frank B. Hu, "The Mediterranean Diet and Mortality—Olive Oil and Beyond," *New England Journal of Medicine* 348 (2003): 2595-96

32. Antonia Trichopoulou, Tina Costacou, et al, "Adherence to a Mediterranean Diet

and Survival in a Greek Population," *New England Journal of Medicine* 348 (2003): 2600. See also Kim T.B. Knoops, Lisette C.P.G.M. de Groot, et al, "Mediterranean Diet, Lifestyle Factors, and 10-Year Mortality in Elderly European Men and Women: The HALE Project," *JAMA* 292 (2004): 1434; and Hu, "The Mediterranean Diet and Mortality—Olive Oil and Beyond," pp. 2595-96.

33. Dr. Roger Blumenthal, "Status of Statins," seminar in "A Woman's Journey," presented by Johns Hopkins Medicine, Nov. 17, 2012, Baltimore, Md.

34. See Knoops, et al, "Mediterranean Diet, Lifestyle Factors, and 10-Year Mortality in Elderly European Men and Women: The HALE Project," pp. 1433-39 and citations therein; and Trichopoulou, Costacou, et al, "Adherence to a Mediterranean Diet and Survival in a Greek Population," pp. 2599-2608.

Long-lived elders in these studies engaged in moderate alcohol consumption and moderate to high physical activity and either did not smoke or quit smoking more than 15 years before the respective study. See Michel, Newton, and Kirkwood, "Medical Challenges of Improving the Quality of a Longer Life," pp. 689-99.

35. Hu, "The Mediterranean Diet and Mortality—Olive Oil and Beyond," p. 2596. The Mayo Clinic describes the DASH diet in "DASH Diet: Healthy Eating to Lower Your Blood Pressure," at http://www.mayoclinic.com/health/dash-diet/HI00047.

36. Agree, "Population Aging and Population Health," endnote 23, *supra.*

37. The quote comes from John W. Rowe, "The New Gerontology," *Science* 278 (1997): 367.

The complete title of Drs. Rowe and Kahn's book is "Successful Aging: MacArthur Foundation's Study Shows You How the Lifestyle Choices You Make Now—More Than Heredity—Determine Your Health." At the time of its publication, Dr. Kahn, Ph.D., was an 80-year-old professor emeritus of psychology and public health at the University of Michigan.

For their explanation of "usual aging," see Rowe and Kahn, *Successful Aging* (New York: Pantheon Books, 1998), pp. 54-58.

38. Paulo H.M. Chaves, M.D., Ph.D., "Addressing the Well-Being of Older Adults: Millions and More at a Time," lecture in "Aging and Health," Johns Hopkins University Mini-Medical School, Oct. 20, 2011. See also "A Profile of Older Americans: 2010," Administration on Aging, U.S. Dept. of Health & Human Services, at http://www.aoa.gov/aoaroot/aging_statistics/Profile/2010/14.aspx; Lamberts, et al, "The Endocrinology of Aging," p. 423; and John W. Rowe, "The New Gerontology," *Science* 278 (1997): 367.

39. Snustad, "Aging: Know Old With Me," endnote 11, *supra.*

40. Chaves, "Addressing the Well-Being of Older Adults: Millions and More at a Time," endnote 38, *supra.*

41. Hayflick, "The Future of Aging," p. 267; and Matteo, Tosato, Zamboni et al, "The Aging Process and Potential Interventions to Extend Life Expectancy," p. 402.

42. The *New England Journal* report is Daniel Rudman, Axel G. Feller, et al, "Effects of Human Growth Hormone in Men Over 60 Years Old," *New England Journal of Medicine* 323 (1990): 1-6.

43. In 1993, in response to the Rudman study (see ibid) and the medical uproar it caused, two osteopathic physicians formed the American Academy of Anti-Age Medicine, a non-profit organization known as A4M. In 1998, A4M co-founder Ronald Klatz wrote the book, "Grow Young With HGH: The Amazing Medically Proven Plan to Reverse Aging," in which he exhorted that the fountain of youth "lies within the cells of each of us." Since the Rudman study, other studies have appeared that document significant risks associated with HGH therapy, especially among older people.

According to historian Carole Haber, "the leaders of the A4M have had their practices and credentials assailed by the medical and legal communities." Whether you consider them quacks or visionaries, anti-ageists preach a message that many people are eager to hear. A4M has about 26,000 members from 110 countries and sponsors an annual World Congress on Anti-Aging Medicine.

For more about the A4M, see Carole Haber, "Anti-Aging Medicine: The History. Life Extension and History: The Continual Search for the Fountain of Youth," *The Journals of Gerontology Series A: Biological Sciences Medical Sciences* 59 (2004): 515-522; and Hayflick, "'Anti-Aging' Is an Oxymoron," p. 576.

Wikipedia, which has been sued by A4M founders Klatz and Robert Goldman for defamation, provides a thorough overview of the organization's history, beliefs, promotion of anti-aging products, and disputes with the medical establishment at http://en.wikipedia.org/wiki/American_Academy_of_Anti-Aging_Medicine.

A4M's website is www.A4M.com.

44. Weinert and Timiras, "Invited Review: Theories of Aging," pp. 1706-07.

45. For my information about basic physiology, I consulted *Essentials of Anatomy & Physiology,* ed. Rod R. Seeley, Trent D. Stephens, and Philip Tate (New York: The McGraw Hill Cos., 2007), and *Encyclopedia of Gerontology: Age, Aging, and the Aged,* endnote 2, *supra.*

46. According to *Brocklehurst's Textbook of Geriatric Medicine & Gerontology*: "[T]he term allostasis, coined and introduced by Peter Sterling and J. Eyer in 1988, has been gaining recognition and use. According to the allostasis model, stability through change is the most realistic situation for living biological systems. The allostasis model also takes into account characteristics such as reciprocal tradeoffs between various cells, tissues, and organs, accommodative sensing and prediction with respect to the severity of a potential stressor, and the final cost of making a response and readjustment to bring about necessary change. Every act of allostasis adds to the allostatic load in terms of, for example, unrepaired molecular damage, reduced energy deposits, and progressively less efficient or less stable structural and functional components."

S.I.S. Rattan, "Homeostasis, Homeodynamics and Aging," *Brocklehurst's Textbook of Geriatric Medicine & Gerontology*, ed. Howard M. Fillit, Kenneth Rockwood, Kenneth Woodhouse, and J.C. Brocklehurst (Philadelphia: Saunders Elsevier, 7th ed., 2010), p. 696 [hereinafter cited in endnotes as *Brocklehurst*].

47. See Robin Holliday, "Aging Is No Longer an Unsolved Problem in Biology," *Annals of the New York Academy of Science* 1067 (2006): 2.

48. See Denham Harman, "Aging: A Theory Based on Free Radical and Radiation Chemistry," *Journal of Gerontology* 11 (1956): 298-99, the first article Dr. Harman wrote about his theory; and Harman, "Free Radical Theory of Aging: An Update," pp. 11-17.

Dr. Harman chronologically summarized his research and thinking about the free radical theory in Denham Harman, "Origin and Evolution of the Free Radical Theory of Aging: A Brief Personal History, 1954-2009," *Biogerontology* 10 (2009): 773-81.

ATP is chemically expressed as $C_{10}H_{16}P_3O_{13}N_5$.

49. Denham Harman, "The Biologic Clock: The Mitochondria?" *Journal of the American Geriatrics Society* 20 (1972): 145-47; and Denham Harman, "Free Radical Theory of Aging: Consequences of Mitochondrial Aging," *Age* 6 (1983): 86-94.

The dietary antioxidants that Harman gave to mice did not decrease the deleterious effects of free-radical reactions in their mitochondria.

50. See Tomohiro Nakamura, Malene Hansen, et al, "The Neurobiology of Aging: Free Radical Stress and Metabolic Pathways," pp. 150-52, and John E. Morley, Ligia J. Dominguez, and Mario Barbagallo, "Antiaging Medicine," p. 148, both in *Brocklehurst,* endnote 46, *supra*; and S. Alvarez, G.J. Lithgow, and M. Muranjan, "Oxidative Stress and Aging," in *Encyclopedia of Gerontology: Age, Aging, and the Aged,* pp. 512-13; and Mayo Clinic, "Red Wine and

Resveratrol: Good for Your Heart?," at http://www.mayoclinic.com/health/red-wine/ HB00089.

51. For the basics, see "Telomere," at http://en.wikipedia.org/wiki/Telomeres, and *Gerontology for the Health Care Professional*, ed., Regular H. Robnett and Walter C. Chop, (Boston: Jones and Bartlett Publishers, 2nd ed. 2010), p. 66.

The 1978 article is E.H. Blackburn and J.C. Gall, "A Tandemly Repeated Sequence at the Termini of the Extrachromosomal Ribosomal RNA Genes in *Tetrahymena*," *Journal of Molecular Biology* 120 (1978): 33-53.

52. Dr. Harman's "basic cause" quote comes from Harman, "Origin and Evolution of the Free Radical Theory of Aging: A Brief Personal History, 1954-2009," p. 774.

For Holliday's contributions, see Holliday, "Aging Is No Longer an Unsolved Problem in Biology," p. 3; and Robin Holliday, "Aging: The Reality. The Multiple and Irreversible Causes of Aging," *The Journals of Gerontology Series A: Biological Sciences Medical Sciences* 59 (2004): 568-69.

53. Holliday, "Aging Is No Longer an Unsolved Problem in Biology," p. 3. Holliday also expressed these thoughts in Holliday, "The Multiple and Irreversible Causes of Aging," pp. 568-71.

54. Holliday, "Aging Is No Longer an Unsolved Problem in Biology," pp. 3-4.

55. Ibid, 4-5; and Holliday, "The Multiple and Irreversible Causes of Aging," p. 569.

56. Holliday, "The Multiple and Irreversible Causes of Aging," pp. 569-71; and Holliday, "Aging Is No Longer an Unsolved Problem in Biology," p. 8.

57. Hayflick, "Aging: The Reality. 'Anti-Aging' Is an Oxymoron," pp. 573-75. See also Hayflick, "The Future of Ageing," pp. 267-69; and Leonard Hayflick, "How and Why We Age," *Experimental Gerontology* 33 (1998): 640-41.

Scientists working on the genetics of longevity point to a body of evidence suggesting that "the intricate genetic pathways of metabolism and stress resistance" are key. This means that the number of genes involved in aging and longevity is likely to be quite large. Jens Weibel, Morten Draeby Sorensen, and Peter Kristensen, "Identification of Genes Involved in Healthy Aging and Longevity," *Annals of the New York Academy of Sciences* 1067 (2006): 317.

58. "Centenarians," *Encyclopedia of Gerontology: Age, Aging, and the Aged*, pp. 271-74. Scientifically rigorous centenarian studies only began in the 1980s.

59. See Weibel, et al, "Identification of Genes Involved in Healthy Aging and Longevity," pp. 317-18, 320-21; Miriam Capri, Stefano Salvioli, et al, "The Genetics of Human Longevity," *Annals of the New York Academy of Sciences* 1067 (2006): 252-53, 258-60; Amandine Cournil and Thomas B.L. Kirkwood, "If You Would Live Long, Choose Your Parents Well," *Trends in Genetics* 17 (2001): 233-35; and Caleb E. Finch and Rudolph E. Tanzi, "Genetics of Aging," *Science* 278 (1997): 407-11

60. "Centenarians," *Encyclopedia of Gerontology: Age, Aging, and the Aged*, p. 275.

CHAPTER EIGHT. MEMORY LOSS, Normal Aging, MCI, or Dementia?

1. Dr. Frank Lin, M.D., Ph.D., "Hear, Hear: The Effect of Hearing Loss on Your Health and What to do About It," Johns Hopkins University Mini-Medical School, Oct. 27, 2011.

2. Constantine G. Lyketsos, "The Interface Between Depression and Dementia: Where Are We With This Important Frontier?," *American Journal of Geriatric Psychiatry* 18 (2010): 95; Guy G. Potter and David C. Steffens, "Contribution of Depression to Cognitive Impairment and Dementia in Older Adults," *The Neurologist* 13 (2007): 105, 108-09; and Martin G. Cole, "Delirium in Elderly Patients," *American Journal of Geriatric Psychiatry* 12 (2004): 11.

3. Ronald C. Petersen, "Mild Cognitive Impairment," *New England Journal of Medicine*

364 (2011): 2227. See also Richard Mayeux, "Early Alzheimer's Disease," *New England Journal of Medicine* 362 (2010): 2195. Dr. Mayeux is with the Taub Institute for Research on Alzheimer's Disease and the Aging Brain and the Gertrude H. Sergievsky Center at Columbia University, New York, NY.

4. "Normal Cognitive Aging," by Jane Martin and Michelle Gorenstein, in *Brocklehurst,* endnote 46, Chapter Seven, *supra,* pp. 170-77.

5. Ibid, 170; Patrick Rabbitt, Amanda Chetwynd, and Lynn McInnes, "Do Clever Brains Age More Slowly? Further Exploration of a Nun Result," *British Journal of Psychology* 94 (2003): 63-71 (especially pp. 69-70).

6. *Brocklehurst,* p. 171; Victoria J. Bourne, Helen C. Fox, Ian J. Deary, and Lawrence J. Whalley, "Does Childhood Intelligence Predict Variation in Cognitive Change in Later Life?," *Personality and Individual Differences* 42 (2007): 1551-59; and Yaakov Stern, Christian Habeck, et al, "Brain Networks Associated with Cognitive Reserve in Healthy Young and Old Adults," *Cerebral Cortex* 15 (2005): 394-402.

7. See Timothy A. Salthouse, "Mental Exercise and Mental Aging: Evaluating the Validity of the 'Use It or Lose It' Hypothesis," *Perspectives on Psychological Science* 1 (2006): 68-87. Dr. Salthouse writes: "Although my professional opinion is that at the present time the mental-exercise hypothesis is more of an optimistic hope than an empirical reality, my personal recommendation is that people should behave as though it were true. . . . [Mentally stimulating activities] are often enjoyable and thus may contribute to a higher quality of life, and engagement in cognitively demanding activities serves as an existence proof—if you can still do it, then you know that you have not yet lost it." Ibid, 84-85.

8. *Brocklehurst,* pp. 171-72.

9. Ibid.

10. Ibid.

11. Ibid, 173-74.

12. Ibid. See Jason Brandt, Eleni Aretouli, et al, "Selectivity of Executive Function Deficits in Mild Cognitive Impairment," *Neuropsychology* 23 (2009): 607, citing A. Miyake, N.P. Friedman, et al, "The Unity and Diversity of Executive Functions and Their Contributions to Complex 'Frontal Lobe' Tasks: A Latent Variable Analysis," *Cognitive Psychology* 41 (2000): 50.

13. *Brocklehurst,* pp. 174-75.

14. Ibid, 172-73.

15. Ibid, 172.

16. For example, Raeford E. Brown, Jr., "A Piece of my Mind: A Door Closes," *JAMA* 305 (2011): 977.

17. The American Psychiatric Assn. published the fourth edition of *Diagnostic and Statistics Manual for Psychiatric Disorders,* known as *DSM-IV,* in 1994; a guidebook to its use came out in 1995. See Allen Frances, Michael B. First, and Harold Alan Pincus, "Delirium, Dementia, Amnestic, and Other Cognitive Disorders," in *DSM-IV Guidebook* (Washington, D.C.: American Psychiatric Assn., 1995) [hereinafter cited as *DSM-IV Guidebook*].

In 2000, the APA published a revision to *DSM-IV,* which medical authors cite as *The DSM-IV-TR* (TR signifying text revision). Because the text revision did not affect diagnostic criteria related to delirium, dementia, and depression, I have elected to cite the 2000 revision as *DSM-IV,* not *DSM-IV-TR.* For that same reason, I use the *DSM-IV Guidebook,* which came out in 1995, to amplify the 2000 text.

18. Peter V. Rabins and Constantine G. Lyketsos, *Diagnosing and Treating Alzheimer's Disease,* (New York: MediZine, LLC, 2010), p. 15. I purchased this publication online from the Johns Hopkins Medicine Library.

19. Petersen, "Mild Cognitive Impairment," p. 2227. In accord with Petersen is Brenda L.

Plassman, Kenneth M. Langa, et al, "Prevalence of Cognitive Impairment Without Dementia in the United States," *Annals of Internal Medicine* 148 (2008): 427. For the Duke estimate, see Potter and Steffens, "Contribution of Depression to Cognitive Impairment and Dementia in Older Adults," p. 105.

20. Petersen, "Mild Cognitive Impairment," pp. 2227-29.

See also Ronald C. Petersen, Rosebud O. Roberts, et al, "Mild Cognitive Impairment: Ten Years Later," *Archives of Neurology* 66 (2009): 1447-49; Bradford C. Dickerson, Reisa A. Sperling, et al, "Clinical Prediction of Alzheimer Disease Dementia Across the Spectrum of Mild Cognitive Impairment," *Archives of General Psychiatry* 64 (2007): 1443-45; Ronald C. Petersen, Joseph E. Parisi, et al, "Neuropathologic Features of Amnestic Mild Cognitive Impairment," *Archives of Neurology* 63 (2006): 665; R.C. Petersen, "Mild Cognitive Impairment as a Diagnostic Entity," *Journal of Internal Medicine* 256 (2004): 183-93; and Ronald C. Petersen, Glenn E. Smith, et al, "Mild Cognitive Impairment: Clinical Characterization and Outcome," *Archives of Neurology* 56 (1999): 303-08.

It is safe to say that MCI is a heterogeneous cognitive state that *sometimes* signals the onset of progressive dementia. See Brandt, Aretouli, et al, "Selectivity of Executive Function Deficits in Mild Cognitive Impairment," pp. 607-18.

21. Petersen, "Mild Cognitive Impairment," pp. 2228-29.

"Milder cognitive syndromes," write Drs. Rabins and Lyketsos of Johns Hopkins, "usually affect only memory or the executive [function, and] have very limited functional effects day-to-day." Half of people with mild impairment, they add, experience other psychiatric symptoms, such as depression, but not delusions or hallucinations.

Peter V. Rabins and Constantine G. Lyketsos, "A Commentary on the Proposed DSM Revision Regarding the Classification of Cognitive Disorders," *American Journal of Geriatric Psychiatry* 19 (2011): 203.

22. Petersen, "Mild Cognitive Impairment," p. 2229, and Petersen's reply to letters about his article, "Mild Cognitive Impairment," *New England Journal of Medicine* 365 (2011): 1358. See also Petersen, Roberts, et al, "Mild Cognitive Impairment: Ten Years Later," p. 1449; Brenda L. Plassman, Kenneth M. Langa, et al, "Prevalence of Cognitive Impairment Without Dementia in the United States," *Annals of Internal Medicine* 148 (2008): 427; Liana G. Apostolova, Rebecca A. Dutton, et al, "Conversion of Mild Cognitive Impairment to Alzheimer Disease Predicted by Hippocampal Atrophy Maps," *Archives of Neurology* 63 (2006): 693-94; and Petersen, Smith, et al, "Mild Cognitive Impairment: Clinical Characterization and Outcome," pp. 303, 307.

A six-year longitudinal study on aging and dementia that started Oct. 1, 1987, and included all residents 75 and older in the Kungsholmen district of Stockholm, Sweden, showed that 35 percent of those with MCI progressed to dementia within three years. Those who improved usually reported cognitive dysfunctions other than memory loss. Katie Palmer, Hui-Xin Wange, et al, "Differential Evolution of Cognitive Impairment in Nondemented Older Persons: Results From the Kungsholmen Project," *American Journal of Psychiatry* 159 (2002): 436-41. See also Potter and Steffens, "Contribution of Depression to Cognitive Impairment and Dementia in Older Adults," p. 107.

23. Petersen, "Mild Cognitive Impairment," pp. 2228-29; and Rabins and Lyketsos, *Diagnosing and Treating Alzheimer's Disease*, p. 23.

24. Rabins and Lyketsos, *Diagnosing and Treating Alzheimer's Disease*, pp. 5, 77.

25. For 75 percent, see Potter and Steffens, "Contribution of Depression to Cognitive Impairment and Dementia in Older Adults," p. 108. I obtained the Alzheimer's Assn.'s prevalence figures from the association's website, "What is Alzheimer's?" at http://www.alz.org/alzheimers_disease_what_is_alzheimers.asp.

For other comments about AD's prevalence, see Susan Okie, "Confronting Alzheimer's

Disease," *New England Journal of Medicine* 365 (2011): 1070; Rabins and Lyketsos, *Diagnosing and Treating Alzheimer's Disease*, pp. 4, 26, and 28; and Rob Stein, "Early Diagnosis of Alzheimer's Risk Is Urged," *The Washington Post*, April 19, 2011, p. A4.

26. Stephen G. Post, "Genetics, Ethics, and Alzheimer Disease," *Journal of the American Geriatrics Society* 42 (1994): 782.

27. This mistake accompanied all of the press coverage that I read in late August 2011 about 59-year-old University of Tennessee women's basketball Coach Pat Summitt's Alzheimer's disease diagnosis. The Mayo Clinic's Dr. Petersen, one of my chief authorities in this chapter, diagnosed Coach Summitt.

28. Rabins and Lyketsos, *Diagnosing and Treating Alzheimer's Disease*, pp. 6-8, 87-88.

29. The APOE gene provides instructions for making apolipoprotein E, a protein that combines with fats (lipids) in the body to form lipoproteins. Lipoproteins play a role in maintaining normal levels of cholesterol in the bloodstream. For more detail about the APOE gene and the APOE e4 allele, see "Genetics Home Reference," National Library of Medicine, National Institutes of Health, at http://ghr.nlm.nih.gov/gene/APOE; Rabins and Lyketsos, *Diagnosing and Treating Alzheimer's Disease*, pp. 9-10; and Post, "Genetics, Ethics, and Alzheimer Disease," pp. 782-86.

30. George S. Alexopoulos, Barnett S. Meyers, et al, "Clinically Defined Vascular Depression," *American Journal of Psychiatry* 154 (1997): 562; and K. Ranga Rama Krishnan, Judith C. Hays, and Dan G. Blazer, "MRI-Defined Vascular Depression," *American Journal of Psychiatry* 154 (1997): 497.

31. Rabins and Lyketsos, *Diagnosing and Treating Alzheimer's Disease*, p. 75.

32. Johns Hopkins Health Alerts: "Memory, Recognizing the Signs of Lewy Body Dementia," published online Sept. 5, 2011. See http://www.johnshopkinshealthalerts.com. In LBD, patients experience a loss of dopamine-producing nerve cells similar to that seen in Parkinson's disease, as well as a loss of acetylcholine-producing nerve cells, similar to Alzheimer's.

According to Dr. Peter V. Rabins, "Some experts identify two types of LBD: *dementia with Lewy bodies*, in which cognitive symptoms appear within a year of neurological problems, such as slowness of movement and impaired balance, and *Parkinson's disease dementia*, in which cognitive symptoms appear more than a year after the onset of movement problems. . . . As a result, there's disagreement among experts whether the presence of Lewy bodies is a unique disease or a variant of Alzheimer's or Parkinson's. They develop Alzheimer's-like cognitive problems and Parkinsonian symptoms." Peter V. Rabins, M.D., M.P.H., Johns Hopkins Medicine, "Understanding Lewy Body Dementia," *Health After 50*, vol. 26, issue 1, March 2014, p. 3.

For more information on LBD, see the Lewy Body Dementia Assn.'s website at www.lbda.org.

33. Rabins and Lyketsos, *Diagnosing and Treating Alzheimer's Disease*, p. 14; and Mayeux, "Early Alzheimer's Disease," p. 2195. Adverse effects of prescription medicines, head trauma, and alcohol abuse are other common causes of non-AD dementia.

According to the Alzheimer's Assn., more than half of the estimated 5.4 million people living with AD today do not know they have the disease: They have not been diagnosed.

34. Rabins and Lyketsos, *Diagnosing and Treating Alzheimer's Disease*, pp. 4-5, 79. For the rate of decline in the first five years, see Stephanie Desmon, "Blood Tests May Hold Clues to Pace of Alzheimer's Disease Progression," *The JHU Gazette*, Oct. 10, 2011, p. 3.

35. Rabins and Lyketsos, *Diagnosing and Treating Alzheimer's Disease*, pp. 5-6, 80. See also Regula H. Robnett and Walter C. Chop, *Gerontology for the Health Care Professional* (Boston/Toronto/London/Singapore: Jones and Bartlett Publishers, LLC, 2010), pp. 130-31; and Mayeux, "Early Alzheimer's Disease," pp. 2195-96.

36. "Dementia," by Mayo Clinic staff, at http://www.mayoclinic.com/health/dementia/DS01131.

37. Rabins and Lyketsos, *Diagnosing and Treating Alzheimer's Disease*, pp. 32-36.

38. Ibid, 36-37. Dr. R. Scott Turner, director of the Georgetown University Memory Disorders Program, described memantine as add-on therapy in a Mini-Medical School lecture at Georgetown University April 27, 2010.

39. Petersen, "Mild Cognitive Impairment," pp. 2228-29; and Petersen, Roberts, et al, "Mild Cognitive Impairment: Ten Years Later," p. 1450-53.

40. *DSM-IV*, p. 148. See endnote 17, *supra*.

41. Ibid, 148-49. See also Rabins and Lyketsos, *Diagnosing and Treating Alzheimer's Disease*, p. 14; and Nancy S. Wecker, Amy Wisniewski, et al, "Age Effects on Executive Ability," *Neuropsychology* 14 (2000): 409-14. For a simple explanation, see "Executive Function," in Encyclopedia of Mental Disorders, at http://www.minddisorders.com/Del-Fi/Executive-function.html.

42. *DSM-IV*, p. 149; and Rabins and Lyketsos, *Diagnosing and Treating Alzheimer's Disease*, p.14.

43. Mary Ganguli, Deborah Blacker, et al, "Classification of Neurocognitive Disorders in DSM-5: A Work in Progress," *American Journal of Geriatric Psychiatry* 19 (2011): 206.

44. American Psychiatric Assn., "About DSM-5," Neurocognitive Disorders, at http://www.dsm5.org/ProposedRevision/Pages/proposedrevision.aspx?rid+419. See also Rabins and Lyketsos, "A Commentary on the Proposed DSM Revision Regarding the Classification of Cognitive Disorders," p. 201; Ganguli, Blacker, et al, "Classification of Neurocognitive Disorders in DSM-5: A Work in Progress," p. 205; and Petersen, "Mild Cognitive Impairment," p. 2232.

I purchased a copy of *DSM-5* in late 2013. For diagnoses of "Major or Mild Neurocognitive Disorder Due to Alzheimer's Disease," see American Psychiatric Assn., *Diagnostic and Statistical Manual of Mental Disorders Fifth Edition* (Washington, D.C.: American Psychiatric Assn., 2013), pp. 611-14. Dr. Ronald Petersen was a co-chair of the *DSM-5* work group on neurocognitive disorders.

45. Pursuant to *DSM-5*, dementia must be evidenced by "significant cognitive decline from a previous level of performance in one or more cognitive domains" and cognitive deficits sufficient to "interfere with independence in everyday activities." *DSM-5*, p. 602.

46. *DSM-IV*, p. 158-61; and *DSM-IV Guidebook*, pp. 111-12.

47. *DSM-5*, p. 621.

48. Lecture by Dr. Peter V. Rabins, "The 36-Hour Day: Guidance in Caring for Dementia," Oct. 16, 2012, Johns Hopkins University, Baltimore, Md.

49. *DSM-IV*, p. 155; and Rabins and Lyketsos, *Diagnosing and Treating Alzheimer's Disease*, p. 14.

The Alzheimer's Assn. (AA) and the National Institute of Neurological and Communicative Disorders and Stroke at the National Institutes of Health (NIH) first published their own diagnostic criteria for Alzheimer's disease in 1984.

Twenty-seven years later, in April 2011, an international workgroup formed by the AA and the National Institute on Aging (NIA), also of the NIH, jointly published new criteria and guidelines for diagnosing Alzheimer's disease. They are relevant today principally to research, not to patient evaluation and care.

Significant in the changes recommended by the AA-NIA commission for the diagnostic criteria are:

1) The identification of three revised stages of the disease, the first of which begins before symptoms of memory loss occur and ADL function is affected; and

2) The incorporation of biomarker tests (which do not yet exist)

The three stages the workgroup proposed are: 1) preclinical Alzheimer's disease; 2) MCI due to Alzheimer's disease; and 3) dementia due to Alzheimer's disease. Its emphasis reflects what it considers to be the "current thinking" about the timing of measurable changes in the brain caused by Alzheimer's—thus its push back to a preclinical stage.

Any biomarker tests associated with Alzheimer's disease would have to measure biological changes in the brain. Two categories identified by the AA-NIA commission are:

1) Biomarkers showing the level of beta-amyloid accumulation in the brain; and

2) Biomarkers showing that nerve cells in the brain are injured or actually degenerating.

Studies to assess and possibly validate Alzheimer's disease biomarkers are expected to take at least a decade or more.

You can read about the workgroup's criteria and guidelines on the websites of the Alzheimer's Assn. and the NIA: www.akz.org and www.nia.nih.gov/Alzheimers, respectively. The workgroup also has elucidated its recommendations in a number of articles published in *Alzheimer's & Dementia*, a journal of the AA, including:

"Toward Defining the Preclinical Stages of Alzheimer's Disease: Recommendations from the National Institute on Aging-Alzheimer's Association Workgroups on Diagnostic Guidelines for Alzheimer's Disease," *Alzheimer's & Dementia* 7 (May 2011): 280-92;

"The Diagnosis of Mild Cognitive Impairment Due to Alzheimer's Disease: Recommendations from the National Institute on Aging-Alzheimer's Association Workgroups on Diagnostic Guidelines for Alzheimer's Disease," *Alzheimer's & Dementia* 7 (May 2011): 270-79;

"The Diagnosis of Dementia Due to Alzheimer's Disease: Recommendations from the National Institute on Aging-Alzheimer's Association Workgroups on Diagnostic Guidelines for Alzheimer's Disease," *Alzheimer's & Dementia* 7 (May 2011): 263-69; and

"Introduction to the Recommendations from the National Institute on Aging-Alzheimer's Association Workgroups on Diagnostic Guidelines for Alzheimer's Disease," *Alzheimer's & Dementia* 7 (May 2011): 257-62.

50. Rabins and Lyketsos, *Diagnosing and Treating Alzheimer's Disease*, pp. 20-22; and Petersen, "Mild Cognitive Impairment," pp. 2229-31. See, e.g., C.R. Jack, Jr., F. Barkhoff, et al, "Steps to Standardization and Validation of Hippocampal Volumetry as a Biomarker in Clinical Trials and Diagnostic Criterion for Alzheimer's Disease," *Alzheimer's & Dementia* 7 (2011): 474-85; Clifford R. Jack, Jr., Heather J. Wiste, et al, "Brain Beta-Amyloid Measures and Magnetic Resonance Imaging Atrophy Both Predict Time-To-Progression From Mild Cognitive Impairment to Alzheimer's Disease," *Brain* 133 (2010): 3336-48; and Linda K. McEvoy, Christine Fennema-Notestine, et al, "Alzheimer Disease: Quantitative Structural Neuroimaging for Detection and Prediction of Clinical and Structural Changes in Mild Cognitive Impairment," *Radiology* 251 (2009): 195-205.

In an effort to ensure consistency in diagnosis, *DSM-5* emphasizes objective evidence and incorporates imaging, biomarkers, and genetic tests into its definition of early or mild Alzheimer's disease. A patient's cognitive decline, it advises, must be confirmed by an objective patient assessment, whether by standardized tests or by a more formal neuropsychological evaluation. See American Psychiatric Assn., "About DSM-5," Neurocognitive Disorders, endnote 44, *supra*; Rabins and Lyketsos," A Commentary on the Proposed DSM Revision Regarding the Classification of Cognitive Disorders," p. 201; and Okie, "Confronting Alzheimer's Disease," pp. 1069-72.

51. Rabins and Lyketsos, *Diagnosing and Treating Alzheimer's Disease*, p. 14.

52. Marshal R. Folstein, Susan E. Folstein, and Paul R. McHugh, "'Mini-Mental State': A Practical Method for Grading the Cognitive State of Patients for the Clinician," *Journal of Psychiatric Research* 12 (1975): 189-98. Drs. Folstein, Folstein, and McHugh developed the MMSE® because older patients, particularly those with dementia, could cooperate with testing

only for short periods, and most of the then-available batteries were lengthy. The MMSE is also known as the Folstein test. See also Rabins and Lyketsos, *Diagnosing and Treating Alzheimer's Disease*, pp. 18, 85.

53. Dr. Peter V. Rabins of Johns Hopkins explains the scoring on the MMSE as follows:
25 to 30: indicates normalcy
21 to 24: may indicate mild cognitive impairment
10 to 20: suggests moderate impairment
9 or below: suggests severe impairment.
Rabins and Lyketsos, *Diagnosing and Treating Alzheimer's Disease*, p. 40.
See also Petersen, "Mild Cognitive Impairment," p. 2229. According to Petersen, the Short Test of Mental Status and the Montreal Cognitive Assessment provide more useful measures than the MMSE.

54. Rabins and Lyketsos, *Diagnosing and Treating Alzheimer's Disease*, pp. 18-19, 30.

55. Thomas E. Finucane, "Viewpoint: Why Alzheimer's Medications Should *Not* Be Prescribed," within Rabins and Lyketsos, *Diagnosing and Treating Alzheimer's Disease*, p. 43.

56. Rabins and Lyketsos, *Diagnosing and Treating Alzheimer's Disease*, p. 58. Dr. Lyketsos is also chairman of the Johns Hopkins-Bayview psychiatry department.

57. Petersen's comments on the "Functional Activities Questionnaire" are in the Supplementary Appendix to his article, "Mild Cognitive Impairment," *New England Journal of Medicine* 364 (2011): 2227-34, available at www.nejm.org to subscribers of the NEJM. The FAQ was developed by a research team in the neurology department at the University of California at Irvine Medical Center. See R.I. Pfeffer, T.T. Kurosaki, et al, "Measurement of Functional Activities in Older Adults in the Community," *Journal of Gerontology* 37 (1982): 323-29. See also Rabins and Lyketsos, *Diagnosing and Treating Alzheimer's Disease*, pp. 18-20; and Jane M. Thibault and Robert William Steiner, "Efficient Identification of Adults with Depression and Dementia," *American Family Physician* 70 (2004): 1101-10, available at the time of my research at http://www.aafp.org/afp/2004/0915/p1101.html?printable+afp. (Please note: The printout I obtained of this article, available free online, ran 14 pages, not 10, and did not indicate page breaks. I could not find a hard copy of the article in a medical-school library and, therefore, do not cite to pages in subsequent references.)

CHAPTER NINE. 2010-11: A PLUMBING NIGHTMARE
The High Price of Botched Repair

1. H. Ballentine Carter, M.D., Johns Hopkins Medicine, "Should You Be Tested for Prostate Cancer?," *Health After 50*, vol. 23, issue 11, January 2012, p. 5. Carter is director of adult urology at Johns Hopkins.

2. Even the over-the-counter drug ibuprofen can elevate a man's PSA level, according to Richard J. Albin, "The Great Prostate Mistake," *The New York Times,* March 9, 2010, at http://www.nytimes.com/2010/03/10/opinion/10Albin.html.

3. Timothy J. Wilt, Michael K. Brawer, et al, "Radical Prostatectomy Versus Observation for Localized Prostate Cancer," *New England Journal of Medicine* 367 (2012): 204. See also Albin, "The Great Prostate Mistake," endnote two, *supra*; and "Assessment of the Prostate," *Brocklehurst's Textbook of Geriatric Medicine & Gerontology*, pp. 704-05 [first reference, endnote 46, Chapter Seven, *supra, hereinafter referred to as Brocklehurst*].

4. My principal sources for anatomy and physiology in this chapter are 1) *Essentials of Anatomy & Physiology* (2007), first cited in endnote 45, Chapter Seven. The description of the ureters, urinary bladder, and urethra is ibid, 514-15; 2) *Brocklehurst*, pp. 112-15; 3) Arthur C. Guyton and John E. Hall, *Textbook of Medical Physiology* (Philadelphia: Elsevier

Saunders, 11th ed., 2006), pp. 311-14; and 4) Elaine Marieb, *Human Anatomy and Physiology* (Menlo Park, CA: Addison Wesley, 1998), pp. 990-92.

See also "Prostate Anatomy 101," Johns Hopkins Health Alert, at http://www. johnshopkinshealthalerts.com/alerts/enlarged_prostate/prostate-gland-anatomy_6157-1. html?ET=johnshopkins:e82096:182592a:&st=email&s =W2R_120421_001.

5. "Outlet Function and Structure," *Brocklehurst*, p. 115.

6. Aruna V. Sarma and John T. Wei, "Benign Prostatic Hyperplasia and Lower Urinary Tract Symptoms," *New England Journal of Medicine* 367 (2012): 248; and David R. Paolone, "Benign Prostatic Hyperplasia," *Clinics in Geriatric Medicine* 26 (2010): 223-24. Dr. Paolone, a urologist at the University of Wisconsin medical school, offers an excellent overview of BPH, pp. 223-39.

See also Clinical Key, "Benign Prostatic Hyperplasia," at https://www.clinicalkey.com/ topics/urology/benign- prostatic-hyperplasia.html.

7. Brian R. Matlaga, Johns Hopkins Medicine, "The Best Treatment Strategies for BPH," The Johns Hopkins Library, 2009, p. 13. I purchased this publication.

8. Ibid, 6-7. See also Paolone, "Benign Prostatic Hyperplasia," pp. 223-24.

9. "Assessment of the Prostate," *Brocklehurst*, p. 702; Sarma and Wei, "Benign Prostatic Hyperplasia and Lower Urinary Tract Symptoms," p. 251; and C.G. Roehrborn, C.J. Girman, et al, "Correlation Between Prostate Size Estimated by Digital Rectal Examination and Measured by Transrectal Ultrasound," *Urology* 49 (1997): 548-56. According to Roehrborn, et al: "DRE is well known to underestimate large and overestimate small glands." Ibid, 554.

10. John T. Wei, Elizabeth Calhoun, and Steven J. Jacobsen, "Benign Prostatic Hyperplasia," ch. 2, pp. 45-48, in *Urologic Diseases in America*, ed. Mark S. Litwin and Christopher S. Saigal (Bethesda, Md.: National Institute of Diabetes & Digestive & Kidney Diseases 2007), hereinafter cited as "NIDDK, 'Benign Prostatic Hyperplasia.'"

11. The questions relate to 1) incomplete emptying; 2) frequency; 3) intermittency; 4) urgency; 5) weak stream; 6) straining; and 7) nocturia.

The IPSS is reproduced at Matlaga, "The Best Treatment Strategies for BPH," p. 10; and Paolone, "Benign Prostatic Hyperplasia," p. 226. Their source is the American Urological Assn., whose "Clinical Guidelines" for "Management of BPH (Revised 2010)," can be accessed at http://www.auanet.org/content/clinical-practice/guidelines/clinical-guidelines. cfm?sub+bph. I hereinafter refer to this source as "AUA Clinical Guidelines: Management of BPH." The AUASI appears in Appendix 6, p. 277 in "Final Appendices" of "AUA Clinical Guidelines: Management of BPH." See also Julie K. Gammack, "Lower Urinary Tract Symptoms," *Clinics in Geriatric Medicine* 26 (2010): 249-51.

12. Matlaga, "The Best Treatment Strategies for BPH," p. 10.

13. Sarma and Wei, "Benign Prostatic Hyperplasia and Lower Urinary Tract Symptoms," p. 248. When BPH is accompanied by enlargement of the prostate gland, it can lead to "static bladder-outlet obstruction," which is "the most commonly cited basis for LUTS," say Drs. Sarma and Wei. Ibid, 249.

14. Matlaga, "The Best Treatment Strategies for BPH," pp. 8-9; and Gammack, "Lower Urinary Tract Symptoms," pp. 249-53.

15. Sarma and Wei, "Benign Prostatic Hyperplasia and Lower Urinary Tract Symptoms," pp. 250-51, 255. The website address for "AUA Clinical Guidelines: Management of BPH" appears in endnote 11, *supra*. The European Assn. of Urology's "Guidelines on the Management of Male Lower Urinary Tract Symptoms (LUTS), Including Benign Prostatic Obstruction (BPO)," appear at http://www.uroweb.org/gls/pdf/12_Male_LUTS_LR%20 May%209th%202012.pdf. I hereinafter refer to them as "2012 EAU Guidelines" with a page citation to a printout of this pdf.

See also Agency for Healthcare Research and Quality, "Guidelines on the Treatment of

Non-Neurogenic Male LUTS," 2011, Rockville, Md., at http://www.guideline.gov/content. aspx?id=34066&search=luts.

16. Paolone, "Benign Prostatic Hyperplasia," p. 225.

17. Gammack, "Lower Urinary Tract Symptoms," pp. 250-55; and Paolone, "Benign Prostatic Hyperplasia," pp. 224-27. A neurogenic bladder is one that becomes dysfunctional because of damage by neurological injury or disease, such as diabetes, Parkinson's disease, or multiple sclerosis.

See Victor W. Nitti, "Pressure Flow Urodynamic Studies: The Gold Standard for Diagnosing Bladder Outlet Obstruction," *Reviews in Urology* 7 (2005, Supp. 6): S14-S15.

18. Matlaga, "The Best Treatment Strategies for BPH," p. 13.

19. Gammack, "Lower Urinary Tract Symptoms," p. 253.

20. According to *Brocklehurst*, researchers who studied urological disorders in the past too often selected symptomatic, rather than asymptomatic elders as subjects. They also typically failed to report on important influencing factors, such as estrogenization status in women and pelvic-floor support and function status in both sexes. *Brocklehurst*, p. 115.

See also Guyton and Hall, *Textbook of Medical Physiology*, pp. 311-12, and Marieb, *Human Anatomy and Physiology*, pp. 990-91, *supra*, endnote 4.

21. Gammack, "Lower Urinary Tract Symptoms," pp. 249-50, 257. (See Chapter Twelve for details about age-related changes in tissue and muscle.)

22. *The Merck Manual of Geriatrics*, endnote 9, Chapter Two, *supra*, p. 965.

23. Ibid.

24. For an easy-to-understand overview, see "Stress Incontinence," Mayo Clinic, at http://www.mayoclinic/health/stress-incontinence/DS00828; and "Urinary Incontinence," Mayo Clinic, at http://www.mayoclinic.org/urinary-incontinence/types.html. For more detail, see "Outlet Incompetence" and treatment thereof in *The Merck Manual of Geriatrics*, p. 968, 977-79.

25. Ann G. Sjoerdsma, *Starting With Serotonin: How a High-Rolling Father of Drug Discovery Repeatedly Beat the Odds* (Silver Spring, Md.: Improbable Books, 2008), pp. 312, 378.

26. "FDA Requests Boxed Warnings on Fluoroquinolone Antimicrobial Drugs: Seeks to Strengthen Warnings Concerning Increased Risk of Tendinitis and Tendon Rupture," at http://www.fda.gov/NewsEvents/Newsroom/PressAnnouncements/2008/ucm116919. htm; "Information for Healthcare Professionals On Fluoroquinolone Antimicrobial Drugs," at http://www.fda.gov/cder/drug/InfoSheets/HCP/fluoroquinolonesHCP.htm; and "Black Box Warnings: Box Denotes a Drug's Possible Serious Side Effects or Risks," at http://drugs.about.com/od/medicationabcs/a/BlackBoxWarning.htm.

27. For Kegel basics, see Mayo Clinic, "Kegel Exercises for Men: Understand the Benefits," at http://www.mayoclinic/health/kegel-exercises-for-men/MY01402; and WebMD, "Kegel Exercises: Treating Male Urinary Incontinence," at http://men.webmd.com/kegel-exercises-treating-male-urinary-incontinence.

28. Sarma and Wei, "Benign Prostatic Hyperplasia and Lower Urinary Tract Symptoms," p. 251; and Debra A. Schwinn and Claus G. Roehrborn, "α1-Adrenoceptor Subtypes and Lower Urinary Tract Symptoms," *International Journal of Urology* 15 (2008): 193-94.

29. Matlaga, "The Best Treatment Strategies for BPH," pp. 19-21, 40, and 44.

30. "2012 EAU Guidelines," pp. 11-30.

31. Matlaga, "The Best Treatment Strategies for BPH," p. 44. See also "2012 EAU Guidelines," pp. 30-39; "AUA Clinical Guidelines: Management of BPH," pp. 8-12; and NIDDK, "Benign Prostatic Hyperplasia," pp. 57-60. The discussion in "2012 EAU Guidelines" is especially useful.

32. Matlaga, "The Best Treatment Strategies for BPH," p. 40; and Kevin T. McVary, Claus

G. Roehrborn, et al, "Update on AUA Guideline on the Management of Benign Prostatic Hyperplasia," *Journal of Urology* 185 (2011): 1796-97.

33. Matlaga, "The Best Treatment Strategies for BPH," pp. 31-35, 40; "2012 EAU Guidelines," pp. 48-54; and "AUA Clinical Guidelines: Management of BPH," Chapter One, pp. 17-18.

34. Of the 120,000 BPH prostatectomies performed in the United States in 2007, the majority were not TURPs: Sarma and Wei, "Benign Prostatic Hyperplasia and Lower Urinary Tract Symptoms," pp. 249, 252-53; and X Yu, S.P. Elliott, T.J. Wilt, et al, "Practice Patterns in Benign Prostatic Hyperplasia Surgical Therapy: The Dramatic Increase in Minimally Invasive Technologies," *Journal of Urology* 180 (2008): 242-44.

In 1999, the TURP represented 81 percent of all BPH surgery in the United States; by 2005, only 39 percent of such procedures were TURPs. And yet, during this period, the total number of BPH surgeries increased by 44 percent. Several factors account for this increase, including the increased number of older men in the U.S. population, but the most significant is the explosion in BPH laser procedures and minimally invasive treatments. Yu, Elliott, Wilt et al, "Practice Patterns in Benign Prostatic Hyperplasia Surgical Therapy," p. 243.

According to Yu, et al, clinical experience with the pioneering laser surgical techniques of the early 1990s was "unsatisfactory." A decade later, however, new techniques were developed that enabled this type of surgery to take off. Ibid, 243-44.

35. No less an authority than Dr. P. Roy Vagelos, retired CEO and Chairman of the Board of Merck & Co., predicted that BPH medications—in particular, Merck's finasteride—would relegate the TURP to history. This did not occur, but TURP rates have been declining since their introduction.

Steven A. Kaplan, "Re: Impact of Medical Therapy on Transurethral Resection of the Prostate: Two Decades of Change," *Journal of Urology* 187 (2012): 2160. See the original article, Jason Izard and J. Curtis Nickel, "Impact of Medical Therapy on Transurethral Resection of the Prostate: Two Decades of Change," *BJU International* 108 (2011): 89-93.

36. Sarma and Wei, "Benign Prostatic Hyperplasia and Lower Urinary Tract Symptoms," pp. 249, 252-53.

For early history of the TURP, see Charles E. Hawtrey and Richard D. Williams, "Historical Evolution of Transurethral Resection at the University of Iowa: Alcock and Flocks," *Journal of Urology* 180 (2008): 55-61; and "2012 EAU Guidelines," p. 40.

37. "AUA Clinical Guidelines: Management of BPH," Chapter One, p. 22; and "2012 EAU Guidelines," p. 41.

38. For a summary and clinical assessment of BPH treatment options available as of 2012, see "2012 EAU Guidelines," pp. 40-68. The open prostatectomy is p. 47. See also "AUA Clinical Guidelines: Management of BPH," Chapter One, pp. 18-22, and Matlaga, "The Best Treatment Strategies for BPH," pp. 35-40.

39. Paolone, "Benign Prostatic Hyperplasia," p. 234; "AUA Clinical Guidelines: Management of BPH," Chapter One, pp. 20-21; and "2012 EAU Guidelines," pp. 40-41.

40. McVary, Roehrborn, et al, "Update on AUA Guideline on the Management of Benign Prostatic Hyperplasia," p. 1800.

41. For an easy-to-understand explanation of "Prostate Laser Surgery," see the Mayo Clinic at http://www.mayoclinic.com/health/prostate-laser-surgery. The EAU gives an excellent overview of laser treatments at "2012 EAU Guidelines," pp. 55-59.

42. In a May 2011 article, the AUA cites five laser surgeries: transurethral holmium laser ablation of the prostate (HoLAP); transurethral holmium laser enucleation of the prostate (HoLEP); holmium laser resection of the prostate (HoLRP); photoselective vaporization of the prostate (PVP); and transurethral vaporization of the prostate (TUVP). McVary, Roehrborn, et al, "Update on AUA Guideline on the Management of Benign Prostatic Hyperplasia," p. 1797.

The HoLRP technique, first described in 1995, evolved into the HoLEP technique. See Douglas C. Kelly and Akhil Das, "Holmium Laser Enucleation of the Prostate Technique for Benign Prostatic Hyperplasia," *The Canadian Journal of Urology* 19 (2012): 6131-34.

43. Matlaga, "The Best Treatment Strategies for BPH," p. 41. See also Jean Nicolas Cornu, "Benign Prostatic Hyperplasia and Lower Urinary Tract Symptoms, " *New England Journal of Medicine* 367 (2012): 1668.

CHAPTER TEN. 2011: CONCURRENT PROBLEMS, Lung Nodules and Fatigue

1. Thomas Bodenheimer, "Coordinating Care—A Perilous Journey through the Health Care System," *New England Journal of Medicine* 358 (2008): 1064.

2. Nancy Gibbs and Amanda Bower, "Q: What Scares Doctors? A: Being the Patient . . . What Insiders Know About Our Health-Care System That the Rest of Us Need to Learn," *Time*, April 23, 2006, at http://content.time.com/time/magazine/article/0,9171,1186553m00. html.

3. Bodenheimer, "Coordinating Care—A Perilous Journey through the Health Care System," p. 1064.

4. Ibid, 1065.

5. See American Cancer Society, "Frequently Asked Questions About Lung Cancer," at http://www.cancer.org/cancer/news/features/frequently-asked-questions-about-lung-cancer.

6. Re malpractice and the fear of being sued, see: Heber MacMahon, John H.M. Austin, et al, "Guidelines for Management of Small Pulmonary Nodules Detected on CT Scans: A Statement from the Fleischner Society," *Radiology* 237 (2005): 399; and Leonard Berlin, "Malpractice Issues in Radiology: Failure to Diagnose Lung Cancer: Anatomy of a Malpractice Trial," *American Journal of Roentgenology* 180 (2003): 37-45.

7. American College of Chest Physicians, "Evaluation of Patients With Pulmonary Nodules: When Is It Lung Cancer?/ACCP Evidence-Based Clinical Practice Guidelines (2nd ed.)," *Chest* 132 (Suppl. 3, 2007): 110S.

8. For basic information about CT scans and contrast material, see UCLA Lung Cancer Program, Patient Education, "Educating Yourself About Lung Cancer: Tests and Studies: Chest CT," at http://lungcancer.ucla.edu/adm_tests_chest_ct.html; Mayo Clinic staff, "CT Scan," at http://www.mayoclinic.com/health/ct-scan/MY00309; WebMD, "Computed Tomography (CT) Scan of the Body," at http://www.webmd.com/a-to-z-guides/computed-tomography-ct-scan-of-the-body?page=4; Medical News Today, "What is a CT Scan? What is a CAT Scan?," at http://www.medicalnewstoday.com/articles/153201.php; and ehealthMD, "When is a Contrast Agent Required?," at http://ehealthmd.com/content/when-contrast-agent-required.

9. Thomas Bodenheimer, "Primary Care—Will It Survive?" *New England Journal of Medicine* 355 (2006): 861. Bodenheimer cites a Jan. 30, 2006 public policy report by the ACP titled "The Impending Collapse of Primary Care Medicine and Its Implications for the State of the Nation's Health Care." I accessed the report on June 30, 2013, at http://www.acponline. org/advocacy/advocacy_in_action/state_of_the_nations_healthcare/assets/stateheco6_1. pdf.

10. See Allan H. Goroll, "Reforming Physician Payment," *New England Journal of Medicine* 359 (2008): 2087; Thomas H. Lee, Thomas Bodenheimer, Allan J. Goroll, Barbara Starfield, and Katharine Treadway, "Redesigning Primary Care," *New England Journal of Medicine* 359 (2008): e24 [transcript of video roundtable discussion available on www.nejm. org.]; Bodenheimer, "Coordinating Care—A Perilous Journey Through the Health Care System," pp. 1064-71; Thomas Bodenheimer and Brian Yoshio Laing, "The Teamlet Model of

Primary Care," *Annals of Family Medicine* 5 (2007): 457-61; Bodenheimer, "Primary Care–Will It Survive?," pp. 861-64; Elizabeth A. McGlynn, Steven M. Asch, et al, "The Quality of Health Care Delivered to Adults in the United States," *New England Journal of Medicine* 348 (2003): 2635-45; and K. Grumbach and Thomas Bodeheimer, "A Primary Care Home for Americans: Putting the House in Order," *JAMA* 288 (2002): 889-93.

11. Bodenheimer uses the phrase, "the tyranny of the 15-minute visit," in Lee, Bodenheimer, et al, "Redesigning Primary Care," cited in endnote 10, *supra*, on p. 2 of the video transcript. The 23-second interruption study is M.K. Marvel, R.M. Epstein, et al, "Soliciting the Patient's Agenda: Have We Improved?" *JAMA* 281 (1999): 283-87, cited in Bodenheimer and Laing, "The Teamlet Model of Primary Care," p. 457.

12. Hoff, *Practice Under Pressure*, endnote 28, Chapter Three, *supra*, pp. 2-3, 6-8. See also Roni Caryn Rabin, "With Marcus Welby Out of the Picture, Every Hospital Patient Needs An Advocate," *The Washington Post*, Health/Science, April 30, 2013, p. E5.

13. American College of Physicians, "A Two-Pronged Strategy to Improve American Health Care: Make the Health System More Effective and Remove Barriers to the Patient-Physician Relationship," a report, Feb. 20, 2013, accessible at http://www.acponline.org/advocacy/advocacy_in_action/assets/snhcreport13.pdf. The income gap is reported on p. 16 of the pdf.

14. Roundtable discussion, "Redesigning Primary Care," endnote 10, *supra*, transcript pp. 1-2, 8. See generally Susan Okie, "The Evolving Primary Care Physician, " *New England Journal of Medicine* 366 (2012): 1849-53; and Thomas Bodenheimer, Kevin Grumbach, and Robert A. Berenson, "A Lifeline for Primary Care," *New England Journal of Medicine* 360 (2009): 2693-96.

15. Hoff, *Practice Under Pressure*, p. 3.

16. The choices for the eighth "degree of bother" question and their add-on scores are:
• Delighted (score zero)
• Pleased (score one)
• Mostly Satisfied (two)
• Mixed (three)
• Mostly Dissatisfied (four)
• Unhappy (five)
• Terrible (six)

See Paolone, "Benign Prostatic Hyperplasia," p. 226, endnote 6, Chapter Nine, *supra*; and "AUA Clinical Guidelines: Management of BPH," p. 4, endnote 11, Chapter Nine, *supra*.

17. Nitti, "Pressure Flow Urodynamic Studies: The Gold Standard for Diagnosing Bladder Outlet Obstruction," pp. S14-S15, S20-S21, endnote 17, Chapter Nine, *supra*.

18. National Cancer Institute, "Fact Sheet: Metastatic Cancer," at http://www.cancer.gov/cancertopics/factsheet/Sites-Types/metastatic/print.

Although rare, blood and lymphatic-system cancers can metastasize to the lungs, the heart, the central nervous system, and elsewhere. Ibid.

19. Ibid.

20. UCLA Lung Cancer Program, Patient Education, "Educating Yourself About Lung Cancer: Signs and Symptoms: Pleural Effusion," at http://lungcancer.ucla.edu/adm_signs_pleural.html and links therein; and National Cancer Institute, "Non-Small Cell Lung Cancer Treatment (PDQ®)," at http://www.cancer.gov/cancertopics/pdq/treatment/non-small-cell-lung/Patient. Other classic symptoms of lung cancer are bloody sputum (coughing up bloody mucus), loss of appetite, unexplained weight loss, voice hoarseness, and frequent lung infections. Ibid.

21. NCI, "Nuclear Imaging (PET and SPECT)," at http://imaging.cancer.gov/patientsandproviders/cancerimaging/nuclearimaging.

For more general information about PET scans, see Mayo Clinic staff, "Positron Emission

Tomography (PET) Scan," at http://www.mayoclinic.com/health/pet-scan/MY00238; Cleveland Clinic, "Diagnostics & Testing: PET Scan," at http://my.clevelandclinic.org/services/pet_scan/hic_pet_scan.aspx; Medical News Today, "What is a PET Scan? How Does a PET Scan Work?," at http://www.medicalnewstoday.com/articles/154877.php; and Radiographics, "An Introduction to PET-CT Imaging," at http://radiographics.highwire.org/content/24/2/523.full.

22. NCI, "Metastatic Cancer," at http://www.cancer.gov/cancertopics/factsheet/Sites-Types/metastatic/print. In 2011, cancer of unknown primary sites ("CUP") or so-called occult primary tumors accounted for about 2 percent of all malignancies diagnosed in the United States. Kyung Won Kim, Katherine M. Krajewski, et al, "Cancer of Unknown Primary Sites: What Radiologists Need to Know and What Oncologists Want to Know," *American Journal of Roentgenology* 200 (2013): 484.

CHAPTER ELEVEN. DEPRESSION & DELIRIUM, A Complicated Picture

1. MedlinePlus, U.S. National Library of Medicine, National Institutes of Health, "Depression–Elderly," at http://www.nlm.nih.gov/medlineplus/ency/article/001521.htm.

2. GMHF, *Depression in Late Life: Not a Natural Part of Aging*, at www.GMHFonline.org. According to clinical researchers at the University of Rochester School of Medicine, the prevalence of major depression in the 65-and-over age group in primary-care settings is 6 to 9 percent and that of clinically significant depressive symptoms in this group in the same setting is as high as 37 percent. Chunyu Li, Bruce Friedman, et al, "Validity of the Patient Health Questionnaire 2 (PHQ-2) in Identifying Major Depression in Older People," *Journal of the American Geriatrics Society* 55 (2007): 596.

3. *DSM-IV*, p. xxxi; and *DSM-5*, p. 20.

4. Jeffrey M. Lyness, Moonseong Heo, et al, "Outcomes of Minor and Subsyndromal Depression Among Elderly Patients in Primary Care Settings," *Annals of Internal Medicine* 144 (2006): 496-97, 502; and Robert M. Carney and Kenneth E. Freedland, "Depression, Mortality, and Medical Morbidity in Patients with Coronary Heart Disease," *Biological Psychiatry* 54 (2003): 243.

5. This seems like common sense to me, but if you have any doubts, look up GMHF, *Depression in Late Life: Not a Natural Part of Aging*, at www.GMHFonline.org; National Institute of Mental Health, "Older Adults: Depression and Suicide Facts," at http://www.nimh.nih.gov/health/publications/older-adults-depression-and-suicide-facts-fact-sheet/index.shtml; and MedlinePlus, "Depression–Elderly," endnote 1, *supra.*

6. Martha L. Bruce, "Psychosocial Risk Factors for Depressive Disorders in Late Life," *Biological Psychiatry* 52 (2002): 175, 180; and Krishnan, Hays, and Blazer, "MRI-Defined Vascular Depression," endnote 30, Chapter Eight, *supra,* p. 500.

7. *DSM-5*, p. 161. For a superb discussion of this change, see Richard A. Friedman, "Grief, Depression, and the DSM-5," *New England Journal of Medicine* 366 (2012): 1855-57. Dr. Friedman predicts that *DSM-5*'s elimination of *DSM-IV's* bereavement exclusion "will no doubt be a boon to the pharmaceutical industry, because it will encourage unnecessary treatment with antidepressants and antipsychotics, both of which are increasingly used to treat depression and anxiety." Ibid, 1856.

8. National Institute of Mental Health, "Older Adults: Depression and Suicide Facts," endnote 5, *supra.* The NIMH advises that you can reach crisis counselors at the National Suicide Prevention Lifeline 24 hours a day every day at 1-800-273-TALK (8255).

For 25 percent, see Geriatric Mental Health Foundation, *Depression in Late Life: Not a Natural Part of Aging* (Bethesda, Md.: GMHF, 2005), p. 6. This booklet is available at www.GMHFonline.org.

9. *DSM-IV*, p. 356.

For a discussion about the risk of "pathologic grief" developing, see Bruce, "Psychosocial Risk Factors for Depressive Disorders in Late Life," p. 179.

10. *DSM-IV*, pp. 356, 376. See also Jurgen Unutzer, "Late-Life Depression," *New England Journal of Medicine* 357 (2007): 2279; and Jeffrey C. Huffman, Lawrence T. Park, et al, "Case 14-2008: A 78-Year-Old Man with Anergia and Anhedonia Associated with Cardiovascular Surgery," *New England Journal of Medicine* 358 (2008): 2054.

11. *DSM-5*, pp. 160-61.

12. GMHF, "Am I Depressed?" and "What Is Late-Life Depression—The Facts" in "Recognizing and Overcoming Depression: A Guide to Mental Wellness in Older Age," available at www.GMHFonline.org. See also Unutzer, "Late-Life Depression," p. 2269.

13. Rabins and Lyketsos, *Diagnosing and Treating Alzheimer's Disease*, endnote 18, Chapter Eight, *supra*, p. 54.

14. Potter and Sheffens, "Contribution of Depression to Cognitive Impairment and Dementia in Older Adults," endnote 2, Chapter Eight, *supra*, p. 107; and Rabins and Lyketsos, *Diagnosing and Treating Alzheimer's Disease*, p. 70.

On the flip side, however, Rabins observes that ". . . [L]ifelong depression, starting at early to midlife, might influence the onset of Alzheimer's 25-30 years later." Recent long-term studies, he says, suggest that mild *behavioral* impairment, such as irritability, anxiety, anhedonia, and social withdrawal, might be associated with an acceleration to Alzheimer's disease, even in the absence of cognitive impairment.

Rabins and Lyketsos, *Diagnosing and Treating Alzheimer's Disease*, pp. 66-68.

15. Rabins and Lyketsos, "A Commentary on the Proposed DSM Revision Regarding the Classification of Cognitive Disorders," endnote 21, Chapter Eight, *supra*, pp. 202-03. The two dementia experts also believe that a major depression can cause dementia—a controversial idea—and note that some clinicians use the term, pseudodementia, to refer to older depressed patients with cognitive disturbances.

16. Health problems can create a depression "chain" effect, according to Bruce, "Psychosocial Risk Factors for Depressive Disorders in Late Life," p. 182.

17. In the 1930s, several studies documented a higher incidence of coronary heart disease-related death among depressed psychiatric patients than among control patients. Carney and Freedland, "Depression, Mortality, and Medical Morbidity in Patients with Coronary Heart Disease," p. 241. See also Huffman, Park, et al, "Case 14-2008: A 78-Year-Old Man with Anergia and Anhedonia Associated with Cardiovascular Surgery," pp. 2051-52, 2054.

18. George S. Alexopoulos, Dimitris N. Kiosses, et al, "Clinical Presentation of the 'Depression-Executive Dysfunction Syndrome' of Late Life," *American Journal of Geriatric Psychiatry* 10 (2002): 98-99, 102-05.

19. Huffman, Park, et al, "Case 14-2008: A 78-Year-Old Man with Anergia and Anhedonia Associated with Cardiovascular Surgery," pp. 2053-54. See also Potter and Steffens, "Contribution of Depression to Cognitive Impairment and Dementia in Older Adults," p. 107; and Bruce, "Psychosocial Risk Factors for Depressive Disorders in Late Life," p. 178-79.

For more about the symptoms and underlying brain anatomy of vascular depression, see:

• Krishnan, Hays, and Blazer, "MRI-Defined Vascular Depression," pp. 497-501.

• Alexopoulos, Meyers, et al, "Clinically Defined Vascular Depression," pp. 562-65.

• Carney and Freedland, "Depression, Mortality, and Medical Morbidity in Patients with Coronary Heart Disease," pp. 241-47.

• Alexopoulos, Kiosses, et al, "Clinical Presentation of the 'Depression-Executive Dysfunction Syndrome' of Late Life," pp. 98-105.

20. For an excellent summary of risk factors for depression in older people, see Bruce, "Psychosocial Risk Factors for Depressive Disorders in Late Life," pp. 175, 178-82; and

MedlinePlus, endnote 1, *supra*.

21. Huffman, Park, et al, "Case 14-2008: A 78-Year-Old Man with Anergia and Anhedonia Associated with Cardiovascular Surgery," p. 2055; and Carney and Freeland, "Depression, Mortality, and Medical Morbidity in Patients with Coronary Heart Disease," pp. 241-47.

22. Huffman, Park, et al, "Case 14-2008: A 78-Year-Old Man with Anergia and Anhedonia Associated with Cardiovascular Surgery," p. 2055.

23. With the high volume of patients they see, family doctors do not linger over problems not raised. See Thibault and Steiner, "Efficient Identification of Adults with Depression and Dementia," endnote 57, Chapter Eight, *supra*, pp. 1101-10.

24. Your Mom's PCP can fall back on a short standardized depression questionnaire. See John W. Williams Jr., Polly Hitchcock Noel, et al, "Is This Patient Clinically Depressed?" *JAMA* 287 (2002): 1160-69; and Kurt Kroenke, Robert L. Spitzer, and Janet B.W. Williams, "The Patient Health Questionnaire–2: Validity of a Two-Item Depression Screener," *Medical Care* 41 (2003): 1284.

Many exist, but one of the easiest to administer is the Patient Health Questionnaire 2 (PHQ-2), which consists of two questions:

1) Over the past month, have you often had little interest or pleasure in doing things? (This is *DSM-IV's* anhedonia criterion.)

2) Over the past month, have you often been bothered by feeling down, depressed, or hopeless? (*DSM-IV's* mood criterion.)

Either your Mom answers yes or no, or, under an alternate, more refined scoring scheme of the questionnaire, "not at all" (computed as zero); "several days" (one point); "more than half the days" (two); and "nearly every day" (three).

The obvious appeal of the PHQ-2 is its brevity. But it also has proved to be quite reliable. When compared with a structured interview-derived diagnosis in people 65 and older, the PHQ-2 is a useful *first-stage* screening tool for identifying probable major depression. It should not substitute for a more comprehensive diagnostic process. See Li, Friedman, et al, "Validity of the PHQ-2 in Identifying Major Depression in Older People," pp. 596-602.

If PHQ-2 results suggest your Mom is depressed, the doctor may administer the popular PHQ-9, a series of nine questions that ask her to answer "how often" she has been "bothered" during the past two weeks by problems that incorporate *DSM* symptoms.

For example: Have you been bothered by "trouble concentrating on things such as reading the newspaper or watching television?" or by "Feeling tired or having little energy?" Your parent chooses from the zero-to-three time-frame responses detailed above, and numerical scoring allows for a calculation of the severity of her depression. See Thibault and Steiner, "Efficient Identification of Adults with Depression and Dementia," endnote 23, *supra*; Kroenke, Spitzer, and Williams, "The Patient Health Questionnaire-2: Validity of a Two-Item Depression Screener," pp. 1284-92; and Kurt Kroenke, Robert L. Spitzer, and Janet B.W. Williams, "The PHQ-9: Validity of a Brief Depression Severity Measure," *Journal of General Internal Medicine* 16 (2001): 606-13.

For primary-care doctors: Williams, Noel, et al, "Is This Patient Clinically Depressed?" pp. 1160-69.

25. Regarding medications: Martin Pinquart, Paul R. Duberstein, and Jeffrey M. Lyness, "Treatments for Later-Life Depressive Conditions: A Meta-Analytic Comparison of Pharmacotherapy and Psychotherapy," *American Journal of Psychiatry* 163 (2006): 1493-94, 1498-1500; and Lyness, Heo, et al, "Outcomes of Minor and Subsyndromal Depression Among Elderly Patients in Primary Care Settings," p. 502.

Regarding ECT: Cecilia A. Peabody, Harvey A. Whiteford, and Leo E. Hollister, "Antidepressants and the Elderly," *Journal of the American Geriatrics Society* 34 (1986): 869-73. The authors endorse ECT at ibid, 869.

Dr. Steve Epstein, chair of the psychiatry department at the Georgetown University School of Medicine, endorsed ECT for intractable major depression in all age groups, during a Mini-Medical School lecture at Georgetown on April 12, 2011.

26. Lyness, Heo, et al, "Outcomes of Minor and Subsyndromal Depression Among Elderly Patients in Primary Care Settings," pp. 496-97; and Jeffrey M. Lyness, Eric D. Caine, et al, "Psychiatric Disorders in Older Primary Care Patients," *Journal of General Internal Medicine* 14 (1999): 249.

27. Sharon K. Inouye, "Delirium in Older Persons," *New England Journal of Medicine* 354 (2006): 1157. Inouye also reports that 1 to 2 percent of *all* people in the community at large, regardless of age, experience delirium.

28. Ashish K. Jha, Kaveh G. Shojania, and Sanjay Saint, "Forgotten but Not Gone," *New England Journal of Medicine* 350 (2004): 2399.

29. These characteristics are drawn from "Delirium," *DSM-IV*, pp. 136-47, and the *Confusion Assessment Method (CAM) Diagnostic Algorithm*, another diagnostic aid. See Inouye, "Delirium in Older Persons," pp. 1158-61, and pp. 1-2 of Supplementary Appendix to article, available with the full text at www.nejm.org (provided you have a subscription). The CAM is nicely summarized in Camilla L. Wong, Jayna Holroyd-Leduc, et al, "Does This Patient Have Delirium? Value of Bedside Instruments," *JAMA* 304 (2010): 784.

See also Frances, First, and Pincus, "Delirium, Dementia, Amnestic, and Other Cognitive Disorders," in *DSM-IV Guidebook*, endnote 17, Chapter Eight, *supra,* p. 105; and Janet M. Torpy, "JAMA Patient Page: Delirium," *JAMA* 300 (2008): 2936.

30. Inouye, "Delirium in Older Persons," pp. 1157, 1161.

31. Four excellent overview articles about delirium in older people are:

Wong, Holroyd-Leduc, et al, "Does This Patient Have Delirium? Value of Bedside Instruments," pp. 779-86.

William Breitbart and Yesne Alici, "Agitation and Delirium at the End of Life: 'We Couldn't Manage Him,'" *JAMA* 300 (2008): 2898-2910.

Martin G. Cole, "Delirium in Elderly Patients," *American Journal of Geriatric Psychiatry* 12 (2004): 7-21.

Lynn McNicoll, Margaret A. Pisani, et al, "Delirium in the Intensive Care Unit: Occurrence and Clinical Course in Older Patients," *Journal of the American Geriatrics Society* 51 (2003): 591-98.

32. Wong, Holroyd-Leduc, et al, "Does This Patient Have Delirium? Value of Bedside Instruments," p. 780; Breitbart and Alici, "Agitation and Delirium at the End of Life: 'We Couldn't Manage Him,'" p. 2899; and Cole, "Delirium in Elderly Patients," pp. 7-9.

33. Inouye, "Delirium in Older Persons," p. 1157; and Cole, "Delirium in Elderly Patients," pp. 8-9, 12. For a list of bedside instruments (tests) that healthcare providers can use to assess a patient, see Wong, Holroyd-Leduc, et al, "Does This Patient Have Delirium? Value of Bedside Instruments," p. 782; and Breitbart and Alici, "Agitation and Delirium at the End of Life: 'We Couldn't Manage Him,'" p. 2900.

34. Wong, Holroyd-Leduc, et al, "Does This Patient Have Delirium? Value of Bedside Instruments," p. 780. See Sharon K. Inouye, Marquis D. Foreman, et al, "Nurses' Recognition of Delirium and Its Symptoms," *Archives of Internal Medicine* 161 (2001): 2467-73; and Yngve Gustafson, Benny Brannstrom, et al, "Underdiagnosis and Poor Documentation of Acute Confusional States in Elderly Hip Fracture Patients," *Journal of the American Geriatrics Society* 39 (1991): 760-65.

35. Inouye, "Delirium in Older Persons," pp. 1157, 1159, 1161; and Sharon K. Inouye, Sidney T. Bogardus, Jr., et al, "A Multicomponent Intervention to Prevent Delirium in Hospitalized Older Patients," *New England Journal of Medicine* 340 (1999): 669-70. See also Jane McCusker, Martin Cole, et al, "Environmental Risk Factors for Delirium in Hospitalized Older

People," *Journal of the American Geriatrics Society* 49 (2001): 1327, 1333-34; Agneta Edlund, Maria Lundstrom, et al, "Delirium Before and After Operation for Femoral Neck Fracture," *Journal of the American Geriatrics Society* 49 (2001): 1335; and Breitbart and Alici, "Agitation and Delirium at the End of Life: 'We Couldn't Manage Him,'" p. 2907-08.

36. Joost Witlox, Lisa S.M. Eurelings, et al, "Delirium in Elderly Patients and the Risk of Postdischarge Mortality, Institutionalization, and Dementia: A Meta-analysis," *JAMA* 304 (2010): 443; Inouye, "Delirium in Older Persons," p. 1157; Cole, "Delirium in Elderly Patients," pp. 7, 9-11; and Joseph H. Flaherty, Syed H. Tariq, et al, "A Model for Managing Delirious Older Inpatients," *Journal of the American Geriatrics Society* 51 (2003): 1034.

For the percentage of patients experiencing delirium at different stages of palliative care, see Breitbart and Alici, "Agitation and Delirium at the End of Life: 'We Couldn't Manage Him,'" p. 2899.

37. David S. Jones, "Still Delirious After All These Years," *New England Journal of Medicine* 370 (2014): 399-401. The quote is ibid, 399.

38. Joseph H. Flaherty, Syed H. Tariq, et al, "A Model for Managing Delirious Older Inpatients," *Journal of the American Geriatrics Society* 51 (2003): 1031-35; Inouye, Bogardus, et al, "A Multicomponent Intervention to Prevent Delirum in Hospitalized Older Patients," pp. 669-76; and Inouye, "Delirium in Older Persons," p. 1161.

39. Geriatricians have suggested setting up a special four-bed "Delirium Room" in which patients would receive 24-hour intensive nursing care and have no physical restraints. A dedicated room would cut down on hospital noise, improve patients' orientation, and enhance their sleep. Cole, "Delirium in Elderly Patients," p. 9.

40. Witlox, Eurelings, et al, "Delirium in Elderly Patients and the Risk of Postdischarge Mortality, Institutionalization, and Dementia: A Meta-analysis," pp. 443-51; and Shaun O'Keeffe and John Lavan, "The Prognostic Significance of Delirium in Older Hospital Patients," *Journal of the American Geriatrics Society* 45 (1997): 174-78.

CHAPTER TWELVE. THE AGING BODY
Normal Physiological Changes

For my aging research, I used the following principal sources, listed in alphabetical order:
• *Brocklehurst's Textbook of Geriatric Medicine & Gerontology*, 7th ed., first referenced in endnote 46, Chapter Seven, *supra,* and cited in this chapter's endnotes and text as *Brocklehurst.*
• *Encyclopedia of Gerontology: Age, Aging, and the Aged,* first referenced in endnote 2, Chapter Seven, *supra.*
• *Gerontology for the Health Care Professional,* ed. Regula H. Robnett and Walter C. Chop (Sudbury, Mass.: Jones and Bartlett Publishers, 2nd ed., 2010). Chapter Three, by David A. Sandmire, M.D., covers "The Physiology and Pathology of Aging," pp. 53-104. Dr. Sandmire is an assistant professor in the Department of Life Sciences at the University of New England, which is in Biddeford and Portland, Maine.
• *Hazzard's Geriatric Medicine & Gerontology,* ed. Jeffrey Halter, Joseph Ouslander, Mary Tinetti, Stephanie Studenski, and Kevin High (New York: McGraw-Hill Cos., 6th ed., 2009).
• *The Merck Manual of Geriatrics*, 3rd ed., first referenced in endnote 9, Chapter Two.
• *Primary Care Geriatrics: A Case-Based Approach,* ed. Richard J. Ham, Philip D. Sloane, Gregg A. Warshaw, Marie A. Bernard, and Ellen Flaherty. (Philadelphia: Mosby, Inc., 5th ed., 2007).
1. Where not specifically endnoted, information in the text on aging and the nervous system can be attributed to one or more of the following sources:
"Aging and the Nervous System," *The Merck Manual of Geriatrics*, pp. 380-83.

"Nervous System," *Gerontology for the Health Care Professional*, pp. 71-74.

"Neurologic Signs in the Elderly," *Brocklehurst*, pp. 101-05.

2. *The Merck Manual of Geriatrics*, p. 383.

3. *Brocklehurst*, p. 101.

4. W. Bondareff, "Brain and Central Nervous System," pp. 187-88, in *Encyclopedia of Gerontology: Age, Aging, and the Aged*.

5. *The Merck Manual of Geriatrics*, pp. 380-81.

6. *Encyclopedia of Gerontology: Age, Aging, and the Aged*, p. 187; and *The Merck Manual of Geriatrics*, p. 381.

7. *The Merck Manual of Geriatrics*, p. 381.

8. The primary sources for my section on "The Endocrine System" are:

"Aging and the Endocrine System," by Harvinder S. Chahal and William M. Drake in *Brocklehurst*, pp. 123-26.

"Endocrine Function and Dysfunction," by F.V. Nowak and A.D. Mooradian, in *Encyclopedia of Gerontology: Age, Aging, and the Aged*, pp. 480-94.

Steven W.J. Lamberts, Annewieke W. van den Beld, and Aart-Jan van der Lely, "The Endocrinology of Aging," *Science* 278 (1997): 419-24.

"Endocrine System," in *Gerontology for the Health Care Professional*, pp. 100-03.

"Endocrine System" in *Essentials of Anatomy & Physiology*, pp. 269-99, first cited in endnote 45, Chapter Seven.

9. When neurohormones secreted by the hypothalamus act on cells of the **anterior lobe** of the pituitary, the gland either increases or decreases its output of one of seven hormones: (human) growth hormone, which targets most tissues; thyroid-stimulating hormone (TSH), which targets the thyroid gland; adrenocorticotropic hormone (ACTH), which targets the adrenal cortex; melanocyte-stimulating hormone (MSH), which stimulates melanin synthesis in skin; luteinizing hormone (LH), also known as the interstitial cell-stimulating hormone (ICSH) or gonadotropic hormone, which targets ovaries in women and testes in men; follicle-stimulating hormone (FSH), which targets follicles in female ovaries and seminiferous tubules in males; and prolactin, which has an effect on ovaries and mammary glands in women and testes in men.

The hypothalamus controls hormone secretions by the **posterior lobe** of the pituitary through the stimulation of nerve cells (i.e., the transmission of action potentials). The posterior pituitary releases antidiuretic hormone (ADH), which increases water reabsorption in the kidneys, so less water is lost in urine; and oxytocin, which is a female hormone important during childbirth and breastfeeding.

10. Lamberts et al, "The Endocrinology of Aging," pp. 420-23; and *Brocklehurst*, pp. 123-26.

11. See Rudman, Feller, et al, "Effects of Human Growth Hormone in Men Over 60 Years Old," p. 5, first cited in endnote 42, Chapter Seven.

12. *Brocklehurst*, p. 123.

13. All of the HGH studies have been conducted with ambulatory, community-dwelling, and generally *healthy* older people—a skewed, homogeneous population. A thorough assessment of synthetic HGH's potential and risks among a more diverse population will take decades.

See Marc R. Blackman, John D. Sorkin, et al, "Growth Hormone and Sex Steroid Administration in Healthy Aged Women and Men: A Randomized Controlled Trial," *JAMA* 288 (2002): 2282-84, 2286-89; and Mary Lee Vance, "Can Growth Hormone Prevent Aging?" *New England Journal of Medicine* 348 (2003): 779-80. See also "Aging and the Endocrine System," by Harvinder S. Chahal and William M. Drake, in *Brocklehurst*, p. 123; and "Endocrine Function and Dysfunction," by Nowak and Mooradian, in *Encyclopedia of Gerontology: Age, Aging, and the Aged*, p. 482.

14. *Brocklehurst*, p. 124; Lamberts et al, "The Endocrinology of Aging," p. 421; and *Encyclopedia of Gerontology: Age, Aging, and the Aged*, pp. 487-89.

15. *Brocklehurst*, p. 125. See also Lamberts et al, "The Endocrinology of Aging," pp. 420-22.

16. *Brocklehurst*, pp. 125-26. See also Lamberts et al, "The Endocrinology of Aging," pp. 420-21.
Cortisol increases the breakdown of fats to accelerate their conversion to usable energy. Cortisol also reduces inflammatory and immune responses, enabling the body to cope better with stress, and helps to prevent blood glucose from falling to dangerously low levels during sleep and between meals.

17. U.S. Centers for Disease Control and Prevention, 2011 National Diabetes Fact Sheet, at http://www.cdc.gov/diabetes/pubs/general11.htm. See also *The Merck Manual of Geriatrics*, pp. 624-25.

18. Nahrain Al-Zubaidi, M.D., "Diabetes Mellitus: The Epidemic," Georgetown University Mini-Medical School, March 9, 2010.

19. For a basic description of type 2 diabetes, see the entry in the U.S. National Library of Medicine/NIH's MedlinePlus Medical Encyclopedia at http://www.nlm.nih.gov/medlineplus/ency/article/000313.htm, or the Mayo Clinic at http://www.mayoclinic.com/health/type-2-diabetes/DS00585.

20. Lamberts et al, "The Endocrinology of Aging," p. 420-23; and *Brocklehurst*, p. 126. Although a sometime suspect source, Wikipedia provides a solid explanation of thyroid hormone at http://en.wikipedia.org/wiki/Thyroid_hormones.

21. *Brocklehurst*, p. 126. In older people, says *Brocklehurst*, hyperthyroidism is chiefly characterized by cardiovascular symptoms.

22. Ibid; and Lamberts et al, "The Endocrinology of Aging," p. 420.

23. Irwin H. Rosenberg, "Summary Comments," *American Journal of Clinical Nutrition* 50 (1989): 1232. Rosenberg spoke at the conference, "Epidemiologic and Methodologic Problems in Determining the Nutritional Status of Older Persons," held in Albuquerque, N.M. Oct. 19-21, 1988. For an excellent overview, see Timothy J. Doherty, "Invited Review: Aging and Sarcopenia," *Journal of Applied Physiology* 95 (2003): 1717-27; and Ronenn Roubenoff and Virginia A. Hughes, "Sarcopenia: Current Concepts," *Journal of Gerontology* 55A (2000): M716-24.

24. Roubenoff and Hughes, "Sarcopenia: Current Concepts," p. M716. See generally Doherty, "Invited Review: Aging and Sarcopenia," pp. 1717-24; and Ronenn Roubenoff and Carmen Castaneda, "Sarcopenia—Understanding the Dynamics of Aging Muscle," *JAMA* 286 (2001): 1230-31.

25. Roubenoff and Castaneda, "Sarcopenia: Understanding the Dynamics of Aging Muscle," p. 1230. See also Rudman, Feller, et al, "Effects of Human Growth Hormone in Men Over 60 Years Old," p. 1.

26. John E. Morley, Ruichard N. Baumgartner, Ronenn Roubenoff, et al, "Sarcopenia," *Journal of Laboratory and Clinical Medicine* 137 (2001): 234-35; Roubenoff and Hughes, "Sarcopenia: Current Concepts," pp. M720-21; and Roubenoff and Castaneda, "Sarcopenia—Understanding the Dynamics of Aging Muscle," p. 1230.

27. Roubenoff and Castaneda, "Sarcopenia: Understanding the Dynamics of Aging Muscle," p. 1230.

28. Doherty, "Aging and Sarcopenia," pp. 1721-23.

29. Ibid, 1722-24; Roubenoff and Hughes, "Sarcopenia: Current Concepts," p. M721; and Roubenoff and Castaneda, "Sarcopenia: Understanding the Dynamics of Aging Muscle," p. 1231.

30. Doherty, "Aging and Sarcopenia," p. 1724; Roubenoff and Hughes, "Sarcopenia:

Current Concepts," pp. M720-21; and Roubenoff and Castaneda, "Sarcopenia: Understanding the Dynamics of Aging Muscle," p. 1231. See generally James E. Graves, Michael L. Pollock, and Joan F. Carroll, "Exercise, Age, and Skeletal Muscle Function," *Southern Medical Journal* 87 (1994): S17-S20; and William C. Thomas, Jr., "Exercise, Age, and Bones," *Southern Medical Journal* 87 (1994): S23-S24.

31. Believe it or not, clinical studies have shown a closer nexus between abdominal fat and cardiovascular disease than general obesity, as quantified by body mass index, and CV disease. Cardiologists are now eyeing your Mom's and Pop's waistlines. The risk of developing CV disease appears higher for men with waistlines of 40 or more inches and for women with waistlines of 35 or more inches. As observed by David L. Pearle, M.D., "Cardiology," Georgetown University Mini-Medical School, March 20, 2012. See Abel Romero-Corral, Fatima H. Sert-Kuniyoshi, et al, "Modest Visceral Fat Gain Causes Endothelial Dysfunction in Healthy Humans," *Journal of the American College of Cardiology* 56 (2010): 662-66.

32. "Change in Body Composition with Aging," *Encyclopedia of Gerontology: Age, Aging, and the Aged,* p. 183-84.

33. Michel, Newton, and Kirkwood, "Medical Challenges of Improving the Quality of a Longer Life," endnote 15, Chapter Seven, *supra,* pp. 688-89. See also Walter Bortz, "Understanding Frailty," *Journal of Gerontology and Biological Sciences Medical Sciences* 65A (2010): 255-56. Dr. Bortz writes that "The diverse states of immobility and malnutrition are prime causative agents of frailty." Ibid, 255.

34. See Roubenoff and Hughes, "Sarcopenia: Current Concepts," pp. M719, M721.

35. At birth, total body water typically accounts for more than 80 percent of the fat-free mass. By young adulthood, the "hydration factor" usually averages 72 percent.

Dale A. Schoeller, "Changes in Total Body Water With Age," *American Journal of Clinical Nutrition* 50 (1989): 1176, 1181. See also "Body Fluid Compartments," *Essentials of Anatomy & Physiology*, pp. 326-27.

36. For a summary of the data, see CDC, "Prevalence and Most Common Causes of Disability Among Adults—United States, 2005," at http//www.cdc.gov/mmwr/preview/mmwrhtml/mm5816a2.htm.

The CDC's questionnaire defined disability as a yes response to at least one of the following limitation categories:

1) use of an assistive aid (cane, crutches, walker, or wheelchair);
2) difficulty performing activities of daily living or instrumental activities of daily living, or specified functional activities;
3) one or more selected impairments; or
4) limitation in the ability to work around the house or at a job or business.

The "specified functional activities" in no. 2 above included seeing letters/words in newsprint, hearing normal conversation, having speech understood, walking three city blocks, climbing a flight of stairs, grasping objects, and lifting/carrying 10 pounds. The "selected impairments" in no. 3 included learning disability, mental retardation, other developmental disability, Alzheimer's disease/senility/dementia, or other emotional/mental disability. Ibid. (The CDC, not I, used the term senility.)

37. See Sandmire, *Gerontology for the Health Care Professional*, p. 78, and Arthritis Foundation, "Osteoarthritis: Who Is At Risk?" at http://www.arthritis.org/disease-center.php?disease_id=32&df=whos_at_risk.

The incidence of other forms of arthritis also increases with age, although for different reasons. These diseases include rheumatoid arthritis, gout, and polymyalgia rheumatica, an inflammatory disorder that causes muscle pain and stiffness primarily in the neck, shoulders, upper arms, hips, and thighs.

Sandmire, *Gerontology for the Health Care Professional*, pp. 78-79. See "Polymyalgia rheumatica," at www.mayoclinic.com.

38. Dermatologists at the University of California-Irvine College of Medicine provide an excellent review of skin aging in Jerry L. McCullough and Kristen M. Kelly, "Prevention and Treatment of Skin Aging," *Annals of the New York Academy of Sciences* 1067 (2006): 323-31. Changes caused by chronological, as opposed to environmental aging, are ibid, 323-24.

39. Sandmire, *Gerontology for the Health Care Professional*, pp. 69-70.

40. See Dr. Diana Howard, The International Dermal Institute, "Structural Changes Associated with Aging Skin," at http://www.dermalinstitute.com/us/library/11_article_Structural_Changes_Associated-with_Aging_Skin.html.

41. Mark Stibich, Ph.D., "Understanding Heart Aging and Reversing Heart Disease," at http://longevity.about.com. Georgetown Professor Adam Myers, a cardiovascular physiologist and pharmacologist, provided similar statistics in his lecture on physiology during the Fall 2014 Georgetown University Mini-Medical School, Washington, D.C., Oct. 28, 2014.

42. In writing "The Cardiovascular System," unless otherwise noted, I relied upon information obtained from the following sources, listed in alphabetical order:

• *Brocklehurst*, 7th ed., 2010: Dr. Susan E. Howlett, "Effects of Aging on the Cardiovascular System," pp. 91-96.

• *Brocklehurst's Textbook of Geriatric Medicine & Gerontology*, ed. Raymond C. Tallis and Howard M. Fillit (London: Churchill Livingstone/Elsevier Science Ltd., 6th ed., 2003). Prof. Wilbert S. Arnow, M.D., of the divisions of cardiology and geriatrics at New York Medical College, wrote Chapter 30, "Effects of Aging on the Heart," pp. 341-48.

• *Essentials of Anatomy and Physiology*: The editors examine the heart in Chapter 12, pp. 322-52, and the blood vessels and circulation in Chapter 13, pp. 353-86.

• *Gerontology for the Health Care Professional*: Dr. Sandmire analyzes the cardiovascular system on pp. 79-84.

• *The Merck Manual of Geriatrics*, Ch. 83, "Aging and the Cardiovascular System," pp. 813-22.

And the following articles:

• "Arterial and Cardiac Aging: Major Shareholders in Cardiovascular Disease Enterprises," a multi-part review for *Circulation* by NIH-affiliated physicians Edward G. Lakatta and Daniel Levy. Part I covers "Aging Arteries: A Set Up for Vascular Disease," *Circulation* 107 (2003): 139-146; and Part II covers "The Aging Heart in Health: Links to Heart Disease," 107 (2003): 346-54.

• Alberto U. Ferrari, Alberto Radaelli, and Marco Centola, "Invited Review: Aging and the Cardiovascular System," *Journal of Applied Physiology* 95 (2003): 2591.

43. Lakatta and Levy, Part I, "Aging Arteries: A Set Up for Vascular Disease," p. 141.

44. Ibid, 141-43. See also "Connective Tissues and Aging," by Nicholas A. Kefalides and Zahra Ziaie, in *Brocklehurst*, p. 80.

45. Some researchers view arterial aging as an early stage of atherosclerotic disease, while others consider atherosclerosis a form of accelerated arterial aging, promoted by noxious stimuli such as smoking and high-blood cholesterol. Lakatta and Levy, Part II, "The Aging Heart in Health: Links to Heart Disease," p. 350.

46. Dr. Christopher Wilcox, "Understanding How High Blood Pressure Affects Your Health," Georgetown University Medical Center, March 31, 2012. Compare with Aram V. Chobanian, "Isolated Systolic Hypertension in the Elderly," *New England Journal of Medicine* 357 (2007): 789-91; and *The Merck Manual of Geriatrics*, p. 833.

47. Shryl Sistrunk, M.D., lecture on "Aging," Georgetown University Mini-Medical School, April 20, 2010.

My mini-medical school instructor, Dr. Paulo H.M. Chaves, a geriatrician and epidemiologist in the Johns Hopkins Center on Aging and Health, essentially agrees with

Sistrunk, noting that in the 75-and-older age group, 76.4 percent of women and 64.1 percent of men have hypertension. Paulo H.M. Chaves, M.D., Ph.D., "Addressing the Well-Being of Older Adults: Millions and More at a Time," lecture in "Aging and Health," Johns Hopkins University Mini-Medical School, Oct. 20, 2011.

But contrast Sistrunk's and Chaves's statistics with those of Dr. Wilcox, endnote 46, *supra*, who says that 5 percent of all young adults, 50 percent of all adults age 50 and older, and 80 percent of all adults 80 and older have high blood pressure.

48. Chobanian, "Isolated Systolic Hypertension in the Elderly," p. 789. See also *The Merck Manual of Geriatrics*, p. 833; *Brocklehurst*, p. 288; and Mayo Clinic, "Isolated Systolic Hypertension: A Health Concern?" at http://www.mayoclinic.com/health/hypertension/AN01113.

49. Despite the evidence for diastolic dysfunction—for a change in the filling pattern—left ventricular end diastolic pressure does not decline in older healthy adults when they are at rest. See "Effects of Aging on the Cardiovascular System," in *Brocklehurst*, pp. 94-95; Ferrari et al, "Invited Review: Aging and the Cardiovascular System," p. 2595; and Lakatta and Levy, Part II, "The Aging Heart in Health: Links to Heart Disease," pp. 346, 352.

For an accessible, easy-to-understand explanation about diastolic dysfunction and other cardiovascular physiological changes, see "Cardiovascular Physiology Concepts" at www.cvphysiology.com. This is the website of Richard E. Klabunde, Ph.D., a professor at Ohio University and author of the textbook, *Cardiovascular Physiology Concepts*.

50. Lakatta and Levy, Part II, "The Aging Heart in Health: Links to Heart Disease," p. 348. The afterload would have to increase substantially before it would decrease the cardiac output of a healthy older heart.

See Ferrari et al, "Invited Review: Aging and the Cardiovascular System," p. 2592, wherein the authors state that "Overall, the peak cardiac output attained in response to maximal effort is blunted by some 20-30% in elderly compared with young healthy subjects."

One physician I consulted said you could calculate maximum heart rate by subtracting a person's age from 220. A 65-year-old's heart, therefore, would beat a maximum of 155 times per minute.

51. Lakatta and Levy, Part II, "The Aging Heart in Health: Links to Heart Disease," pp. 348-50; and "Effects of Aging on the Cardiovascular System," in *Brocklehurst*, p. 95.

52. *Brocklehurst*, pp. 95-96.

53. "Aging and the Blood," in *The Merck Manual of Geriatrics*, pp. 672-73.

54. "Aging in the Blood," in *Brocklehurst*, p. 127; and "Hematologic System," in *Gerontology for the Health Care Professional*, pp. 88-90.

According to the World Health Organization, the lower limit of the normal range for hemoglobin concentration in blood is 13 grams per deciliter for men and 12 g/dl for women. *Encyclopedia of Gerontology: Age, Aging, and the Aged*, p. 672.

55. *The Merck Manual of Geriatrics*, p. 674.

56. *Brocklehurst*, p 131. See *The Merck Manual of Geriatrics*, p. 675 (for iron deficiency) and p. 685 (for pernicious anemia).

57. *Brocklehurst*, p. 82.

"[T]he risk of infectious diseases attributable to immune senescence," *Merck* agrees, "is difficult to differentiate from that attributable to the various pathophysiologic structural and functional alterations of different organs, which probably determine the specific location of some infections." *The Merck Manual of Geriatrics*, p. 1358. See also *Encyclopedia of Gerontology: Age, Aging, and the Aged*, pp. 745-47.

58. For an excellent overview, see "Immune System," by N.S. Shah and W. B. Ershler, *Encyclopedia of Gerontology: Age, Aging, and the Aged*, pp. 742-48.

59. *The Merck Manual of Geriatrics*, p. 1351. See also *Encyclopedia of Gerontology: Age,*

Aging, and the Aged, p. 743.

60. *The Merck Manual of Geriatrics*, p. 753.

61. *Brocklehurst*, pp. 97-98; and Sandmire, *Gerontology for the Health Care Professional*, p. 85.

62. Charles Read, M.D., lecture on "The Lung," Georgetown University Mini-Medical School, March 27, 2012. See also Sandmire, *Gerontology for the Health Care Professional*, p. 84.

63. *Brocklehurst*, p. 98; and Sandmire, *Gerontology for the Health Care Professional*, pp. 85-86. The loss of alveolar wall surface area is estimated to be about 4 percent per decade after age 30.

64. *Brocklehurst*, p. 98.

65. Ibid, 100: "Immunosenescence explains a large part of the increased susceptibility to lower respiratory tract infection in the elderly. However, causes which contribute to pneumonia risk in this population are multifactorial."

66. Ibid, 99. Other age-related deficits that contribute to an elder's susceptibility to pneumonia occur at a cellular level and are well beyond my scope of review here.

67. *The Merck Manual of Geriatrics*, pp. 758-62; Paul E. Marik and Danielle Kaplan, "Aspiration Pneumonia and Dysphagia in the Elderly," *Chest* 124 (2003): 328-34; and Paul E. Marik, "Aspiration Pneumonitis and Pneumonia: A Clinical Review," *New England Journal of Medicine* 344 (2001): 665-72.

The prevalence of dysphagia in stroke patients is reported to be between 40 and 70 percent: Marik and Kaplan, "Aspiration Pneumonia and Dysphagia in the Elderly,"p. 329; and Marik, "Aspiration Pneumonitis and Pneumonia: A Clinical Review," p. 667, with citations to other articles.

About 50 percent of all healthy adults reportedly aspirate small amounts of oropharyngeal secretions during their sleep. See Marik and Kaplan, "Aspiration Pneumonia and Dysphagia in the Elderly,"p. 329; and Marik, "Aspiration Pneumonitis and Pneumonia: A Clinical Review," p. 666.

68. Phillip P. Smith and George A. Kuchel, "Aging of the Urinary Tract," in *Brocklehurst*, p. 111. See also *The Merck Manual of Geriatrics*, p. 951.

69. Unless otherwise noted, my facts for this section come from one or more of the following sources, listed alphabetically:

• *Brocklehurst*, 7th ed., 2010: "Aging of the Urinary Tract," by Phillip P. Smith and George A. Kuchel, pp. 111-16.

• *Brocklehurst*, 6th ed., 2003: "Aging of the Urinary Tract," by Sarbjit Vanita Jassal and Dimitrios G. Oreopoulos, pp. 108-86.

• *Essentials of Anatomy & Physiology*: Ch. 18, "Urinary System and Fluid Balance," pp. 507-35.

• *Gerontology for the Health Care Professional*, "Genitourinary System," pp. 97-100.

• *The Merck Manual of Geriatrics*, 3rd ed.: "Aging in the Kidney," pp. 951-54; and "Urinary Incontinence," pp. 965-80.

70. *Essentials of Anatomy & Physiology*, p. 515. But see Jassal and Oreopoulos, in *Brocklehurst* 6th ed., p. 1083.

71. *Brocklehurst*, p. 111; and *The Merck Manual of Geriatrics*, p. 952.

72. GFR is calculated using a mathematical formula that compares a person's age, sex (women have less muscle mass than men), race (blacks generally have more muscle mass than non-blacks), and size to serum creatinine levels. According to the National Kidney Foundation, normal GFR results, without adjusting for individual factors, range from 90 to 120 mL/min/1.73 m2, which translates to 120 millileters per minute per 1.73 meters squared. The meters-squared measurement takes into account the body surface area (height, weight,

and mass) of the person being tested. See National Kidney Foundation at http://www.kidney. org/kidneydisease/understandinglabvalues.cfm, and "Glomerular Filtration Rate," the U.S. National Library of Medicine/NIH at MedlinePlus, http://www.nlm.nih.gov/medlineplus/ ency/article/007305.htm. A GFR of 60 or below for three or more months indicates chronic kidney disease, and a GFR of 15 or below signals kidney failure. Ibid. at MedlinePlus.

According to *Brocklehurst*, a blood-level test of cystatin C, a protein secreted by most cells in the body, has been suggested as an improved marker of reduced GFR in older people who have normal creatinine levels. Cystatin reflects kidney function independent from muscle mass and protein consumption. According to textbook writers, "[T]he precise role of cystatin C measurements in clinical decision-making remains to be defined." *Brocklehurst*, p. 111.

BUN and serum creatinine levels are expressed in milligrams per deciliter (mg/dL) or millimoles per liter (mmol/L), representing the amount of the product cleared by the kidneys per minute in a deciliter or liter of plasma.

The Duke Medical Center laboratory that tested my father's blood in February 2012 gave the following normal value ranges: 7.0 to 20.0 for urea nitrogen and 0.6 to 1.3 for creatinine.

73. *The Merck Manual of Geriatrics*, p.1000; and "Geriatric Gastroenterology: Overview," *Brocklehurst*, p. 106.

74. Unless otherwise noted, all of my information about the digestive system comes from Sandmire, *Gerontology for the Health Care Professional*, pp. 93-97 and "Geriatric Gastroenterology: Overview," by Richard C. Feldstein, Robert E. Tepper, and Seymour Katz in *Brocklehurst*, pp. 106-10.

75. "Geriatric Gastroenterology: Overview," *Brocklehurst*, p. 106. See K.R. DeVault, "Presbyesophague: A Reappraisal," *Current Gastroenterology Reports* 4 (2002): 193-9.

76. *The Merck Manual of Geriatrics*, pp. 1141-42.

77. Konner, *Becoming a Doctor*, endnote 1, Preface, *supra*, p. 347.

78. My facts about diverticulosis, diverticulitis, their symptoms, treatments, and potential consequences come from "Diverticulosis and Diverticulitis," by the National Digestive Diseases Information Clearinghouse of the National Institute of Diabetes and Digestive and Kidney Diseases at http://digestive.niddk.nih.gov/ddiseases/pubs/diverticulosis/.

CHAPTER THIRTEEN. 2012: THE "RESCUE" COMES
With Pain and Atrial Fibrillation

1. See A. Kumar, E.R. Litt, et al, "Artificial Urinary Sphincter Versus Male Sling for Post-Prostatectomy Incontinence—What Do Patients Choose?" *Journal of Urology* 181 (2009): 1231-35.

2. Charles Read, M.D., lecture on "The Lung," Georgetown University Mini-Medical School, March 27, 2012.

3. Edward C. Rosenow III, Mayo Clinic, "Can Lung Nodules Be Cancerous?" at http://www.mayoclinic.com/health/lung-nodules/AN01082/METHOD=print.

4. World Health Organization, International Agency for Research on Cancer, *Reversal of Risk After Quitting Smoking* (Lyon, France: IARC, 2007), p. 15.

5. Ibid, 107. For more about the genetic damage that persists, see ibid, pp. 29-44. According to the IARC, there are several thousand "constituents of smoke," whose metabolism and excretion from the human body differ. Ibid, 7-8.

The IARC also says: "Cigarette smoking causes relatively few deaths before 35 years of age, but it causes many deaths in middle age (here defined as 35-69 years) and at older ages. Although some of those killed by tobacco in middle age might have died soon anyway, many could have lived on for another 10, 20, 30 or more good years. Those who stop smoking in early middle age, however (before they have incurable lung cancer or some other fatal disease), avoid most of their risk of being killed by tobacco, and stopping before middle age is even more effective, gaining on average about an extra 10 years of life." Ibid, 16.

There have been scores of epidemiological studies done on the impact of smoking cessation on the risk of lung cancer. Among the most often cited is a British study of male doctors: Richard Doll, Richard Peto, et al, "Mortality in Relation to Smoking: 50 Years' Observations on Male British Doctors," *British Medical Journal* 328 (2004): 1519, published at http://www.bmj.com/content/bmj/328/7455/1519.full.pdf.

6. IARC, *Reversal of Risk After Quitting Smoking*, p. 10.

7. For a discussion about the use of beta blockers in rate-control strategy, see Johns Hopkins Medicine, "Atrial Fibrillation," p. 34-35, endnote 1, Chapter Five, *supra*.

8. Ibid, 40-41. See also "Flecainide," on the U.S. National Library of Medicine/NIH's MedlinePlus at http://www.nlm.nih.gov/medlineplus/druginfo/meds/a608040.html.

9. Johns Hopkins Medicine, "Atrial Fibrillation," pp. 12-13.

10. Ibid, 5, 13. See also Mayo Clinic, "Atrial Fibrillation: Complications," at http://www.mayoclinic.org/disease-conditions/atrial-fibrillation/basics/complications/con-20027014.

11. Johns Hopkins Medicine, "Atrial Fibrillation," p. 43; National Heart, Lung, and Blood Institute, "What Is Catheter Ablation?" at http://www.nhlbi.nih.gov/health/health-topics/topics/ablation/; Mayo Clinic, *Discovery's Edge,* "New Treatment for Atrial Fibrillation: Catheter Ablation Procedure Avoids Drugs and Surgery," at http://discoverysedge.mayo.edu/atrial-fibrillation-treatment/index.cfm; and Mayo Clinic, "Perspectives on the Evolution of Therapy for Atrial Fibrillation," at http://www.mayoclinic.org/medicalprofs/atrial-fibrillation.html.

In this type of ablation, the cardiologist inserts a catheter into a blood vessel, often in the patient's groin, threads it to the heart, and then sends radiofrequency energy (heat) through it to the target heart tissue.

According to Drs. Calkin and Berger, AF can run in families. "The presence of a first-degree relative with AF," they say, doubles "the likelihood" that other members of a family will develop it. Johns Hopkins Medicine, "Atrial Fibrillation," p. 10.

According to a 2003 Mayo Clinic study, "lone" atrial fibrillation, which is AF "not caused by underlying heart disease," can run in families. Investigators in Mayo's Cardiovascular Genetics Research Laboratory are reportedly "searching for specific genetic mutations that can lead to atrial fibrillation." Mayo Clinic, *Discovery's Edge,* "New Treatment for Atrial Fibrillation: Atrial Fibrillation and Inheritance," at http://discoverysedge.mayo.edu/atrial-fibrillation-treatment/index.cfm.

CHAPTER FOURTEEN. 2013: A RUNAWAY TRAIN
With Too Many Station Stops

1. Richard E. Klabunde, Ph.D., "Cardiovascular Physiology Concepts: Electrocardiogram (EKG, ECG)," at http://www.cvphysiology.com/Arrhythmias/A009.htm.

2. Randy Jones, M.D., "Atrial Flutter, Fibrillation and Ablation," at http://blog.ercast.org/2011/04/atrial-flutter-fibrillation-ablation/; Heart Rhythm Society, "Atrial Flutter," at http://www.hrsonline.org/Patient-Resources/Heart-Diseases-Disorders/Atrial-Flutter#axzz2YlPkMZqL; Mayo Clinic, "Atrial Flutter," at http://www.mayoclinic.org/atrial-flutter/treatment.html; and Johns Hopkins Medicine, "Atrial Fibrillation," endnote 1, Chapter Five, *supra*, p. 52.

3. National Heart Lung and Blood Institute, "Diseases and Conditions Index: Heart & Vascular Diseases: Heart Block," at http://www.nhlbi.nih.gov/health/dci/Diseases/hb/hb_types.html. See also Heart Rhythm Society, "Heart Block," at http://www.hrsonline.org/Patient-Resources/Heart-Diseases-Disorders/Heart-Block#axzz2YlPkMZqL; and

Klabunde, "Cardiovascular Physiology Concepts: Electrocardiogram," endnote 1, *supra.*

4. Johns Hopkins Medicine, "Atrial Fibrillation," pp. 23-24. For a contrast, see Wikipedia, "CHADS2 Score," at http://en.wikipedia.org/wiki/CHADS2_score.

Researchers clinically validated the $CHADS_2$ stroke-risk classification scheme in Brian F. Gage, Amy D. Waterman, et al, "Validation of Clinical Classification Schemes for Predicting Stroke: Results From the National Registry of Atrial Fibrillation," *JAMA* 285 (2001): 2864-70.

Dabigatran, approved by the FDA in 2010, directly inhibits an enzyme involved in the formation of blood clots. It came on the market amid claims that it does not cause increased bleeding, like other anticoagulants do, and is much easier to use than warfarin. Johns Hopkins Medicine, "Atrial Fibrillation," p. 29, 32.

In 2011, Drs. Calkins and Berger described dabigatran (Pradaxa®) as a "game changer." Taken twice daily, dabigatran, they said, "has proven much easier to use than warfarin, does not cause increased bleeding, and does not require constant monitoring to make sure therapeutic goals are achieved. Everyone takes the same dose of this medicine, independent of body weight, sex, and diet. The drug has no known interactions with foods (such as green, leafy vegetables rich with vitamin K [a reference to warfarin]) and minimal interactions with other drugs. Dabigatran reaches an effective level within a few hours, which makes it simpler to schedule patients for a cardioversion or ablation because we know for sure that the patients will be in the therapeutic range and have minimal stroke risk. . . . [T]he drug can easily be stopped 24 hours before any elective surgery to prevent bleeding risks." Ibid, 29.

I have heard anecdotally from physicians that dabigatran does cause increased bleeding and is not the wonder drug that it originally seemed to be.

5. Johns Hopkins Medicine, "Atrial Fibrillation," p. 24; and University of Pittsburgh Medical Center (UPMC), "Atrial Fibrillation," *Heart and Vascular Grand Rounds* (Winter 2014), p. 2. For a slightly different computation of $CHADS_2$ scores correlated with stroke risk and rate per 100 patient-years, see Gage, Waterman et al, "Validation of Clinical Classification Schemes for Predicting Stroke," p. 2867.

6. The University of Pittsburgh Medical Center cites 4.7 percent in "Atrial Fibrillation," endnote 5, *supra,* p.3. For a different percentage calculation, see QxMD, "Calculate by QxMD: $CHA_2 DS_2$-VASc," at http://qxmd.com/calculate-online/calculate.

7. Johns Hopkins Medicine, "Atrial Fibrillation," pp. 34-35.

CHAPTER FIFTEEN. 2013: (SUB)ACUTE WRECKAGE
Dad Loses Ground

1. Howard Spiro, "The Practice of Empathy," *Academic Medicine* 84 (2009): 1177.

2. See, e.g., "Howard Marget Spiro, M.D. Obituary," at http://www.legacy.com/obituaries/bostonglobe/obituary.aspx?pid=156526465.

3. Spiro, "The Practice of Empathy," p. 1177.

4. Dr. Verghese is quoted in Okie, "The Evolving Primary Care Physician," endnote 14, Chapter Ten, *supra,* pp. 1850-51.

5. Michelle J. Naidich and Sam U. Ho, "Case 87: Subacute Combined Degeneration," *Radiology* 237 (2005): 102-03. The turn-of-the-century citation is J.S. Risien Russell, F.E. Batten, and James Collier, "Subacute Combined Degeneration of the Spinal Cord," *Brain* 23 (1900): 39.

6. Niranjan N. Singh and Florian P. Thomas, "Vitamin B-12 Associated Neurological Diseases," at http://emedicine.medscape.com/article/1152670-overview; and Naidich and Ho, "Case 87: Subacute Combined Degeneration," p. 103. A copper deficiency produces a clinical picture like subacute combined degeneration.

7. Naidich and Ho, "Case 87: Subacute Combined Degeneration," p. 103. The Babinski

sign, named for French neurologist Joseph Francois Babinski (1857-1932), is a big-toe reflex that can be elicited by stroking the sole of a person's foot.

8. Ibid.

9. Victor R. Fuchs, "Major Trends in the U.S. Health Economy Since 1950," *New England Journal of Medicine* 366 (2012): 976, quoting physician-economist David Meltzer of the University of Chicago.

10. Robert M. Wachter and Lee Goldman, "Sounding Board: The Emerging Role of 'Hospitalists' in the American Health Care System," *New England Journal of Medicine* 335 (1996): 514-17.

11. All of the following articles are from *The New England Journal of Medicine*, abbreviated here as *NEJM*: Victor R. Fuchs, "Major Trends in the U.S. Health Economy Since 1950," endnote 9, *supra*, pp. 973-77; Mary Beth Hamel, Jeffrey M. Drazen, and Arnold M. Epstein, "The Growth of Hospitalists and the Changing Face of Primary Care," *NEJM* (2009): 1141-43; Yong-Fan Kuo, Gulshan Sharma, et al, "Growth in the Care of Older Patients by Hospitalists in the United States," *NEJM* 360 (2009): 1102-12; Laurence F. McMahon, Jr., "The Hospitalist Movement—Time to Move On," *NEJM* 357 (2007): 2627-29; Peter K. Lindenauer, Michael B. Rothberg, et al, "Outcomes of Care by Hospitalists, General Internists, and Family Physicians," *NEJM* 357 (2007): 2589-2600; and Wachter and Goldman, "Sounding Board: The Emerging Role of 'Hospitalists' in the American Health Care System," endnote 10, *supra*.

CHAPTER SEVENTEEN. 2013: FAILING TO THRIVE
"Ticky-Tack" Doctoring

1. Dupuytren's contracture is named for the 19th century French surgeon who first corrected the condition, Baron Guillaume Dupuytren. Dupuytren gained fame for treating Napoleon Bonaparte's hemorrhoids. The contracture is 10 times more likely to develop in men than women. Although surgery will correct it, repeat surgeries are usually necessary. See "Guillaume Dupuytren" and "Dupuytren's contracture" on http://wikipedia.org.

2. The American Geriatrics Society 2012 Beers Criteria Update Expert Panel, "American Geriatrics Society Updated Beers Criteria for Potentially Inappropriate Medication Use in Older Adults," *Journal of the American Geriatrics Society* 60 (2012): 626.

3. See Mayo Clinic, "Lumbar Puncture (Spinal Tap)," at http://www.mayoclinic.org/tests-procedures/lumbar-puncture/basics/definition/prc-20012679.

4. See National Institutes of Neurological Disorders and Stroke, "Peripheral Neuropathy Fact Sheet," *How is peripheral neuropathy diagnosed?*, at http://www.ninds.nih.gov/disorders/peripheralneuropathy/detail_peripheralneuropathy.htm#266753208.

CHAPTER EIGHTEEN. 2013: NEVER EVENTS, Killing Him Slowly

1. Dennis Brady, "Painkillers to Get New Warning Labels," *The Washington Post*, Sept. 11, 2013, p. A2.

2. See, e.g., Howard Brody, "Medicine's Ethical Responsibility for Health Care Reform—The Top Five List," *New England Journal of Medicine* 362 (2010): 285.

3. For the basics about Clostridium difficile, see Mayo Clinic Staff, "C. Difficile Infection," at http://www.mayoclinic.org/diseases-conditions/c-difficile/basics/treatment/com-20029664?p=1; WebMD Digestive Disorders Health Center, "C. Diff," at http://www.webmd.com/digestive-disorders/clostridium-difficile-colitis#; and National Library of Medicine-NIH, "Clostridium Difficile Infections," and citations therein, at http://www.nlm.nih.gov/medlineplus/clostridiumdifficile.html.

4. Michael W. Kessler, M.D., "Orthopeaedic Surgery," Georgetown University Mini-

Medical School, Nov. 19, 2013.

5. Mayo Clinic Staff, "C. Difficile Infection," endnote 3, *supra.*

6. See, e.g., Consumer Reports, "A Bacterium That Can Be Lethal," *The Washington Post,* Dec. 17, 2013, p. E3.

According to the U.S. Centers for Disease Control and Prevention, C. difficile causes 14,000 deaths per year, up from about 3,000 deaths just 10 years ago. A 30-percent reduction in the use of those antibiotics that can lead to C.-diff infections would result in 25 percent fewer infections, says the CDC. See CDC, "Healthcare-Associated Infections (HAIs): Clostridium Difficile Infection," and links therein, at http://www.cdc.gov/hai/organisms/cdiff/cdiff_infect.html; Dennis Brady and Brian Vastag, "Drug-Resistant Bacteria Take Toll," *The Washington Post,* Sept. 17, 2013, p. A3; and Steven Reinberg, *HealthDay,* "U.S. Hospitals Overuse, Misuse Antibiotics, CDC Says," at http://consumer.healthday.com/infectious-disease-information-21/antibiotics-news-30/hospitals-overuse-antibiotics-cdc-685478.html.

7. According to the CDC's 2011 Healthcare-Associated Infections (HAI) survey, 722,000 HAIs, affecting 648,000 patients, occurred in acute-care hospitals nationwide, more than half of them outside of the ICU. About 75,000 patients with HAIs died during their hospitalizations. The survey estimated infection totals as follows:

Pneumonia:	157,500 (22 percent)
Surgical-site infections from any inpatient surgery:	157,500 (22 percent)
Gastrointestinal infections:	123,100 (17 percent)
Urinary tract infections:	93,300 (13 percent)
Primary bloodstream infections:	71,900 (10 percent)
Other types of infections*:	118,500 (16 percent)

*These include eye, ear, nose, or mouth; lower respiratory-tract; skin and soft-tissue; cardiovascular-system; bone and joint; central-nervous-system; reproductive-tract; and systemic infections.

8. See, e.g., Peter Jaret, WebMD, Digestive Disorders Health Center, "What Are Probiotics?" at http://www.webmd.com/digestive-disorders/features/what-are-probiotics?

9. Mayo Clinic Staff, "Vasovagal Syncope," at http://www.mayoclinic.org/diseases-conditions/vasovagal-syncope/basics/symptoms/con-20026900, et seq.

10. Ibid. See also Maw Pin Tan and Steve Parry, "Vasovagal Syncope in the Older Patient," at http://www.medscape.com/viewarticle/577022.

11. Jeffrey T. Chapman, "Interstitial Lung Disease," at http://www.clevelandclinicmeded.com/medicalpubs/diseasemanagement/pulmonary/interstitial-lung-disease/.

12. Ellen Meredith Stein, Johns Hopkins Medicine, "Solving a C. Difficile Problem: If Antibiotics Fail, a Stool Transplant Can Help Cure a Severe Infection," *Health After 50,* vol. 25, issue 13, January 2014, p. 4. See also Kim Meeri, "You'll Never Believe This Infection Fighter," *The Washington Post,* Jan. 7, 2014, p. E1.

CHAPTER NINETEEN. MY ENDING, There's No Place Like Home

1. R.A.C. Hughes, T. Umpathi, et al, "A Controlled Investigation of the Cause of Chronic Idiopathic Axonal Polyneuropathy," *Brain* 127 (2004): 1723-30. Hughes, et al identified exposure to environmental toxins and hypertriglyceridaemia as risk factors that "deserve further investigation as possible causes of CIAP in both clinical practice and research." Ibid, 1729.

Two years later, Charlene Hoffman-Snyder of the Mayo Clinic in Arizona and colleagues observed that abnormal glucose metabolism is twice as common among patients with CIAP than among the general population. "Peripheral Neuropathy with Impaired Glucose

Intolerance," *Archives of Neurology* 63 (2006): 1055-56.

In 2008, Dr. Anthony wrote in his exam notes that Dad had hyperlipidemia, which, again, is excess fat in the blood.

2. See, e.g, BioMed Health Technology Co-operative, "Catheter Encrustation," at http://www.biomedhtc.org.uk/EncrustationClinical.htm; Ann Yates, "The Causes and Management of Catheter Encrustation," *Continence Essentials* at www.continence-uk.co.uk/.../Continence_Essentials_2008_Catheter _Encrustation.pdf; Kathryn Getliffe, "How to Manage Encrustation and Blockage of Foley Catheter," *Nursing Times,* at http://www.nursingtimes.net/how-to-manage-encrustation-and-blockage-of-foley-catheter/205481; and Kathryn Getliffe, "Managing Recurrent Urinary Catheter Encrustation," *British Journal of Community Nursing* at http://www.ncbi.nlm.nih.gov/pubmed/12447119.

3. You may view the Durable Do Not Resuscitate Order form and instructions at http://www.vdh.virginia.gov/OEMS/Files_Page/DDNR/AuthorizedDurableDNRForm.pdf. Virginia enacted its DDNR order in 2011.

4. Celexa is associated with *torsades de pointes*, which is a ventricular tachycardia that has a distinctive wave pattern (undulation) on an ECG, as well as with a more common v-tach. For the definition in the text, see "Ventricular Tachycardia," U.S. National Library of Medicine/NIH, MedlinePlus, at http://www.nlm.nih.gov/medlineplus/ency/article/000187.htm. My father was very familiar with *torsades de pointes*.

5. The articles I read about Celexa mostly summarized a Jan. 29, 2013 article published by the online *British Medical Journal*: Victor M. Castro, Caitlin C. Clements, et al, "QT Interval and Antidepressant Use: A Cross-Sectional Study of Electronic Health Records," at http://www.bmj.com/content/346/bmj.f288.

The FDA reports are: "FDA Drug Safety Communication: Abnormal Heart Rhythms Associated With High Doses of Celexa (Citalopram Hydrobromide)" at http://www.fda.gov/Drugs/DrugSafety/ucm269086.htm; and "FDA Drug Safety Communication: Revised Recommendations for Celexa (Citalopram Hydrobromide) Related to a Potential Risk of Abnormal Heart Rhythms With High Doses," at http://www.fda.gov/Drugs/DrugSafety/ucm297391.htm.

6. See "Transcript of Afib Chat with Cleveland Clinic Atrial Fibrillation Experts on March 2, 2012," at http://www.stopafib.org; search "Cleveland Clinic."

7. There is evidence that bupropion (Wellbutrin®, Zyban®), which was developed by another of Dad's young NIH charges, shortens the QT interval. Wellbutrin inhibits the reuptake of dopamine, serotonin, and norepinephrine, especially dopamine. See the 2013 *British Medical Journal* article, *supra,* endnote 5.

8. Jason S. Chinitz, Jonathan L. Halperin, et al, "Rate or Rhythm Control for Atrial Fibrillation: Update and Controversies," *The American Journal of Medicine* 125 (2012): 1049.

9. "Transcript of Afib Chat with Cleveland Clinic Atrial Fibrillation Experts on March 2, 2012," *supra,* endnote 6.

10. Chinitz, Halperin, et al, "Rate or Rhythm Control for Atrial Fibrillation: Update and Controversies," pp. 1054-55. See also Wilbert S. Aronow, "Atrial Fibrillation Management in Elderly," *Current Cardiovascular Risk Reports* 6 (2012): 431-42; and Andrew J. Krainik and Jane Chen, "Atrial Fibrillation in the Elderly," *Current Cardiovascular Risk Reports* 4 (2010): 354-60

11. Kenneth R. Hess, Gauri R. Varadhachary, et al, "Metastatic Patterns in Adenocarcinoma," *Cancer* 106 (2006): 1624-25. The Paget article is "The Distribution of Secondary Growths in Cancer of the Breast," *The Lancet* 133 (1889): 571-73.

12. Hess, Varadhachary, et al, "Metastatic Patterns in Adenocarcinoma," pp. 1625-32.

13. Guy diSibio and Samuel W. French, "Metastatic Patterns of Cancers: Results From a Large Autopsy Study," *Archives of Pathology & Laboratory Medicine* 132 (2008): 931-39.

14. Ibid, 939.

15. Richard L. Byyny, "AΩA and Professionalism in Medicine," *The Pharos* (Summer 2011): 1.

16. Ibid, 2.

17. Maxine A. Papadakis, Arianne Teherani, et al, "Disciplinary Action by Medical Boards and Prior Behavior in Medical School," *New England Journal of Medicine* 353 (2005): 2676.

18. David T. Stern and Maxine Papadakis, "The Developing Physician—Becoming a Professional," *New England Journal of Medicine* 355 (2006): 1794.

19. Abigail Zuger, "Dissatisfaction with Medical Practice," *New England Journal of Medicine* 350 (2004): 69.

20. Duke Signature Care, at http://www.dukemedicine.org/treatments/duke-signature-care. See also Lisa Gerstner, "6 Things to Know About Concierge Medicine," at http://www.kiplinger.com/article/spending/T027-C000-S002-6-things-to-know-about-concierge-medicine.html.

21. Bodenheimer and Laing, "The Teamlet Model of Primary Care," endnote 10, Chapter Ten, *supra,* pp. 457-61. For more details about Bodenheimer's teamlet concept, including studies of the concept in actual practices, see the articles listed in Dr. Bodenheimer's UCSF profile at http://profiles.ucsf.edu/thomas.bodenheimer.

22. Dr. Paul Rothman, "Humanism in Medicine," lecture at Johns Hopkins University, Baltimore, Md., March 27, 2014. Dr. Rothman asked the class of about 20 people how many thought that physicians care about patients. Only about five raised their hands. He was stunned.

Index

A

ablation, cardiac. See atrial fibrillation
Accreditation Council for Graduate Medical
    Education (ACGME), 513, 514–15
acetaminophen (Tylenol®), 119, 389, 411
acetylcholine, 189, 190, 275, 550n32
ACGME. See Accreditation Council for
    Graduate Medical Education
Achilles' heel tendon, torn, and Levaquin®,
    222
ACP. See American College of Physicians
ACTH. See adrenocorticotropic hormone
action potentials. See neurons
Active Disability-Free Life Expectancy, 158–59
activities of daily living (ADL), 106–7, 112, 113,
    138, 179, 187–88, 538n11
adenosine triphosphate (ATP), 164–65,
    546n48
ADH. See antidiuretic hormone
adipose tissue (fat), 280, 281-2, 284–85, 296,
    566n31
ADL. See activities of daily living
ADmark Assays, 196
adrenaline. See epinephrine
adrenocorticotropic hormone (ACTH), 564n9
adrenal cortex, glands. See kidneys
adrenopause, 280
ADRs. See Affective Dispositions to Respond
advance directives, 123
adverse drug "events," 505
adverse events caused by medical management,
    503–4
adverse reactions to drugs, 262, 266–67, 505
AF. See atrial fibrillation
affective dispositions to respond (ADRs), 87
African trypanosomiasis (tryps), 37–39
afterload, cardiac, 292, 294, 568n50
Agatha (Dr. Terse's PA), 401, 403, 405, 432,
    458–59
age spots, 288–89
ageism
    among physicians, 146, 147–48, 150,
        541–42n5
    among resident physicians, 146, 147
    as ascertainment bias, 86, 88
    avoiding, 527
    body odors, 543n13
    Butler's research and writing on, 144–46

childhood, old age compared to, 148, 151
dementia and, 268
depression and, 256
Dr. Al and, 144, 170
Konner on, xi–xii
LOL. See Little Old Lady Syndrome
in medical schools, 147, 541–42n5
in medicine and medical culture, xi–xii,
    147–48, 150–51, 272
at OBH, 224
offensive language and humor, 31, 144, 145,
    147, 150–51, 542–43nn9–10
origin of geriatrics and, 146, 147–48
origin of term, 144–45
patronizing speech to elders, 5, 6, 11, 17
racism compared to, 145
speculations on, 4, 8, 24, 33, 224
in U.S. culture, 145–46
aging. See chapters 7 and 12, generally
    17 ways to do it well, 526–27
    anti-aging movement, 161, 165, 545–46n43
    arterial, 290–94, 567n45
    of body systems, 152-53, 543n15. See indi-
        vidual systems
    cell division and, 154
    cognitive, normal, 174–79, 277, 548n7
    environment and, 162, 302–3
    error theory of, 161, 162
    free radical theory of, 164–65, 167,
        546nn48–49
    genes and, 547n57
    height, loss of, 67
    "Grow Young with HGH" (Klatz), 545n43
    heterogeneity of, 152–53, 154
    Inborn Aging Process (IAP), 543n15
    International Club for Research on Aging,
        148
    kitchen-sink theory of, 166–68
    LUT, normal, 212–14
    mitochondrial theory of, 167
    normal, usual, and successful, 159–60. See
        also normal aging
    physiology of, 152–54
    programming theory of, 161–62
    reproductive success and, 153–54, 168
    sexual maturation and, 153–54
    somatic mutation theory, 167
    stroke risk and, 342, 343